WITHDRAWN

Orthopaedic Manual Therapy Diagnosis

SPINE AND TEMPOROMANDIBULAR JOINTS

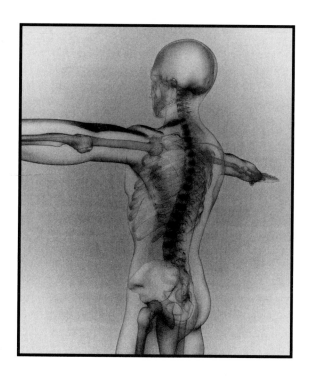

Aad van der El, BPE, BSc PT, Dip. MT, Dip. Acupuncture

First English Edition

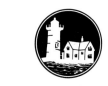

JONES AND BARTLETT PUBLISHERS
Sudbury, Massachusetts
BOSTON   TORONTO   LONDON   SINGAPORE

World Headquarters
Jones and Bartlett Publishers
40 Tall Pine Drive
Sudbury, MA 01776
978-443-5000
info@jbpub.com
www.jbpub.com

Jones and Bartlett Publishers Canada
6339 Ormindale Way
Mississauga, Ontario L5V 1J2
Canada

Jones and Bartlett Publishers International
Barb House, Barb Mews
London W6 7PA
United Kingdom

Jones and Bartlett's books and products are available through most bookstores and online booksellers. To contact Jones and Bartlett Publishers directly, call 800-832-0034, fax 978-443-8000, or visit our website at www.jbpub.com.

Substantial discounts on bulk quantities of Jones and Bartlett's publications are available to corporations, professional associations, and other qualified organizations. For details and specific discount information, contact the special sales department at Jones and Bartlett via the above contact information or send an email to specialsales@jbpub.com.

The authors, editor, and publisher have made every effort to provide accurate information. However, they are not responsible for errors, omissions, or for any outcomes related to the use of the contents of this book and take no responsibility for the use of the products and procedures described. Treatments and side effects described in this book may not be applicable to all people; likewise, some people may require a dose or experience a side effect that is not described herein. Drugs and medical devices are discussed that may have limited availability controlled by the Food and Drug Administration (FDA) for use only in a research study or clinical trial. Research, clinical practice, and government regulations often change the accepted standard in this field. When consideration is being given to use of any drug in the clinical setting, the health care provider or reader is responsible for determining FDA status of the drug, reading the package insert, and reviewing prescribing information for the most up-to-date recommendations on dose, precautions, and contraindications, and determining the appropriate usage for the product. This is especially important in the case of drugs that are new or seldom used.

Production Credits

Publisher: David Cella
Production Director: Amy Rose
Associate Editor: Maro Gartside
Senior Production Editor: Renée Sekerak
Production Assistant: Jill Morton
Senior Marketing Manager: Barb Bartoszek
Manufacturing and Inventory Control Supervisor: Amy Bacus

Cover Design: Kristin E. Parker
Cover Image: © Sebastian Kaulitzki/Dreamstime.com
Composition: Atlis Graphics
Illustrations: P.F. de Stigter, Rotterdam, The Netherlands
Photography: J.A.M. Donckers, Lage Zwaluwe, The Netherlands
Printing and Binding: Courier Westford
Cover Printing: Courier Westford

Library of Congress Cataloging-in-Publication Data
El, Aad van der.
   [Manuele diagnostiek wervelkolom. English]
   Orthopaedic manual therapy diagnosis: Spine and Temporomandibular Joints / by Aad van der El.
      p. ; cm.
   Includes bibliographical references and index.
   ISBN-13: 978-0-7637-5594-2
   ISBN-10: 0-7637-5594-X
   1. Orthopaedics—Diagnosis.   2 Manipulation (Therapeutics)   I. Title.
   [DNLM: 1. Musculoskeletal Diseases—diagnosis.   2 Manipulation, Orthopaedic—methods.
   3. Physical Examination—methods.   WE 141 E37m 2010a]
   RD734.E413 2010
   616.7'075--dc22
                                                                         2008047474

6048

Printed in the United States of America
13 12 11 10 09   10 9 8 7 6 5 4 3 2 1

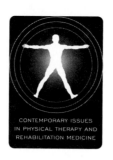

CONTEMPORARY ISSUES
IN PHYSICAL THERAPY AND
REHABILITATION MEDICINE

Jones and Bartlett's
Contemporary Issues in Physical Therapy and
Rehabilitation Medicine Series

Series Editor
Peter A. Huijbregts, PT, MSc, MHSc, DPT, OCS, MTC, FAAOMPT, FCAMT

Other books in the series:

Tension-Type and Cervicogenic Headache: Pathophysiology, Diagnosis, and Management
César Fernández-de-las-Peñas, PT, DO, PhD
Lars Arendt-Nielsen, DMSci, PhD
Robert D. Gerwin, MD

Wellness and Physical Therapy
Sharon Fair, PT, PsyD, PhD

Contents

Introduction by the Series Editor

Although admittedly diverse with regard to concepts and techniques, orthopaedic manual therapy (OMT) has never been the unique domain of any single profession. Whether by way of interprofessional cooperation, adoption of techniques and concepts developed within one profession by others active in this field, or at times through true parallel development, OMT clinicians will agree that current-day OMT consists of an amalgam of concepts and techniques stemming from varied professions including but not limited to physical therapy, manual medicine, osteopathy, chiropractic, massage therapy, and athletic training. Perhaps nowhere is this confluence of professional contributions more evident than in the unique system of OMT diagnosis and management developed in The Netherlands, the diagnostic component of which is presented in this textbook.

Although preceded by developments in Sweden, where physical therapy started as a direct-access, university-educated profession in 1813, when Ling founded the *Kungliga Gymnastiska Centralinstitutet* or Royal Central Institute for Gymnastics in Stockholm (Ottoson, 2005), Dutch physical therapists were among the first in western Europe to establish a professional association, the *Genootschap ter Beoefening van de Heilgymnastiek in Nederland*, or Society for Practicing Remedial Gymnastics in The Netherlands in 1889. This was closely followed by a standardized national entry-level examination (Terlouw, 2007). Heavily influenced by developments in Germany, Sweden, but also within The Netherlands itself, from its very beginning OMT—albeit in a now likely considered unsophisticated form—always was part of the diagnostic and management options within physical therapy in The Netherlands (Kellgren, 1890; Terlouw, 2007).

In the 1960s, OMT in The Netherlands received a unique infusion of new ideas with the concepts developed by Van der Bijl, Sr. (1909–1977), a Dutch-trained physical therapist and French-trained osteopath, who opened the first postgraduate institute for education in manual therapy in Utrecht in 1964. In 1967, the engineer Philips, founder of the international electronics manufacturing company—impressed with the chiropractic care he had received while in New Zealand—invited a chiropractor, Pheleps, to The Netherlands to teach in a school of manual medicine in Eindhoven. This school was later divided into separate training institutes for physicians and physical therapists; the latter was called the *Stichting Opleiding Manuele Therapie* (SOMT) or Manual Therapy Training Foundation (www.somt.nl), for which this text was initially developed as a training manual in 1983. Other influential figures within Dutch OMT were physical therapist Marsman (1918–1992) and physician Sickesz (1923), who developed variants on the Van der Bijl method named the Marsman method and orthomanual medicine. The establishment of separate training institutes for the Nordic and Maitland systems and the development of the first graduate program in manual therapy at the Free University of Brussels further illustrated the diversity of OMT in The Netherlands.

Also influential within Dutch OMT were the postwar developments in Germany. With chiropractic adjudicated there to the medical domain, chiropractors Peper and Sandberg were instrumental in the establishment of the *Forschungs- und Arbeitsgemeinschaft für Chiropraktik* in 1953. In 1955, a second OMT institute that exclusively trained medical physicians opened under the direction of the physician Sell in Isny. Indicating the acceptance within the medical world unlike the situation in, for example, the

United States at this time, university chairs in manual medicine followed in the neurology department at the University of Graz in Austria and in the orthopaedic department at the University of Münster in Germany.

OMT had its early roots in developments in Sweden, Germany, and The Netherlands in the early to late 19th century. Influences from chiropractic, French and English osteopathy, and German and English manual medicine further added to its development, as did concepts and techniques developed by Dutch therapists and physicians. Early authority- and experience-based knowledge was supplemented as of the 1990s by an active research program in OMT, perhaps best exemplified by and discussed by Oostendorp (2007), and also illustrated by the professional master's degree now offered at SOMT. However, because of language barriers most of this knowledge and the unique concepts and techniques developed within this comprehensive system of diagnosis and management until now has not been available to English-language OMT clinicians. It is my hope and expectation that this book will find a welcome reception in both entry-level and postgraduate programs in OMT in the varied professions active in this field.

Peter A. Huijbregts, PT, MSc, MHSc, DPT, OCS,
MTC, FAAOMPT, FCAMT
Series Editor, *Contemporary Issues in Physical
Therapy and Rehabilitation Medicine*
Victoria, British Columbia, Canada, 2008

Acknowledgments

I would like to express my gratitude to colleagues Rob Sillevis, PT, DPT, and Peter Huijbregts, PT, DPT: In their capacity as translation supervisors, they have been instrumental in presenting this first English edition in a technically correct format. In addition, Peter Huijbregts has added significantly to this first English edition in both a quantitative and qualitative sense by updating the eighth Dutch edition, upon which this edition is based, with recent research references throughout, thereby illustrating the increasingly scientific basis for orthopaedic manual therapy (OMT) clinical practice. Further additions by Peter Huijbregts include the section "Orthopaedic Manual Therapy Diagnosis" in Chapter 4; the sections titled "Circulation" and "Reflexes" in Chapter 7; and the section titled "Clinical Research into Lumbar Segmental Instability" in Chapter 14. He has also added Chapter 5, Introduction to Test Psychometric Properties, discussing the psychometric properties of reliability, validity, and responsiveness and also explaining confidence intervals, thereby allowing the reader—where psychometric data are available—a research-based interpretation of test findings as required under the current evidence-informed practice paradigm. In all, the contributions by this co-author have greatly added to *Orthopaedic Manual Therapy Diagnosis,* for which, once again, I'd like to express my gratitude. I would also like to thank David Cella, Publisher at Jones and Bartlett Publishers, and his editorial staff, for their unwavering assistance and for the trust placed in us during the production of this first English edition.

Contributors

John M. Bos, PT, MT, MSc
Instructor, Hogeschool voor Fysiotherapie Rotterdam, The Netherlands
Instructor, Professional Master in Manual Therapy, Transfergroep Rotterdam, The Netherlands
Editor-in-Chief, *Tijdschrift voor Manuele Therapie*
Private practice for Orthopaedic Manual Physical Therapy (OMPT), Zwijndrecht, The Netherlands

Peter A. Huijbregts, PT, MSc, MHSc, DPT, OCS, MTC, FAAOMPT, FCAMT
Assistant Professor, University of St. Augustine for Health Sciences, St. Augustine, Fla., USA
Advisory Faculty Member, North American Institute of Orthopaedic Manual Therapy, Eugene, Ore., USA
Consulting Editor and Immediate-Past Editor-in-Chief, *Journal of Manual and Manipulative Therapy*
Scientific Board Member, *Rehabilitacja Medyczna Journal*
Consulting Editor, Jones and Bartlett Publishers

Consultant Physiotherapist, Shelbourne Physiotherapy and Massage Clinic, Victoria, BC, Canada
Educational Consultant, Dynamic Physical Therapy, Cadillac, Mich., USA

Rob Langhout, PT, MT
Instructor, Manual Therapy Training Foundation (SOMT), Amersfoort, The Netherlands
Private practice for OMPT, Nijmegen, The Netherlands

Roel Wingbermühle, PT, MT
Instructor, Manual Therapy Training Foundation (SOMT), Amersfoort, The Netherlands
Private practice for OMPT, Krimpen aan de IJssel, The Netherlands

PART I

Introduction

CHAPTER 1

Introduction to Spinal Anatomy

MORPHOLOGY

With a newborn infant, the spine as a whole exhibits a dorsal-facing convexity in the sagittal plane. During the first few years of life, this convexity diminishes in the cervical and lumbar regions of the spine, and after the third year this initial kyphosis develops into an opposite curvature, the cervical and lumbar lordosis. The spine attains its definitive morphology after the 10th year, when the curvatures become set. The morphology is determined by the fact that the intervertebral disks—and to a lesser extent the vertebral bodies—are wedge shaped. In lordotic areas, these structures are higher on the ventral side than on their dorsal aspect; in the thoracic area, the opposite is true.

The lordotic morphology of the cervical and lumbar spine helps bear the weight of the head and the torso, respectively, thereby unloading the dorsal anular fibers. In terms of movement, the S-shaped curved and articulated spine has certain advantages over a totally straight spine (**Figure 1–1**). Because the individual vertebrae can move in relation to each other, movements in the lumbopelvic region can be compensated for by movements in the more cranial segments. Without these compensatory abilities, a small range of caudal movement would require a significantly greater range of cervical movement. The formula $R = N^2 + 1$ proposed by Kapandji (1974), in which he indicates that the load-bearing capacity is directly proportional to the number of curvatures squared plus one, appears incorrect. A straight column is always more stable than a curved column is. However, the S-shaped curved spine can absorb more energy because of its greater resistance to deformation.

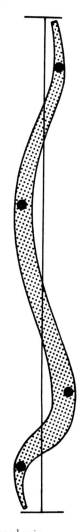

Figure 1–1 The S-shaped spine.

JOINTS BETWEEN INDIVIDUAL VERTEBRAE

The articulation between individual vertebrae is composed of the following components, as shown in **Figure 1–2**:

- Intervertebral disk (a)
- Intervertebral joint (b)
- Ligaments and the joint capsule (c)
- Uncovertebral cervical joint (d)
- Intrinsic lower back musculature
- Intervertebral disk (**Figure 1–3**)

The intervertebral disk is made up of cartilaginous endplates, anulus fibrosus, and nucleus pulposus.

Cartilaginous Endplates

The cartilage plates that form the upper and lower boundaries of the disk are connected to the vertebral bodies. They are composed of hyaline cartilage and are attached circumferentially to the inner rim of the fused ring apophysis of the bony vertebral body. According to Schmorl (1932), these endplates are attached to the vertebral body by a layer of calcium. This layer of calcium has small nutritional pores. The vertebral body is connected to the carti-

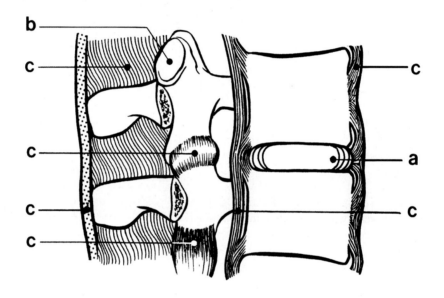

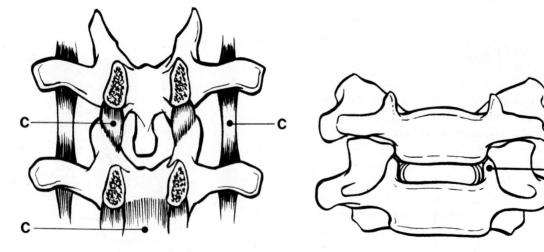

Figure 1–2 Joints between individual vertebrae.

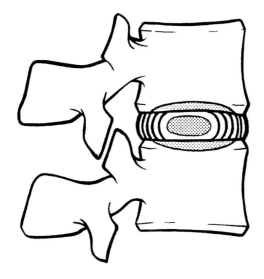
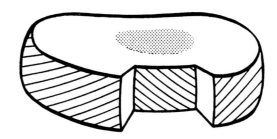

Figure 1–3 Intervertebral disk.

laginous endplate by its sieve-like surface (lamina cribrosa). The greatest part of the metabolic processes within the disk takes place by diffusion through this cartilaginous endplate.

Anulus Fibrosus

The anulus is primarily composed of fibers that are interwoven, like the thread on a screw, connecting one vertebra to the next. The Sharpey's fibers, which radiate outward into the bony outer wall of the vertebral body to which they are anchored, are located in the outermost boundary of the anulus. The ring-shaped lamellae making up the anulus are more numerous and stronger at their ventral and lateral aspect than they are dorsally and dorsolaterally. Whatever the direction of movement, one part of the fibers is tensed and another part is relaxed. The outer anulus bears 25% of the weight (Nachemson, 1966).

At birth, the cervical disks are not distinct from the disks in other regions of the spine—but a pseudodegenerative process occurs in the cervical intervertebral disk in late childhood (roughly from the ninth year onward), which causes tearing in the fibers of the outer anulus. This tearing progresses, and, in many cases, the fibers in the middle between two vertebral bodies appear completely torn in later life (Töndury, 1974; Hoogland, 1988). According to examinations carried out by Bogduk (1990), the ventrally located anular fibers appear to remain intact.

This tearing of the cervical anular fibers causes the disk to split into two parts: caudal and cranial. This cranial and caudal portion consisting of torn anular fibers appears to function as two brushes with the bristles opposing each other.

Nucleus Pulposus

The nucleus pulposus constitutes the central portion of the intervertebral disk between the two vertebral bodies and is considered a remnant of the notochord. The tissue is made up of bladder-shaped notochord cells and notochord strands, which together form the chorda reticulum.

The mesh of this network is filled with a jelly-like substance produced by connective tissue cells. This extensive and widely branched hollow space is initially filled with a synovial-like fluid and later with Gallert tissue. Later in life, this Gallert tissue becomes less homogeneous, leading to a decrease in elasticity. The nucleus pulposus is responsible for bearing 75% of the weight (Nachemson, 1966).

INTERVERTEBRAL JOINT

The intervertebral (or zygapophyseal) joints are synovial joints. The articular facets are covered with hyaline cartilage, and the capsule is made up of two membranes: synovial and fibrous. The hyaline cartilage covering of the superior articular process is thickest in the center, thinning out toward its periphery. This rim is cranially thicker in the cervical and thoracic sections of the spine; in the lumbar section, it is laterally thicker. In both cases, this extra thickness is made up of smooth hyaline cartilage. The thickness of the cartilage on the joints decreases from the caudal to the cranial aspects of the spine—the only exception being the atlanto-occipital joints.

On the inferior articular process, the cartilage covering is also thickest in the center, generally thinning out closer to its periphery. In the lumbar section of the spine, there is a noticeable thickening on the caudal aspect of articular facets; there is often a cartilaginous rim on their cranial aspect. The cartilaginous surfaces of the lumbar inferior articular processes are split in two parts: the thin medial section is located at an obtuse angle to the wider lateral section.

In a movement segment, the articular facets cover each other completely only in certain positions. In most cases, this occurs in the normal physiologic position. In the joints of the cervical and lumbar spine, partial loss of contact can be caused by various kinds of movement. In the end range position, there is often a wedge-shaped opening in the joint. According to Stofft and Müller (1971), corresponding articular facets differ slightly in size; the more they differ, the greater the mobility of a segment. The greatest difference exists in the C5–C6 joint.

In general, concave articular facets are slightly larger than their convex counterparts. In the cervical and thoracic spine, the more caudal articular facets are larger than the more cranially located ones.

In the lumbar area, the superior articular facets are larger than the inferior ones. More information about the intervertebral joints in each region of the spine can be found in the chapters concerning functional aspects of the lumbar, thoracic, and cervical spine.

Spongiosa Structure

The spongiosa structure of the vertebral processes must be able to withstand the stress of both compression and bending. With regard to the superior articular process, the organization of the spongiosa is the same in the sagittal plane of all vertebrae. Short struts of bone stand perpendicular to the articular facets and are attached to each other by struts set at perpendicular angles. In the transverse plane, these bony struts are not arranged in the same way for every articular facet. In the cervical and thoracic areas, they are arranged as they are in the sagittal plane. In the lumbar area and the sacrum, the spongiosa struts form a "pointed arch structure" (Putz, 1981). This implies they are at times exposed to a bending stress in the transverse plane.

Transverse forces are caused by rotation resulting from local pressure of the inferior articular process of the vertebra above and from tensile stress of ligaments and muscles whose insertion is on the mamillary process. These are mainly the transverse reinforcing fibers of the joint capsule and the short (segmental) rotator muscles.

For the inferior articular process, the spongiosa structure in the sagittal plane is generally constructed similarly throughout the entire spine. Pointed arch structures extend from the roots of the vertebral arch, implying bending stress in the sagittal plane. This arrangement is most obvious in the lumbar section, which corresponds to the change in joint space morphology required during extreme flexion. Determining the spongiosa structure of the inferior articular process in the transverse plane with any degree of certainty has proven difficult.

Joint Capsule

The joint capsule, as shown in **Figure 1–4**, is composed of the following structures:

- Synovial membrane
- Synovial folds and protrusions
- Fibrous membrane

Synovial Membrane

The synovial membrane is attached to the periphery of the articular facet, on the outside edge of the cartilage. Because the cartilage covering ends abruptly, there is a deep split, largely covered by the adjacent synovial membrane. This membrane also completely covers the articular cavity, with the exception of the joint cartilage, and is at times separated by an interstitial tissue from the overlying fibrous membrane. On the top and bottom of the articular cavity, the synovial membrane exhibits extensive bulging; these

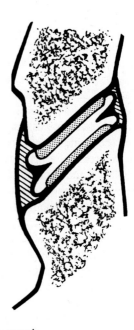

Figure 1–4   Joint capsule.

bulges are somewhat smaller on the lateral aspects of the articular cavity. This recess serves as reserve space for extreme movements. The synovial and fibrous membranes are separated by adipose and connective tissue.

Meniscoid Folds

Between the articular facets of all intervertebral joints, there are also folds and protrusions of variable shapes and sizes. These often extend a significant distance into the joint cavity. According to Putz (1981), they can be arranged in many different ways and are mostly found in the lordotic areas of the spine, where they are both numerous and ubiquitous.

In the cervical spine, there are large synovial folds in the caudal and cranial aspects of the joints, and smaller ones laterally. In the thoracic spine, there are small folds throughout the joints. In the medial aspect of the thoracic joints, these folds can be somewhat larger. The lumbar spine contains many synovial folds of varied composition. They are predominantly situated in the cranial and medial part of the joint cavity. In the cervical and thoracic spine, the folds are broad extensions of the joint capsule. In the lumbar spine, they are more pointed and can intrude up to 6 mm into the joint space.

Attempts have been made to explain the function of these protrusions in histological terms. Schminke and Santo (1932) described them as articular disks. In reference to the cervical spine, Töndury (1940, 1958) described them as meniscoid folds. According to Kos and Wolf (1972) and Benini (1978), meniscoid folds are all constructed in the same way. They are composed of a peripheral adipose tissue section that is fixed to the capsule, a blood-vessel-rich middle section, and a relatively blood-vessel-free rim that is composed of compact collagenous connective tissue containing cartilage cells.

According to examinations by Putz (1981), large and strong folds can be found in the cervical spine, especially in the atlantoaxial joint. These folds are mostly composed of compact connective tissue and extend at their base into the fibrous membrane. Adipose tissue can be found at the base. In the thoracic spine, the folds are mostly composed of connective tissue. In the lumbar spine, these folds vary in structure and morphology. They are predominantly composed of adipose tissue, rich in blood vessels.

The T12, L1, and L2 folds are almost exclusively composed of connective tissue that is extensively attached to the fibrous membrane. Their free rims are often frayed. The joint cavity often contains particles that have been torn off.

The meniscoid folds are not spare folds for extreme movements, as is the function of the capsular recess. They remain present during large movements. They are tissues that by way of limited deformation adapt to changes of the joint cavity. Sometimes the folds fill the space left behind when cartilage has been lost. They play a role in pressure transfer in the joints. The ligaments and muscles bordering on the meniscoid folds can exert pressure from the outside, depending on the position of the spine.

The meniscoid folds also have another function: the prevention of capsular impingement in the joint.

Fibrous Membrane

A number of authors have described the fibrous membrane as generally flaccid; others as either flaccid or firm, depending on the level of mobility in a specific area. The collagenous connective tissue of the joint capsule extends beyond the adjacent periosteum. Depending on the spinal region, membranes of different sizes can develop. Here, reinforcement fibers can exist that cannot be distinguished as independent capsular ligaments. According to Putz (1981), the differentiation of the fibrous membrane in the various spinal regions has to do with the thickness, the orientation of the reinforcement fibers, and the relation to the adjacent ligaments and muscles. The insertion site for the fibrous membrane is more or less the same in every region of the spine.

The fibrous membrane originates at the base of the articular process. In the thoracic and lumbar area, the place of attachment is farthest from the periphery of the articular surfaces. This leaves the innermost aspects of the articular processes exposed within the articular cavity.

At its medial aspect, the fibrous membrane is very thin, so it appears as though the intracapsular tissue is connected to the extracapsular tissue. The development of the fibrous membrane's bandlike reinforcement fibers mentioned earlier determines both the firmness of the capsule and the degree of mobility of the joint. In the lumbar spine, the highly developed fibers run from the lateral aspect of the inferior articular process to the mamillary process and the parts of the superior articular process located caudally to these mamillary processes. They run in the transverse plane and are particularly well developed in the middle.

They often diverge laterally (**Figure 1–5**). These transverse reinforcement fibers can also be found in the lower thoracic vertebrae where the joint cavity orientation corresponds to that found between the lumbar vertebrae. They serve to inhibit flexion and—to a lesser extent—extension and rotation. In the cervical and thoracic joints, the capsule is thinner and there are no bandlike reinforcement fibers.

In the cervical spine, the outer fibers of the fibrous membrane course almost longitudinally and are slightly more

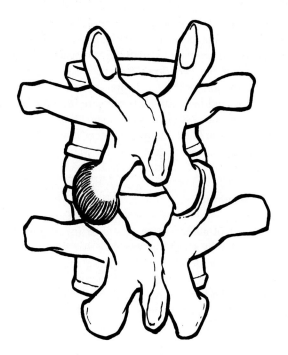

Figure 1–5   Fibrous membrane (Transverse reinforcing fibers).

developed. In the thoracic spine, they have less tensile strength and a less orderly arrangement, exerting little influence on mobility.

Ligamentous Relationships

In the cervical and lumbar spine, the intertransverse ligaments are close to the joint capsule—in the lumbar spine, there is even direct contact, whereas in the thoracic spine, these ligaments and the fibrous membrane are clearly separated. In each of the spinal regions, the intertransverse ligaments differ in strength, size, and orientation.

In the cervical spine, the thin intertransverse ligaments border on the ventrolateral part of the fibrous membrane. Small foramina allow blood vessels and nerves access to the outer surface of the vertebral arches.

In the thoracic spine, the intertransverse ligaments run more or less along the front of the transverse process, leaving space in their midsection for blood vessels and nerves.

In the lumbar spine, the intertransverse ligaments form the medial edge of an aponeurosis that extends laterally into the deep lamina of the lumbar dorsal fascia. They contain large openings through which course the dorsal branches of the spinal nerves and blood vessels. The ligaments have a protective function for these tissues.

In the cervical spine, the lateral portion of the flaval ligaments is attached at an angle to the joint capsules in the form of a small vertical sheet. A small space, filled with loose tissue, is left between the joint capsule and the flaval ligament.

In the thoracic spine, the flaval ligaments diverge cranially. At their medial aspect, they partially enclose the tops of the superior articular processes and lie close to the joint capsules.

In the lumbar spine, the superior articular processes are surrounded by the lateral surfaces of the flaval ligaments all the way to the base of the inferior articular process. The ligaments have a thicker portion at the level of the superior articular process. In the thoracolumbar and lumbosacral transitional area, sharp bony ridges can often be found in the attachment area for the flaval ligaments. Junghanns (1954) sees these as an expression of a general chronic degenerative change.

The most lateral bony ridges can be found at the level of the anterior-most part of the joint capsule of the intervertebral joints. They can cause dysfunctions and pain in the intervertebral joints.

Not directly adjacent to the joint capsules, the interspinous ligaments are relevant to spinal function because of their fiber orientation.

According to Heylings (1978), they run dorsally from the root of the caudal vertebra's spinous process to the underside of the cranial vertebra's spinous process in a fanlike S shape (**Figure 1–6**). This structure allows the spinous processes to separate and inhibits the dorsal translation of the cranial vertebra in relation to the caudal vertebra.

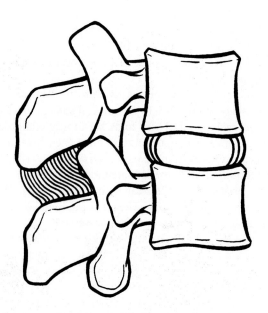

Figure 1–6   S-shape fiber structure.

Muscular Relationships

In the cervical and thoracic spine, the deepest fascicles of the intrinsic musculature are not interconnected with the joint capsules. When contracting with the thoracic spine in a flexed position, the long rotator muscles use the inferior articular process and the adjacent joint capsules as their fixed point against which to exert force. In the lumbar spine, fascicles of the multifidi muscles originate from the joint capsules and the mamillary processes and can, therefore, increase capsular tension.

During global contractions of the intrinsic back musculature, pressure increases in its surrounding osseofibrous structures. As a result, the meniscoid folds of the joint capsule are forced to move into the joint cavity, which causes the weight-bearing surface to enlarge. This occurs particularly with forceful flexion, side bending, and rotation.

Arterial Circulation

In the different spinal regions, the arterial blood supply to the intervertebral joints and surrounding area is organized in different ways.

In the lumbar and thoracic spine, articular branches originate from the segmental arteries (lumbar and posterior intercostal arteries). A branch originating in the iliolumbar arteries supplies the most lumbosacral joint (**Figure 1–7A** and **1–7B**).

In the cervical spine, branches from the vertebral artery and the cervical ascending pharyngeal artery supply arterial

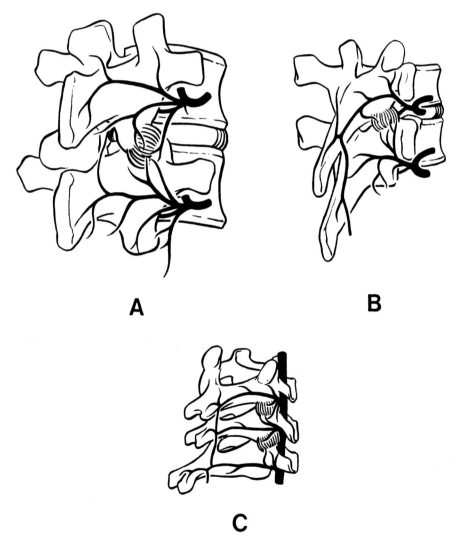

A

B

C

Figure 1–7   Arterial circulation of the lumbar (A), thoracic (B), and cervical (C) intervertebral joints.

blood to the joints. The lower cervical joints are also supplied by branches from the deep cervical artery (Kos, 1969) and the supreme intercostal artery (Jellinger, 1966) (**Figure 1–7C**).

In the cervicothoracic transitional area, blood is also supplied by way of the inferior thyroid artery (Yu Che, 1966). All arteries mentioned lead into the dorsal ramus at the lateral exit of the respective intervertebral foramen. This dorsal ramus then gives rise to the spinal ramus and the medial and lateral cutaneous ramus.

The medial cutaneous arterial ramus is primarily responsible for the arterial supply to the superior and inferior articular processes. Runge and Zippel (1976) named the sub-branches extending laterally from this medial cutaneous ramus the superior and inferior lateral vertebral arch arteries. These provide arterial supply to the superior and inferior articular processes, respectively. The lateral and caudal part of the joint capsule is supplied by sub-branches that originate from these branches or from the medial cutaneous branch itself. The cranial part of the joint capsule is supplied by a branch directly derived from the dorsal ramus. The medial cutaneous branch runs over the base of the relevant spinous process both caudally and cranially, forming—together with the branches above and below it—intersegmental anastomoses.

Their branches reach the medial part of the joint capsule (Lewin, 1968b). The branches of the medial cutaneous branch are unlikely to supply enough blood. It is, therefore, assumed that branches of the dorsal ramus supply the cranial part of the joint capsule as well as the medial part. The branches leading to the intervertebral joint also supply the adjacent periosteum and the bone in which the fibrous membrane originates. Thin arterial branches enter the marrow space of the bone via large foramina located on the lateral and caudal part of the base of the superior articular process and on the lateral surface of the inferior articular process. They partially originate in the dorsal ramus and the medial cutaneous ramus (Yu Che, 1966).

According to Clemens (1961), the bone is supplied from the periosteum by way of Volkmann's canals. Throughout the entire spine, the intervertebral joints' arterial network of dorsal rami is connected to the networks above, below, and on the opposite side (Ferguson, 1950; Louis, 1978). As is the case with the intervertebral joints of the other cervical vertebrae, the arterial needs of the atlanto-occipital joints are met by branches of the vertebral artery (Fischer, Garret, Gonan, and Sayfi, 1977). These branches form anastomoses with the frontal deep neck arteries. The branches from the vertebral artery, which supply the dorsal parts of the joint capsules, correspond to the dorsal rami of the segmental arteries. The anterior ascending artery, which supplies the frontal parts of the joint capsules, originates below the level

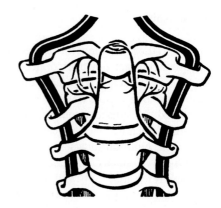

Figure 1–8   Apical arch of the axis. *Source:* Schiff and Parke, 1973.

of the axis out of the vertebral artery and runs cranially along the ventral aspect of the axis (Schiff and Parke, 1973). Together with the branch from the other side, this artery forms the apical axis arch (**Figure 1–8**).

The superior articular processes of the axis are supplied from the dorsal side; a direct branch of the vertebral artery enters the axis arch on the lateral side of the vertebral foramen.

Venous Circulation

The two dense venous plexuses, which can be found near the spinal column, are described in detail by Batson (1957) and Clemens (1961).

The posterior external vertebral venous plexus lies between the base of the spinous process and the transverse process, against the vertebral arches and the posterior aspect of the joints. The posterior internal vertebral venous plexus courses longitudinally within the spinal canal.

Here, the veins are connected to each other by transverse anastomoses. Bone veins of the vertebral arches and the articular processes flow into the adjacent plexus. According to Clemens (1961), the absence of valves can alter the direction of the flow in the vertebral plexus. Depending on the current local pressure ratio, the blood from the vertebral arches and the articular process can flow into either the dorsal or ventral plexus.

According to research by Putz (1981), small veins connect the plexus veins to the vertebral, intercostal, and lumbar veins. These veins run parallel to the arteries that supply the joint capsule. From the base of the skull to the sacrum, the vertebral venous system forms a chain of anastomoses. According to Ghazwinian and Kramer (1974), the filling of the lumbar epidural veins is dependent on the central venous pressure, which is dependent on position. A crawling position causes the least pressure. Coughing, sneezing, or pushing causes a pressure increase in the skull, thorax, and abdomen, which can also cause an increase in the venous pressure.

Innervation

The intervertebral joints are supplied by branches of the spinal nerves coursing through the respective intervertebral foramina. As shown in **Figure 1–9**, the dorsal ramus (a) and the meningeal ramus (b) branch off these spinal nerves before leaving the intervertebral foramen.

Running in a gutter between the superior articular process and the transverse process, the dorsal ramus courses around the base of the articular process and reaches the base of the spinous process via the arch of the lamina. Along with the relevant blood vessels, the dorsal ramus is closely connected to the medial fibers of the intertransverse ligament (Braus and Elze, 1921, 1954). According to Putz (1981), these medial fibers often ossify.

The joint capsule, the musculature, and the skin are innervated by the dorsal ramus and its branches, the medial (c) and lateral rami (d). Emminger (1954), Clemens (1971), Frick, Leonhardt, and Starck (1977) state that the dorsal ramus is solely responsible for innervation of the intervertebral joints. Loeweneck (1966) reports that the dorsal branch of the respective spinal nerves is solely responsible for innervation of the joint capsules of the lumbar joints. The meningeal ramus (Luschka, 1862) or sinuvertebral nerve, also known as the recurrent or dural ramus (Clara, 1959), returns into the intervertebral foramen and the vertebral canal, where it creates a neural plexus.

The meningeal ramus sometimes originates from the dorsal ramus (Stofft, 1977). According to Luschka (1862), it originates distally in the spinal ganglion and absorbs a number of the fibers from the sympathetic trunk before returning to the intervertebral foramen.

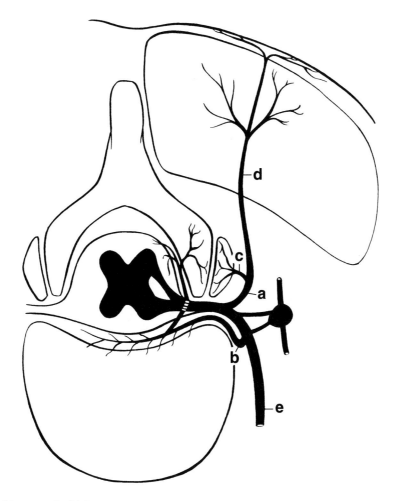

Figure 1–9 Innervation of intervertebral joints.

Grieve (1975) observes a close correlation between the meningeal ramus and the sympathetic system. In the cervical area, the meningeal branch originates in the plexus of sympathetic fibers surrounding the vertebral artery; in the thoracic area, it originates in the ganglia of the sympathetic trunk.

According to Krämer (1978), the meningeal ramus (together with its branches) supplies the innermost part of the joint capsule, periosteum, and posterior longitudinal ligament, as well as the meninges, with efferent, afferent, and sympathetic fibers.

With regard to pain in the spinal area, Vélé (1968) and Tilscher (1982) attribute a special significance to the meningeal ramus; the nerve branches for the dorsal parts of the atlanto-occipital joint capsule emerge from the ventral ramus (e) of the C1 and C2 spinal nerves (Loeweneck, 1966). Direct branches from the meningeal ramus also supply these capsules, in particular the ventral part of the atlantoaxial joint.

Schmorl and Junghanns (1968) point out that a motion segment is never supplied in a monoradicular way. Anastomoses between dorsal rami above and below occur predominantly in the cervical and lumbar area. The current view is that each segment helps meet the needs of adjacent superior and inferior segments (Paris, 1982) (**Figure 1–10**).

The outermost connective tissue layer of the ventral nerve root is probably innervated by sub-branches of the meningeal ramus; the dorsal nerve root is supplied by fibers from the spinal ganglion.

The peri- and epineurium of the ventral and dorsal ramus are supplied by branches of the nerve's own axons and by sub-branches of the perivascular nerve. The blood vessels inside and outside the vertebral canal and the intervertebral foramen are surrounded by plexi of unmyelinated, autonomic afferent and efferent nerve fibers. Running independently from the peripheral nerves, these nerves are hypothesized to provide the primary joint innervation of capsule and ligaments. From this, one might conclude that

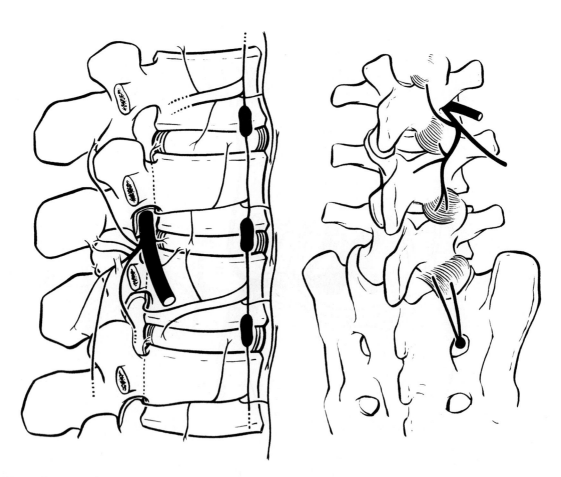

Figure 1–10   Multisegmental innervation. *Source:* Paris, 1982.

these nerves conduct nociceptive impulses (among others) from both blood vessels and the joint.

Ligaments

The anterior longitudinal ligament (a in **Figure 1–11**) runs as a broad band over the front of the vertebral bodies and anulus fibrosus, becoming the anterior atlanto-occipital membrane above the level of C2. The ligament is firmly attached to the intervertebral disk, the middle portion of the vertebral body, leaving free the ring apophyses (where osteophytes sometimes form).

The posterior longitudinal ligament (b) runs over the posterior aspect of the vertebral bodies and anulus fibrosus.

This ligament is firmly attached to the intervertebral disk and the upper- and lowermost sections of the vertebral bodies, leaving the vertebral body mid portions free for the venous plexus. This ligament grows thinner as it courses from cranial to caudal.

In the lumbar section, it presents as a thin cord that does not cover the dorsolateral surfaces of the disk. At the same level as the disk, a few fibers of the ligament run obliquely in a caudal direction toward the roots of the vertebral arches. In disk pathology, these fibers can become tensioned and cause periosteal pain, which must be differentiated from joint pain.

The flaval ligament (c) extends between two adjacent arches over the entire dorsal side of the spine and is,

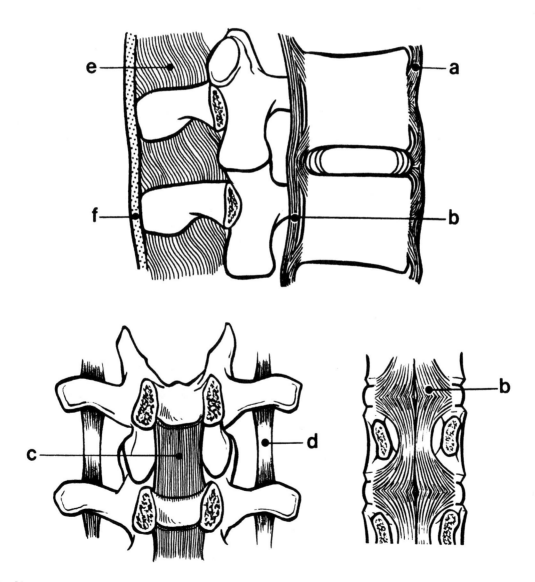

Figure 1–11 Ligaments.

therefore, a component of the spinal canal. The ligament thickens caudally—it is also highly elastic, which is of extreme functional importance to the spinal cord. When flexion occurs, its length increases by 40% (Penning, 1978). All the way down the spine, the intertransverse ligament (d) and interspinous ligament (e) extend between two adjacent transverse and spinous processes, respectively.

The supraspinous ligament (f) connects the posterior-most aspects of the adjacent spinous processes along the whole length of the spine and, at the level of the C7 spinous process, becomes the elastic nuchal ligament, which connects the cervical spinous processes from T2 to C5 inclusive with the posterior tubercle of the atlas, the external occipital crest, and the external occipital protuberance. The ligaments referred to here guarantee both the stability of the spine and its mobility. In terms of movement, they have a guiding and movement-limiting function in keeping with their position relative to the axis of movement.

UNCOVERTEBRAL JOINT

As well as intervertebral joints, the cervical spine contains uncovertebral joints (Luschka's joints; Luschka, 1862). These joints are located on the dorsolateral aspect of the cervical vertebral bodies (**Figure 1–12**). They are bony ridges that articulate with each other and provide lateral stability. These uncovertebral joints are the first place where decompensation caused by excessive strain will show up in X-rays (Penning, 1978)—this is known as uncarthrosis.

Because the axis of rotation is located below the plane of the disk, the movement of flexion/extension results in a translatory movement between adjacent vertebrae and consequently a functional disk deformation, which is greatest at the location of the uncovertebral joints. As a result of the vertical position of the uncinate process, this is where the distance between two vertebral bodies is smallest, while the distance to the axis of rotation is largest.

The load on the uncovertebral joints increases as the disk grows thinner with age. Usually, the thinning of the disk begins in segment C5–C6, where the average level of mobility is greatest.

JOINTS BETWEEN THE OCCIPUT, ATLAS, AND AXIS

The joints between the occiput, atlas, and axis (**Figure 1–13**) can be classified as follows:

• Atlanto-occipital joint (a)
• Atlanto-odontoid joint (b)
• Atlantoaxial joint (c)

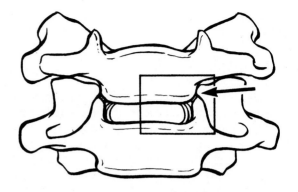

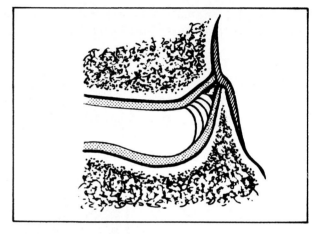

Figure 1–12   Uncovertebral joint.

These joints are constructed differently from any other intervertebral joints. There is no intervertebral disk between the atlas and the occiput and between the atlas and the axis, and the dens of the axis takes the place of the body of the atlas. On the superior aspect of the lateral masses of the atlas, there are two oval articular facets that are concave in both the sagittal and the frontal planes. The longitudinal axes converge medioventrally. The convex occipital condyles articulate with these articular facets.

The connection between atlas and axis is composed of three joints: the atlantoaxial joints are located laterally and are made up of biconvex articular facets both on the lower side of the atlas and on the upper side of the axis.

In the center is the median atlantoaxial joint, the joint composed of the dens of the axis, the anterior arch of the atlas, and the transverse atlantal ligament. The transverse atlantal ligament and the anterior arch of the atlas have an articular facet (cava articularis) on their inner surface.

The individual joints are reinforced by a number of ligamentous structures. The transverse atlantal ligament is

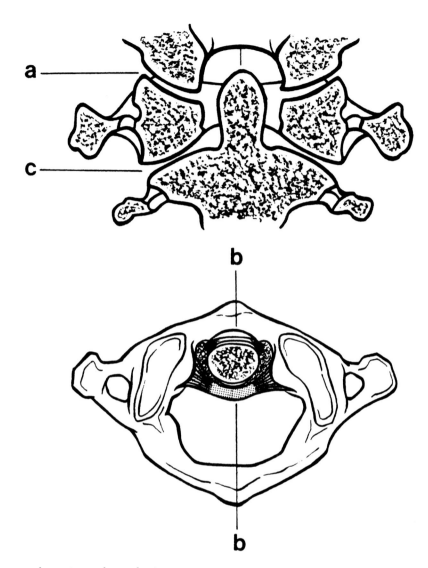

Figure 1–13 Joints between the occiput, atlas, and axis.

complemented by longitudinal fibers running cranially toward the anterior aspect of the foramen magnum and caudally toward the body of the axis. Together, they form the cruciate ligament of the atlas.

From the tip of the dens, the apical ligament of dens also runs toward the anterior aspect of the foramen magnum.

The alar ligaments extend between the back and the front of the tip of the dens and the lateroventral side of the foramen magnum and the medial side of the occipital condyles. Furthermore, in many of the cases mentioned previously, they form a connection between the dens and the lateral masses of the atlas. All ligaments noted previously course

within the vertebral canal and are covered by the tectorial membrane. The anterior atlanto-occipital membrane is located on the front between the occiput and the atlas; the posterior atlanto-occipital membrane is located posteriorly.

The anterior and posterior atlantoaxial membranes are located between atlas and axis. The specific motion characteristics of the C0–C2 complex are determined by the variations in morphology and the ligamentous structure as well as by the absence of an intervertebral disk.

With their local musculature, the atlanto-occipital and atlantoaxial joints are the only joints in the entire spine capable of independent movement.

COSTOVERTEBRAL JOINTS AND COSTOSTERNAL CONNECTIONS

Costovertebral Joints

Costovertebral joints are made up of two synovial joints, the costovertebral and the costotransverse joint (**Figure 1–14**).

The costovertebral joints 1, (in some subjects 10), 11, and 12 are formed by the head of the rib and the superior costal facet of the thoracic vertebra of the same number.

For ribs 2 to 9 (10) inclusive, the superior costal facet of the vertebra of the same number, the intervertebral disk above, and the inferior costal facet of the vertebra above combine to form the joint cavity. These ribs contain a bony crest on the head of the rib, connected to the outermost layers of the anulus fibrosus by way of the intra-articular ligament of the head of the rib (a). This ligament divides the joint cavity into two incompletely separated compartments.

The capsular radiate ligament of the head of the rib (b) radiates from the head of the rib over the periphery of the corresponding joint. Three sections—superior, intermediate, and inferior—can be distinguished in this ligament. Their

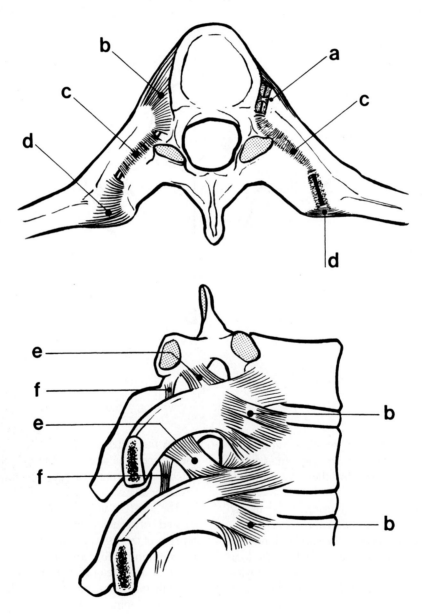

Figure 1–14   Costovertebral joints.

respective attachment places are the vertebra above, the intervertebral disk, and the vertebra of the same number.

The costotransverse joint is formed by the articular facet of the tubercle of rib and the costal facet on the transverse process. This joint is absent in the 11th and 12th ribs. Relatively loose, the capsule is strengthened by a few extracapsular ligaments.

The costotransverse ligament or ligament from the neck of the rib (c) extends from the dorsal side of the neck of the rib to the ventral side of the transverse process, completely filling the space between them. The lateral costotransverse ligament or ligament from the tubercle of the rib (d) connects the tubercle of the rib with the tip of the transverse process.

The anterior costotransverse ligament (e) connects the bony crest on the neck of the rib with the ventrocaudal aspect of the transverse process above. The posterior costotransverse ligament (f) connects the neck of rib with the dorsocaudal side of the transverse process above and the base of the lamina above. The lumbocostal ligament connects the caudal side of the 12th rib with the tips of the costal processes of the first and second lumbar vertebrae.

The two costovertebral joints form a mechanical entity with the axis of movement (axis of rotation) running through the middle of both joints. The axis of the upper costovertebral joints runs in more or less a frontal orientation.

The axis of the middle thoracic costovertebral joints runs obliquely at an angle of 45° to the sagittal plane. The axis of the lower costovertebral joints runs in a sagittal orientation.

Costosternal Connections

The costosternal connections consist of synovial joints called the sternocostal joints (**Figure 1–15**). These joints are formed where the costal notches of the sternal body join the cartilaginous tips of the true ribs 2 to 7 inclusive.

The first rib, which has no joint cavity, is a synchrondosis and is attached to the manubrium. This rib is attached to the clavicula by way of the costoclavicular ligament. The costal notch of the second rib is located at the transitional area between the manubrium and the body of the sternum (**Figure 1–16**).

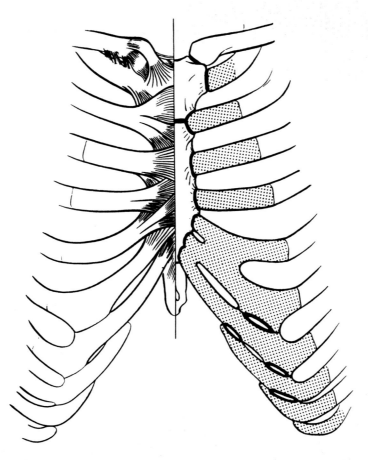

Figure 1–15 Costosternal connections.

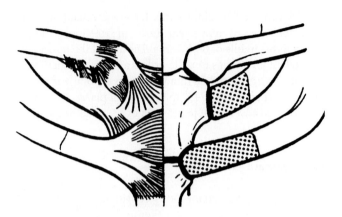

Figure 1–16   Costosternal connection of ribs 1 and 2.

The interarticular sternocostal ligament attaches the tip of the second rib's cartilage with the cartilage between the manubrium and the body of the sternum. The relatively tight capsules of the costosternal joints are strengthened at the front by the radiate sternocostal ligament, which radiates into the ventral aspect of the sternum, where it strengthens the periosteum of the sternum. Together they are called the sternal membranes.

Finally, the costoxiphoid ligaments attach the ventral aspect of the xiphoid process to the cartilaginous tips of the sixth and seventh ribs. The cartilage components of ribs 8 to 10 inclusive, the vertebrochondral ribs, are attached to each other and have indirect contact with the sternum by way of the cartilage of the seventh rib. These cartilaginous joints, also located between the fifth, sixth, and seventh ribs, are called interchondral joints.

The internal and external intercostal membranes, with fibers that take the same path as those of the internal and external intercostal muscle, are located in between the cartilaginous parts of the ribs. They are considered syndesmoses.

Sternum

The sternum (**Figure 1–17**) is composed of the sternal manubrium, the body of the sternum, and the xiphoid process.

At its superior aspect, the sternal manubrium has a jugular notch; bilaterally, it has a clavicular notch and a costal notch for the first and second ribs. The joint between manubrium and body of the sternum is called the sternal synchondrosis, and the angle between the two bones is the sternal angle. The body of the sternum contains the costal notch of ribs 2 to 7 inclusive. The ventral aspect of the body of the sternum is called the sternal plane.

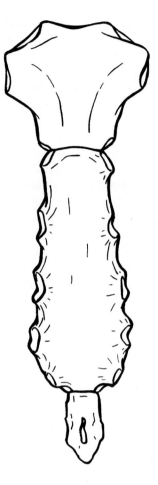

Figure 1–17   Sternum.

The efficient functioning of the costovertebral and costosternal joints is important not only to the breathing process, but also to the movement of the thoracic spine and everything related to it (see Chapter 15, "Examination of the Thoracic Spine").

PELVIS

Together with the diaphragm and the abdominal, back, and pelvic floor muscles, the pelvis (**Figure 1–18**) forms the abdominal and pelvic cavity and connects the spine to the lower extremities. The pelvis is a closed bony ring, composed of three joints and three bones—the two innominates and the sacrum. The innominates (**Figure 1–19**) are formed by the union of three initially separate bones: the ilial bone, the ischial bone, and the pubic bone.

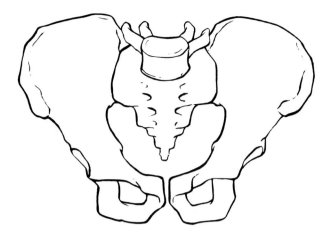

Figure 1–18   Pelvis.

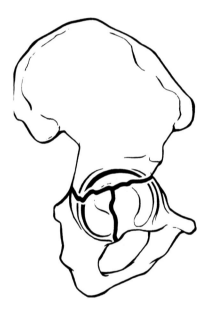

Figure 1–19   Innominates.

Ilial Bone

The components of the ilial bone are the ilial body; the ilial wing; ventromedially, the arcuate lines on the ilial wing; cranially, the ilial crest, with the superior and inferior anterior ilial spines on the ventral aspect, and the posterior superior and inferior ilial spines on the dorsal aspect; the ilial fossa on its ventral aspect; on the dorsal aspect, the gluteal surface with the anterior, posterior, and inferior gluteal line and the auricular surface on its medial aspect.

Ischial Bone

The ischial bone is composed of the ischial body, the superior and inferior ischial branches, the ischial tuberosity, the ischial spine, and the greater and lesser ischial notches.

Pubic Bone

The pubic bone is formed by the pubic body, the superior and inferior pubic branches, the pubic arch (made up of both inferior pubic branches), the symphyseal surface, the pubic crest, the pectineal line, the pubic tubercle, the iliopectineal eminence, and the posterior obturator crest.

Acetabulum

The acetabulum is made up of the bodies of the three bones described previously and the following: the acetabular fossa, the acetabular notch, and the lunate surface.

The obturator foramen is composed of the bodies of the innominate bones and branches from the pubic bone and the ischial bone.

Sacrum

The sacrum (**Figure 1–20**) is formed by the union of five initially separate sacral vertebrae and articulates caudally to the coccyx. The elements of the sacrum are, cranially, the sacral base, the sacral promontory, and the superior articular processes with the mamillary processes; caudally, the sacral apex, and the sacral hiatus with the sacral horns; ventrally, the pelvic surface, the pelvic sacral foramina, and the transverse lines; dorsally, the dorsal surface, and the dorsal sacral foramina; laterally, the lateral part with the auricular surface on the side of its uppermost portion. The lateral mass is located craniolaterally.

From medial to lateral, there is on the dorsal side the median sacral crest, the intermediate sacral crest, and the lateral sacral crest.

Coccyx

The coccyx is composed of three or four coccygeal vertebrae.

Pelvic Parameters

The pelvis is composed of the pelvic inlet, the pelvic midplane, and the pelvic outlet (**Figure 1–21**).

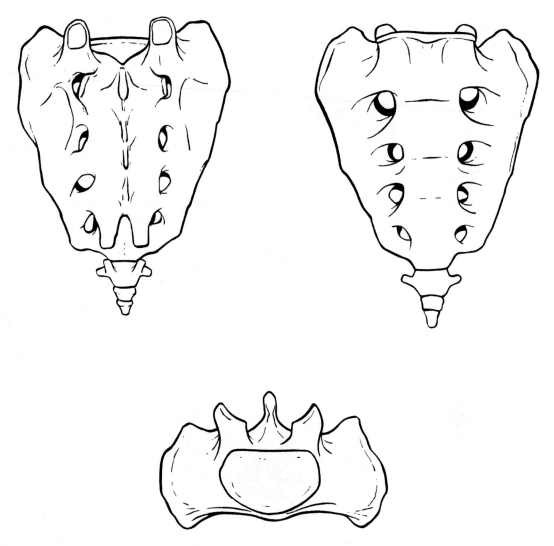

Figure 1–20   Sacrum.

The pelvic inlet is defined by the arcuate line, which extends to the pubic crest and the promontory, thus forming the iliopectineal line (a). This line divides the pelvis into the false and true pelvis. The pelvic midplane is the level defined by an imaginary line between the middle of the posterior aspect of the pubic symphysis and the middle of the connection of the ischial spines.

The pelvic outlet is defined by the pubic arch, the ischial tuberosities, and the coccygeal apex.

Other morphologic characteristics of the pelvis include the true conjugate diameter (b) between the sacral promontory and the superior aspect of the symphysis, the diagonal conjugate diameter (c) between the inferior aspect of the symphysis and the sacral promontory, the transverse diameter (d) between the left and right sections of the il-

iopectineal line, where the distance between these sections is the greatest, the sagittal diameter (e) between the coccygeal apex and the inferior aspect of the symphysis, and the oblique diameter (f) between the sacroiliac joint and the iliopectineal eminence.

Pelvic Joints

The four joints of the pelvis are the following:

- Two sacroiliac joints
- Pubic symphysis
- Sacrococcygeal joint

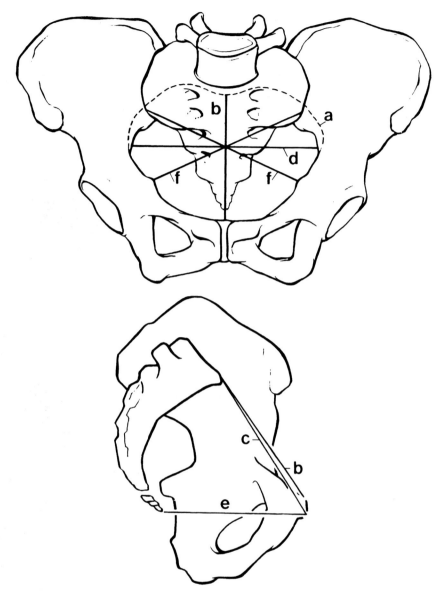

Figure 1–21 Pelvic parameters.

Sacroiliac Joint

The sacroiliac joint (**Figure 1–22**) is composed of the auricular surfaces of the ilial bone and of the sacrum. The articular facets are covered with fibrocartilage. Although these joint surfaces are largely irregular, some researchers have attempted to establish a relationship between a specific morphology and its function. Faraboef (Kapandji, 1974) described a long crest along the length of the auricular surface of the ilial bone, which he considered part of a circle with its midpoint situated on the S2 sacral tuberosity. Strong sacroiliac ligaments are also attached here. In the center of the auricular surface of the sacrum there are two crests, which are also part of a circle with a center located at the S1 transverse tubercle. Here, too, strong sacroiliac ligaments are attached.

According to Faraboef (Kapandji, 1974), the crests mentioned here are matching—although research based on a few dissections indicated that this is not entirely true. Delmas (1950) established that in the dynamic type with a

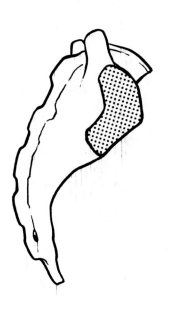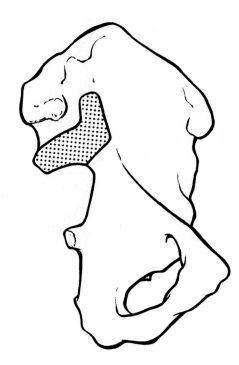

Figure 1–22   Sacroiliac joint.

horizontal pelvis, the sacroiliac joints allow more movement than is allowed by the joints in the static type that are longer in a vertical direction.

Weisl (1955) specifically studied the surface contours of the articular surfaces. He established that of the two segments the cranial is normally longer and thinner than the caudal. He also described a small depression in the center where the two segments of articular surface of the sacrum meet, and two small bulges near the corners of both segments. On the ilial articular surface, the center of the transition between the two segments exhibits a small prominence, known as Bonnaire's tubercle (Kapandji, 1974). Weisl suggested that it may correspond to the depression in the center of the sacral joint surface.

The ligamentous structure of the sacroiliac joint consists of the following structures, as shown in **Figure 1–23**:

- The superior iliolumbar ligament (a) extending from the inner rim of the ilial bone to the L4 transverse process
- The inferior iliolumbar ligament (b) extending from the inner rim of the ilial bone (and the sacrum) to the L5 transverse process
- The superior interosseous sacroiliac ligament (c) extending from the ilial crest to the S1 transverse sacral tuberosity

- The posterior sacroiliac ligaments (d) extending from the dorsal rim of the ilial bone to the sacral tuberosity
- The superior (e) and inferior (f) anterior sacroiliac ligaments between the ventral rim of the ilial bone and the ventral side of the sacrum
- The sacrospinous ligament (g) extending obliquely from the lateral rim of the sacrum and the coccygeal bone to the ischial spine
- The sacrotuberous ligament (h) extending between the dorsal rim of the ilial bone, the sacrum, the first two vertebrae of the coccyx, and the ischial tuberosity and ramus of the ischial bone

These last two ligaments form the superior and inferior ischial foramina. The obturator foramen is covered by the obturator membrane.

Pubic Symphysis

The pubic symphysis (**Figure 1–24**) is composed of the two cartilage-covered symphyseal surfaces of the pubic bone and the fibrocartilaginous interpubic disk. The disk has a fissure in the center and is connected to the pubic bone by the interosseous ligament (a). It is a secondary cartilaginous joint (amphiarthrosis) and not very mobile.

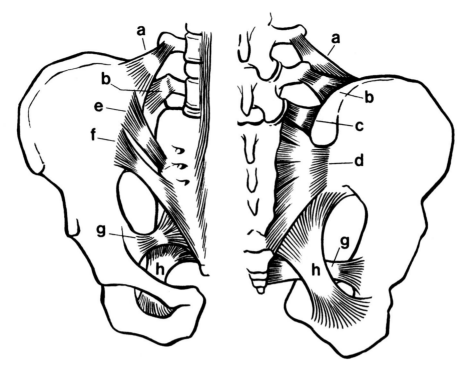

Figure 1–23 The ligamentous structure of the sacroiliac joint.

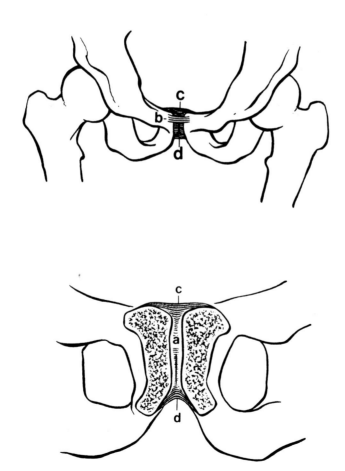

Figure 1–24 Pubic symphysis connections.

The following ligaments are part of this joint:

- The anterior pubic ligament (b), a thick ligament covering the joint at the front and composed of diagonal and oblique fibers.
- The extensions of the aponeurosis of the transverse abdominis, rectus abdominis, pyramidalis, internal oblique, and adductor longus muscles that run obliquely over the anterior aspect of the joint, together forming a tight fibrous network.
- The posterior pubic ligament (d), a fibrous membrane that represents an extension of the periost at the back.

- The posterior pubic ligament (c), a thick fibrous ligament on the superior aspect of the joint. The arcuate pubic ligament turns into the interosseal ligament on the inferior aspect of the joint.

Sacrococcygeal Joint

The sacrococcygeal joint (**Figure 1–25**) is a secondary cartilaginous joint (amphiarthrosis). The sacral articular facet is convex and the coccygeal one is concave. The joint has an interosseous ligament (a), an anterior sacrococcygeal

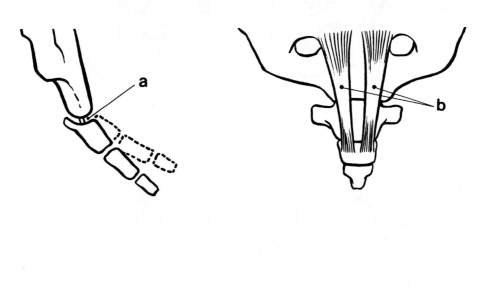

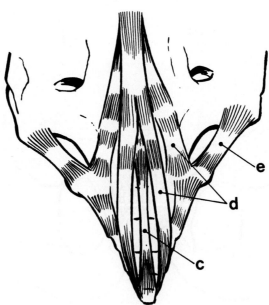

Figure 1–25   Sacrococcygeal joint and ligaments.

ligament (b), deep (c) and superficial (d) posterior sacrococcygeal ligaments, and a lateral sacrococcygeal ligament (e).

Lumbopelvic Angles

De Sèze (1961) provides some average angular values (measured while at rest) in relation to the lumbosacral junction, as shown in **Figure 1–26**:

- The lumbosacral angle, formed by the L5 to sacrum transition, is 140° (α).
- The sacral inclination angle, formed by the base of the sacrum and the horizontal plane, is 30° (β).
- The pelvic inclination angle, formed by the true conjugate diameter and the horizontal plane, is 60° (γ).

The lumbar lordosis is considered normal if the line between the posterior border of the superior aspect of L1 and the superior border of the inferior aspect of L5 coincides with a plumb line descending from the back of the superior aspect of L1. The apex of the lordosis should be at L3 (a).

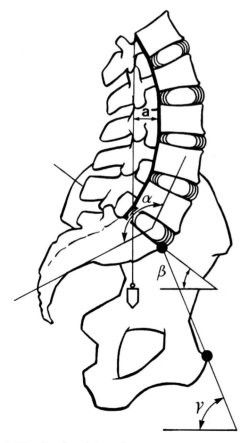

Figure 1–26   Lumbopelvic angles.

SPINAL MUSCULATURE

Muscle Location

The muscles responsible for maintaining the shape of the spine and for carrying out movements are represented schematically in **Figure 1–27**. They are largely part of the erector muscles of the spine. Although it is often hard to distinguish the individual muscles of the erector of the

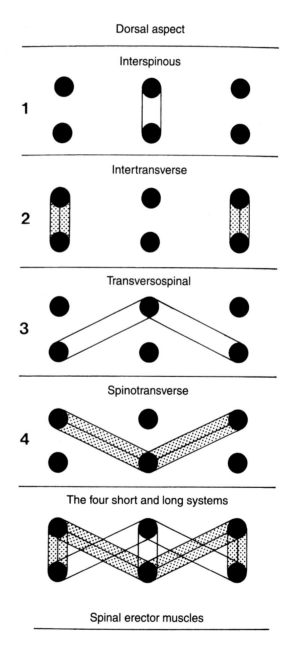

Figure 1–27   Schematic functional outline of spinal erector muscles.

spine in tissue preparations, it is functionally useful to make a distinction between short and long elements within this group.

The short muscles are medially located and fill the space between the spinous processes and the costal angles. The interspinous, intertransverse, and transversospinous muscles belong to this group.

The transversospinous muscles run between the transverse process and the higher spinous processes and include the rotatores muscles (which insert one or two spinous processes higher up), the multifidi muscles (which span four vertebrae), and the semispinalis muscles (which as a group span six vertebrae).

The semispinalis muscle is divided into the semispinalis thoracis, the semispinalis cervicis, and the semispinalis capitis, which inserts into the superior nuchal line of the back of the head. Of the long muscles, only the spinalis muscle is positioned medially. The short fibers of this muscle lie deep and connect a few adjacent vertebrae; the long fibers connect more remote spinous processes with each other. The lateral long muscles are composed of the longissimus and the iliocostalis muscles positioned lateral to the longissimus. The longissimus muscle runs both cranially and laterally from the sacrum and also from the transverse processes to the costal angles. The uppermost section, the longissimus capitis, inserts into the back of the mastoid process.

The lumbar part of the iliocostalis muscle originates from the pelvis and attaches laterally to the costal angles of the lowermost ribs. The thoracic part of the iliocostalis runs from the lowest ribs to the costal angles of the more cranial ribs. The cervical part of the iliocostalis runs from the rib angles of the uppermost ribs to the transverse processes of the cervical vertebrae. In the cervical portion of the spine, the erector muscles of the spine are complemented by the more superficially located splenius muscles. The splenius cervicis muscle originates from the spinous processes of the uppermost thoracic and lower cervical vertebrae and inserts into the transverse processes of the upper cervical vertebrae.

The splenius capitis muscle originates from the lateral portion of the nuchal ligament and from the four uppermost cervical spinous processes. The muscle inserts into the superior nuchal line and into the mastoid process.

As shown in **Figure 1–28**, The sternocleidomastoid muscle (a), the scalene muscles (b), and the short suboccipital muscles (c) also belong to the group of muscles that perform an important function with regard to movements of the head and neck.

The sternocleidomastoid muscle has a sternal origin at the ventral surface of the sternal manubrium and a clavicular origin at the sternal end of the clavicle. The two heads join and insert into the mastoid process.

The anterior, middle, and posterior scalene muscles originate from the anterior tubercles, the spinal grooves, and the posterior tubercles of the transverse processes of the third to seventh cervical vertebrae, respectively.

The anterior and middle scalene muscles insert into the tubercle of the anterior scalene muscle and the subclavian artery groove of the first rib, respectively.

The posterior scalene muscle inserts into the second rib.

The brachial plexus and the subclavian artery run through the triangular foramen formed by the anterior and middle scalene muscles.

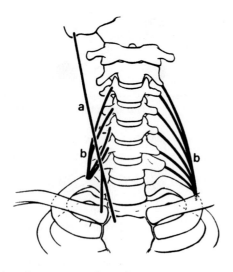
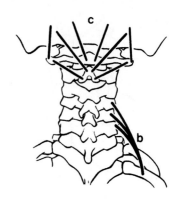

Figure 1–28   Mid- and upper-cervical muscles.

The suboccipital muscles connect the upper two cervical vertebrae with the occipital bone. The rectus capitis posterior major muscle lies dorsally, running from the spinous process of the axis to the lateral part of the inferior nuchal line. The rectus capitis posterior minor muscle originates from the posterior tubercle of the atlas and inserts into the middle portion of the inferior nuchal line.

The obliquus capitis inferior muscle connects the spinous process of C2 with the transverse process of the atlas; the obliquus capitis superior muscle connects the transverse process of the atlas with the lateral part of the inferior nuchal line.

On the ventral aspect, the rectus capitis anterior muscle runs from the lateral mass of the atlas to the basilar portion of the occipital bone, and the rectus capitis lateralis muscle runs from the transverse process of the atlas to the jugular process of the occipital bone.

CHAPTER 2

Introduction to Applied Biomechanics

Understanding how the spine works requires some knowledge of mechanics and the use of clearly defined terminology. Biomechanics is a branch of mechanics that studies structure and function within biological systems, using methods from mechanics. Biomechanics, like other disciplines of mechanics, can be subdivided into the following subdisciplines:

- *Kinematics.* The study of motion, and only motion—not its causes.
- *Dynamics.* The study of the relationship between the action of forces on a body and the motion of that body. Dynamics can, in turn, be subdivided into the following two fields:
  - *Statics.* The study of bodies at rest. The sum of forces is zero, so no motion occurs. In other words, equilibrium.
  - *Kinetics.* The study of bodies in motion in relation to the forces acting on them.

Within mechanics, a distinction is made between solid and fluid mechanics. Both are often combined in the body. Solid mechanics is involved in the loading on a joint; fluid mechanics in the lubrication of that joint. In the context of this book, we limit ourselves to solid mechanics. To understand this aspect of mechanics properly, it is of the utmost importance to clearly define the terminology used.

Scalar. A quantity that has only magnitude—temperature, for example.

Vector. A quantity determined and characterized by both magnitude and direction—a speed or a force, for exam-

ple. A vector is represented by an arrow, the length and direction of which indicate magnitude and direction. Of the many calculations using vectors, the most common are addition and subtraction by way of parallelogram constructions (**Figure 2–1**). The F_1 and F_2 forces together can be replaced by the R force without changing anything in the load situation. Conversely, a force can also be separated into two or more different forces using this method.

Movement. The distance traveled by an object, whether linear or angular. In the first case, this distance is expressed in meters or parts thereof (centimeters, millimeters); in

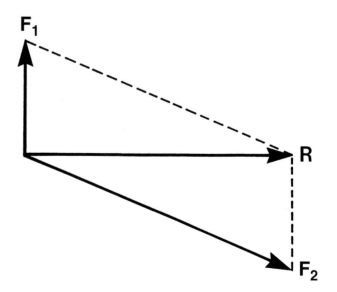

Figure 2–1   Parallelogram construction for vector calculation.

the second case, in degrees or radians. A radian is the angle at which the arc of a circle has the same length as the radius (**Figure 2–2**). The circumference of the circle is $2\pi R$ and, therefore, equal to 2π times the radian or 360°. Thus, 1 radian = 360°/2π = 57°.

Speed. The distance traveled per unit of time, expressed in meters per second, kilometers per hour, and so forth for linear speeds. For angular speeds, it is defined as the change of angle per unit of time, expressed in degrees or radians per second.

Acceleration. The change in speed per unit of time; it can be either linear or angular. These are expressed in m/s², cm/s² and °/s², and rad/s², respectively. Negative acceleration is called deceleration (braking, for example).

Force. Every action that imparts (or tries to impart) linear acceleration to an object. Friction and gravity are examples of external forces. The relationship between the net force and the acceleration in the same direction is represented by the following formula:

$$F = ma$$

where *m* is the object's mass. The unit of force is the Newton (N).

Moment (torque). The effect of a force in relation to a point that does not lie on that force's line of action. The magnitude of the moment is the product of the magnitude of the force and the perpendicular distance between the point and the force's line of action. A moment will cause (or try to cause) an angular rotation. If this angular rotation is around the longitudinal axis, then the accompanying moment is called a torsion or bending moment.

Equilibrium. A situation where the sum of all forces and moments exerted on an object equals zero.

Stress. The force per unit of surface area. Stress indicates the intensity of the force exerted on an object. When the force is exerted on a small surface area, the intensity is larger than when the same force is exerted on a large surface area. We can divide stress into compressive, tensile, and shear stress. The first two work in an axial direction relative to the surface area of the body and cause contraction and elongation, respectively. Elongation is called strain and is expressed in percentages of the original, non-weight-bearing measurement or length. Shear stresses work tangentially to this surface area. Tensile and compressive stresses are expressed with σ; shear stresses with τ. The difference between force and stress is important. When you look at the material's mechanical load, the stress exerted plays the most important role. In general, forces are related to the total load of an object and to the accompanying movement pattern.

Centroid. The point in the body where the body weight is concentrated. When all weights of the body parts are represented by vectors, the centroid forms the point of application of the resultant of all these weight vectors. To study motion and calculate the forces involved, we use the total body centroid and the partial centroids of the body's component parts. In this whole, the weight must be defined as the force that the Earth exerts on a body. This is expressed in Newton (N) and is, through the acceleration of gravity, linked to the body's mass (expressed in kilograms):

$$\text{Weight} = \text{Mass} \times \text{Acceleration of gravity}$$

Curvature. The extent to which an object is curved at a certain point; its value is equal to the reciprocal value of the radius of curvature:

$$C = 1 / R$$

The radius of curvature is the radius of the circle that, at the point in question, corresponds with the curvature of the actual object at that point (**Figure 2–3**). At point 1, the radius of this circle is larger than it is at point 2. The curvature at point 1 is therefore smaller than it is at point 2, where the curve is flatter.

With all biomechanical considerations, we start with an abstract representation of the anatomic and physiologic reality. Even when we look at small parts of it, the body is so

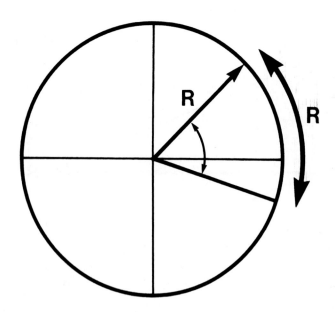

Figure 2–2   Radian.

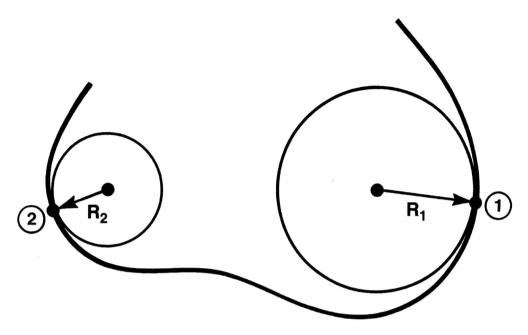

Figure 2–3   Radius of curvature R_1 and R_2 at points 1 and 2, respectively.

complex that an exact representation of all relevant parameters is unattainable. Consideration of the factors believed to be most important must suffice. At all times, we must therefore be cautious in interpreting the data obtained through biomechanical analyses, whether qualitative or quantitative. With the latter, we must always take into account the individual differences between different people and the unknowns related to spatial geometries and material properties. In addition, these theories are usually applied to patients who, by definition, do not have a normal, healthy constitution.

STATICS

Statics is defined as the study of situations in which no motion occurs. The bodies or body parts in question are at rest. The sum of the load is zero, or in other words, the sum of both moments and forces is zero. The body is in equilibrium. Static load situations can be calculated with the assistance of the two given conditions of equilibrium. A few examples follow:

Example 1

In a joint, the two forces F_2 and F_3, as shown in **Figure 2–4**, exerted by ligaments on the sides of the joint compensate for the vertical load force F_1, which is applied from a

craniocaudal direction on the superior aspect of the inferior joint partner in a static situation. The magnitude of F_2 and F_3 and the position of the force F_1 can be determined from this static equilibrium. This is described in **Figure 2–5**. In

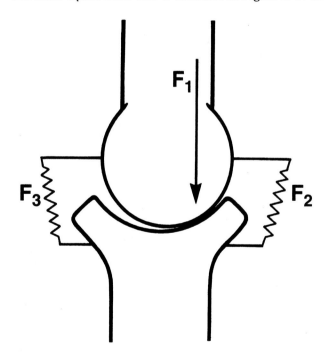

Figure 2–4   Schematic representation of a joint with loading force F_1.

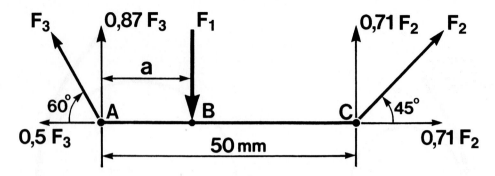

Figure 2–5   Forces on the lower joint partner.

the figure, the geometry indicated is applied. The forces are separated into two components: one horizontal and one vertical.

The fact that the sum of the horizontal forces is zero implies the following:

$$0.5F_3 - 0.71F_2 = 0$$

The fact that the sum of the vertical forces is zero implies the following:

$$0.87F_3 + 0.71F_2 - F_1 = 0$$

The fact that the sum of the moments around point A is zero implies the following:

$$F_1 \text{ times } a - 0.71F_2 \text{ times } 50 = 0$$

When F_1 is equal to 600 N, the preceding equations produce the following values:

$$F_2 = 308 \text{ N}$$

$$F_3 = 438 \text{ N}$$

$$a = 18 \text{ mm}$$

The forces exerted on the ligaments create stress in these structures that is equal to the force divided by the surface area of a cross section of the ligament. This stress determines the behavior of the ligament. Under normal circumstances, an elongation of the ligament will occur that is dependent on the current stress. **Figure 2–6** shows the relationship between the elongation ($^{\Delta L}/_L$) and stress (σ). When a stress is excessive, the ligament ruptures. This stress is called the *ultimate* or *maximum stress*. In this example, the ultimate stress is 60 N/mm². The strain induced by this ultimate stress is approximately 10%. In daily life, the normal loads remain well below that limit and tend to fall within an order of magnitude of 10 N/mm² with a strain of 4%.

The compressive force on the point of contact between the joint partners is turned into a compressive stress. Theoretically, there is one point of contact with an extremely small contact surface area. Because of this, the compressive stress increases enormously. The effect is a deformation of the hyaline cartilage, which results in an increase in the contact surface area and, as a consequence, a lower compressive stress on average. Equilibrium is established between the compressive force F_1 and the compressive stress in the cartilage of the contact surface area (A) between the articular segments (**Figure 2–7**).

The synovial fluid present also plays a part in the distribution of the compressive stress. This is something we do not investigate further here. The stress field is shown in Fig-

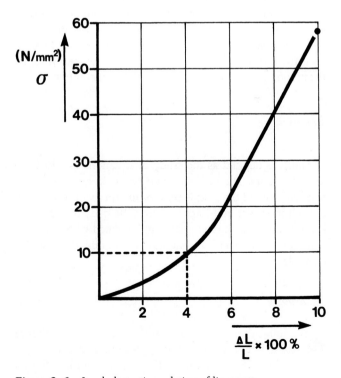

Figure 2–6   Load-elongation relation of ligaments.

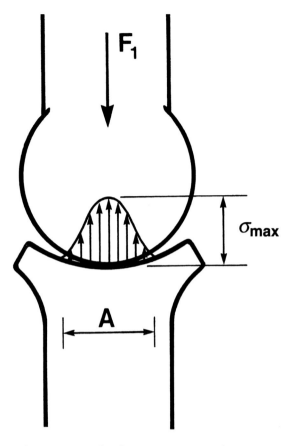

Figure 2–7   Pressure distribution in joint area of contact.

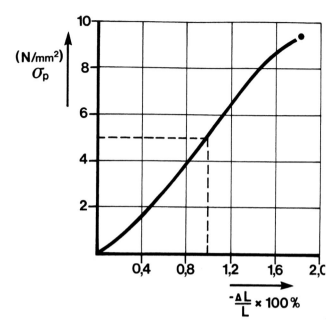

Figure 2–8   Load-deformation relation for hyaline cartilage.

ure 2–7. The cartilage also has a maximum weight-bearing capacity; if the compressive stress exceeds the ultimate stress, the cartilage tears.

Figure 2–8 shows the load-deformation relation for hyaline cartilage. Hyaline cartilage can tolerate loads that reach 50% of its ultimate strain. The solution to the problem presented previously could also have been described graphically.

In an equilibrium situation, two criteria must be met:

- The line of action of every force must run through one point. This determines the position of the joint force F_1, with a line of action that must always pass through the point of intersection of the lines of action of F_2 and F_3, and with the directions determined by the orientation of the ligaments.

- When we lay out all the force vectors in sequence, the result must be a closed figure. This determines the magnitude of F_2 and F_3. With the known magnitude of F_1, and the known directions of F_2 and F_3, a triangle representing the force can thus be drawn (**Figure 2–9**).

Example 2

The loading of the spine when lifting a weight in a bent-forward position is shown in **Figure 2–10**. When a person in this position lifts a weight (B) of 200 N and we assume the following:

- The centroid of this joint is located 400 mm (a) ventrally from the center of rotation of the fourth lumbar vertebra.

- The weight of the person's upper body (G) amounts to 400 N, and its centroid is located 200 mm (b) ventrally from the center of rotation of L4.

- In this position, the vertebral body is angled at 30° from the horizontal.

- The forces on the vertebra can be divided into an axial force (R) perpendicular to the endplates (compressive force originating in the nucleus), and a shearing force (A) in the intervertebral joints and the anulus.

- The muscle activities on the dorsal side of the spine can be described by means of one total muscle force (S) parallel to the spine at a distance of 50 mm— then, when the person maintains this position, all forces acting on the spine can be calculated from this situation of equilibrium. If we consider the equilibrium in the direction of the vertebral body and perpendicular to it, then both load forces must be separated in these directions (**Figure 2–11**).

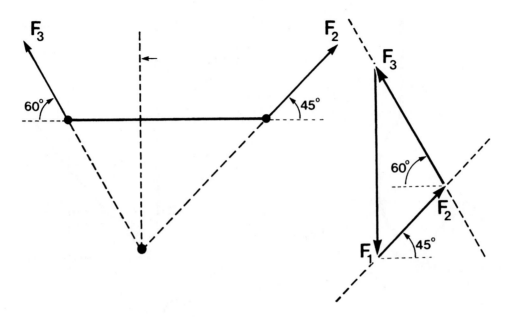

Figure 2–9   Graphic representation of joint forces.

From the fact that there is equilibrium in a sagittal direction, it follows:

$$A - 0.5G - 0.5B = 0$$

The shearing force to be carried over amounts to this:

$$A = 0.5G + 0.5B = 200 \text{ N} + 100 \text{ N} = 300 \text{ N}$$

From the equilibrium of applied torque about the center of rotation of the vertebral bodies, it follows:

$$S50 - G200 - B400 = 0$$

$$S = 4G + 8B = 1600 \text{ N} + 1600 \text{ N} = 3200 \text{ N}$$

This is the muscle force that must be delivered on the dorsal side of the spine.

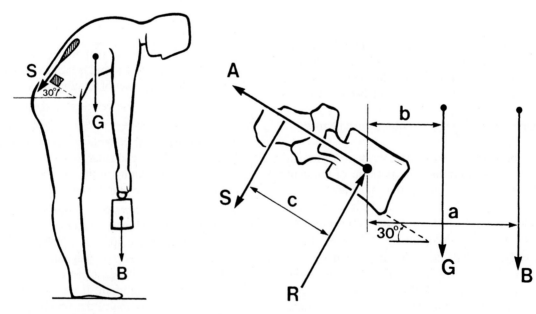

Figure 2–10   The loading of the spine when lifting a weight in a bent-forward position.

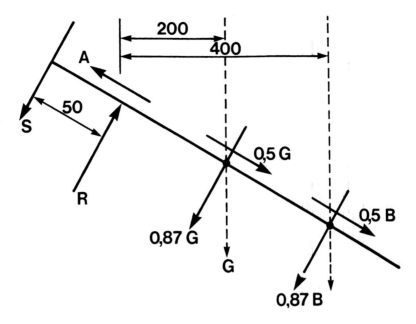

Figure 2-11 Equilibrium of forces at the level of the individual vertebra.

From the force equilibrium in an axial direction, it follows:

$$R - S - 0.87G - 0.87B = 0$$

$$R = 3200\,N + 175\,N + 350\,N = -3725\,N$$

This is the compressive force that must be handled by the nucleus. Within the nucleus, this compressive force is spread out among all structures in every direction. This systematic sharing process is called *hydrostatic pressure*. Both the endplates (axially) and the anular tissue (radially) must process this pressure. As shown in the previous example, this pressure depends strongly on the external load and the position assumed. **Figure 2-12** shows the pressure change as a consequence of changes to position and load.

The load on the spine, and particularly on the disk, results in distortions. With an axial compression load, the disk will be compressed, and its height will decrease. The extent of the compression is dependent on the load and is called its *stiffness* or *elasticity*. Elasticity is not always uniform (**Figure 2-13**).

The viscous nucleus pulposus is considered incompressible. Any decrease in height will, therefore, cause an increase in diameter (**Figure 2-14**).

When a certain pressure is applied, fluid is forced out of the nucleus and into the body, meaning that the decrease in

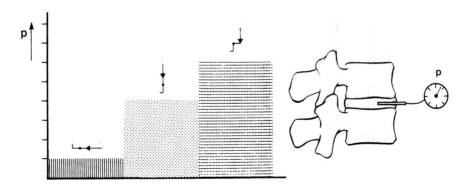

Figure 2-12 Nuclear pressure in different positions.

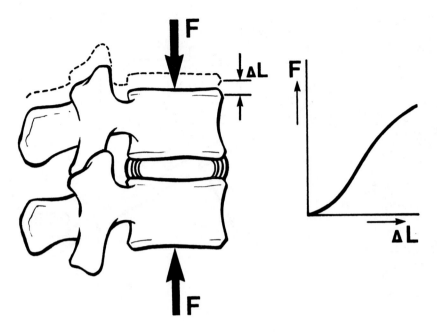

Figure 2–13   Stiffness of the complete intervertebral disk.

height and the increase in diameter are no longer proportional. The disk structures can also only be loaded to a limited extent. The values described in the first example also apply to the compressive tolerance of the hyaline endplates of the vertebral bodies. In the anular tissue, the off-center radial pressure is converted into tensile stresses in the anular fibers (**Figure 2–15I**). Naturally, this tensile stress should not exceed the ultimate stress.

To a limited extent, the anular tissue is capable of absorbing shear forces and shear stresses. **Figure 2–15II** shows the maximum load-bearing capacity of anular fibers

in a transverse (diagram A) and longitudinal (diagram B) direction. In daily life, the stresses should not be more than 25–30% of the ultimate stresses.

The anulus and the articular facets absorb the sagittal plane force. In the articular facets of the intervertebral joints, when both articular facets remain reasonably parallel, the shear force exerted—which works axially on the intervertebral joints—is distributed hydrostatically over all structures by the synovial fluid. The maximum compressive load of the hyaline cartilage and the maximum tensile load of the capsular fibers are grossly equal to the values calcu-

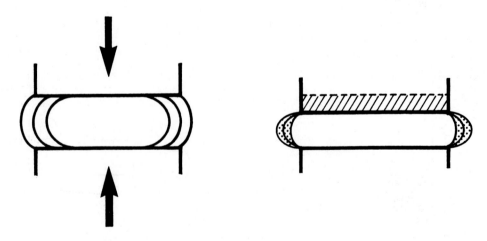

Figure 2–14   Increase in diameter with pressure on the intervertebral disk.

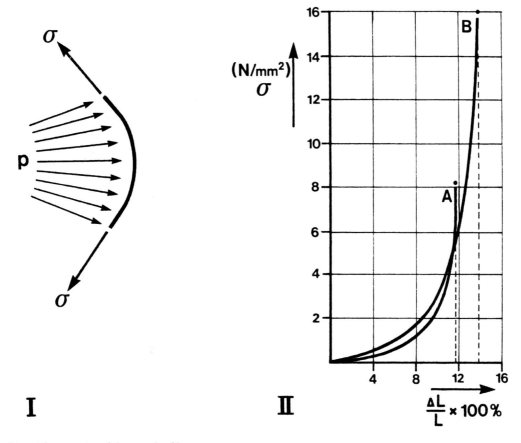

I   **II**

Figure 2–15   Material properties of the annular fibers.

lated earlier. However, focal joint loading may occur when extreme angular rotations in the disk mean that the articular facets are no longer in parallel alignment (**Figure 2–16**).

With the morphology of the intervertebral joints rather pointed at their periphery, the shear forces are then transferred over a very small surface area. In this scenario, the resulting stresses can be very large and may even exceed the ultimate stress of the hyaline cartilage. In addition, the situation described here influences the segmental movement behavior. The center of rotation, which normally lies within the contours of the disk, moves to this new center of rotation located in one of the intervertebral joints, which—in addition to an increase in stress in this joint—will also cause changes in the structural stresses exerted elsewhere.

The loading situation described in this example occurs not only at the level of L4, as is the case in the example we used, but in all other intervertebral disks as well. The magnitude of the individual loads is dependent on the position of the disk in question in relation to the primary load, which in the earlier example is provided by the extra weight in the hand, gravity, and the compensatory muscle force. At every level, this load will cause an angular rotation in the disk. Together with the initial shape of the spine in its non-weight-bearing state, the sum of these angular rotations will determine the spinal posture during loading.

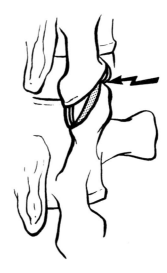

Figure 2–16   Focal joint loading in the intervertebral joint.

Mathematically, this posture can best be expressed in terms of its curvature because in the sagittal and frontal planes, that is, when the spine is bent, a mathematical relation exists between this curvature (C) and the accompanying load, namely:

$$\Delta C = M \, / \, EI$$

The change in curvature (ΔC) is the ratio between the resultant flexion torque M and the bending stiffness of EI. This bending stiffness can be seen as the resistance to bending. With a specific flexion torque, only a slight curvature will occur when this EI is large. This bending stiffness consists of two components:

E: *The modulus of elasticity.* For industrial-grade materials, the modulus of elasticity is fixed. For a complex, composite, nonlinear structure such as the intervertebral joint, it is an average of all elasticity moduli of the various structures, which is, moreover, dependent on the amount of loading and the speed with which the loading has taken place.

I: *The surface area moment of inertia determined by the cross-sectional measurements.*

Taking into account the relationship mentioned previously, we can also learn more about the loading of the spine by studying its shape with methods such as X-rays and outline photos, which can then be described mathematically. This description of its shape can be optimized using known mathematical techniques, and the curvatures can be calculated. When additional facts are known about the bending stiffness of the spine, we can better understand the loading.

Within one individual, greater spinal curvature always means greater load. Determining the exact spinal curvature is an extremely difficult process, and one that can be seriously complicated by positioning and by changes to the contours caused by contracting musculature and movements in the adjacent joints, such as the hip joint. In summary, this second example shows clearly that the lifting technique has an enormous influence on spinal loading, as illustrated in **Figure 2–17**.

KINEMATICS

Kinematics is the study of motion. It does not deal with the forces that cause motion. We can distinguish between linear (or translational) motion and angular (or rotational) motion. In translational motion, all points of a moving body move simultaneously at the same velocity (speed). The path taken is the same for every point, forming a pattern of parallel straight paths. When a body moves from position I to

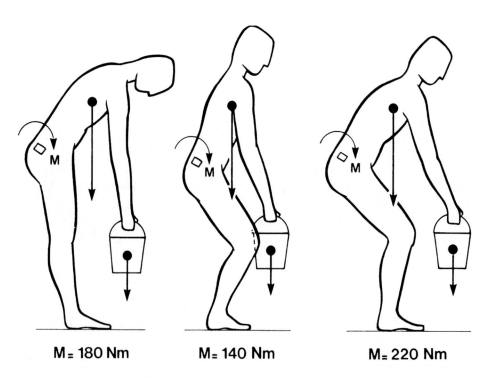

M = 180 Nm   M = 140 Nm   M = 220 Nm

Figure 2–17   Influence on spinal loading of different lifting techniques.

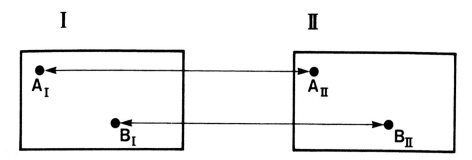

Figure 2–18 Translational motion.

position II, the path taken by point A is exactly equal and parallel to the path taken by point B (**Figure 2–18**).

With a pure rotational motion, each point executes an identical angular rotation at the same angular velocity (**Figure 2–19**). When a body rotates from situation I to situation II, the angular rotation of point A and point B are both equal to α—this angle is also α for all other points of the body. Because this occurs at the same time for all points, they all have the same angular velocity, represented by ω. The velocity of every point is equal to the product of the angular velocity and the distance from the center of rotation O. Point A, therefore, has a greater velocity (V_A) than point B (V_B) has because it is farther from the center of rotation. Point A also covers a greater length of arc in the same time—the time over which angular rotation α takes place.

The position of the center of rotation does not have to be constant. When this position changes from one instant

to the next, we call it an *instantaneous center of rotation*. This is the point of the body that is motionless—around which all rotations take place—at the time in question. A moment later, it may be a different point. The points mentioned do not have to lie within the physical borders of the body in question, but can be virtual points outside the body. With three-dimensional bodies, we talk of *axes of rotation* rather than centers of rotation. When angular or rotational motion takes place, a *centripetal acceleration* effect always occurs.

When a point moves through the arc of a circle at a constant velocity—and thus has a constant angular velocity—the direction of the velocity changes constantly. In situation I, the velocity is directed toward the upper right; in situation II, the lower right. This change in the direction of velocity requires acceleration (**Figure 2–20**), which is always directed toward the instantaneous center of rotation and is

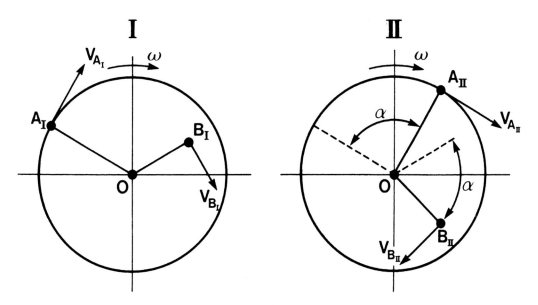

Figure 2–19 Rotational motion.

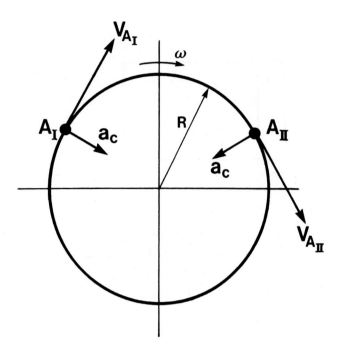

Figure 2–20   Centripetal acceleration in the case of circular movements.

thus called centripetal acceleration. This is represented by the following equation:

$$a_c = V^2 / R$$

where $V = \omega R$.

So, we can also represent the centripetal acceleration by this:

$$a_c = \omega^2 R$$

This centripetal acceleration is responsible for the centrifugal force we all know from merry-go-rounds—the force that (for example) expels water out of the perforations in a centrifugal dryer. In the human body, pure translational and rotational motion hardly ever occurs. In general, standard motion in a joint is made up of translational and rotational motions working together to create a rolling effect.

With a pure roll, the movement of the contact point A_I over the circle arc from situation I to situation II (a_1) is equal to both the movement (a_2) of the center point M and the movement (a_3) of the temporary point of contact (**Figure 2–21**).

A pure roll should be seen as a combination of pure translational motion of the center point M and a pure rotational motion around this center point. The translational velocity (V_T) of the center point is equal to the maximum velocity as a result of the rotational motion (V_R) in the outer shell. The sum of both velocity patterns gives the velocity pattern of pure rolls, whereby the translational velocity can be found at the center point M (**Figure 2–22**).

At every instant, the uppermost point B has twice the translational velocity, while the contact point A is stationary and so forms the instantaneous center of rotation. However, pure rolls such as these do not occur in real life. Depending on the discrepancy between the translational and rotational velocities, rolls will be combined with either skidding or sliding, which means the instantaneous center of rotation is located inside or outside the moving body, respectively.

The number of motion possibilities is described by the *degrees of freedom*. Technically speaking, this term is defined as the minimum number of coordinates that can be used to describe the position of a body. In a flat plane, a body can execute two translational motions and one rotational. With three coordinates, we can describe every position of that

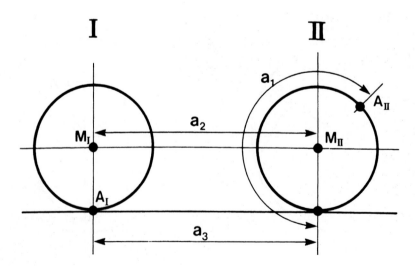

Figure 2–21   Pure roll.

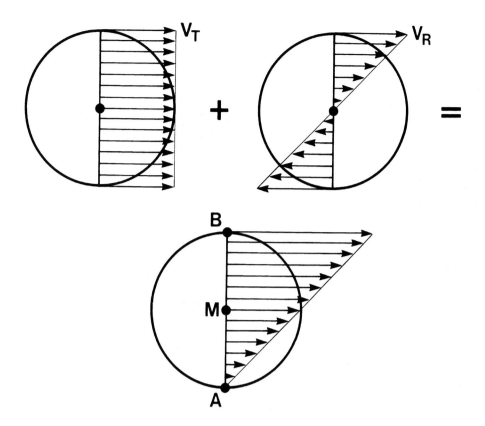

Figure 2-22   Pure roll = Translation + Rotation.

body in this two-dimensional plane: x, y, and φ (**Figure 2-23**).

Changes of position can also be described with three coordinates; there are three degrees of freedom. In a three-dimensional situation, there are six degrees of freedom: three translational motions and three rotational. It is characteristic of every connection between two bodies, and therefore in a joint, that a number of these degrees of freedom are limited or obstructed by (in this case) the structure of the joint and the surrounding ligament complex. The remaining degrees

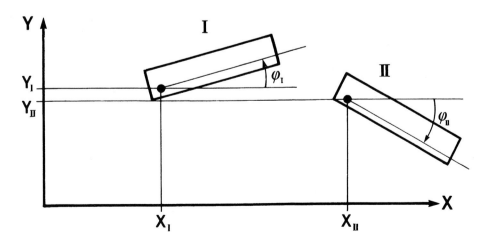

Figure 2-23   Degrees of freedom in two-dimensional motion.

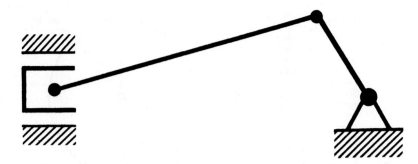

Figure 2–24   The piston/connecting rod principle as a kinetic chain.

of freedom determine the motion possibilities of the joint—when they are rotational, we are dealing with axes of rotation.

In the body, it is often hard to determine the exact degrees of freedom (or motion possibilities) because elastic deformations, ligament structures, and passive or active motion can all exert an influence. When a number of connected joints in a series (each with its own specific characteristics) exhibit, as a whole, one particular motion pattern that differs from the sum of the individual motion possibilities, these connected joints constitute what is called a *kinetic chain*. The most common technical example is the piston/connecting rod principle (**Figure 2–24**).

The whole has one defined motion pattern with reciprocating piston and rotating shaft. There are various kinematic chains in the body—as in the palm of the hand and sole of the foot, among others.

KINETICS

Kinetics is the study of the relationship between motion and loading. If we assume that every motion is caused by a mechanical load, then a number of formulas can be used to describe these relationships. The relationship between force and linear acceleration has already been mentioned:

$$F = ma$$

A force always causes a linear acceleration, the direction of which corresponds with the direction of the force. By *force*, we mean the resultant of all forces working on the body, including the compensatory reactions of muscles and/or ligaments. A moment—and in this case, we mean the resulting moment—always causes an angular accelera-tion. The relationship between moment and actual angular acceleration is this:

$$M = I\omega$$

where I is the mass moment of inertia and ω is the accompanying angular acceleration.

This book does not intend to examine this subject in depth. Studies on human dynamic behavior are carried out by specialized research establishments. Film or video recordings are used to measure the paths of the body—or body parts—centroids. Mathematical calculations are employed to determine linear and angular accelerations, providing information about dynamic loading of the human body.

ASPECTS OF SYNDESMOLOGY

Joints

The term *joint* is understood to mean the connection between two or more bones. Some have structures called joint cavities; others do not.

Joints Without a Joint Cavity or Synarthroses

Synarthroses include the following:

- Synostosis
- Synchondrosis
- Syndesmosis

Within the context of this book, which excludes the skull, only the synchondrotic joints are considered relevant.

Joints With a Joint Cavity or Diarthroses

A diarthrosis or synovial joint possesses a number of obligatory and some optional features. The obligatory features are these:

- Bone ends: two (simple joint) or more (composite joint)
- Joint cartilage
- Joint lubrication
- Joint cavity
- Capsule: synovial and fibrous membrane

The optional features are as follows:

- Cartilage structures (meniscus, disk)
- Capsular reinforcement fibers or capsular ligaments
- Capsular folds
- Meniscoid folds

Morphology

The morphology of a distal end of a bone that makes up a joint can be one of the following:

- Biconcave
- Biconvex
- Concave-convex

The condyloid joint (biconvex or biconcave) and the saddle joint (concave-convex) represent, therefore, the two basic morphologies of joints. Flat joints are theoretically possible, and the ball-and-socket joint is a derivative of the condyloid joint. The cylindrical joint is structurally somewhat similar to the saddle joint. Cylindrical joints come in two types: hinge joints and pivot joints. In these joints, movement can occur around or along imaginary axes. The degrees of freedom available for movement can be converted into a number of axes of rotation. We can distinguish the following:

- Two axes for the condyloid joints
- Two axes for the saddle joints
- Two axes for the cylindrical joints
- Three axes for ball-and-socket joints

As a rule, the cylindrical joint does not utilize one of its degrees of freedom. This is a result of limitations imposed by bony, structural, physiologic, and/or ligamentous restrictions.

Whether highly complex or relatively simple, the articulations between two vertebrae (odontoid, intervertebral disk, intervertebral joints, and uncovertebral joints) from the atlanto-occipital joints down to and including the sacroiliac joints have three degrees of freedom. Movement along any of these degrees of freedom is limited by bone or ligament.

Literature dealing with movement mentions three separate planes and an average range of motion expressed in angular degrees. However, as with all physiologic movements, no motion is a pure uniplanar movement. This point is clearly demonstrated by the relationship between the intervertebral joints in the cervical spine and their inability to move in a purely transverse plane and a purely frontal plane.

Basic Movement Types

Theoretically, there are two basic movement types: rotational and translational. For explanatory text and drawings, see Chapter 2 on "Kinematics" on pages 37–38.

To a significant extent, every component in the joint mechanism plays a role in determining the following:

- The shape of the peripheral movement trajectory
- The intra-articular movement behavior

Peripheral Movement Trajectory

A peripheral movement trajectory can be broken down into a swing and a rotational movement (spin or conjunct rotation).

Swing. A movement is described as a swing when a change occurs in the angular relationship between the longitudinal axes of the bones belonging to the joint in question. If a swing movement occurs around one axis, it is called a pure swing or a cardinal swing (**Figure 2–25**). If, during a swing movement, a secondary movement occurs around another axis, it is called an impure swing or arcuate swing. This arcuate swing is significant in achieving the close-packed position.

Spin. By *spin*, we mean the movement of a bone around a fixed mechanical axis that coincides in its location with the normal (N in **Figure 2–26**) in the point of contact between the two joint surfaces. A single point on one of the joint surfaces remains in contact with a single point

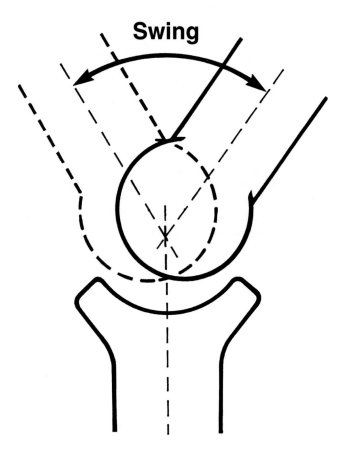

Figure 2–25   Swing movement.

on the other. A pure spin movement is both intra-articularly and peripherally equal with regard to form and direction.

The terms defined earlier are generally used to describe peripheral joint movement behavior. In the spine, the terms *flexion*, *extension*, and *sidebending* are generally considered swing movements, and *rotation* is considered a spin movement. However, as we show later in this book, these movements never occur separately, but always in combination.

Intra-Articular Movement Behavior

From an intra-articular perspective, every movement involving an angular change between joint partners breaks down into a combined roll/slip movement (**Figure 2–27**).

Roll. The direction of roll is always the same as that of the change in angular relationship.

Slip. The direction of slip is determined by the articular surface shape of the moving joint partner.

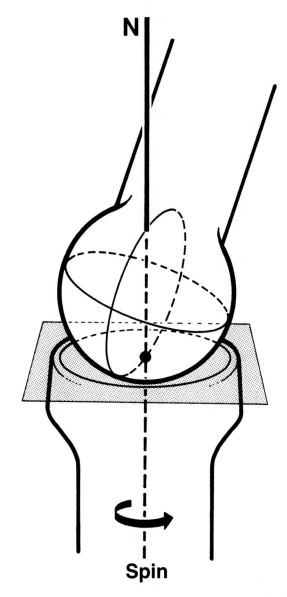

Figure 2–26   Spin movement.

With a moving convex articular partner, the instantaneous center of rotation is located within the moving bone. So, from an intra-articular perspective, the direction of slip is opposite to that of the angular rotation of the roll component. The movement's instantaneous center of rotation is the point that is not moving at any specific moment (**Figure 2–28**).

With a moving concave joint partner, the instantaneous center of rotation is located outside of the confines of the moving bone. So, from an intra-articular perspective, the direction of slip is the same as that of the angular rotation of the roll component (**Figure 2–29**).

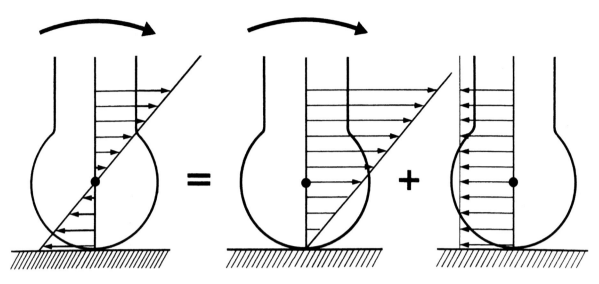

Figure 2–27   Combined roll/slip movement.

Note that convex-concave and concave-convex movements are not the only types of movement in the spine—there is also convex-convex (C1–C2) (**Figure 2–30**). Theoretically, the convex-convex movement is kinematically unstable. In real life, its movement behavior is determined by the surrounding structures and generally matches the convex-concave principle of movement. Kinematically, the axis is located between both articular facets.

With regard to the spine, we have the following:

- *Convex-concave.* The C0–C1 level, where the direction of slip is opposite to the direction of roll

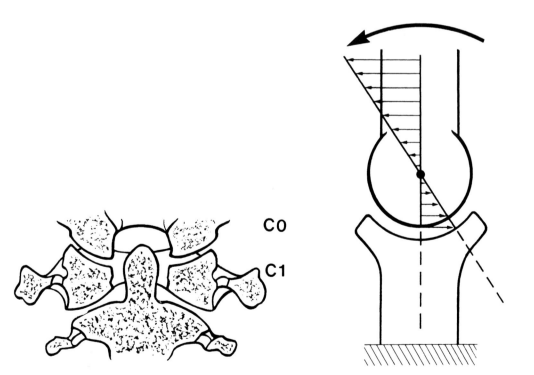

Figure 2–28   Convex-concave movement pattern.

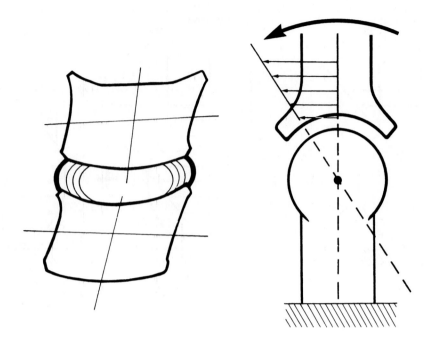

Figure 2–29   Concave-convex movement pattern.

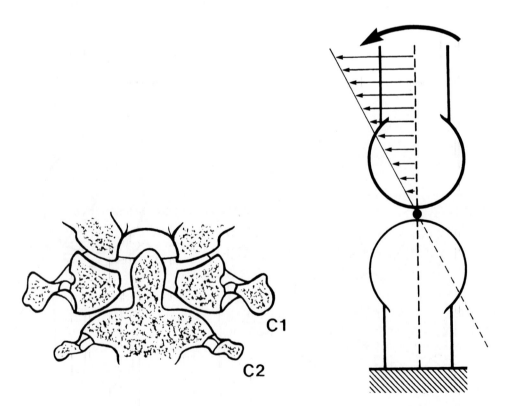

Figure 2–30   Convex-convex movement pattern.

- *Convex-convex*. The C1–C2 level, where the direction of slip is opposite to the direction of roll
- *Concave-convex*. The levels below C2, where the direction of slip is the same as the direction of roll

The slip component increases in line with the distance between the instantaneous center of rotation and the actual joint surface (see the section titled "Examination of the Lower and Mid-Cervical Spine" in Chapter 16). Where the articular facets of the intervertebral joints have a limited radius of curvature, there is a relatively large translational component. Therapeutically, in mobilization of the C0–C1 joint and with traction mobilization in general, the movement focus is mostly on the translational component.

Joint Positions

In examination and therapy, knowledge of the joint positions is important. The following joint positions can be identified:

- Maximally close-packed position
- Close-packed position
- Maximally loose-packed position
- Loose-packed position

Maximally Close-Packed Position

The *maximally close-packed position* is a three-dimensional endrange position of the joint, where there is bone restriction and/or maximal capsular or ligamentous tension. This is caused by conjunct rotation.

The implication of the maximally close-packed position is threefold:

- Mobilization is physiologically impossible.
- There is optimal stability.
- It can be used as a locking technique to create a lever function during mobilization and manipulation techniques.

Close-Packed Position

The *close-packed position* is all one- or two-dimensional endrange positions of the joint where bony restriction occurs and/or a part of the capsule and certain ligaments are maximally tensed. In both cases, the capsular and ligamentous tension and gravity cause a compression of the joint surfaces relative to each other. During active motion, the muscle tone also plays a role.

Maximally Loose-Packed Position

The *maximally loose-packed position* here means the capsule and the ligamentous and muscular complex are maximally relaxed. The joint is in the so-called physiologic or pathologic resting position.

The importance of the maximally loose-packed position is threefold:

- Unloading of joint, capsule, and ligaments
- Examination of the movement possibilities in the physiologic directions starting from this position
- Traction examination from this position

Loose-Packed Position

The *loose-packed position* is a position between close-packed and maximally loose-packed.

Interpretation of the aforementioned terminology with regard to the spine

Maximally close-packed position

Extension, sidebending, and contralateral or ipsiexternal rotation. Flexion, sidebending, and contralateral or ipsiexternal rotation.

Close-packed position

All other endrange positions.

Maximally loose-packed position

Midposition between flexion and extension, left and right sidebending and left and right rotation.

Loose-packed position

All positions where the total capsule and ligamentous complex is neither maximally tensed nor maximally relaxed. In these positions, some capsule structures and ligaments will exhibit more tension than others.

CHAPTER 3

Function and Dysfunction of the Spine

Humans are physically different from animals because of—among other things—their balanced vertical position with straightened knees. The human spine guarantees both a wide range of movement possibilities and the necessary strength and stiffness. In the vertical position, limited muscle power is sufficient to maintain balance. Spine function depends on three factors:

- Material properties of bone, cartilage, intervertebral disk, meniscoid folds, joint capsule, and ligaments
- Load imposed by gravity and muscle power
- Coordination, carried out by the neural adaptation and coordination system

The spine has four functions:

- Static
- Kinematic
- Balance
- Protective

STATIC FUNCTION

To comprehensively understand the static function we need to accurately define certain parameters. We need to discuss some of the required definitions as provided by, among others, Putz (1981) and illustrated in **Figure 3–1**:

- *Angle of inclination (α).* The sagittal plane angle between the cranial surface of the vertebral body and the articular facets of the superior articular processes.

- *Opening angle (β).* The transverse plane angle between the surfaces of both articular facets of the superior articular processes.
- *Vertebral body angle of inclination (γ).* The sagittal plane angle between the cranial surface of the vertebral body and the horizontal plane. The angle is positive in the direction indicated.
- *Loading triangle (A).* The triangle formed by the three lines connecting the two joint centers to the center of the vertebral body.

The static loading of the human spine, predominantly made up of axial pressure, is maintained by the ligaments and muscles connecting the vertebrae. This axial load can be reduced only by raising the intra-abdominal and intrathoracic pressure or through the support of the arms.

The disk and both intervertebral joints play a role in load transfer between two vertebrae. As a result of the orientation of the anular fibers, the intervertebral disk is able to absorb both compressive and shear forces. In a healthy intervertebral disk, the presence of the round nucleus pulposus allows compressive or peak load to be dispersed evenly throughout all surrounding tissues (Schlüter, 1965). With a damaged intervertebral disk, uneven load transfer occurs, and portions of the hyaline cartilaginous structure can be overloaded. When calculating the loading in young people, we can theoretically represent the compressive force as a force acting on a single point. As a person ages and the intervertebral disk decreases in height, the peripheral areas become more loaded and a segment can become unstable (Junghanns, 1954).

The daily fluctuations in disk height play a role in the distribution of load within the segment, as do these lasting

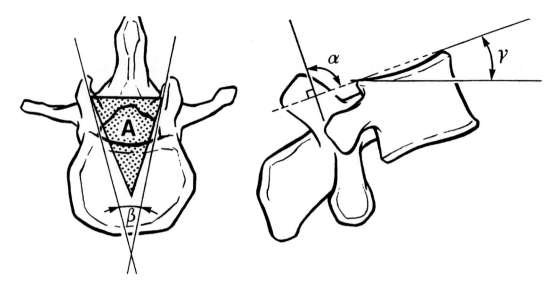

Figure 3–1   Characteristic parameters of the vertebra.

age-related morphologic changes. The cartilage surfaces and the synovial fluid between them ensure that there is barely any friction during load transfer in the intervertebral joints. The load transfer is free of any shear force, and the synovial fluid distributes all loads evenly over the joint surface. In every segment of the spine, except the C0–C2 joints, there is a loading triangle that increases in size progressing in a caudal direction. The load in the corners of this triangle depends on the magnitude and direction of the total loading in the segment and on the position of the point of application of the loading resultant force. The morphology of the loading triangle is dependent on the relationship between the transverse dimension of the intervertebral articular facets and their sagittal distance to the center of the vertebral body. From C3–T3, the transverse dimension of the triangle is larger than the sagittal; from C7–L3, the transverse dimension decreases and the sagittal increases.

When the resultant compressive force is located within the loading triangle, a stable balance is established in the movement segment. Of the tension-resistant structures the muscles, both mono- and multisegmental in relation to the movement segment, play a major role in maintaining balance. The flexion load exerted on the spine is converted into axial compressive load. The angles of the loading triangle function as rotational points. In the thoracic spine, where the ribs form long lever arms, attaining balance of moments requires significant force production in the back muscles, which are attached to the vertebral arches and processes, making use of these short lever arms. The tensile force of the ligaments plays a part predominantly in the endrange of movements.

Within the movement segment, the compressive forces are absorbed by all available structures capable of dealing with pressure transfer. Quantitatively, the portion of the compressive load handled by the vertebral body and intervertebral articular facets is determined by the magnitude and direction of the resulting compressive force, the angle of inclination of the articular facets, and the angle of inclination between the vertebral endplate and the transverse plane. The portion of the compressive load handled by the articular facets also depends on the distance from their center point to the point of application of the resultant loading force.

In any movement segment, the disk absorbs the bulk of the compressive load (F_d) (**Figure 3–2**) if the following conditions are present:

- The angle between the cover plate and the superior articular processes (angle of inclination) is 40°.
- The angle between the cover plate and the transverse plane (vertebral body angle of inclination) is 5°.
- The distance from the point of application of the resultant loading force to the center of the vertebral endplate is 4 mm.

Because they are farther away from the point of application of the resultant loading force, the intervertebral articular facets absorb a lower portion of the compressive load (F_j).

The resultant compressive force on the endplate has two components, one axial in direction (F_{dN}) and the other sagittal in direction (F_{dS}), respectively. Because of the verte-

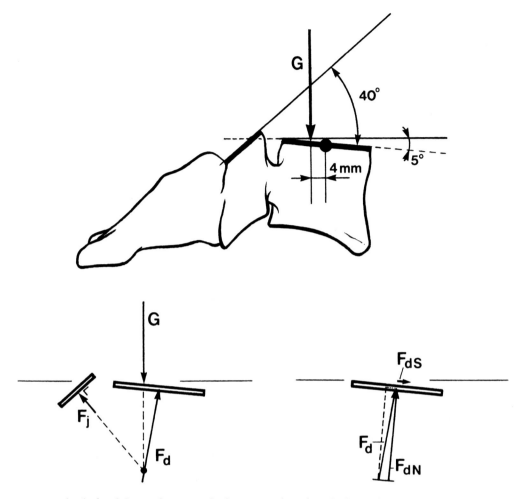

Figure 3–2 Compressive load of endplate and intervertebral joints resulting from body weight.

bral body angle of inclination that is inclined 5° downward and ventrally, this sagittal component is directed ventrally. As a result, the intervertebral articular facets absorb more compressive loads. The tensile stress of the muscles, ligaments, and anulus compensate for this ventrally directed force.

From C3 to T1, the increase in the angles of inclination is near linear, so the compressive loads on the intervertebral articular facets increase caudalward. The position of the compressive force's line of action determines the distribution of the compressive force within the loading triangle of every vertebra. The position of this line of action can be defined only for the upper cervical spine (Putz, 1981).

It is important that the facets that absorb pressure are positioned in such a way—relative to the longitudinal axis of the spine—as to keep the contents of the vertebral canal from being exposed to compressive load when the compres-

sive forces are dispersed. The intervertebral foramen is also located in an area of reduced stress.

In their endrange positions, the intervertebral joints can function as centers of rotation, changing the way the compressive forces are distributed. Together with the relatively long lever arm of the thoracic vertebrae's spinous process, the almost vertical orientation of the intervertebral joints that serve as a center of rotation ensures that the resulting compressive force is transmitted perpendicular to the joint surfaces.

In addition, the structure and arrangement of the lumbar intervertebral articular facets enable them to absorb forces working in a sagittal direction. If the articular facets in the lumbar spine had been located purely in the sagittal plane, the compressive force would have been transmitted exclusively to the intervertebral disk.

The meniscoid folds also play a role in transfer of segmental compression loads; some people consider them a protection against overload. When impinged, they can cause a segmental fixation (Kos and Wolf, 1972).

In most cases, the meniscoid folds are attached to the joint capsule by a broad base and are located only between the outermost rims of the joints. Depending on the position of the joint, they will adapt themselves to any changes in the shape of the joint space (**Figure 3–3**).

At rest, the pressure in the joint space is equal to the pressure of its surroundings, that is, atmospheric pressure. In certain positions, the pressure in the intervertebral joints can drop because the joint contact has been temporarily lost, the so-called vacuum phenomenon or Fick syndrome (Fick, 1911; Ravelli, 1955). Because the intervertebral articular facets become partly or wholly separated, there is a temporary increase in volume. After a while, the low pressure that this causes is compensated for, and the balance between the pressure within the joint space and the joint capsular tension is restored. In all intervertebral joints, the opening of the joint space is part of normal joint function. In extreme joint positions, in the enlarged section of the joint space, only the bases of the meniscoid folds are pressed against the fibrous membrane to absorb joint loading. When the joint space does not open, the entire meniscoid fold can sometimes transfer pressure. The large, robust meniscoid folds of the cervical and thoracic spine often contain cartilaginous tissue, so they can handle this load.

The tension of the joint capsule is very important to the normal pressure-transfer function of the meniscoid folds (Putz, 1981), but so is the association with the adjacent lig-

aments and muscles. When flexion occurs in the lumbar spine, an increase in stress causes the flaval ligaments to press the meniscoid folds into the joint space. The deep musculature of the spine is located directly adjacent to the joint capsule—in the event of forceful flexion and rotation, it uses the upper rims of the superior articular processes as hypomochlea or fixed points. During powerful contractions of the intrinsic lower back musculature, the pressure increases in the osseofibrous tunnel where this musculature is located.

This dorsal-to-ventral force pushes the meniscoid folds attached to the joint capsule into the joint space. In general, the pressure-transfer function of the meniscoid folds is mostly seen as important during the extreme positions that various movements can cause. There are reported nerve fibers in various folds—fibers that appear firmly embedded in the fat and connective tissue, protecting them from direct pressure or damage.

KINEMATIC FUNCTION

Kinematic function of the spine depends on the following conditions:

- The orientation of the intervertebral articular facets
- The extensibility of the joint capsule
- The elasticity (stiffness) of the intervertebral disk

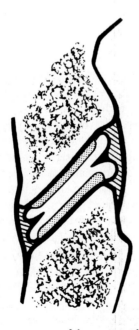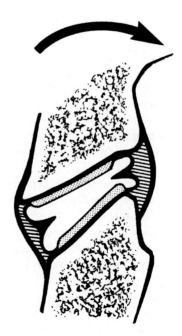

Figure 3–3 Adaptation to movement of the meniscoid folds.

- The condition of the ligamentous complex
- The tone of the musculature
- The coordination function of the nervous system

The mobility of the spine is based on the displacement potential of any one vertebra in relation to another. The significance of segmental stability is twofold: first, manifold movements are possible; and second, many stable positions can be assumed, in which impact, tensile, and shear loading can be efficiently processed. Although all components within the movement segment (Schmorl and Junghanns, 1968) influence the potential movement in all directions, the position of the intervertebral joints' articular facets is essentially the decisive factor. Every pair of adjacent vertebrae has a specific movement quality and quantity, and thus influences the total movement quality and quantity of the spine. In terms of quality, the transitional segments play a special role; as for quantity, the spinal region and the location of the segment within this spinal region are important factors.

In terms of movement quantity, we need to distinguish between the following:

- Constitutional hypo- or hypermobility
- General pathologic hypo- or hypermobility
- Local pathologic hypo- or hypermobility

Local pathologic hypo- or hypermobility involves one or a small number of segments and should be viewed in terms of their relationship to the adjacent segments. The rhythm and sequence of movement can be disturbed as a consequence of local pathologic hypo- or hypermobility (van Mameren, 1988). "The most efficient movement" means that all segments are free to move optimally in all directions and in the correct sequence.

If the endfeel in a segment appears to be disrupted in one or more directions, it is very important to ascertain the causal relationship—this will help to clarify whether it is the result of a pathologic situation or of a functional adaptation.

Every individual has his or her own unique optimal functional movement potential. When this is altered, functional or afunctional adaptation is possible. Distinguishing between the two requires an objective analysis of the individual movement pattern, and that in turn requires knowledge of—and insight into—the movement mechanism. The fact that an objective analysis of the individual movement pattern can only ever be approximate indicates the level of caution that must be taken when interpreting possible dysfunctions.

In cases of segmental pathology, the functional mechanism as a whole must be examined, as well as the actual structures in the movement segment. When analyzing the segmental movement mechanism, we must distinguish between active and passive movement. Active movement is determined not just by the more or less intrinsic segmental lower back musculature, but also by the musculature that works at a distance from the specific segment. This further complicates the process of understanding the three-dimensional functioning of the spine. When unilateral contraction occurs, the rotatores muscles cause rotation in the spine; when these muscles contract bilaterally, they cause extension.

The most important function of these muscles, as with all other muscles attached to the spinous processes, lies in their ability to initiate, stabilize, and support the segmental movements. These muscles prevent sudden sliding in starting positions at the extremes of range and ensure that a full range of movement is possible as part of normal function of the spine. Passive movement is predominantly controlled by the morphology of the bone, by the capsule, and by the ligaments. The bone needs the right morphology and the ability to absorb sufficient loads. The capsule needs sufficient extensibility and—in the lumbar area and other regions—sufficient stiffness. The ligaments must be oriented in the correct anatomic position and must be long enough to respond efficiently to elongation stresses.

Different movements have their own instantaneous centers of rotation, which shift position during the course of the movements. Depending on morphologic characteristics, the shift in location of the instantaneous center of rotation can be jerky—especially near the endrange of certain movements. This is particularly true when the intervertebral joints are blocked in endrange of rotational movements and suddenly function as a new instantaneous center of rotation.

This displacement of the center of rotation depends on the morphology of the intervertebral joints in combination with the intervertebral disk and the ligaments. Some intervertebral articular facets, acting as centers of rotation, are exposed to extreme focal load this way.

The limits of the intervertebral joints' movement range are determined by the restraints imposed by bones and ligaments. Within each movement segment, the ligaments that promote the balance of moments are tautened in the endrange of each individual movement. The nature and extent of this tautening are partly determined by the morphology of the articular processes.

Together, the articular surface morphology, ligaments, and muscles determine the endrange load. A segment's maximal movement range is determined by the balance between the forces working in the same direction as the movement and the counterforces caused by the stress on the ligaments. Locking of a joint in the terminal position is determined by the displacement of the center of rotation and the accompanying change to the force lever arms.

The magnitude of the load in the contact area of the intervertebral articular facets can be calculated based on the balance of moments and forces. Before we can determine the lever arm of a force, we need to ascertain the location of the center of rotation for each of the movement phases. In the terminal phase of flexion and extension, a gapping of the joint spaces can occur.

The joint spaces of most intervertebral joints are oblique in relation to the concentric circles surrounding the instantaneous center of rotation in the plane of movement. During flexion and extension, therefore, the distance between the cranial segmental articulations and the center of rotation changes. This is what causes the gapping of the joint space during extension and flexion (**Figure 3–4**).

The endrange position of sidebending is also determined by the balance between the forces working in the direction of movement and the tensile stress developed by the contralateral ligaments and muscles. The movement takes place on a sagittal axis of rotation, which in the endrange is localized differently depending on the region.

In the cervical spine, the axis lies in the uncovertebral joint; in the thoracic spine, in the intervertebral joint; and in the lumbar spine, on the line connecting the intervertebral disk's rim and the adjacent intervertebral joint (**Figure 3–5**).

The position of the axis also determines the length of the force's lever arm. The load on the intervertebral joints as centers of rotation in sidebending depends on the angle of inclination of the intervertebral articular facets. The smaller the angle, the greater the axial pressure that can be absorbed by the intervertebral joints. The angle of inclination also limits the range of the coupled rotation, which occurs in the same direction as the sidebending (Putz, 1981).

During sidebending movement, the tensile forces that work sideways pull on the vertebral processes on the concave side, while compressive forces occur in the lateral aspect of the disks, intervertebral joints, or uncovertebral joints. On the contralateral (convex) side, tensile stresses occur in the ligaments that connect the processes and in the anular fibers. The longitudinal and flaval ligaments on the contralateral side also become loaded. Depending on the intervertebral articular facets' angles of inclination, varying compressive and tensile forces occur during rotational movement.

The greater the angle of inclination, the greater the pressure component applied perpendicularly at the intervertebral articular facet joint surface. This compression restricts the segmental deviation potential into sidebending.

The movement process in the intervertebral joints, especially at endrange, differs from that of other joints because it involves a partial separation occurring in the joint cavity, limiting joint contact to a small portion of its entire surface.

The loading triangle of each vertebra enables the muscles to work together to carry out nuanced movements of the vertebrae. The individual vertebra acts as a partner to the adjacent vertebra as a result of passive pressure transfer, passive strain in the capsule and ligaments, and active muscle tension. So, in functional terms, the intervertebral joints of the individual movement segments cannot be considered in isolation because every displacement influences the initial position of the segmentally adjacent joints.

Apart from the disk, the ligaments, and the muscles, the most important element in determining the range of the various movements per region is the position of the intervertebral articular facets. In all movement areas, the oblique orientation of these facets causes an enforced combination of movements whose axes are perpendicular to each other.

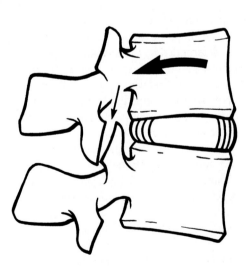 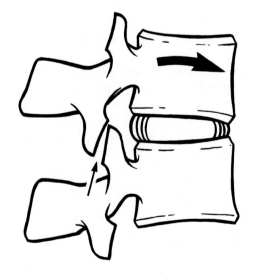

Figure 3–4   Gapping of the joint space during extension and flexion.

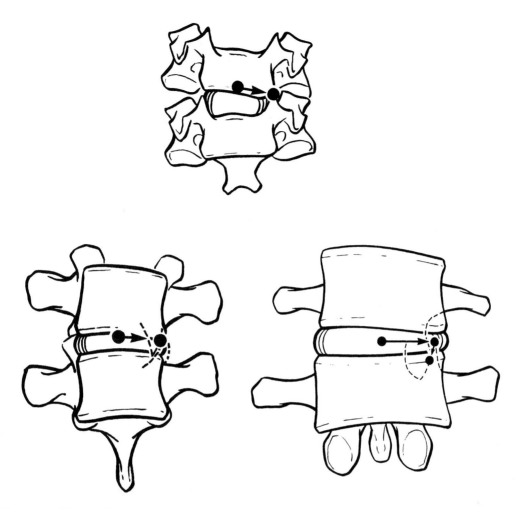

Figure 3–5   Movement of the axis during sidebending.

In the endrange of movements in the frontal plane, the center often shifts its position to the residual thin contact zone of the intervertebral or uncovertebral joints, which can expose these structures to heavy loading. In the endrange position, the ligaments on the contralateral side should be under tension, which results in a balance of moments and forces. The summation of these forces and counterforces at work in the movement segment acts at the centers of rotation. The joints are locked by the abrupt shifts in position of the axes of rotation in the endrange of the various movements and by the corresponding change of moments.

The mechanism is most sensitive to disturbances during the final degrees of displacement in the endrange of a movement. In most cases, functional overload occurs because the disk becomes unstable, increases or decreases in volume, or undergoes an irreversible change.

In conclusion, we can state that the spine is composed of individual segments, which, per region and sometimes per segment, have their own typical characteristics and properties. To comprehend how the segment functions, we need to understand the interrelation of all structures involved in that segment. We also need to understand the linked joints and the influence they mutually exert on each other. It follows that the movement mechanism cannot be deduced purely from the morphology of the intervertebral articular facets—it is rather a compromise of every structure involved in movement within that segment. Interpreting the function of these structures demands knowledge of biomechanics as well as anatomy.

The average ranges of motion of the entire spine are as follows:

- Flexion-extension: 250°
- Sidebending: 73°–85°
- Rotation: 90°

BALANCE FUNCTION

The spine, as the central axis for the body, plays an important role in maintaining balance. Because the body's center of gravity is at the level of S2, the majority of the spine is located cranial to it. In normal posture, both ends—pelvis and head—are maintained in a horizontal position: the pelvis by the lower extremities and the head by the reflex circuits involving the vestibular and ocular system. On the input side for these reflex circuits, the propriosensory afferent information of the intervertebral joint capsule is important, as is the input that the vestibular organ receives during every change in position. The flexibility of the spine enables the output to be efficiently processed, achieving and maintaining balance.

McCouch, Deering, and Ling (1951) described the propriosensory influence of the upper cervical joints years after Magnus and de Kleyn (1912) mentioned the tonic neck reflexes present in both children and adults.

Through tests carried out on rabbits, Komandatow (1945) defined the tonic reflexes originating in the lumbar intervertebral joints; he described the eye–coccyx and head–coccyx reflexes. During sidebending of the lumbar spine, the head will rotate in the opposite direction—unless the upper body and neck are in a fixed position, in which case the eyes will rotate. Komandatow's tests also showed that the coccygeal and cervical reflexes can influence each other, with the cervical reflex seeming to impart the predominant input to the balance systems. According to Cramer (1958), when the terminal portions of the spine change their positions, a reflexogenic influence is exerted on the musculature of the spine that controls posture. Alongside the significant mechanosensory influence of the intervertebral joints at the terminal portions of the spine, the mechanosensors of the other intervertebral joints also play a role in posture and balance. The key to efficient balance is an optimally functioning spine.

PROTECTIVE FUNCTION

The protective function of the spine is of vital importance. Its morphology ensures that—in a healthy spine—the impact load can be absorbed and structures can be protected from the potentially harmful stretching and compressive forces to which they could otherwise be subjected. Absorption of impact concerns all structures, including the contents of the skull. The spine's protective function is clearly differentiated per area.

In the lumbar area, it is predominantly the cauda equina and the spinal nerve roots that must be protected. In the thoracic and cervical area, the structures that need protection are the spinal cord with its membranes and the cerebrospinal fluid-filled cavities, the spinal nerve roots with their ganglia, the recurrent nerve, the arteries and veins, the sympathetic cord with its ganglia, and finally—in the cervical spine—the vertebral artery and the accompanying vertebral nerve.

DYSFUNCTION

The functions of the spine described earlier are so interwoven that dysfunction in any one of them directly influences the others. The dysfunctions of the spine can be classified as general dysfunction and segmental dysfunction.

General dysfunction can involve either the entire spine or a specific region (for instance Bechterew (ankylosing spondylitis) or Scheuermann disease).

Segmental dysfunction can be caused by dysfunctions or pathologies that are located in the segment (as a result of trauma, tumor, herniations of the nucleus pulposus) or that are located outside the segment, including those with an etiology in other segments (hypo-/hypermobility, protective fixation) or in segmentally related tissues: peripheral elements (skin, muscles, joints, ribs), internal organs, or the tissues receiving sympathetic innervation originating in the dysfunctional segment.

FUNCTIONAL ASPECTS OF THE CONNECTIVE TISSUES
John M. Bos

Collagenous Tissue, Cartilaginous Tissue, and Bone Tissue

There are three types of connective tissue: collagen (an extremely dynamic tissue), cartilage, and bone tissue. These tissues are mesenchymal in origin and exhibit—as a result of their common embryological origin—a comparable morphologic make-up, composed of cells and an extracellular matrix (de Morree, 1993; van Wingerden, 1997; Culav, Clark, and Merrilees, 1999; van den Berg, 1999). See **Figures 3–6** and **3–7**.

The extracellular matrix is made up of an amorphous gelatinous mass, ground substance, and fibers. There are three types of fibers: elastin, collagenous, and reticular. The reticular fibers are actually a type of collagenous fiber because they are made up of similar proteins, although thinner and arranged in a different pattern. The cells can be seen as "tissue producers." The three types of connective tissues differ

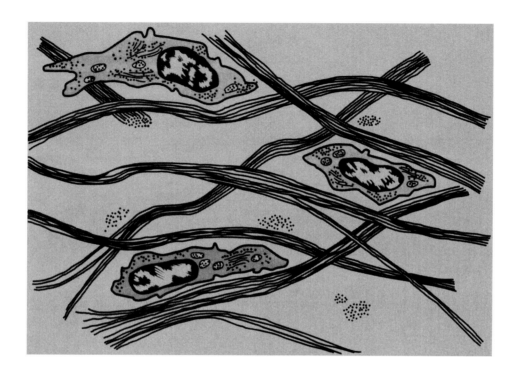

Figure 3–6

in terms of the functional properties of the cells and the composition of the extracellular matrix.

Of the three connective tissues mentioned, we discuss the functional characteristics and adaptive processes of collagenous connective tissue and—to a lesser extent—cartilaginous tissue. Bone tissue is not examined. This primary focus on collagenous connective tissue is because of its presence in every organ. All organs are an organized complex of multiple tissues with a number of common functions; collagenous connective tissue is ubiquitous and has an organizing function.

Connective tissue forms a mechanical support skeleton that contains the parenchymal tissue. The division into organized and loose connective tissue refers to a difference in macroscopic structure (Viidik, 1990; Josza, Kannas, Balint, and Reffy, 1991). This difference concerns a variation in cellular density, the differences in proportions of ground substance and collagenous fibers, and the degree of organization of the extracellular matrix. In loose connective tissue, the matrix contains an extensive capillary vascular bed and lymphatic system. In addition to the fibroblasts (fibrocytes), there are also other types of cells in connective

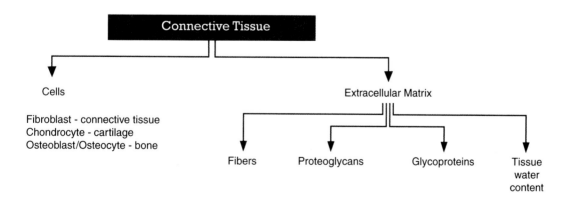

Figure 3–7

tissue, such as adipose cells, macrophages, histiocytes, and mastocytes.

This means that the collagenous connective tissue not only provides support and mechanical consistency but also fulfills a circulatory function (Currier and Nelson, 1992; de Morree, 1993). As a result, the collagenous tissue ground substance is also referred to as an *interstitium*. This ground substance is made up of water that is bound, thereby forming a gelatinous substance. This high water content makes the interstitium an excellent exchange medium between the cells and the capillary vascular bed.

At the proximal aspect of the capillary vascular bed, there is a net filtration pressure of approximately +10 mmHg, which means that water is pushed through the single-walled capillary vessels into the interstitium: a hydrostatic pressure of approximately +35 mmHg and a colloid osmotic pressure of approximately +25 mmHg, results in a net filtration of water. At the distal end of the capillary bed, the hydrostatic pressure drops to approximately +15 mmHg, which, combined with the ambient colloid-osmotic pressure of approximately +25 mmHg, results in a net resorption pressure of approximately 10 mmHg. In net terms, water is filtered and resorbed in equal amounts, causing—under normal conditions—an interstitial fluid exchange.

As stated, the water in the ground substance is bound into a gelatinous form. Negatively charged sugar–protein compounds, called proteoglycans, bind water by way of electrovalent bonds (de Morree, 1993; van den Berg, 1999). A proteoglycan consists of a central protein chain to which glycosaminoglycans (GAGs) are connected on either side. This results in a large bonding surface to which positively charged molecules can attach via electrovalent bonds. In the collagenous tissues, water behaves like a bipolar molecule and bonds to the proteoglycans with its positively charged hydrogen elements (**Figure 3–8**).

In hyaline joint cartilage, these binding molecules are even larger because a great many proteoglycans are bound to a long central chain consisting of hyaluronic acid (Heerkens, 1989); these chains are called proteoglycan aggregates. Because of the negative charge of the glycosaminoglycans, the molecules exhibit maximal spatial dispersion in the ground substance. As with equally charged magnets, the negative charges repel each other (van den Berg, 1999). See **Figure 3–9**.

The proteoglycans bind not only the water in the extracellular matrix, but also the positively charged collagenous fibers. A collagenous fiber is built up of a triple helix structure of collagen fibrils joined together by stable hydrogen bridges. A collagen fibril, in turn, consists of a series of connected stable proteins, called tropocollagen molecules. These tropocollagen molecules are produced by the fibro-

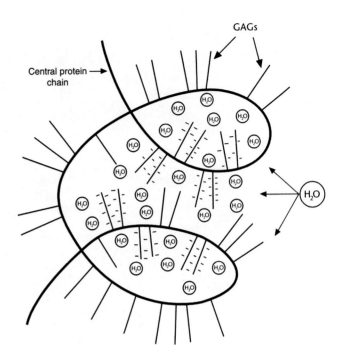

Figure 3–8   Proteoglycan unit with hydrophilic glycosaminoglycans.

blasts (-cytes) in the form of the so-called soluble procollagen. Only once outside the cell, the stable protein molecules are polymerized into a fibril (**Figure 3–10**). Vitamin C is extremely important to the production of collagenous fibers (de Morree, 1993; Culav et al., 1999).

The collagenous fibers are stabilized in a wavelike formation in the ground substance, and as a result the tissue offers hardly any initial resistance to extension. When further extended, the collagenous fibers are pulled out of this wavelike arrangement, thereby breaking the electrovalent bonds between these fibers and the ground substance (de Morree, 1993; van den Berg, 1999).

Collagenous fibers can be deformed much less than can the elastin fibers, allowing for a maximum elongation of only 7% to 10% of their original length. This elongation is not the result of any actual elongation of the individual collagenous fibers, but rather of a combined elongation within the three-dimensional organization of the individual fiber (Viidik, 1990; Josza et al., 1991; Culav et al., 1999). Further elongation causes proportionate intrinsic plastic damage to a collagenous fiber, until it reaches its breaking point.

As the name suggests, elastin fibers are elastic, capable of elongating up to approximately 150% of their original length (Viidik, 1990; de Morree, 1993). There are many elastin fibers in the connective tissue of the skin, but hardly any in the ligaments. Two exceptions to this rule are the

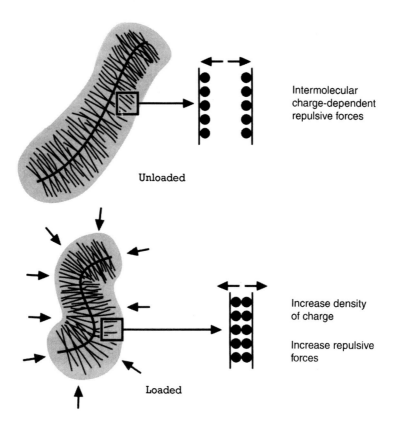

Figure 3–9

nuchal and flaval ligaments. For the flaval ligament, which spans the vertebral arches, the percentage of elastin fibers is approximately 80%. This ligament forms the posterior wall of the spinal canal. It allows for flexion and extension of a movement segment without resisting the movement or forming an obstruction within the spinal canal. In the event of structural loss of elastin fibers, this ligament can play an important role in the pathophysiology of the lateral and central lumbar canal stenoses. Structural loss of elastin fibers after trauma is characterized by a biological inability to synthesize these fibers. With trauma irreparable, the relevant ligaments can no longer function optimally (Josza et al., 1991; Woo and Buckwalter, 1991).

Although there are a great many different types of collagenous fibers, for practical reasons we divide them here into type I and type II collagen (Currier and Nelson, 1992; Culav et al., 1999). Type I collagen is predominantly found in the collagenous connective tissue of the capsuloligamentous structures in joints, the striated muscles, and in the skin. Type II collagen is present in hyaline joint cartilage. Both types are found in lumbar intervertebral disks. This is a necessary distinction that will allow us to clarify the adap-

tive possibilities for dealing with lesions in different locations, as described later on. The structural organization of collagenous fibers varies depending on the functional characteristics of connective and cartilage tissues. In hyaline joint cartilage, many collagenous fibers exhibit a specific pattern. Anchored in the subchondral bone, these fibers form an arcade (de Morree, 1993; Cohen, Foster, and Mow, 1998), and when they suffer structural lesions, this pattern affects the joint cartilage's ability to adapt (**Figure 3–11**).

We summarize that collagenous connective tissue and cartilage tissue have a comparable functional-morphologic construction in terms of cells with an extracellular matrix. The constituents of this matrix vary for each tissue and the functional demands placed upon this tissue. The matrix is made up of fibers and a ground substance that is predominantly composed of proteoglycans and glycoproteins. The characteristics of the proteoglycans are the ability to bind water, to stabilize collagenous fibers, and to determine the functional morphology of the matrix. The matrix's ability to bind water is limited both by the number of glycosaminoglycans and by the spatial hydration restriction placed upon it by the network of stabilized collagenous fibers. Because of

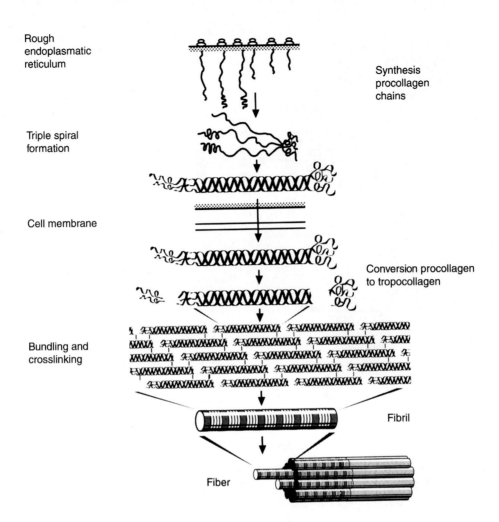

Rough endoplasmatic reticulum

Synthesis procollagen chains

Triple spiral formation

Cell membrane

Conversion procollagen to tropocollagen

Bundling and crosslinking

Fibril

Fiber

Figure 3–10

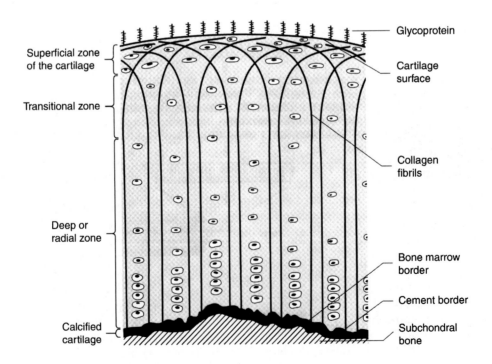

Glycoprotein

Superficial zone of the cartilage

Cartilage surface

Transitional zone

Collagen fibrils

Deep or radial zone

Bone marrow border

Cement border

Calcified cartilage

Subchondral bone

Figure 3–11

its unique arcade morphology, particularly in hyaline joint cartilage, this network of collagenous fibers limits the extent to which the cartilaginous surface will swell.

Mechanical forces cause connective tissues to dehydrate; the extent to which this happens depends on the binding forces between water and the proteoglycans. As dehydration increases, dehydration itself is impeded by the diminishing spaces within the extracellular matrix. This phenomenon is called *hydraulic permeability* (Heerkens, 1989; Cohen et al., 1998). (See **Figure 3–12**.) It is important to note that the mechanical characteristics of connective tissues—such as their ability to withstand tensile and compressive forces—are determined by the composition of the extracellular matrix. Furthermore, the preservation of the properties of the matrix (as well as its functional organization) is determined by the nature and extent of the mechanical loading of the connective tissue (Currier and Nelson, 1992; Lederman, 1997).

Functional Characteristics of the Connective Tissues

The load-bearing capacity of connective tissues is determined by the interrelationship between individual components. This capacity is the result of a balance between form and function, a relationship that reflects the average loading on the tissues (Hagenaars, Bernards, and Oostendorp, 1996; Bernards, 1997). It is therefore a composite term that indicates how much mechanical, thermal, and chemical loading a tissue is able to bear.

Within the limitations set by heredity, age, gender, and constitution, connective tissues exhibit considerable plastic-

ity in terms of their functional characteristics and morphologic composition. *Load-bearing capacity*, as a term, provides a temporal dimension that can be expressed in terms of conditional properties, also known as the *level of training*. The ongoing process of attuning these conditional properties is a function of the average degree of biological loading and originates in the adaptive properties of living organisms, known as *adaptation*. Adaptive capacity is primarily a characteristic of cells that defines the extent to which they are capable of executing a range of adjustments and repairs. This capacity is cell-specific. In connective tissues, the individual cells are therefore responsible for maintaining the extracellular matrix and its conditional properties. In this respect, the tissue maintenance should be considered one expression of adaptability.

There is sufficient evidence that maintaining the conditional properties of connective tissues requires physiologic mechanical loading. Connective tissues adjust their morphologic characteristics to compensate for fluctuations in the mechanical forces to which they are exposed (Currier and Nelson, 1992; Bernards, 1997; Lederman, 1997; Walker, 1998). So, for example, it follows that for a synovial joint, movement is essential to the maintenance of proteoglycans in the hyaline joint cartilage, and also to their replacement rate. On the other hand, underuse (immobilization or disuse) results in atrophy of the cartilage as a result of a loss of proteoglycans. It should be noted that atrophy caused by immobilization could be corrected by restoring movement in the joint in question.

In connective tissue, note that although fibroblasts can be seen as "fiber formers," they are responsible for the

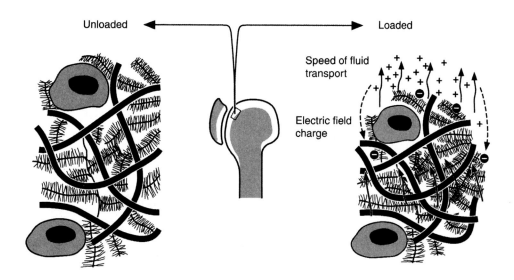

Figure 3–12

ongoing production of not only procollagen molecules but also glycosaminoglycans and glycoproteins (de Morree, 1993; Culav et al., 1999; van den Berg, 1999).

Trainability indicates the extent to which this adaptive capacity can be exploited. The carrying out of such tissue maintenance, where the constant replacement of material is not preceded by cell mitosis, is called *restoration* (Harff, 1998). *Adaptation* is a composite term that covers all adjustment and reparatory processes. *Restoration* implies the ongoing replacement of "tissue product" by cells, the need for which is determined by the average biological usage. The replacement of tissues is dependent on the cells' functional metabolic process. By *functional metabolic*, we mean any metabolic activity that serves the specific function of a cell. For fibroblasts and chondroblasts, this means producing components of the extracellular matrix.

As well as maintaining the extracellular matrix, cells must also maintain their own morphology and function through constructive metabolization. Functional metabolic processes alternate with *constructive metabolic processes*, a term that applies to any metabolic activity that addresses the cell's own needs—that is, maintenance of the cell condition. Restoration processes are cell- and tissue-specific, and the level they achieve is a function of training (Bernards, 1997).

The speed at which the processes take place is expressed by the term *turnover rate*. The biological half-life indicates the time required for a 50% replacement. Functionally, both biodegradation and functional loading stimulate the biosynthesis of proteins. Fluctuations in the balance between biosynthesis and biodegradation are expressed in the morphologic tissue properties and, therefore, also alter the mechanical properties. A net biodegradation of the extracellular matrix's components results in a degenerative condition (Culav et al., 1999).

In collagenous connective tissue, the biological half-lives of restoration of collagenous fibers and glycosaminoglycans vary greatly. For the former, they can range from 200 to 500 days. For the latter, they are a factor of 100 shorter—that is, between 1.9 and 9.2 days (de Morree, 1991; van Wingerden, 1997). In collagenous connective tissue, therefore, the restoration of both proteoglycans and collagenous fibers never ends. Type I collagen is produced more rapidly than type II is. Chondroblasts in the hyaline joint cartilage and fibrochondroblasts in the lumbar intervertebral disk function under anaerobic conditions (Buckwalter, 1998; Cohen et al., 1998) because there is no capillary vascular bed at the surface of the endplate hyaline cartilage. The circulatory support for chondroblasts' metabolic activities is determined by the synovia and the vascular bed in the subchondral bone (Walker and Helewa, 1996; van den Berg 1999). Similarly, there is no capillary vascular bed in the central part of a lumbar intervertebral disk. Here, the cells' meta-

bolic activities are supported indirectly by diffusion from the surrounding areas, that is, through the vertebral capillary vascular bed via the vertebral endplates and from the disk's peripheral vascularized components. The adaptive capacity of cells is totally dependent on effective circulation and adequate circulatory maintenance of tissue.

The restorative capacity of damaged hyaline joint cartilage depends on the number of chondroblasts available, the condition of each individual cell, and the scale of the damage. When the collagenous fibers in joint cartilage are structurally intact, restorative processes take place through appositional accumulation of collagenous fibrils. Under normal conditions, in other words, collagenous fibers are never replaced entirely. Type II collagenous fiber can be reproduced only under optimal conditions (Walker, 1998; Newman, 1998; Buckwalter, 1998).

When damage to the collagenous fibers is so extensive that it destroys their structural arrangement, it becomes virtually impossible to reestablish the collagenous arcade formation. In hyaline joint cartilage, therefore, the limiting factor is not the adaptive capacity itself, but rather the local presence of something that disrupts this process. In this case, this is an anatomic disposition because the pressure in the hyaline joint cartilage inhibits the reorganization and reintegration of the restored collagenous fibers. The term *degeneration* refers to a failure in the adaptive processes, which could be caused by a diminished adaptive capacity or by the presence of any local or general obstacles.

Viscoelasticity

The mechanical, thermal, and chemical load-bearing capacity of collagenous connective tissue is determined by the quality of the individual components and their interaction. Expressed in such terms as *creep*, *stress relaxation*, and *hysteresis*, viscoelasticity is an important mechanical property of connective and cartilaginous tissues. Viscoelasticity expresses the manner in which specified tissues react to mechanical loads over time (Lederman, 1997). For both kinds of tissue, this viscoelastic behavior is determined by four factors.

First, both tissues contain a relatively large quantity of water in a bound state. Water is noncompressible and therefore highly resistant to compressive loads. However, it can change shape—in this case, that means displacement, which requires space and time. Because water is electrovalently bound to the glycosaminoglycans, and the matrix of collagenous fibers restricts the space available for displacement, water exhibits inertia to rapid displacement in the aforementioned tissues. The dehydration and hydration curve of hyaline cartilaginous tissue (**Figure 3–13**) schematically represents this mechanical behavior (Heerkens, 1989).

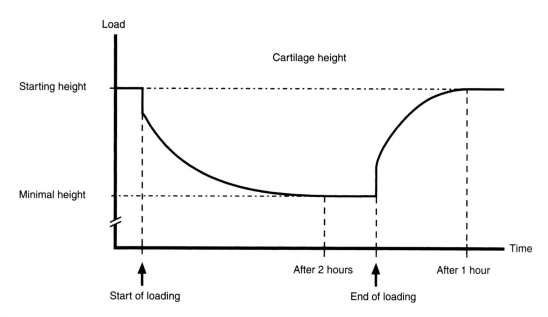

Figure 3–13

Joint cartilage offers a great deal of resistance to sudden compressive load because the mass of water is simply too great to be displaced quickly. The faster the load is applied, the greater the resistance offered. When the compressive load peaks, the joint cartilage gradually dehydrates, until equilibrium is achieved between the forces of repulsion and attraction based on electrovalent bonds and osmotic pressure. As the joint cartilage dehydrates, the intrinsic displacement capacity of water within the tissue, known as *hydraulic permeability*, decreases. Because the water content is lower, therefore, it follows that the permeability of the extracellular matrix rapidly decreases (Heerkens, 1989; van den Berg, 1999). When the load is taken off the tissue, the joint cartilage once again becomes saturated with water—the number of electrovalent binding points and the arcade structure of the collagenous fiber network serving as limiting factors here (de Morree, 1993).

As mentioned earlier, the substratum has a function reminiscent of similarly charged magnets, with the negatively charged glycosaminoglycans repelling each other. As compressive loads increase, so does the mutually repulsive force. As a result, connective tissue has a certain "spring function" (de Morree, 1993; van den Berg, 1999).

The electrovalent bonds between the water and the glycosaminoglycans also play an important role in the viscoelastic behavior of connective tissues. The collagenous fibers are kept in place by electrovalent bonds with the glycosaminoglycans. When collagenous connective tissue is stretched or deformed by external mechanical forces, the internal forces are initially transferred to the substratum by

way of the collagenous fibers' electrovalent bonds. In this way, collagenous connective tissue can absorb a great deal of kinetic energy, converting it into potential energy. Under normal conditions, forces exerted on the collagenous fibers are transmitted to the substratum. The stress–strain diagram (**Figure 3–14**) shows the viscoelastic behavior of collagenous connective tissue (Viidik, 1990; de Morree, 1993; van den Berg, 1999).

This figure shows that there is relatively little initial resistance to deformation or elongation of the tissue, and when the collagenous fibers are pulled taut in the direction of the elongation, the stress increases linearly with elongation. Further stretching places a strain on the intrinsic bonds of the collagenous fiber structure and leads to plastic deformations that are—in the short term—irreversible. If the elongation continues, the individual collagenous fibers reach their ultimate strain point and an anatomic deformation occurs; the fibers break and lose their continuity.

Circulatory Disorders

Physiologic disorders in the circulatory system exert considerable influence on the load-bearing capacity of connective tissues in both the short and the long term, and can affect the following:

- Water balance
- Circulatory environment
- pH levels

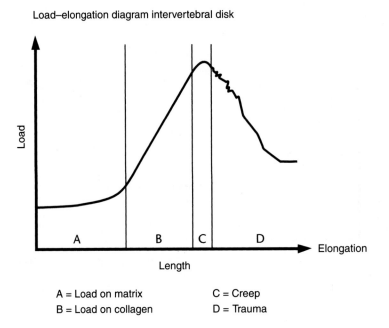

Figure 3-14

Later we give a systematic description of the effects of these disorders. Please note that our conclusions are speculative in nature, based on experimental research into the consequences of immobilization, as shown in the stress–strain diagram for connective tissue (Viidik, 1990; Lederman, 1997). Specifically, we are dealing with ligaments and hyaline joint cartilage, based on clinical data with which manual therapists are familiar. We have, with a degree of caution, drawn a number of conclusions about the pathophysiology of connective tissue disorders.

First of all, when a circulatory disorder occurs, less and less water is filtered per unit of time in the proximal portion of the capillary vascular bed, leading to a deterioration of the interstitial fluid flow. In the event of a segmental dysfunction, circulation will worsen as a result of a vasoconstriction under the influence of heightened tonic activity in the sympathetic nervous system. The tissues that depend directly on this circulation will be the first to be affected by the disorder in fluid equilibrium. In fact, connective tissues can be left "dry." Less water is filtered at the proximal portion of the capillary vascular bed while the quantity reabsorbed at its distal end remains virtually the same.

Water balance disorders make connective tissue physically stiffer because water loss in the extracellular matrix frees up glycosaminoglycan binding points, which then bond more strongly to collagenous fibers. The viscoelastic behavior of connective and cartilaginous tissues varies and can be determined clinically by examining the changes in the mechanical behavior of connective tissue in various organs. Resistance to deformation and elongation increases, elongation range decreases, and the endfeel becomes stiffer. These are known as connective tissue–specific disorders. A *segmental disorder* is one that is specific to connective tissues and organs with a segmental relationship based on an ongoing or previous segmental dysfunction (Bernards, 1991; Hagenaars et al., 1996).

The stress–strain diagram shows disorders in the dynamics of fluid equilibrium. The curve levels off, indicating that a small strain is associated with substantial internal tension or stress (**Figure 3–15**).

The fact that connective tissues become physically stiffer does not mean that they can tolerate greater mechanical forces. In fact, the opposite is true: their load to failure decreases. This is because under normal circumstances, mechanical loading can be transferred to the water-rich substratum by means of the collagenous fibers. Less water in the substratum means that connective tissues can absorb less potential energy. As a result, any mechanical load will cause damage to the connections between the collagenous fibers and the glycosaminoglycans, and within the biological structure of the fibers themselves (Viidik, 1990; de Morree, 1993), earlier than it would otherwise have done. In this situation, the intervertebral disk (a particular form of connective tissue) exhibits comparable changes in visco-

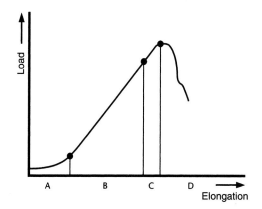
Load–elongation diagram
with normal loading

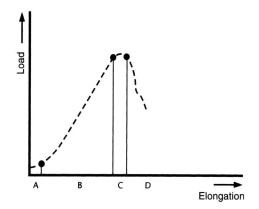
Load–elongation diagram
after immobilization

Figure 3–15

elastic behavior. Under the conditions described here, connective tissue does retain the capacity to bind water to glycosaminoglycans.

This may explain the rapid reversibility of disorders in viscoelastic behavior when segmental dysfunction ceases to exist. Some authors have also suggested the existence of a "reflex tone" in collagenous tissue to explain the rapid reversibility frequently observed in physiotherapy clinical practice (Hagenaars, Bernards, Bos, and Oostendorp, 1991; de Morree, 1991).

Circulatory disorders also have considerable consequences for the circulatory environment, which can reduce oxygen supply (ischemia) in the tissues concerned. The first tissues to suffer from this are those with high metabolic demands, such as muscle tissue (McComas, 1996). In the long term, the metabolic properties of the fibroblasts in connective tissue are also adversely affected by ischemia, and the first process to suffer is the current biosynthesis of glycosaminoglycans. This means that water- and collagen-binding capacity drops significantly when production of these glycosaminoglycans decreases. Consequently, the collagenous fibers become less stable and in effect "come loose" (de Morree, 1993; van den Berg, 1999).

The viscoelastic behavior of connective and cartilaginous tissues changes again, but this time the tissue becomes more flaccid physically. The change from a curve into an inverted parabola, shown in **Figure 3–16**, illustrates this.

Under these circumstances, a slight extension of connective tissue will barely lead to a transfer of mechanical forces to the substratum, but it will lead directly to an internal elongation of the collagenous fibers. The mechanical load-bearing capacity is also considerably reduced. The effect on the absorption of mechanical forces is considerable,

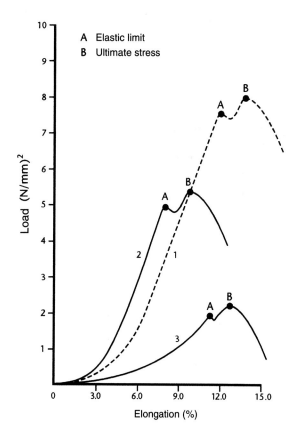
Load–elongation diagram

1. Normal
2. Increased stiffness
3. Decreased stiffness

Figure 3–16

especially for hyaline joint cartilage. A small peak load will damage the biological structure of the collagenous fiber.

A third consequence of impaired circulation, especially when accompanied by stasis in tissues, is an exacerbation of ischemia. For the metabolic properties of certain cells (eg, especially muscle tissue and the intervertebral disk) this means a shift from aerobic to anaerobic processes. The formation of the anaerobic metabolic by-product lactic acid results in extreme acidification of the tissues involved. This has two consequences. First, metabolic processes are all pH-dependent (Currier and Nelson, 1992; Culav et al., 1999). For the intervertebral disk, production of glycosaminoglycans by the fibrochondroblasts deteriorates if the pH is too low. In muscle tissue, this affects the functional metabolism in the short term and constructive metabolism in the long term. A lower level of ATP resynthesis for the individual muscle fibers leads to loss of function as the excitation–contraction coupling is disrupted. Alternating groups of muscle fibers contract to maintain the muscle's rest tone. Once in a state of contraction, metabolization of ATP is required to break up the relationship between actin and myosin. The calcium incorporated during the contraction coupling must be pumped back to the endoplasmatic reticulum, and this mechanism also requires energy. A cramp is the result of a persistent state of contraction. Rigor mortis is a common example of this (McComas, 1996). In connective tissue, the H+ ions (originating in lactic acid) repel the bound water and the collagenous fibers of the glycosaminoglycans and claim the binding points for themselves. This also leads to a change in the viscoelastic behavior that can be illustrated graphically in a stress–strain diagram. Apart from causing the aforementioned changes to the viscoelastic behavior of connective and cartilage tissues, circulatory disorders also reduce the efficiency and effectiveness of essential repair processes.

Restoration, Regeneration, and Repair

If damage causes tissue loss but does not lead to necrosis, a slight increase in cell metabolism can accelerate replacement of the damaged material. In the case of collagenous connective tissue, this means damage to the extracellular matrix without cell death. An increase in the fibroblasts' functional metabolism is all that is required to restore this damaged product. As mentioned earlier, this process is called *restoration* (Harff, 1998). Maintenance of the properties of the extracellular matrix is regulated and controlled by a balance of biosynthesis and biodegradation processes. This balance is controlled by a great many local factors. When the cells' functional metabolism increases, a

number of circulatory conditions (predominantly vascular support in the form of local vasodilation) have to be met to enable the restoration process (Culav et al., 1999). Polymodal nociceptive nerve fibers play an important role in regulation of the local homeostasis by local release of substance P. This local tissue reaction is also classified as an axon response.

If tissue loss is accompanied by damage to capillary veins, even cells that do not normally directly depend on this vascular bed suffer an oxygen shortage. The ischemia this provokes will cause necrosis (Spector, 1980; Harff, 1998).

In addition to hematoma that occurs as a result of capillary damage, the tissue necrosis causes a physiologic reaction in the damaged tissue, known as the inflammatory process (Spector, 1980; Harff, 1998). This reaction allows the physiologic and morphologic properties to be restored within a certain time frame. To restore the functional characteristics, damaged tissue must be replaced; depending on its nature, it may or may not be replaced with identical tissue. When connective tissue is damaged, *regeneration* takes place: the replacement of damaged cells and product with identical tissue, based on mitotic reactions (Evans, 1980; McComas, 1996; Harff, 1998). This suggests that collagenous connective tissue has a mitotic property and, like bone, belongs in the recurrent mitotic group.

If the damaged tissue cannot be replaced with identical tissue, the process that takes place is known as *repair* (McComas, 1996; Harff, 1998). One example is necrosis of striated muscle tissue, in which connective tissue is used to replace damaged muscle. It is the tissues' mitotic properties that determine whether regeneration or repair takes place. Taking this into account, the tissues can be classified as mitotic (blood, epithelial, and endothelial cells), postmitotic (muscle and nerve tissue), and recurrent mitotic (connective, bone, and cartilaginous tissue) (Currier and Nelson, 1992; Burgerhout, Mook, de Morree, and Zijlstra, 1995).

Stages in the Inflammatory Process

The inflammatory process is a physiologic reaction of tissues to damage. A capillary network is often present in collagenous connective tissue. Damage to this tissue triggers a repair process, in which a number of the reactions are determined by the extent of the damage to the capillary network. The inflammatory process consists of a number of phases (**Figure 3–17**).

In collagenous connective tissue that contains blood vessels, the phases in the inflammatory process are as follows

Trauma **Repair after injury**

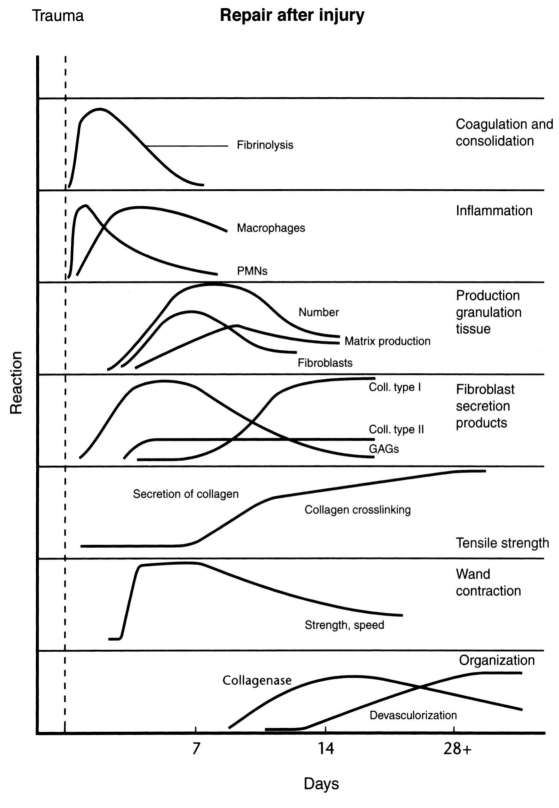

Figure 3–17

(de Morree, 1991; Woo and Buckwalter, 1991; Davidson, 1998; van den Berg, 1999):

- Bleeding phase (extravasation of blood, hemostasis, blood coagulation)
- Vascular phase, often called the inflammatory phase because of the symptoms that occur then, namely, calor, dolor, rubor, tumor, and decreased function
- Cellular phase, which can be further divided into an infiltration phase and a proliferation phase
- Production phase
- Organization phase (repair of organ characteristics)
- Integration phase (restoration of the functional characteristics within an organ system)

The duration of each individual phase, and therefore of the whole process, is determined by the extent as well as the location of the damage (Spector, 1980). The time taken depends on which tissue.

There is a large body of evidence with regard to the healing processes in the skin. In the following text, rough indications of the length of time taken by the different phases in the process are based on this body of evidence with regard to skin healing. The data can be cautiously extrapolated to connective tissue lesions in other organs.

The first phase of the inflammatory process is called the *bleeding phase*. Blood escapes from the torn capillary vessels. It accumulates in the interstitium, causing a lump known as the primary swelling. If there is damage inside a joint, the synovial fluid becomes mixed with blood (hemarthrosis). If the primary swelling is in an anatomically delineated location, it can cause eccentric pressure in and around the damaged area. The escape of blood from the vascular system triggers the hemostasis and coagulation responses. Blood platelets degranulate as soon as they are outside the vascular system, giving off serotonin and platelet-derived growth factor (PDGF). The PDGFs cause fibroblasts to produce an extracellular matrix. Serotonin (perhaps this function is best remembered by: serum and tone) stimulates vasoconstriction in the distal portions of the damaged capillary bed, leading to hemostasis. In addition, a reflex supports this vasoconstriction. The blood platelets then stick together (this is called thrombocyte aggregation) and form a plug that closes the damaged vessels. A complex cascade of reactions results in the conversion of fibrogen into the active substance fibrin, which has adhesive properties. The fibrin threads stick to the thrombocyte plug, causing coagulation; this process takes about 15 minutes (Evans, 1980; Spector, 1980).

It is known that a cold stimulus can aid hemostasis because rapid and brief cooling of the damaged area promotes vasoconstriction in the local blood vessels. This is the basis of the ICE rule used in traumatology (ice, compression, and elevation) (Spector, 1980; Hardy and Woodall, 1998). The sooner hemostasis occurs, the smaller the primary swelling.

When the bleeding phase is over, the inflammatory process moves into the *vascular phase*. During this phase, the intact part of the vascular system is the source of a number of processes that occur in and around the damaged tissue. Various tissue mediators cause vasodilatation and changes in permeability in the intact system of blood vessels. These mediators—such as prostaglandin E2—are set free by damaged cells or formed from them; bradykinin comes from damaged endothelial cells, and substance P from polymodal nociceptives. During this process, the blood supply to the damaged area increases, which raises the local tissue temperature (calor). This provides the best conditions for breakdown by enzymes. If the damage is close to the surface of the body, the increase in the blood supply causes visible redness of the skin (rubor) (Spector, 1980; Evans, 1980; Woo and Buckwalter, 1991; Davidson, 1998).

Because of the increased permeability of the single-wall capillary vessels, large proteins, including albumin, leave the vascular system, causing the ambient colloid osmotic pressure there to fall. This in turn causes osmotic pressure in the interstitium to rise, thereby attracting water. The damaged area swells once more; this is called the secondary swelling. The swelling or tumor that can be seen or felt in the local tissues after a few hours is, therefore, a result of both the primary and the secondary swelling. If the secondary swelling forms in a joint cavity, it is called a *synovial effusion*. It is essential to realize that the secondary swelling is not influenced by the application of local stimuli: the reaction is caused by the influence of various tissue mediators on the capillary vessel bed. However, it is possible to influence the degree to which secondary swelling develops in the first place. If the damage is to one of the limbs, the prevailing hydrostatic pressure in the vascular system can be minimized by elevation.

The secondary swelling facilitates access to the area by cells that play an important part in dealing with debris. Cells of various kinds release their contents, allowing (proteo)lytic enzymes to break down cell and tissue remnants into smaller fragments. This allows the phagocytosing cells to take up the fragments and remove them via the lymph vessels. The fall in the colloid-osmotic pressure means that the tissue debris (remnants of cell and tissue products mixed with water and released lytic enzymes) are removed, however not by way of the vascular system, but via the lymphatic drainage system (Spector, 1980; Harff, 1998). In this way sepsis is avoided. The swelling causes a rise in pressure in the area of the damage, causing the lymphatic vessels to open. Pressure differences in the tissues make for efficient drainage. Additionally, the application of graded mechanical stresses to the tissue can promote drainage via the lymphatic system.

During the vascular phase, the stasis of blood in the vascular system allows leukocytes to creep along the walls of the blood vessels, after which they leave the vascular system through the fenestrations in the capillaries. Most important, the damaged area is infiltrated by neutrophil granulocytes. Through the action of various tissue mediators, this group of leukocytes is transported chemically to the damaged area, where they leave the vascular system. This process is called *chemotaxis* and *diapedesis* (Evans, 1980; Spector, 1980).

When a joint undergoes a severe inflammatory process, the raised temperature in the synovial fluid, combined with the presence of large quantities of released lytic enzymes, can have a destructive effect on proteins, which have a thermolabile structure. Proteins are the basis of the proteoglycan aggregates in the hyaline cartilage of the joint. An increase in enzyme activity can occur if the temperature in the joint cavity is too high, resulting in possible damage. This damage will surely occur if the vascular reaction continues too long (Walker, 1998). To prevent this the area then needs to be cooled. If the joint is near the surface of the body, local application of a cold stimulus can draw heat from the joint cavity.

In addition to the symptoms of calor, rubor, and tumor, there will also be pain in the damaged area, also known by the Latin term *dolor*. This is an increased sensitivity to pain at the site of the damage. This phenomenon is called *primary hyperalgesia* (Bernards, 1991). The nociceptives are chemically stimulated by the action of the various algogenic substances. The free nerve endings will already have been made more sensitive to such stimuli. This increased sensitivity to pain means that the damaged area is protected from further injury.

The vascular phase reaches its peak about 1 to 1½ days after the injury. Because of the symptoms described earlier,

the vascular phase is also called the inflammatory phase. This is somewhat confusing because the term *inflammatory process* denotes the whole sequence of events, whereas the *inflammatory phase* is part of that sequence (de Morree, 1993).

During the vascular phase, the area is increasingly infiltrated by phagocytosing cells, and the vascular phase slowly gives way to the *cellular phase*. The infiltration by phagocytes ensures that the damaged area around the wound is cleared and cleansed. After about 2 to 3 days, neutrophil granulocytes, monocytes, and macrophages will have reached the whole area. The clearing of the debris can thus be completed. This stage in the cellular phase is called the *infiltration phase*. Functionally, it is part of the clearing activities (Evans, 1980; Spector, 1980; Davidson, 1998).

After 3 to 4 days, if the damaged tissue area is completely cleansed, the infiltration phase gives way to the *proliferation phase*. The local growth factors that were released at an earlier stage, together with other factors that promote proliferation, stimulate a proliferative response of the surrounding fibroblasts. The fibroblasts will move to the area of the injury by means of chemotaxis. Substance P, released by polymodal nociceptive neurons, plays an important part in inducing proliferation. Fibroblasts start cell division as soon as they have penetrated the area. In addition, some fibroblasts develop into contractile cells, called myofibroblasts (de Morree, 1993; Davidson, 1998; van den Berg, 1999). The myofibroblasts are important in closing the wound. Chains of linked cells bond with the two edges of the wound and contract, drawing them together (**Figures 3–18** and **3–19**).

When the damaged area is fully infiltrated by fibroblasts, the mitotic process stops. Contact inhibition is an important mechanism in stopping cell division: physical contact between newly formed cells triggers the production of cellular signaling substances that stop the division process

Interaction of myofibroblast, proteoglycans, fibronectin, and collagen

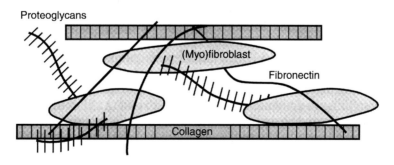

Figure 3–18

Contraction of the wound

A. Myofibroblast in resting position

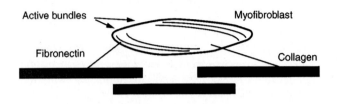

B. Myofibroblast and collagen position after contraction

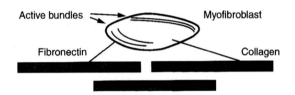

Figure 3–19

(Spector, 1980; Evans, 1980; Woo and Buckwalter, 1991). As new cells grow, the proliferation phase slowly gives way to the *productive phase*. Fibroblasts start to produce proteoglycans and collagen material. At the same time, to support the process of cell division and cell production, capillaries grow into the area from the surrounding tissues. A new vascular bed is formed by division of endothelial cells (Spector, 1980; Davidson, 1998).

The yellow tissue with small red spots that can be seen about a week after the injury is called granular tissue. It is rich in fibroblasts, basic substances, remaining fibrin threads, and inward-growing blood vessels (Spector, 1980). The duration of the productive phase depends on the amount of material to be produced and the relationship between the basic substance, the collagen material, and the site of the damaged tissue. Calculated from the time of the injury, the time needed for repair generally varies between 2 and 4 weeks. The load-bearing capacity of the recovering tissue initially increases sharply because of the increased formation of tissue products. The extracellular formation of type I collagen fibers contributes to this. The load-bearing capacity increases in proportion to tissue product formation (de Morree, 1993; Davidson, 1998; van den Berg, 1999) (**Figure 3–20**).

When sufficient material has been produced, the productive phase gives way gradually to the *organization phase*. The load-bearing capacity of the tissue continues to increase despite the fact that there is no further increase in the number of collagen fibers. The increase in strength is a result of the proper arrangement of the collagen fibers in the basic substance and an increase in the internal stability of the collagen fibers caused by *crosslinking* (Evans, 1980; de Morree, 1993; Davidson, 1998). The application of mechanical stress to the tissue causes differences in electrical potential, called the piezoelectric effect. These mechanical stresses enable the level of organization in the tissue to be restored (Lederman, 1997; van Wingerden, 1997; van den Berg, 1999). In addition, the number of type III collagen fibers slowly increases during the organizational phase; this also contributes to the increase in tissue strength (Woo and Buckwalter, 1991).

After a few weeks, this phase ends, and the *integration phase* begins. During the integration phase, the damaged tissue once more becomes a functional part of an organ within an organ system. Depending on the severity of the injury and on its location, it can sometimes take as long as 6 to 9 months for the inflammatory process to be completed (Lederman, 1997).

When connective tissue in joint capsules or joint capsule ligaments is damaged, mechanoreceptors and nerve fibers are also damaged. Reinnervation must, therefore, be part of the inflammatory process, as well as revascularization (Spector, 1980; Lederman, 1997). The damaged nerve fibers sprout and form a new peripheral receptive field with new mechanoreceptors. This process is known as *direct sprouting*. Whether the mechanoreceptors appear in their proper places, that is, whether the level of organization is identical to that existing prior to the injury, is determined by the functional demands placed on the joint during the repair process. The application of graded mechanical stress during the productive phase determines whether the newly formed collagen fibers and sensors develop the proper architecture. During the organizational phase, this functional loading must continue to restore the strength of the joint (Woo and Buckwalter, 1991; van Wingerden, 1997). If the stress is excessive or applied too early, the newly formed connective tissue will be elongated, and the consequence for the joint is hypermobility in a particular direction. Once the organization phase is complete, the tissues have reached their new permanent state. Functional demands on the newly formed connective tissue that are too little, too late, or too unidirectional will result in a suboptimally organized extracellular matrix and in deficiencies in the architecture and density of the mechanoreceptors. This leads to hypomobility and active instability. The arthrokinetic reflexes are

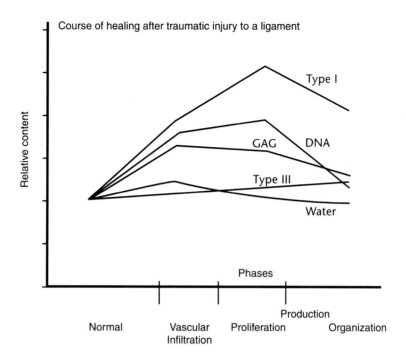

Figure 3–20

not sufficiently restored and integrated for the joint to play its full part in the sensorimotor control of more complex movement sequences. Functional training is needed during the integration phase. The initially used specially designed exercises should slowly give way to more functional forms of exercise.

Once the inflammatory process is complete, achieving a reorganization through the remodeling and reintegration phases of the newly formed tissue is much more difficult from a physiologic point of view. The structure of the newly formed tissue is not so quickly reversible because the normal laws of recovery once again apply. If there are adhesions as a result of crosslinking within and between collagen fibers, remodeling is virtually impossible without introducing a new injury.

The inflammatory reaction in hyaline joint cartilage proceeds through different time phases (Buckwalter, 1998; Walker, 1998). Hyaline joint cartilage lacks both blood vessels and nerve fibers. Despite the fact that cartilage tissue cannot be restored, it undergoes an inflammatory process when damaged (Cohen et al., 1998). This process is characterized by the absence of a bleeding phase and a vascular phase. When the damage to the cartilage is relatively serious, the local reaction can spread via the synovial fluid to other joint tissues. This can result in inflammation of the synovial membrane of the joint capsule. The membrane

contains a dense capillary network and plays an important part in the vascular phase of the joint inflammatory process. A joint inflammation of this kind, which causes internal inflammation, is called *synovitis*. Inflammation in joints leads to a disturbance of the balance between the synthesis and the degradation of proteoglycans, which are then unable to bind themselves to hyaluronic acid and form large aggregates with it (Walker and Helewa, 1996; Culav et al., 1999). As a result, the joint cartilage is no longer able to withstand compressive forces effectively. This results in the cartilage becoming much more vulnerable to new damage. As discussed earlier, a lasting disturbance in physiologic turnover, with degradation as the net result, can cause cartilage tissue to degenerate (Walker, 1998; Culav et al., 1999). In relatively young people, moderate cell death and damage to the extracellular matrix in the joint cartilage can still be followed by regeneration. In young people, hyaline joint cartilage can be regarded as a recurrently mitotic tissue (Currier and Nelson, 1992; Buckwalter, 1998; Walker, 1998).

In summary, it is clear that knowledge of the processes of recovery, regeneration, and repair in connective tissues is of enormous importance for the manual physical therapist. It directly affects the treatment choice. The manual physical therapist's strategy—be it local adaptation, or intrinsic or extrinsic compensation—is based on clinical judgments with regard to the ability of the damaged tissues to adapt locally.

THE INTERVERTEBRAL DISK
Rob Langhout and Roel Wingbermühle

Morphology

The intervertebral disks consist of a unique type of connective tissue and a highly specialized form of cartilage (Gosh, 1988). Their main constituents are cells and the extracellular matrix. The latter consists of a proteoglycan gel containing a structurally complex three-dimensional network of collagen fibers. The functional characteristics of the intervertebral disk depend on the interactions among its constituents. The strength of the disk is determined by the quality and quantity of its constituent parts.

Cells

The cells have a functional role in both constructive metabolism and product metabolism. Product metabolism serves to create and maintain the extracellular matrix, which supports the collagen fibers and the proteoglycan component. Cells can exert subtle influences on changes in the matrix via specific cell membrane receptors and transmembrane glycoproteins; this permits coordination of the growth and repair processes. Under normal circumstances, the metabolism of the intervertebral disk appears to be slow; nevertheless, the disk cells seem able to react rapidly to changes in their environment. This applies, for example, in immobilization and chemonucleolysis (Gosh, 1988). After the fourth year of life, most of the original notochordal cells have disappeared and have been replaced by a population of cells that are comparable with fibroblasts and chondrocytes (Bogduk and Twomey, 1991).

In the adult intervertebral disk, the cell population of the nucleus pulposus is the lowest to be found in any type of connective tissue, and the vertebral endplate contains a quantity of cells similar to those in hyaline cartilage. Some authors argue that at an early stage in the degeneration of the intervertebral disk, a shift takes place in the cell population of the nucleus pulposus that is not yet detectable in the annulus fibrosus. This impedes the synthesis of molecules in the nucleus pulposus and is thought to increase the vulnerability of the matrix (Oegema, 1993).

Collagen Fibers

The collagen fibers are bundles of stabilized collagen fibrils that consist of tropocollagen arranged in a zigzag pattern. A tropocollagen unit is made up of three polypeptide chains, each forming a triple helix (**Figure 3–21**).

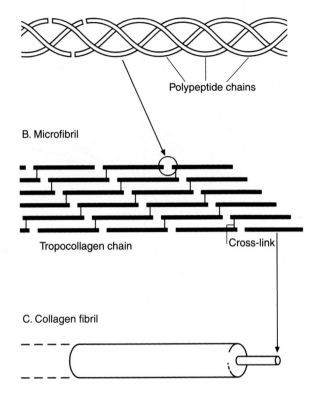

Figure 3–21

Seventeen types of collagen with different functional characteristics have been identified. The fibrils that form the collagen fibers in the intervertebral disk are collagen types I, II, III, V, and XI. The intervertebral disk fibers that consist of short helices are of types VI, IX, and XI (**Figure 3–22**). The fibrous forms of collagen have great tensile strength and are not elastic: they will only stretch by 3% of their original length.

The main purpose of type I collagen is to withstand tensile forces. Accordingly, it is found mainly in the outer zone of the annulus fibrosus. Type II collagen is found in all parts of the intervertebral disk, especially in the nucleus pulposus. Its main function is to absorb pressure. The smaller collagen types seem to be important in structuring the collagen network because they control the organization of the larger collagen fibers. Type IX collagen seems to work as a kind of glue between type II collagen and the proteoglycan gel. Type VII collagen forms an extracellular network that anchors the disk cells in the matrix (Roberts et al., 1991).

Collagen classification

A. Fibril formation

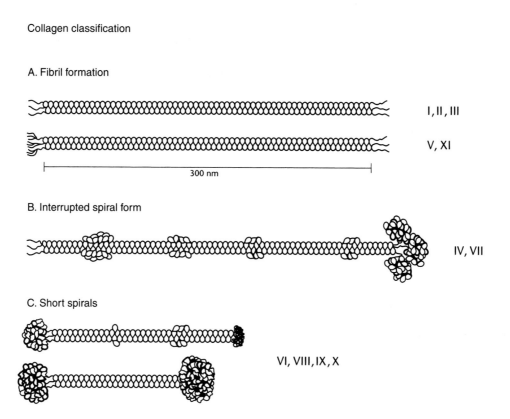

I, II, III

V, XI

300 nm

B. Interrupted spiral form

IV, VII

C. Short spirals

VI, VIII, IX, X

Figure 3–22

Proteoglycans

The proteoglycans are long molecules containing a central protein chain to which many glycosaminoglycans (GAGs) are attached (**Figure 3–23**). The proteoglycans can occur both as single units and in aggregated form. In the latter case, the proteoglycans are linked by small binding proteins to a hyaluronic acid chain. The glycosaminoglycans of the intervertebral disk are keratan sulphate and chondroitin sulphate. They are negatively charged because of the sulphate and the carboxyl groups that they contain. These two GAGs give the matrix its net negative charge. The concentration and proportions of the keratin sulphate and the chondroitin sulphate determine the fixed charge density (FCD) of the intervertebral disk (Urban and Maroudas, 1980; de Morree, 1989).

Nutrition and Function

The main constituent of the intervertebral disk is water (80–85%), together with the substances that are dissolved in it. These include oxygen, nutrients, waste products, glycoproteins, hormones, and enzymes. The nucleus pulposus contains more water and also has a greater concentration of proteoglycans than the anulus fibrosus does.

The mechanical functioning of the intervertebral disk is determined by the concentration, arrangement, and quality of its components. Interactions among the proteoglycans with their glycosaminoglycans, the water, and the collagen network give the intervertebral disk a certain flexibility that allows it to function as a joint. It is able to withstand the tensile and compressive forces exerted upon it in the course of daily activities. The intervertebral disk functions as a closed compression/expansion system. Pressures are transmitted from the body of the vertebra via the vertebral endplate to the nucleus pulposus and annulus fibrosus; they are then transformed by the nucleus pulposus into centrifugal forces and directed toward the annulus fibrosus and the vertebral endplates. This is possible because of the hydrophilic properties of the proteoglycan gel, which cause the collagen network to swell. The high osmotic pressure exerted by the proteoglycan solution is primarily a result of the relative distribution of ions between the intervertebral

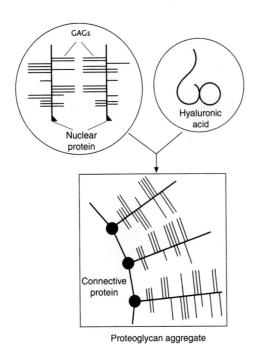

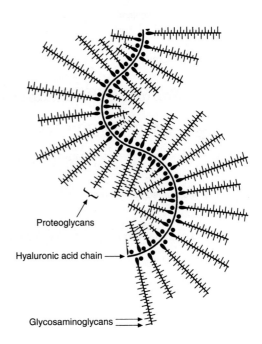

Figure 3–23

disk and the plasma in the local blood vessels. In osmosis, water moves through a semipermeable wall in the direction of the highest concentration of dissolved particles. Because of its net negative charge, the number of ions in the intervertebral disk is always greater than in the blood plasma. The fixed charge density is balanced electrostatically by mobile cations. The mobile anions that penetrate into the intervertebral disk are also compensated for by the mobile cations; therefore, the matrix has a higher concentration of ions than its surroundings. The size and shape of the proteoglycans make a limited contribution to the osmotic pressure gradient (Gosh, 1988) (**Figure 3–24**).

In the intervertebral disk, the tendency to swell as a result of osmosis is countered by two pressure systems. The first is the pressure that arises from the combination of body weight and muscle and ligament tension; the second is the pressure arising from the opposing forces exerted by the collagen network in the intervertebral disk itself. This network adapts to the pressure of the load by changing the water content of the intervertebral disk. An increase in load causes dehydration and as a result the proteoglycan concentration rises, the osmotic pressure increases, and the tension in the collagen network falls (Urban and Maroudas, 1980). According to Krämer (1978), the hydrostatic turning point for absorbing or expelling water probably lies between 700 N and 800 N (**Figure 3–25**). Nachemson (1966) studied

the pressure in the L5–S1 disk in different bodily positions (**Figure 3–26**).

The fine porous structure of the intervertebral disk is primarily determined by the concentration of proteoglycans, which are only separated by a few tens of Ångstroms from each other. The speed with which the fluid streams under pressure through the intervertebral disk depends on its hydraulic permeability. This is determined by size of the pores between the proteoglycans, that is, it depends on the proteoglycan concentration. As the load on the disk increases, water leaves the disk tissue and the hydraulic permeability falls; this combats further dehydration (Urban and Maroudas, 1980).

Electrostatic forces are also involved. Whenever water is driven from the environment of the proteoglycans as a result of the load, negatively charged GAGs are brought into closer proximity and then repel each other (de Morree, 1989).

The spongiosa of the vertebral body is rich in blood vessels. Blood vessels pass through small canals in the subchondral bone and connect via "vascular buds" with the vertebral endplates. Viewed in the transverse plane, the innermost third of the vertebral endplate is richly vascularized, whereas the more peripheral part of the endplate is virtually nonvascularized. The outermost third of the annulus fibrosus, next to the innermost part of the endplate, is

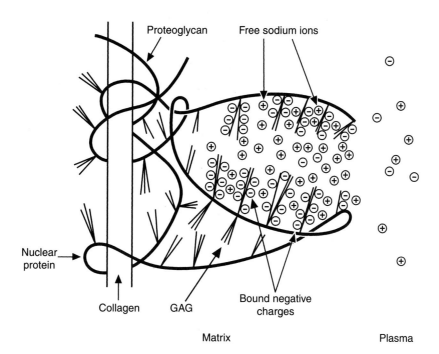

Figure 3–24

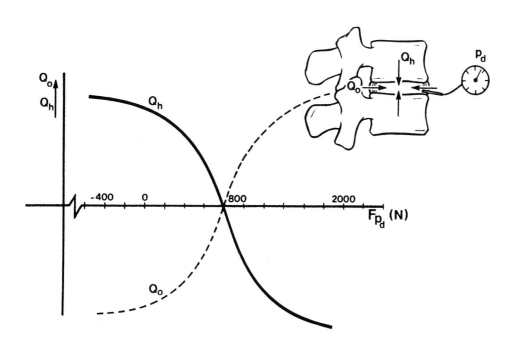

Figure 3–25 Hydrostatic water balance.

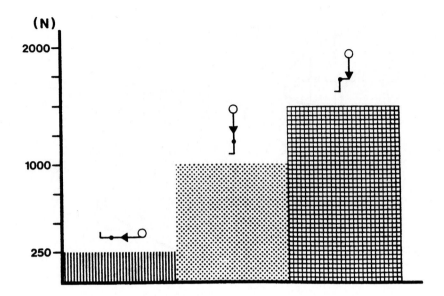

Figure 3–26   Pressure in the L5–S1 disk in different body positions. Reproduced from Nachemson (1966).

also vascularized. The intervertebral disk communicates with the blood plasma via these two routes (**Figures 3–27** and **3–28**).

Oxygen, nutrients, and smaller hormones and enzymes reach the cells of the intervertebral disks by diffusion through the matrix. This is of great importance for the metabolism and renewal of the matrix constituents. The suggested exchange of substances by way of a "pump action" is questionable and should be regarded only as an auxiliary form of transport for larger particles (Urban and Maroudas, 1980; Gosh, 1988).

Local differences in the fixed negative charge of the intervertebral disk determine the concentration of the charged particles. The concentration of positive ions, such as sodium and calcium, is higher in the intervertebral disk than in the surrounding plasma. The concentration of negative ions such as sulphate and chloride, however, is lower than in the plasma. This seems to apply to the nucleus pulposus even more than it does to the annulus fibrosus. The close proximity of the proteoglycans to each other determines the level of permeability for the large molecules. Because of their size, serum albumin, hemoglobulin, and immunoglobulin cannot normally penetrate to the healthy matrix. However, pathologic processes that cause a change in the concentration of proteoglycans can result in these large molecules entering (Urban and Maroudas, 1980).

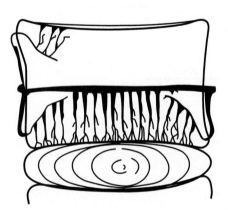
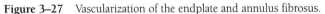
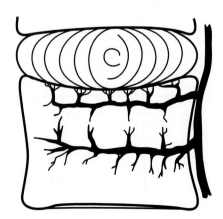

Figure 3–27   Vascularization of the endplate and annulus fibrosus.

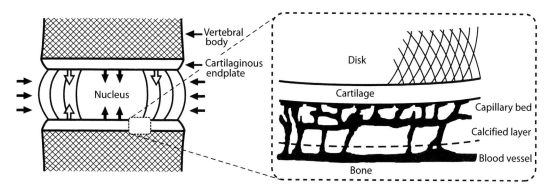

Figure 3–28

The peripheral nutrition route via the anulus fibrosus remains relatively permeable into old age, but the route through the vertebral endplate is vulnerable. As a result of age-related and degenerative processes, the endplate starts to calcify and becomes less permeable. This mainly affects the central part of the intervertebral disk, especially, the nucleus pulposus. The central part of the disk has a very low oxygen concentration and a high lactic acid content, and therefore has a low pH value. If diffusion via the vertebral endplate route decreases, the pH level can fall still further. This increases the activity of the destructive enzymes, thus increasing the vulnerability of the intervertebral disk (Urban and Maroudas, 1980). If the pH level is too low, it can lead ultimately to cell death. This affects the adaptive properties of the disk and will thus lead to further degeneration (Gosh, 1988; Oegema, 1993).

The literature contains little information about the enzyme systems that are responsible for catabolic processes within the intervertebral disk. A number of proteolytic enzymes appear to be responsible for the degradation of the proteoglycans. Collagen is broken down by the synergistic action of collagenase and other proteinases.

Circulatory Disorders

A decrease in effective circulation in the tissues around the intervertebral disk has direct consequences for the metabolism of the disk cells, and thus for the quality and quantity of the extracellular matrix. A change in the total water content may occur within the disk; the process is analogous to that which takes place in connective tissue (see the section titled "Functional Aspects of the Connective Tissues" p. 54). The tissue dries out and is physically less flexible. It therefore becomes more vulnerable, resulting in increased interaction between the collagen network and the proteoglycan gel. The initial signs of damage that may occur in the proteoglycan gel are called cracks (**Figure 3–29**).

The acidity in the disk—especially in the nucleus pulposus, where it is normally already low—falls even further when anaerobic metabolism increases. This causes cells to become distressed. If there is a further decrease in effective peripheral circulation, the disk cells can no longer maintain their productive metabolism at a satisfactory level. Given the speed of synthesis of proteoglycans, the consequences will be noticeable first in the proteoglycan gel. This means a fall in the fixed charge density, and therefore a decrease in affinity for water. This reduces the collagen network's control capabilities, which means that the collagen is damaged sooner. As soon as the acidity level exceeds the critical value, the constructive metabolism cannot be kept up to the required level, and cells can start to die. The research of Kitano et al. (1993) shows that patients with demonstrable disk disorders had significantly lower acidity levels (lower pH values) than the control group did.

The direct consequence of an increase in anaerobic metabolism is a raised concentration of hydrogen. The positive charge of the hydrogen ions affects the balance of forces existing between the negatively charged glycosaminoglycans with their attached water molecules and the positively charged collagen. The hydrogen ions will compete with the water molecules and the collagen network for the negatively charged binding sites of the proteoglycans. The result of this is that the collagen network is less stabilized by the

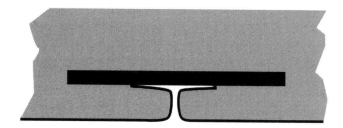

Figure 3–29   A crack in a proteoglycan gel.

proteoglycan gel and the tissue becomes physically weaker. A falling pH value also has implications for the enzyme processes inside the intervertebral disk. In a healthy disk, there is a delicate balance between active and latent enzymes on the one hand and their inhibitors on the other. This balance is sensitive to acidity levels. If the pH value falls, the balance is disturbed and the destructive enzymes gain the upper hand. This results in degradation of the protein and collagen components of the extracellular matrix (Fujita, Nakagawa, Hirabayashi, and Nagai, 1993).

Pathological Consequences

The nucleus pulposus normally translates the compressive forces exerted on the disk by the vertebral bodies by way of the inferior and superior endplates into centrifugal forces that support the wall of the annulus and the endplates from the inside out. When pathologic changes have taken place in the nucleus, it may no longer be able to perform this function adequately. The result is a clinically unstable movement pattern (**Figures 3–30** and **3–31**).

The increase in bonding between the proteoglycan components on the one hand and the hydrogen ions and collagen on the other decreases the bonding of water molecules, resulting in an increase in unbonded water. When the tissues are stressed, especially during static stress, dehydration accelerates, which manifests itself clinically after long periods of sitting, standing, or strolling as stiffness in the lumbar region of the spine. Practitioners call this the *dehydration phenomenon*. It may also be observed in disk disorders seen in clinical practice. The symptoms of the phenomenon are stiffness of the lower back in the mornings and difficulty in bending and putting socks and shoes on.

To understand this, one needs to consider the forces to which the disk is exposed during stress and relaxation. During relaxation, the tendency to swelling as a result of osmosis is countered by two forces: first, the load imposed by body weight and tension of the ligaments and the musculature; and second, the tension that builds up as a result of swelling in the collagen network of the intervertebral disk itself. If the collagen network becomes physically weaker as a result of direct damage or through the acidifying processes described previously, dehydration will be relatively greater during stress compared with the healthy situation (Grieve, 1988).

Therapeutic Aspects

The repair process depends on the presence of viable cells (see the section titled "Functional Aspects of the Connective Tissues). Under ideal circumstances, repair takes place. Recovery is possible from a peripheral annular injury if conditions are favorable and if there is no cell death. Favorable conditions include a sufficient supply of building materials, fuel, oxygen, and normal anatomic relationships within the motion segment. Arthrogenic rigidity or instability in the segment affects its movement pattern and, therefore, influences the structure of the collagen network in terms of length and resistance to tensile forces. Before the recovery process begins, therefore, plans must be made for creating optimal conditions. If during recovery the load on the tissues is kept proportional to their current strength,

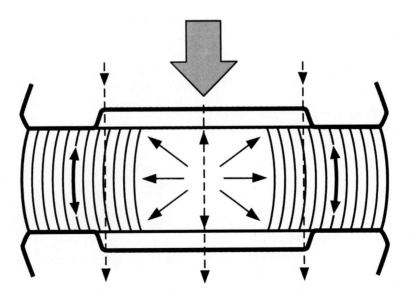

Figure 3–30

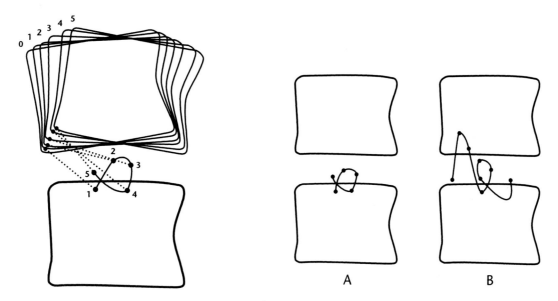

Figure 3–31 Instantaneous axis of rotation in five phases during flexion–extension: (A) centrode of axes in normal disk; (B) centrode of axes in pathologic disk.

complete recovery is possible. The proteoglycans in the tissues of the annulus take a few weeks to recover. For the collagen in the periphery of the intervertebral disk, the literature suggests a recovery time of 3 months (Moore, Vernon-Roberts, and Osti, 1996; Osti, Vernon-Roberts, Moore, and Fraser, 1992; Gosh, 1988).

If the proper conditions cannot be met in full, or if the damage to the disk cells is too great, complete recovery will not take place but will be limited to whatever is possible (Bernards, 1997). Compensatory processes will, therefore, be involved; muscles or bones (spondylosis) may attempt to stabilize, and posture and movement patterns may be adapted.

The restoration of the proteoglycan component of the nucleus pulposus takes significantly longer even under ideal circumstances and depends heavily on age. In animal experiments, the speed of turnover varies from 250 days in rabbits to 680 days in dogs (Urban and Maroudas, 1980; Gosh, 1988). As stated earlier, the central diffusion route seems to be the most vulnerable. This is one of the most significant obstacles to recovery, along with the strong increase in acidity, which can lead to cell death, and thus directly damages the adaptive capability of the nucleus pulposus.

When assessing the potential for recovery, it is useful to make an inventory of the factors that support adaptive capability and of those that limit it. The extent to which these factors can be influenced determines whether we base our therapeutic intervention on an adaptive or a compensatory strategy (Bernards, 1997).

Depending on the therapeutic goals, efforts will be made to encourage the production and strengthening of the ma-

trix, the latter both with regard to its form and its function. The cell reacts to the chemical, thermal, and mechanical changes that are part of homeostasis. These changes will stimulate cell metabolism. The productive and constructive metabolism of the disk cells can, therefore, be influenced by applying appropriate loads. Dynamic loading in the form of graded movement exposure should form a significant part of the treatment strategy because these movements will stimulate cell metabolism. An increase in cell metabolism is associated with the use and consumption of nutrients, building materials, and oxygen. This causes the concentration of these substances to fall short locally in the disk. Diffusion will, therefore, have to increase, according to the principle of supply and demand.

Optimal reestablishment of the matrix architecture is of great importance. The primary aim is to achieve the best possible level of three-dimensional mobility in the segment. If there is segmental fixation or segmental instability, attempts should be made to restore the physiologic axes of rotation and the range of movement. Graded three-dimensional loading is needed to guarantee proper formation of cross-links and resistance to traction in the collagen network, in interaction with the proteoglycan gel.

If optimal recovery is not possible, a compensatory strategy must be devised. The main factors to be taken into consideration are the mobility of the affected segment and the region to which it belongs; the retraining of the musculature of the segment; active stabilization of the segment; and optimizing the arthrokinetic reflex activity or coordination (van der El, 2002). In addition, limits should be set on physical stress, and patient education based on ergonomic principles should be given. Sitting at an angle of 120° with a 5-cm back support at the level of L3 seems to be the least stressful for the lumbar part of the spine. To maintain stability during lifting activities, the patient should be advised to tense the oblique abdominal muscles, thus temporarily raising intra-abdominal and intrathoracic pressure.

The cervical and lumbar intervertebral disks seem to be the most vulnerable. In these regions, the disks are higher in comparison to the vertebral body than they are in the cervical and lumbar regions (**Figure 3–32**). The advantage of this is greater movement range. Therefore, the cervical and lumbar regions are dependent to a significant degree on musculature to maintain stability.

FUNCTIONAL ASPECTS OF THE SPINAL MUSCULATURE

There is little point in analyzing the functions of the individual muscles because they almost always work together in groups. Great demands are placed on the muscles of the back in daily life because they are necessary both for maintaining the upright posture needed for walking and standing and for carrying out movements.

The center of gravity of the whole body and the center of gravity of the trunk lie in front of the spinal column. The trunk and the pelvis tend to tilt forward under the influence of gravity. This tilting is prevented by the isometric contraction of the erector spinae, the pelvic extensor muscles, and the triceps surae. These muscles have a double function when movements are made with the body in an upright position.

Bending the trunk forward requires isometric contraction of some muscles to maintain the position of the spinal column, and eccentric contraction of others to counteract gravity. Returning from this position requires isometric and concentric activity, respectively, in the different muscle groups. With regard to movement, there is a functional difference between the long and the short components of the erector spinae muscle. The long muscles with their long lever arm extending over multiple segments are responsible for the general movement, whereas the short muscles are primarily responsible for distributing this general movement evenly across the different segments. The operation of this mechanism is clearly illustrated during rotation of the trunk. When the trunk is turned to the left, the rotation is brought about primarily by the right external oblique and the left internal oblique. The fibers of these muscles are aligned in extension of each other. When the movement is performed, the oblique abdominal muscles are supported from the left by the longissimus, iliocostalis, and splenii muscles and from the right by the transversospinal system. The ipsilateral rotators on the left and the long muscles on the right work together to ensure that the trunk remains extended during the movement. The transversospinal system on the right side can contribute little rotatory power because of the direction of its muscle fibers relative to the axis of rotation. Its most important function, therefore, is to evenly spread the total rotational movement across the different vertebral segments.

The same mechanism comes into play during movements of the cervical spinal column and the suboccipital joints. Here, too, the short suboccipital muscles are responsible for distributing total movement evenly across the mid- and lower parts of the cervical spine and the suboccipital joints.

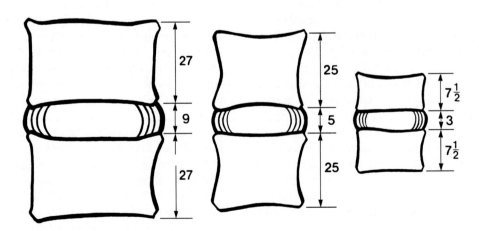

Figure 3–32   Average height of vertebral body and disk in the lumbar, thoracic, and cervical regions.

CHAPTER 4

Terminology and Theories

ORTHOPAEDIC MANUAL THERAPY DIAGNOSIS
Peter A. Huijbregts

Classification of Patients

Diagnosis is classification of patients based on predetermined defining characteristics. Diagnosis requires a classification system. The *Guide to Physical Therapist Practice* (2001) notes three criteria that a classification system must meet to be useful for physical therapy—and as a subset, also orthopaedic manual therapy (OMT)—clinical practice:

- The system must be consistent with boundaries placed upon the profession by law or society.
- The tests necessary for confirming the diagnosis must be within the legal purview of physical therapy.
- The label used to categorize a condition must direct the selection of interventions toward those interventions that are part of the physical therapy scope of practice.

Classification systems are clinimetric indices, that is, rating scales and other expressions used to measure symptoms, physical signs, and other phenomena in clinical medicine (Riddle, 1998). There are four types of clinimetric indices relevant to classification systems used for diagnosis of patients presenting to OMT clinicians:

- Status indices
- Prognostic indices
- Clinical guideline indices
- Mixed indices

Status indices are classification systems used to define patient problems. The most common clinically used example of a status index is the International Classification of Diseases (ICD). This is a taxonomy of diagnostic labels for the purpose of standardizing nomenclature of diagnoses for statistical and administrative reasons. At least in the United States, OMT clinicians are all familiar with ICD-9 codes for insurance reimbursement for their services. Because the ICD manual does not describe the procedures used to apply the diagnostic labels, reliability of assigning ICD-9 codes is low (Riddle, 1998). The traditional medical, structure-based model is also a status index: it assumes a direct correlation between underlying pathology and signs and symptoms and uses a pathoanatomic classification system (Fritz, 1999). As a clear example of its limited value in general and specific to OMT diagnosis, the medical model is unable to provide up to 85% of patients with low back pain a specific diagnosis because of the weak association between symptoms, pathologic changes, and results from imaging tests (Deyo, Rainville, and Kent, 1992; van den Hoogen, Koes, van Eijk, and Bouter, 1995). Despite these drawbacks, OMT diagnosis at times uses diagnostic labels consistent with this structure-based or pathoanatomic model. Examples include diagnoses of facet joint syndrome, sacroiliac joint syndrome, and disk lesions.

A prognostic index is a classification system that allows the clinician to predict the patient's future status; this type of system is mainly designed to aid the clinician in making predictions regarding the chance of a poor outcome and the implied need for referral for other services to optimize outcome. Research into the predictive validity of (clusters of) signs and symptoms is needed to produce prognostic indices. Predictive validity and its statistical expression are discussed in Chapter 5. An example of a prognostic index is provided by the research into prognostic indicators for the efficacy of OMT interventions in patients with cervicogenic headache. Jull and Stanton (2005) aimed to identify those patients with cervicogenic headache who did or did not achieve a 50–79% or 80–100% reduction in headache immediately and 12 months post intervention. Only the absence of lightheadedness indicated higher odds of achieving either a 50–79% (odds ratio, OR = 5.45) or 80–100% (OR = 5.7) reduction in headache frequency in the long term.

The third type of classification system is the clinical guideline index. This type of index is designed specifically to provide instructions regarding treatment. Most relevant to OMT diagnosis are mechanism- and treatment-based classification systems. The mechanism-based classification system is based on the premise that impairments identified during examination are the cause of musculoskeletal pain and dysfunction (van Dillen et al., 1998). In the treatment-based system, a cluster of signs and symptoms from the patient history and physical examination is used to classify patients into subgroups with specific implications for management. In current-day OMT clinical practice, the once predominant mechanism-based system is increasingly supplemented by treatment-based classification systems (Childs et al., 2004b; Delitto, Erhard, and Bowling, 1995; Donelson, 2007; Fritz, Brennan, Clifford, Hunter, and Thackeray, 2006).

The classification developed by the Quebec Task Force on Spinal Disorders is an example of a mixed index, designed to help make clinical decisions, establish a prognosis, as well as evaluate the quality of care for patients with low back pain (Riddle, 1998).

The purpose of OMT diagnosis in cases of neuromusculoskeletal dysfunction is to identify the joint(s) implicated, the damaged tissue, the possible neuroreflexive extension of the local dysfunction, and the levels of reactivity and ability for a targeted or selective response within the nervous system. Paris (1979) defined joint dysfunction as a state of altered mechanics, characterized by an increase or decrease from the expected normal or by the presence of an aberrant motion. However, within the context of OMT diagnosis and with the emphasis placed here on not only structural but also functional aspects of joint function and their associated (or at least assumed) implications on patient function, it is perhaps better to use the terminology of impairment, limitations in activity, and restrictions in participation as proposed by the World Health Organization (2001). (See **Table 4–1**.) This terminology is also increasingly used in a broader sense in physical therapy to standardize communication with regard to diagnosis, management, and outcome measures. The OMT examination strategy depends on the patient's presentation and on how acute the damage is. The examination sequence and choice of examination techniques are characterized by an ongoing decision-making

Table 4–1   Definitions of International Classification of Functioning, Disability, and Health (ICF) Terminology

ICF Terminology	Definitions
Impairment	Any loss or abnormality of body structure or of a physiologic or psychological function.
Activity	The nature and extent of functioning at the level of the person. Activities may be limited in nature, duration, or quality.
Participation	The nature and extent of a person's involvement in life situations in relation to impairments, activities, health conditions, and contextual factors. Participation may be restricted in nature, duration, or quality.

process that determines the appropriate sequence and content of the examination. As such, OMT diagnosis can be seen to predominantly use a mechanism-based and a patho-anatomic classification model. However, as noted earlier this combination is increasingly supplemented by various treatment-based models.

Arguably, within the context of OMT diagnosis the Mechanical Diagnosis and Therapy (MDT) approach as proposed by McKenzie is the most extensively research treatment-based classification system. Donelson (2007) provides an excellent overview of the current state of research with regard to this approach. However, of greater relevance to OMT diagnosis as presented in this book is the treatment-based classification for patients with neck pain and low back pain (Childs et al., 2004b; Delitto et al., 1995) presented in **Tables 4–2** and **4–3**.

There is an increasing body of research that supports aspects of the preceding treatment-based systems with a great many studies producing clinical prediction rules relevant to these proposed diagnostic classification systems. Clinical prediction rules are decision-making tools that contain predictor variables obtained from patient history, examination, and simple diagnostic tests; they can assist in making a diagnosis, establishing prognosis, or determining appropriate management (Laupacis, Sekar, and Stiell, 1997). As Childs and Flynn (2004) point out, if studies included in a systematic review or meta-analysis use no patient classification other than the broad category of nonspecific low back (or neck) pain, the resultant heterogeneous study samples pretty much preclude finding real effects of any specific intervention. In contrast, the recent clinical prediction rules all aim to identify a more homogeneous diagnostic sub-

Table 4–2 Treatment-Based Classification for Patients With Neck Pain

Classification	Examination Findings	Proposed Matched Interventions
Mobility	• Recent onset of symptoms • No radicular or referred symptoms in the upper quarter • Restricted range of motion with rotation and/or discrepancy in sidebending • No signs of nerve root compression or peripheralization of symptoms in the upper quarter with cervical range of motion	• Cervical and thoracic spine mobilization and/or manipulation • Active range of motion exercises
Centralization	• Radicular or referred symptoms in the upper quarter • Peripheralization and/or centralization of symptoms with range of motion • Signs of nerve root compression present • May have pathoanatomic diagnosis of cervical radiculopathy	• Mechanical and/or manual traction • Repeated movements to centralize symptoms
Conditioning and increase exercise tolerance	• Lower pain and disability scores • Longer duration of symptoms • No signs of nerve root compromise • No peripheralization and/or centralization of symptoms with range of motion	• Strengthening and endurance exercises for the muscles of the neck and upper quarter • Aerobic conditioning exercises
Pain control	• High pain and disability scores • Very recent onset of symptoms • Symptoms precipitated by trauma • Referred or radiating symptoms extending into the upper quarter • Poor tolerance for examination or most interventions	• Gentle active range of motion within pain tolerance • Range of motion exercises for adjacent regions • Physical modalities as needed • Activity modification to control pain
Reduce headache	• Unilateral headache with onset preceded by neck pain • Headache pain triggered by neck movement or positions • Headache pain elicited by pressure on posterior neck	• Cervical spine mobilization and/or manipulation • Strengthening of the neck and upper quadrant muscles • Postural education

Source: Adapted from: Childs JD, Fritz JM, Piva SR, Whitman JM. Proposal of a classification system for patients with neck pain. *J Orthop Sports Phys Ther.* 2004b;34:686–696.

group of patients that is expected to respond to manipulative or other OMT intervention.

Diagnostic clinical prediction rules relevant to OMT diagnosis include rules on the diagnosis of cervical radiculopathy and sacroiliac joint pain. Wainner and associates (2003) identify four variables as accurate predictors of cervical radiculopathy:

• Positive median bias upper limb tension test
• Ipsilateral cervical rotation active range of motion less than 60°

• Positive Spurling test A: Patient seated with ipsilateral sidebending of the neck and 7 (kg) of overpressure applied reproducing or aggravating symptoms
• Positive supine cervical distraction test as indicated by a symptom reduction/resolution

The positive likelihood ratio (LR)—a statistic discussed in Chapter 5—for two positive tests was established to be 0.88, for three tests 6.1, and for four positive tests 30.3 (Wainner et al., 2003).

Table 4–3   Treatment-Based Classification for Patients With Low Back Pain

Classification	Examination Findings	Proposed Matched Interventions
Specific exercise	• Strong preference for sitting or walking • Centralization with motion testing • Peripheralization in direction opposite centralization	• Repeated endrange exercises
Stabilization	• Younger age • Increased straight-leg raise range of motion • Aberrant motions present • Positive prone instability test • Hypermobility with spring testing • Increasing episode frequency • Three or more previous episodes	• Trunk strengthening and stabilization exercises
Manipulation	• More recent onset of symptoms • No symptoms distal to the knee • FABQ Work scale score < 19 • Hypomobility with lumbar spring testing	• Manual therapy • Range of motion exercise
Traction	• Leg symptoms • Signs of nerve root compression • Peripheralization with extension movements and/or positive crossed straight-leg raise	• Traction intervention and repeated endrange exercise

Laslett and associates (2003) studied concurrent criterion-related validity of a comprehensive examination consisting of a McKenzie evaluation combined with a cluster of sacroiliac joint (SIJ) provocation tests. The tests used were the distraction, compression, thigh thrust, pelvic torsion, and sacral thrust tests. The rating scale for the individual tests was dichotomous; the subjects were diagnosed with sacroiliac joint disease (SIJD) when three or more tests were positive after exclusion of diskogenic complaints with a McKenzie repeated movement evaluation. The gold standard test was a fluoroscopically guided double SIJ block with at least 80% pain reduction. The authors reported positive LR of 6.97 (95% confidence interval: 2.70–20.27) and a negative LR of 0.11 (95% CI: 0.02–0.44). Excluding the diskogenic patients yielded a positive LR of 4.16 (95% CI: 2.16–8.39) and a negative LR of 0.12 (95% CI: 0.02–0.49). Laslett (2008) recently suggested this examination protocol as a diagnostic sacroiliac clinical prediction rule with Huijbregts (2008) noting the need for additional research before this rule could be converted into a clinical prediction rule relevant to management of this patient group.

Various clinical prediction rules have been produced related to management. Flynn and associates (2002) developed a clinical prediction rule consisting of five predictor criteria to identify a subgroup of patients with nonspecific low back pain who were likely to benefit from thrust manipulation. This rule was subsequently validated by Childs and colleagues (2004b), who calculated an adjusted OR of 114.7 at the 1-week follow-up and one of 60.8 for a positive functional outcome at the 4-week follow-up for patients who were positive on the rule (≥ 4 predictor criteria present) and received manipulation versus those patients who were negative on the rule and received exercise.

Fritz and associates (2005a) derived a subsequent two-factor rule from this prediction rule and reported a positive LR of 7.2 for a positive outcome in patients with low back pain positive on both predictor variables and treated with manipulation. Fritz and associates (2007) reported preliminary evidence that there is a subgroup of patients with low back pain likely to benefit from traction characterized by leg symptoms, signs of nerve root compression, and peripheralization with extension movements or a positive crossed straight-leg raise test.

Hicks and colleagues (2005) identified four variables relevant to predicting success with stabilization exercises: age < 40, average straight-leg raise test > 91°, presence of aberrant motions, and a positive prone instability test. The presence of three or more variables indicated the greatest likelihood of success with a positive likelihood ratio of 4.0 (95% CI: 1.6–10.0). Variables associated with failure were a negative prone instability test, absence of aberrant motions, absence of hypermobility on lumbar spring testing, and a Fear Avoidance Beliefs Questionnaire Physical Activity (FABQ-PA) subscale score of < 9. Two or more of these variables present carried a negative LR of 0.18 (95% CI: 0.08–0.38). Similarly, Fritz and associates (2004) identified longer symptom duration, symptoms in the leg or buttock, absence of lumbar hypomobility, less hip rotation range of motion, less side-to-side discrepancy in hip internal rotation range of motion, and a negative pelvic torsion test as predictors of lack of success with manipulation.

Tseng and associates (2006) identified six predictor variables for an immediate positive response to cervical manipulation in patients with neck pain including patients diagnosed with cervical spondylosis with or without radiculopathy, cervical herniated disk, myofascial pain syndrome, and cervicogenic headache. An increasing number of predictor variables present led to progressively higher positive likelihood ratios of an immediate positive response to manipulation: four predictor variables present yielded an LR of 5.33 and an 89% probability of a successful manipulation (Tseng et al., 2006).

Cleland and colleagues (2007) derived six predictor variables in patients with mechanical neck pain without neurologic involvement, indicating a likely positive response to a combination of three different thoracic thrust manipulations, one simple cervical range of motion exercise, and patient education. They suggested using a criterion of three out of six variables present as a sufficient research-based indication for the use of thoracic manipulation in patients with mechanical neck pain: three of six variables present yielded a positive LR of 5.5 and an 86% probability of a successful outcome. **Table 4–4** provides the predictor variables in the various manipulation-related clinical prediction rules.

Although less relevant to the current proposed classification system for patients with neck pain but likely to be included in updated versions of this treatment-based classification system, Fernández-de-las-Peñas and associates (2008) developed a clinical prediction rule to identify

Table 4–4   Clinical Prediction Rules and Predictor Variables

CPR to identify patients with LBP most likely to benefit from manipulation
- Duration of current episode < 16 days
- No symptoms distal to the knee
- FABQW score < 19
- ≥1 hypomobile segment on lumbar segmental mobility testing
- One or both hips with > 35° of internal rotation range of motion

Abbreviated CPR to identify patients with LBP most likely to benefit from manipulation
- Duration of current episode less than 16 days
- No symptoms distal to the knee

CPR to identify patients with immediate response to cervical manipulation
- Initial NDI < 11.50
- Bilateral involvement pattern
- Not performing sedentary work > 5 hours per day
- Feeling better while moving the neck
- Not feeling worse when extending the neck
- Diagnosis of spondylosis without radiculopathy

CPR to identify patients with neck pain likely to respond to thoracic manipulation
- Symptom duration < 30 days
- No symptoms distal to the shoulder
- Looking up does not aggravate symptoms
- FABQPA score < 12
- Diminished upper thoracic kyphosis
- Cervical extension range of motion < 30°

CPR, Clinical prediction rule; LBP, low back pain; FABQW, Fear Avoidance Beliefs Questionnaire Work Subscale; NDI, Neck Disability Index; FABQPA, Fear Avoidance Beliefs Questionnaire Physical Activity Subscale.

patients with chronic tension-type headache apt to have short-term benefit from manual trigger point therapy consisting of varied combinations of pressure release, muscle energy, and soft tissue techniques combined with progressive, low-load deep cervical flexor and extensor muscle strengthening exercises. Relevant improvement was defined in this study as an at least 50% reduction in either headache intensity, frequency, or duration and an increase of greater than or equal to 5 points on a 15-point global rating of change or patient satisfaction scale. Four variables constituted the clinical prediction rule for benefit at one week after discharge: headache duration < 8.5 hours per day, headache frequency < 5.5 days per week, Short Form (SF)-36 bodily pain domain score < 47, and SF-36 vitality domain score < 47.5. If the patient had three of these four variables, the positive LR for short-term benefit at one week post discharge was 3.4 (95% CI: 1.4–8.0). If all four variables were present, the positive LR increased to 5.9 (95% CI: 0.8–42.9). Two variables made up the clinical prediction rule for benefit one month post discharge: headache frequency < 5.5 days per week, SF-36 bodily pain domain score < 47. With one of these two variables present, the positive LR was 2.2 (95% CI: 1.2–3.8); two variables present yielded a positive LR of 4.6 (95% CI: 1.2–17.9).

The clinical reasoning involved in OMT diagnosis has shifted over time from a pathoanatomic model to the current model where mechanism-based and treatment-based classification systems are integrated. With evidence despite great research efforts in recent years insufficient for a solely treatment-based approach, the OMT clinician still depends heavily on the treatment-based diagnostic classification system that is the main topic of discussion in this text.

SEGMENT

In this context, "a segment is a complex of tissues that is innervated by one spinal nerve in addition to the gray communicating rami, or the vegetative efferent innervation" (Hagenaars, 1987).

MOVEMENT SEGMENT

A *movement segment* is a functional unit of two vertebrae (Junghanns, 1954) (**Figure 4–1**).

A functional unit contains the following structures:

- Intervertebral disk:
  Nucleus pulposus
  Anulus fibrosus

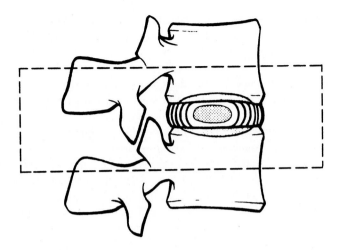

Figure 4–1   The movement segment. *Source:* Junghanns, 1954.

Cartilage endplate
Caudal aspect of the vertebral body that lies above
Cranial aspect of the spinal body that lies below

- Intervertebral joints:
  Cartilaginous surfaces
  Chondrosynovial membrane (gelatin-like membrane)
  Meniscoid folds
  Caudal aspect of the joint surfaces of the vertebra above
  Cranial aspect of the joint surfaces of the vertebra below
  Joint capsule
- Intervertebral foramen
- Anterior longitudinal ligament
- Posterior longitudinal ligament
- Flaval ligament
- Intertransverse ligament
- Inter- and supraspinous ligament
- Musculature that spans the segment and the rotatores brevis muscle
- Tissues that enter and leave the foramen and that are located at the same level in the vertebral canal

In the cervical region:

- Uncovertebral joints

In the upper cervical area:

- Atlanto-occipital joints
- Atlantoepistropheal joints

- Atlantoaxial joints
- Apical ligament
- Alar ligament
- Tectorial membrane
- Transverse ligament
- Cruciform ligament
- Musculature that spans the segment
- Structures that enter and leave the segment
- That part of the vertebral artery that runs alongside the segment

In the thoracic area:

- Rib joints fixed to the segment and connecting structures

INTERVERTEBRAL FORAMEN

The anatomic boundaries for the foramen are formed as follows:

- *Posterior.* The two articular processes and the joint that they form. The processes are joined together by the capsular ligament and the lateral edge of the flaval ligament.
- *Anterior.* The dorsal aspects of vertebral bodies and the intervertebral disk.
- *Cranial.* The pedicle of the vertebra above.
- *Caudal.* The pedicle of the vertebra below.

The organs and vascular-lymphatic structures that pass through the foramen are the following:

- The nerve root
- The spinal artery with its branches
- The veins
- The lymph vessels
- The meningeal ramus
- The cerebrospinal fluid, which passes through the perineural space to the sympathetic capillaries

JOINT

The joint (also known as the *arthron*; in the spinal column as the *vertebron*) as described by Gutzeit (1951) consists of the following structures:

- The joint, which is moved passively
- The muscles, which move actively
- The controlling innervation

JOINT PLAY

Joint play means the amount of movement (play) in a joint that cannot be actively controlled in a selective manner. The amount of joint play can be examined passively from the resting state by pulling the joint partners apart (traction) and by moving the joint partners perpendicular to the plane of traction (translation). Normal joint play is a necessity to achieve normal joint function.

BLOCK VERTEBRA

Block vertebra is a condition in which the mobility in a motion segment is completely and irreversibly lost. It is a pain-free endstate (for example, ankylosis; **Figure 4–2**).

IMMOBILE SEGMENT (FUNCTIONAL BLOCK VERTEBRA)

An *immobile segment* is a condition in which the mobility of a segment is lost completely, but only temporarily. The condition is not painless. The following are examples of circumstances in which it can occur:

- A fracture
- A herniation of the nucleus pulposus
- An inflammatory-type process
- An osteolytic process

INTERVERTEBRAL FIXATION

Intervertebral fixation means restriction of movement in the joint. Mobility is never completely lost but is limited to a greater or lesser extent in one or more directions. In cases of local hypomobility, clinicians should start by exploring possible biomechanical causes.

Etiology of Intervertebral Fixation

It is not known which component is responsible for intervertebral joint fixation. There are a number of working

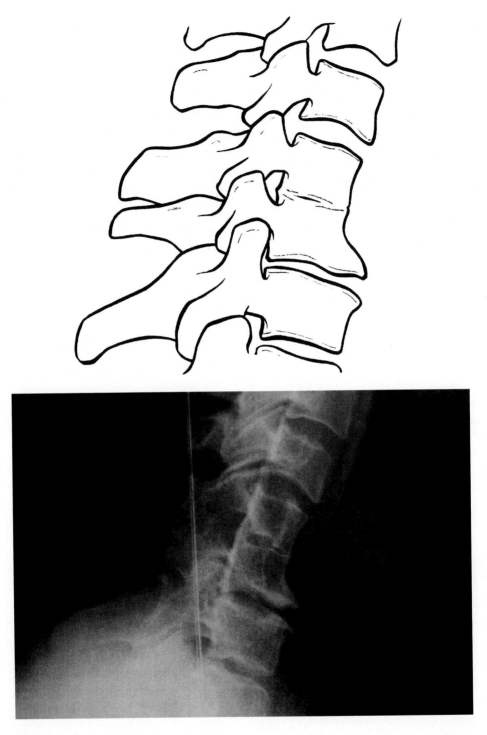

Figure 4–2   Block vertebra.

hypotheses, but no scientific proof. In the case of the vertebron, the three possible elements are the following:

- The joint that can be moved passively (bone, cartilage, circulation, synovial fluid, meniscoid folds, chondrosynovial membrane, capsule, ligaments)
- Segmental musculature
- Segmental innervation

The last two would seem to be not purely segmental.

Hypotheses Regarding Intervertebral Fixation

In the literature we can find various hypotheses with regard to possible causes for this intervertebral fixation.

Subluxation

The subluxation theory was the starting point for chiropractors. It seems to be one of the oldest theories and has not been adopted by many others because of its primitive mechanical assumptions. According to this theory, an intervertebral joint becomes irritated in its physiologic endrange, exerting pressure on the spinal ganglia and thus causing dysfunction. Manipulation is thought to be effective in repositioning the joint to its neutral state. True subluxation seldom occurs except occasionally in the atlantooccipital joint.

Nerve Entrapment

Clinicians must distinguish between a genuine irritation of the nerve root with radicular symptomatology and pseudoradicular symptomatology caused by irritation of the joint capsule. Although irritation of the root can cause an intervertebral joint blockage in the affected segment or neighboring segments, this does not necessarily explain the joint fixation because an intervertebral joint fixation can occur in the absence of irritation of the root.

Rotation

The rotation theory is based on the old osteopathic view that an intervertebral joint fixation is always accompanied by a fixed rotational malposition. This theory does not explain the fixation, and in any case it is inaccurate because fixation can occur when the vertebrae are in other positions relative to each other. Moreover, this theory implies that in a situation such as scoliosis the vertebral column is blocked at almost all levels.

Thixotropy

The thixotropy theory rests on the fact that a substance can change its viscosity in response to mechanical forces exerted upon it. Hyaluronic acid, for example, can move under pressure from a thick, viscous state to a thin, fluid state. This phenomenon is applied to the fluids in the joint to explain the blockage.

Arthrosis

The arthrosis theory is based on the fact that degenerative changes in the joint cartilage can produce certain irregularities in the articular surfaces. A fixation could, therefore, occur in a particular position. It is claimed that this theory can also explain the recurrent nature of a fixation.

Chondrosynovial Membrane

Wolf (1970) shows that the joint cartilage is covered by a gelatin-like layer called the chondrosynovial membrane. Segmental fixation is explained by splits occurring in this thin membrane.

Articular Meniscal Entrapment

Various publications (Emminger, 1967; Wolf, 1970) describe disk, menisci, or cushions of fat in the intervertebral joints that are said to be responsible for absorbing and distributing the forces exerted on the joint. It has been shown that meniscoid folds are present (Putz, 1981) (**Figure 4–3**).

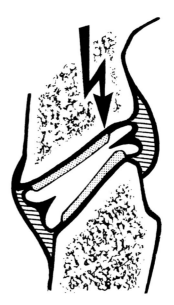

Figure 4–3 Articular meniscal entrapment.

The conclusion has been drawn from this that compression of the meniscoid folds, or damage to them, can cause segmental fixation. This theory also seems inconclusive because rigidity can occur in joints that have no disk or meniscus, such as the sacroiliac joint. Despite repeated attacks on this theory by Penning (1964, 1968, 1978), Emminger (1967) continues to defend it.

Polarity

Charnley (Neuman, 1978) starts from the premise that the two articular surfaces that lie opposite each other in the intervertebral joint have a weak identical charge. This means that they should repel each other weakly, which would counteract gravity and muscular compression. The argument is that a disturbance of this electrical charge leads to fixation.

Prolonged Sympathetic Nervous System Hyperactivity (Related to Inactivity/Immobilization)

Contemporary thought is increasingly influenced by the neuroreflexive model (Hagenaars et al., 1985; Hagenaars, 1987; Bernards and Oostendorp, 1988). Afferent stimuli from the disk, the intervertebral joint, the dermatome, the myotome, the sclerotome, the viscerotome, and the angiotome enter the central nervous system at the segmental level. Here they are evaluated, processed, and stored or passed on. The processing of incoming stimuli seems to depend heavily on the reactivity and ability to produce a targeted or selective response of the nervous system. Stress can have a negative influence here. An increase in input from nociceptors causes an increase in activity in the sympathetic part of the autonomic nervous system. Increased activity in the sympathetic nervous system, when combined with decreased activity or immobilization, can lead to the following: disturbance of effective blood supply to the different parts of the movement apparatus; muscular hypertonicity; changes in the elasticity of connective tissue; lowering of the threshold value of the nociceptive system.

Negative consequences for the intervertebral joint can include changes in synovial production; changes in the elasticity of the capsular connective tissue; and hypertonicity of the segmental musculature. It, therefore, seems possible that a persistent increase in the activity of the sympathetic part of the autonomic nervous system, when combined with inactivity or immobilization, could lead to restriction of movement or fixation in a joint. This hypothesis could also offer an explanation of *Schutzblockierung*, or protective fixation, which arises in arteriosclerosis or other threatening conditions.

In conclusion, we can say that the cause of intervertebral joint fixation has not yet been established scientifically. However, fixations can be identified clinically and treated successfully.

Onset of Intervertebral Joint Fixation

Many factors can lead to fixation of an intervertebral joint. They include the following:

- Temporary overload, quantitative or qualitative (mild fixation)
- An uncontrolled movement
- Pathologic overload, quantitative and qualitative, both static and dynamic
- Faulty control and loading of the musculature

Efficient neural control supports proper functioning of the vertebral column by maintaining an appropriate motor pattern and also by ensuring appropriate compensation if function is disturbed. Inefficient neural control can prolong the disorder by maintaining the pathologic control patterns that have developed.

Other factors leading to intervertebral fixation include the following:

- Trauma of external origin and short duration, which is violent and damaging to the structure of the vertebral column, thus affecting function. The functional disturbance can develop following a single trauma or it can be caused by an accumulation of microtrauma.
- Reflexive processes within the segment resulting from a disorder in another part of the vertebral column (see the section titled "Movement Regions and Transitional Areas" later in this chapter)
- Reflexive processes within the segment resulting from damage outside the vertebral column, such as lesions in the segmentally innervated musculature
- Reflexive processes within the segment resulting from problems outside the movement apparatus, for example, organ disorders

Clinical Presentation of Intervertebral Joint Fixation

The symptoms are as follows:

- Restriction of movement in the segment
- Irritation in the segment

If active and passive movement is restricted in one or more directions, joint play is reduced or lost. The range of physiologic movement is usually examined in three dimensions by way of segmental motion palpation that pays particular attention to the quality of the endfeel.

Segmental irritation occurs regularly as a sign of intervertebral joint fixation. There are both proprioceptors and nociceptors in the joint capsule, ligaments, and tendons of the muscles that belong to the joint. The proprioceptors serve both the static and the dynamic functions of the muscles. The role of the nociceptors, which are also present in internal organs, is to signal damage.

The central nervous system uses information from the proprioceptors and nociceptors to stimulate and maintain the reactions needed to protect against structural and/or functional lesions, or to deal with them if they occur. The nociceptive afferent enters the dorsal horn complex via the spinal ganglion and connects with the ventral motor horn, the sympathetic chain, and the central nervous system via the spinothalamic tract and the spinoreticular tract. The nociceptive-motor efferent connects with the muscular fibers of the striated muscles through alpha and beta motoneurons, and with the fusimotor fibers of the muscle spindles through gamma motoneurons. The nociceptive-vegetative efferents connect with the organs, smooth muscle tissue, glands, and blood vessels. An increase in nociceptive input raises the activity in the sympathetic part of the autonomic nervous system, which can have the following consequences for the movement apparatus:

In the skin:

- Changes in the elasticity of the connective tissue
- Increased sensitivity (decreased threshold to depolarization) of the nociceptors
- Increased tone in the erector pili muscles
- Increased secretion of sweat

In the muscle:

- Hypertonicity
- Changes in the elasticity of the muscle connective tissue
- Less effective circulation in the muscle
- Increased sensitivity in the sensors, including the nociceptors
- Tendomyoses and myofascial *trigger points*

In the intervertebral joint:

- Changes in synovial production
- Changes in the elasticity of the capsular connective tissue

- Increased sensitivity of the nociceptors
- Tendomyoses in the periarticular musculature

Consequences of Intervertebral Joint Fixation

Consequences of intervertebral joint fixation include the reflexive reactions described earlier as part of the clinical picture. Neighboring segments can also be drawn into the fixation, causing the symptom pattern to spread.

If there is insufficient selectivity in the nervous system, the disorder can spread to vegetatively related levels in the segment. Lumbar and cervical disturbances can spread in this way to the thoracic region. A well-known example of segmental spread is the *quadrant syndrome*, which involves spread via the stellate ganglion. Although we have good knowledge of intersegmental relationships, it is not always easy to diagnose the primary cause when the pattern of symptoms spreads to other segments.

From a biomechanical point of view, if one link in the chain does not work well, it will affect the functioning of the whole. If one segment is fixated, then no matter how well the compensatory mechanisms work, the fixation will influence the static, kinetic, protective, and balancing functions of the whole of the vertebral column (see the sections titled "Functional Characteristics of the Vertebral Column" and "Movement Regions and Transitional Areas" later in this chapter).

Local hypomobility is often accompanied by hypermobility in a neighboring segment. Osteophyte formation may occur as a stabilizing reaction to the hypermobility. As a result, this segment also becomes more vulnerable to fixation. As well as prompting osteophyte formation, the compensatory hypermobility can also cause degeneration of the disk, which in turn often results in instability.

HYPOMOBILITY

The following conditions should be distinguished:

- Local pathologic hypomobility
- General pathologic hypomobility
- Constitutional hypomobility

Local Pathologic Hypomobility

Local pathologic hypomobility can occur in one or more segments of the vertebral column. The condition was described earlier in relation to the concept of intervertebral joint fixation. Special attention should be paid in this context to the segments in the transitional areas of the spine.

When examining the patient, one should keep in mind the various biomechanical possibilities. If there are no anomalies, the criterion should be the quality of the endfeel perceived during segmental motion palpation.

General Pathologic Hypomobility

General pathologic hypomobility occurs in various systemic disorders, such as Scheuermann's disease (kyphosis), Bechterew's disease (ankylosing spondylitis), and general osteoarthritic processes.

Constitutional Hypomobility

Constitutional hypomobility is characterized by the fact that all joints are usually affected, although there are no indications of a pathologic process. The range of all movements is reduced in comparison with mobility norms.

Although a decrease in mobility is a physiologic fact of aging, the presence of constitutional hypomobility in young people is difficult to explain. Diagnosing constitutional hypomobility is important both for accurate etiologic analysis of a movement disorder and to determine the most appropriate therapy.

HYPERMOBILITY

The following conditions should be distinguished:

- Local pathologic hypermobility
- General pathologic hypermobility
- Constitutional hypermobility

Local Pathologic Hypermobility

Local pathologic hypermobility can occur in one or more segments of the vertebral column. It results from the presence of excessive laxity in the capsuloligamentous mechanism resulting from overstretching or hormonal influences. The most common location is above or below a hypomobile segment in the vertebral column and in the sacroiliac joint.

Although pathologic hypomobility can exist in an absolute sense, hypermobility is only a relative concept. It means that the segment can move more, in the absence of dysfunction, than neighboring segments that are also not dysfunctional. The additional movement is therefore not pathologic, but should be regarded as extra local mobility. A hypermobile segment can indicate either a pathologic hypo-

mobile disorder or a hypermobile one. To assess functional hypermobility, one needs to understand the morphology. In the literature, one can find ranges of segmental movement measured in degrees (Penning, 1978; Putz, 1981). However, these differ between individuals and across age groups, and differences are difficult to detect clinically because they are so small.

Long-standing pathologic hypermobility may be caused by a spontaneous trauma (whiplash injury), or by movements repeated over time that approach or exceed physiologic limits, or by hormonal influences. This kind of hypermobility is usually associated not only with a high level of segmental mobility, but also with pathologic symptoms and phenomena. In the presence of increased segmental mobility, data from the history taking and the signs and symptoms occurring during terminal movements are important in identifying pathologic hypermobility. Although terms such as *pathologic hypermobility* and *instability* are often confused in clinical practice, an identifying difference is the course and rhythm of movements, which might not be disturbed in local pathologic hypermobility. If the course or rhythm of the movements is disturbed, then it is probably caused by instability.

General Pathologic Hypermobility

General pathologic hypermobility occurs mainly where there is a disturbance of the afferent information, such as in tabes dorsalis (syphilis) and in some polyneuropathies. It also occurs with some central disturbances of regulation of tone, oligophrenia syndrome, and some extrapyramidal disturbances such as athetosis.

Constitutional Hypermobility

Constitutional hypermobility is characterized by the fact that all joints are usually affected, in the absence of a pathologic process. It does not have to be strictly symmetric or present to the same degree in all parts of the body. Its cause is unknown, but it is probably associated with insufficiency of the mesenchymal tissues (Janda, 1979). It is found more frequently in women than in men. Identification of this form of hypermobility is of great importance for assessment and therapy. The constitutionally hypermobile type has, by nature, a lower static load-bearing capacity and is sensitive to dynamic overloading.

MOBILITY RATING SCALE

In a functional examination, the quality of movement is the critical concern. However, the following mobility rating scale

(Stoddard, 1961; Maigne, 1968), which is widely used in manual therapy, is included here for the sake of completeness:

0	Total loss of movement (block vertebra or immobile segment)
1	Major restriction of movement
2	Minor restriction of movement
3	Normal excursion
4	Increased movement excursion (hypermobility)
5	Increased movement excursion with pain (pathologic hypermobility)

STABILITY

Stability or *stable position* can be defined as a position in which there is a clear relationship between the position and the forces needed to maintain it. The end positions of movements of all kinds are stable end positions.

INSTABILITY

As part of the scientific discipline of mechanics, the concept of *instability* can be clearly defined. When it comes to physiologic movement, one can only try to describe what is meant by the vernacular use of this term. In general, it is used to denote a disturbance in the relationship between the load applied and the resulting displacement (movement), such that a small force has a large consequence. A characteristic feature is disruption of the rhythm of the movement: it may consist of a large movement component followed by a small one, or vice versa (**Figure 4–4**).

A distinction can be made between

- Active instability
- Passive instability

Active Instability

Active instability of the spinal column is a consequence of sensorimotor dysfunction. The forces applied to a motion segment are not processed in a coordinated fashion. Coordinative dysfunction, or failure of the musculature to work efficiently, can be an indirect result of the shape, position, and condition of the disk; the condition of the capsule and the ligaments; and general physical condition.

One factor that may be involved is the shape of the articular surfaces. With regard to position, a high assimilation pelvis in relation to L5 is more likely to cause instability than a pelvis more adapted to load bearing. The condition of the disk is the crucial factor that determines whether or not the pressures exerted are evenly distributed. The condition of the capsule and the ligaments, together with the afferent input system, is extremely important for efficient muscular function. The importance of general physical condition in the sense of overall psychosomatic state should also not be underestimated. If the patient is fatigued, the sensorimotor system is likely to work less efficiently.

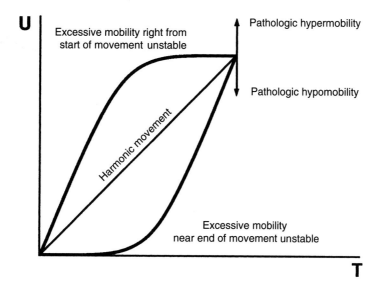

Figure 4–4 Movement diagram illustrating normomobility and instability.

The most important cause of reduced active stability is a disturbance of the arthrokinetic reflex mechanism, that is, the muscular response to changes in joint position and movement. The joint capsule type I, II, and III mechanoreceptors play an important part in coordinating the musculature that belongs functionally to the joint. Together with proprioceptive information from the muscle spindles, tendons, and vestibular organs, and exteroceptive information from the skin, eyes and ears, they determine perception of position and movement (statesthesia and kinesthesia).

Movement is coordinated via a widespread system of feedback loops, involving processing at the spinal level (segmental and multisegmental) and at supraspinal levels. If the sensory feedback to the central nervous system is inadequate or inefficient, this can result in an inadequate muscular response, leading to impaired static and dynamic stability.

Active stability must be assessed during active examination. If there are any indications of active instability, the joint should also be examined for passive instability.

Active instability can be caused by the following factors:

- Disturbance in the central nervous system or a peripheral nerve
- Muscular disease
- Arthritis, arthrosis
- Trauma
- Long periods of inactivity
- Residual postoperative and posttraumatic symptoms

Active instability can lead to

- Disturbance of joint function
- Damage to the joint and the tissues that belong to it
- Change in normal movement patterns, which can lead to overloading of the tissues throughout the whole kinetic chain
- Development or increase of muscular imbalance throughout the whole kinetic chain

Passive Instability

Passive instability of the spinal column is found in the positions in which the inherent osseous stability on one hand and the tension on the capsule and ligaments on the other are not adjusted to a balanced state. In other words, passive instability exists when the harmony of the physiologic movement sequence, which depends on the structural arrangement of bones, disks, capsules, and ligaments, is disturbed, causing the addition of undesirable and uneco-

nomical movement components. Where the structure of the bones, capsules, and ligaments is normal, a passive movement will be harmonious. If passive instability is not actively compensated by the co-coordinating musculature, the situation is known as *uncompensated* instability.

Passive instability in a segment of the vertebral column is usually caused by a disturbance of the balance between the turgor of the nucleus pulposus and the tensile stress on the annular fibers and surrounding ligaments. When instability is present, a reactive process often leads to the formation of osteophytes, which causes passive stability to again increase.

If it seems likely that there is passive instability in a segment, that segment should be examined passively rather than by means of active-assisted movements. For the sake of clarity, it should be said that active instability and passive instability can occur separately or concurrently. Passive instability can be compensated for by the activity of efficient co-coordinating musculature. Under these circumstances, the active stability masks the passive instability, which is then known as *compensated* instability.

Passive instability might be suspected on the basis of data from the history, observation of active movements, and active-assisted regional examination. The segment should then be examined passively to confirm or rule out a suspected passive instability. The section on clinical physical examination (specifically Chapters 13, 14, and 17) contains a more detailed description of instability by region.

LAXITY

Laxity is a term used to signify a greater or lesser degree of slackness in the capsuloligamentous system.

BIOMECHANICAL LESION

A biomechanical lesion is characterized by the following symptoms:

- Pain
- Muscular spasm
- Decreased function

PAIN

Patients with disorders and diseases of the musculoskeletal systems frequently report pain. It is a symptom associated with dysfunction. The degree of pain reported is not directly related to the extent of the tissue damage or threat of tissue damage (Bernards, 1991). Rather, there are three other factors to which it is related:

- The innervation density of the affected tissue
- The degree of sensitivity of the nociceptors in the affected tissue
- The level of selectivity in the central nervous system especially with regard to the processing of the nociceptive input

PRIMARY HYPERALGESIA

The central nervous system receives information about actual, or the threat of, tissue damage from the nociceptors. These can be divided into two groups, namely, unimodal and polymodal. The unimodal nociceptors are the endings of thin, myelinated afferent nerve fibers. Their stimulus threshold is high. They are excited only if there is (the threat of) damage to tissues.

When tissue is damaged, the unimodal nociceptors are sensitized by mediating substances released by the tissues as a result of the damage. One such substance is prostaglandin E2. This sensitizing of the free nerve endings consists of a marked lowering of the stimulation threshold of unimodal nociceptors. This is called *primary hyperalgesia*. The function of this mechanism is to protect the damaged tissues. Because of the pain, the individual avoids using the damaged tissues during activities; this allows catabolic metabolism to be increased in the affected region. The polymodal nociceptors form the endings of unmyelinated afferent nerve fibers. They are sensitive to mechanical, chemical, and thermal stimuli. Their stimulus threshold is very high: they are excited only by tissue damage and serious disturbances in homeostasis (Bernards, 1991).

The unimodal nociceptors adapt quickly. The polymodal nociceptors, however, have a regulatory role in addition to their function as a signaling mechanism: when tissues are damaged, they start a local (neurogenic) inflammatory reaction by releasing tissue mediators called tachykinins. The best-known tachykinin is Substance P, which is produced in the spinal ganglion and stored in the nerve endings of the polymodal nociceptors. If there is a disturbance in homeostasis, Substance P functions as a neurotransmitter at the central endings (in the spinal marrow) to pass nociceptive information from the primary to the secondary neurons. Peripherally, when the nerve endings are stimulated, Substance P is released in the interstitium, causing local vasodilatation. If this does not lead to full restoration of homeostasis, the cells affected by the tissue damage produce Prostaglandin E2,

which lowers the threshold of both unimodal and polymodal nociceptors.

Nociceptors are also stimulated elsewhere in the receptive field because of the lowering of their threshold. This excitation of unimodal and polymodal nociceptors leads in turn to the release of Substance P in areas that are not primarily affected by the actual or threatened tissue damage.

SECONDARY HYPERALGESIA

Secondary hyperalgesia is an increased sensitivity to pain in tissues and organs innervated by the same segment of the spinal cord as the damaged tissue. It is a consequence of spatial and temporal facilitation of secondary neurons in the dorsal horn of the spinal segment. Excitation takes place as a result of the lowering of the threshold of secondary neurons. The location of increased sensitivity to pain in tissues belonging to the same segment is determined by the somatotopical arrangement of the secondary neurons in the dorsal horn of the spinal marrow.

REFERRED PAIN

Referred pain is pain that is perceived not in the location of the actual or threatened tissue damage, but is nevertheless caused by it. It is a consequence of the fact that numerous primary nociceptive neurons from different tissues or organs converge on a shared small group of secondary afferent neurons. The level of referred pain that is experienced is determined by the innervation density of the affected tissues and organs and the somatotopical arrangement of the secondary neurons in the dorsal horn.

DISORDERS IN THE RELATIONSHIP BETWEEN LOAD AND LOAD-BEARING CAPACITY

The body adapts continuously to the load placed on it, or on a part of it. This adaptation takes place through cell substitution. Every cell, tissue, and organ adapts in a particular way and at a particular speed. The extent to which adaptation takes place is partly dependent on the size and type of the load.

The level of fitness of the person, or of the tissue or organ, also helps to determine the speed with which a program of adaptation can be completed. Under favorable conditions, load-bearing capacity increases with regular loading. This applies both to physical and to psychological capacity. If strength has increased, this implies that a controlled and adequate program of adaptation has taken place.

When the load changes at cell, tissue, and/or organ level, metabolism must adapt to maintain homeostasis. It must make optimal adjustments to changing circumstances to keep the vegetative climate constant. If there is insufficient balance between catabolic metabolism and anabolic metabolism, load-bearing capacity decreases. The preservation of homeostasis is thus a fundamental prerequisite for maintaining the relation between load on the one hand, and on the other, the changes in shape that take place in tissues and organs in response to the load. The turnover rate in tissues depends on good circulation and nutrition.

When the load or stress changes, adaptation is needed at the level of the whole person if integrity is to be preserved. Factors that disturb the relationship between stress and adaptation to it are as follows:

- (Persistent) exceeding of capacity through overloading at the cell, tissue, organ, or individual level
- Prolonged reduction of the load at all these levels

Specific factors include the following:

- Psychogenic stress
- Social pressure
- Inadequate circulation in the tissues
- Nutritional deficiencies
- Anabolic metabolism taking (persistent) precedence over catabolic metabolism

The consequences of a faulty relationship between stress and adaptive mechanisms have a particular significance in manual therapy. In describing the consequences of disorders in support and movement systems, manual therapy uses the system introduced in the International Classification of Impairments, Disabilities and Handicaps (ICIDH), where the consequences of illnesses and other afflictions are classified as impairments, disabilities, or handicaps.

SEGMENTAL DYSFUNCTIONS

Nociceptive input arising from actual or the threat of tissue damage is processed initially at the segmental spinal level. The activity of the spinal interneurons in the dorsal horn determines whether the receiving secondary neurons will be excited and the nociceptive input passed on. If there is continuing nociceptive activity combined with an alarm situation in the central nervous system (so-called aspecific arousal), electrical activity in the lateral spinal horn will increase, specifically in the origin segments of the sympathetic

innervation of the structure affected by the actual or threatened tissue damage. This increase in postganglionic sympathetic activity leads to a decrease in effective circulation in the tissues and organs that are segmentally related, and an increase in sensitivity of the peripheral receptors, including the nociceptors. In the ventral horn of the segment, there is also an increase in activity that leads to hypertonicity in the musculature innervated from the segment. A segmental disturbance is suspected when, as a result of persistent increased sympathetic activity in the affected segment, changes specific to organs or connective tissue are found in the form of currently present clinical manifestations, or as earlier trophic disturbances within the segment.

RELEASE PHENOMENON

Cyriax (1947) described the *release phenomenon* in the spinal nerve compression syndromes. If there is light mechanical compression of the spinal nerve, the patient will report a mild prickly sensation, followed by a numb feeling. If the mechanical pressure on the nerve tissue increases, the changes in sensation disappear. If the pressure decreases, the numb feeling and the paraesthesia return. Cyriax calls this reappearance of the paraesthesia and the numb feeling when pressure is reduced on the peripheral nerve tissue the release phenomenon. It is said also to occur as a result of compression of the medial fascicle of the plexus brachialis (Cyriax, 1947).

There are doubts as to whether mechanical pressure on peripheral nerve tissue alone is responsible for the appearance of paraesthesia and anesthesia in the area innervated by the affected nerve tissue (Sunderland, 1978; Rydevik et al., 1991; Olmarker et al., 1990a; Olmarker et al., 1990b) (**Figure 4–5**). It is probable that the main factor causing these symptoms is not the mechanical pressure on the nerve tissue, but the ischemia in the nerve tissue resulting from changes in pressure in the arteriae and venae nervorum.

Sunderland (1978) gives a detailed description of the pathogenesis of partial conductive disturbances in peripheral nerve tissue. Under normal physiologic circumstances, the pressure gradient in the arteriae and venae nervorum is as follows: Part $> P_{cap} > P_{end} > P_{ven} > P_{ext}$, where P_{art} stands for arterial pressure, P_{cap} for capillary pressure, P_{end} for endoneural pressure, P_{ven} for venous pressure, and P_{ext} for the pressure outside the blood vessels.

If there is an aphysiologic increase in the pressure on the peripheral nerve tissue, the external pressure on the system of blood vessels increases. If the external pressure increases above the level of the venous pressure, this decreases the blood flow. The pressure relationships then reverse to $P_{ext} >$

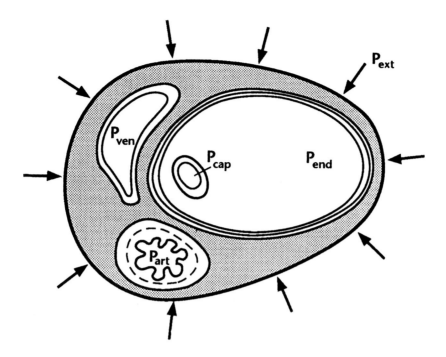

Figure 4–5

$P_{ven} > P_{end} > P_{cap} > P_{art}$. The decrease in flow in the veins will then lead to ischemia in the peripheral nerve tissue.

Olmarker and associates (1990) describe the appearance of spontaneous action potentials in the axons of the cauda equina. Experimentally induced pressure on the cauda equina of pigs led to a significant decrease in intraneural blood circulation, resulting in intraneural edema, ischemia, and conductive disturbances. The paraesthesiae are probably caused by the occurrence of spontaneous action potentials. Because of the partial ischemia, the resting difference in membrane potential in the axons of the thick nerve fibers cannot be maintained. The difference in membrane potential decreases and approaches the limit of –55 mV. When the threshold value is reached, there is a spontaneous depolarization, which the patient experiences as a prickling and tingling in the distal innervation area of the affected peripheral nerve.

A spontaneous depolarization of the thinner nerve fibers can lead to painful paraesthesiae. A numb feeling occurs when there is a block in conduction caused by ischemia or mechanical compression (Lundborg, 1975). If there is a conduction block, the paraesthesiae disappear because the intraneural ion flow of ions is impeded. When the pressure decreases, the flow of ions begins, and the potential falls from 0 to –55 mV. As a result, the paraesthesiae reappear.

PAINFUL ARC

The painful arc is the phase in the movement trajectory during which pain is experienced.

RELATIONSHIP BETWEEN DYSFUNCTION AND MORPHOLOGIC DEGENERATIVE CHANGE

Functional disturbances often seem to precede morphologic changes. This means that the clinical symptoms of the functional disturbances appear before degenerative morphologic changes have taken place.

Degenerative abnormalities such as osteophytosis, spondylosis, spondylarthrosis, and uncovertebral arthrosis develop gradually. Reishauer (1957) concludes that degenerative changes are sequelae of a previous pathologic process. It rarely happens that osteophytes or uncovertebral arthroses narrow the intervertebral foramen to such an extent as to produce clinical symptoms.

The nociceptive stimulation caused by tension or pressure is a warning sign that from a biological point of view needs to be given at the right time. This right time is when the functional disturbance appears, not when degenerative changes have already taken place. From the diagnostic point of view, it is important to know that the nociceptive stimulus can prompt reflexogenic reactions without necessarily exceeding the pain threshold.

In summary, we can say that functional disturbance produces nociceptive activity that leads to reflexogenic change. This may then be followed by degenerative change.

MOVEMENT REGIONS AND TRANSITIONAL AREAS

Every movement region has its own characteristics and features. If we group the segments into regions, we see differences in the relationships between disk and vertebral body; angle of inclination and angle of opening; length and position of the articular, transverse, and spinous processes; and length of the ligaments and muscles.

The following regions can be distinguished, as shown in **Figure 4–6**:

Upper cervical joints: C0–C3
Cervical: C3–T1 (2)
Thoracic: T1(2)–T(11)12
Lumbar: T(11)12–S1

This classification is subject to individual variation depending on the structure of the vertebrae in the transitional areas. Only a general label is given to the transitional areas, namely, craniocervical, cervicothoracic, thoracic-lumbar, and lumbosacroiliac.

In the literature, the segments C3–C4, T4–T5, T7–T8, and L3 are described as transitional areas. C3–C4 is so described because of its connection with the important levator scapulae muscle, which originates from the transverse processes of the uppermost cervical vertebrae. T4–T5 is considered a transitional area because, from a kinematic point of view, the cervical spinal column ends there. T7–T8 is the rotational center during walking. L3 is the relay station between the caudal and cranial parts of the lumbar vertebral column.

The articulatory control mechanisms of the transitional areas seem to exert an important reflexogenic influence within the whole musculoskeletal system. The mechanoreceptive influence described by Wyke (1966) seems to be particularly important in achieving the best possible functioning of the spinal column both during movement and when stationary. Although the capsules of all the intervertebral joints play a part in this, research has indicated that the transitional areas exert a special influence on the working of the whole, both qualitatively and quantitatively.

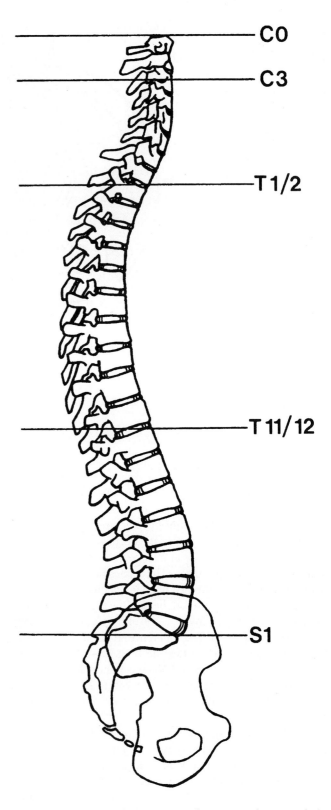

Figure 4–6 Movement regions and transitional areas of the spine.

Magnus (1924) and de Kleyn (1927), who demonstrated the existence of tonic neck reflexes, supposed that the afferent organs responsible for them were situated in the upper cervical muscles. However, McCouch, Deering, and Ling (1951) showed later that afferent stimuli from the joint capsules of the upper cervical intervertebral joints were responsible.

Cramer (1958) and Gutmann and Vélé (1970) used electromyography to measure the influence of the upper cervical intervertebral joints on the tone of the muscles responsible for posture. In experiments with rabbits, Komandatow (1945) showed the reflexogenic effect at a distance by demonstrating the existence of the coccyx–eye and coccyx–neck reflexes. Clinical findings also suggest that the other transitional areas exercise an influence on the whole.

MOVEMENT DIRECTIONS

The following are different systems for naming the three possible directions in which movements can take place, as shown in **Figure 4–7**:

1.
  - Rotation about a frontal plane axis (front to back) (A)
  - Rotation about a sagittal plane axis (left to right) (B)
  - Rotation about a vertical axis (anticlockwise-clockwise) (C)

2.
  - *Flexion*. Movement about a frontal plane axis, with increase in the existing degree of curvature (A)
  - *Extension*. Movement about a frontal plane axis, with decrease in the existing degree of curvature (A)
  - *Lateroflexion (sidebending)*. Movement about a sagittal plane axis, left-right (B)
  - *Concave rotation*. Movement about a vertical axis in the direction of the concavity (ipsilateral rotation) (C)
  - *Convex rotation*. Movement about a vertical axis in the direction of the convexity (contralateral rotation) (C)

3.
  - *Sagittal flexion* (A). Ventral: movement about a frontal plane axis in a ventral direction; dorsal: movement about a frontal plane axis in a dorsal direction
  - *Sidebending*. Movement about a sagittal plane axis, left-right (B)
  - *Left front–right back rotation*. Clockwise rotation about a vertical axis (C)
  - *Right front–left back rotation*. Counterclockwise rotation about a vertical axis (C)

4.
  - *Flexion*. Movement about a frontal plane axis in which the articular surfaces are pushed away from each other (A)
  - *Extension*. Movement about a frontal plane axis in which the articular surfaces are pushed toward each other (A)
  - *Left sidebending*. Movement about a sagittal plane axis in which the left joint surfaces are pushed toward each other and the right articular surfaces away from each other (B)

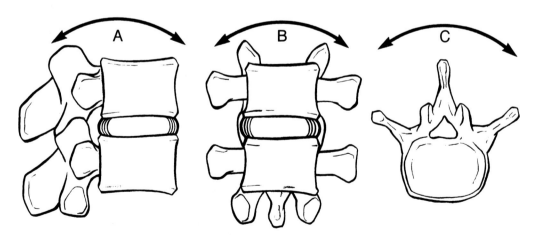

Figure 4–7   Movement directions.

- *Right sidebending.* Movement about a sagittal plane axis in which the right articular surfaces are pushed toward each other and the left articular surfaces away from each other (B)
- *Left rotation.* Movement about the vertical axis in which the left inferior articular process of the vertebra above moves backward and the right inferior articular process of the vertebra above moves forward (C)
- *Right rotation.* Movement about the vertical axis, where the right inferior articular process of the vertebra above moves backward and the left inferior articular process of the vertebra above moves forward (C)

In the preceding descriptions of the rotational movements, *above* means cranial and *below* means caudal.

Note: The terminology provided in section 4 is used throughout this book.

THREE-DIMENSIONAL SPINAL MOVEMENT

It is taken as an established fact in the kinesiology of the human spinal column that asymmetrical movements (sidebending, rotation) do not occur as separate forms of movement. Sidebending is always accompanied by a rotational component. Rotation is always accompanied by sidebending. When working with these concepts, therefore, we need to answer the following questions:

- What is the direction of the accompanying rotation or sidebending?
- Is the accompanying rotation or sidebending in the same direction throughout the vertebral column, or does it differ according to region?
- Does the direction of the accompanying movement differ according to whether the movement is an active or a passive one?
- Is the position of the vertebral column in the symmetrical plane (flexion or extension) important for the direction of accompanying rotation or sidebending?
- Does the direction of the accompanying movement differ in the loaded positions (sitting, standing) as against the unloaded position (lying) of the vertebral column?

We may start by looking at the literature to see whether it gives us the answers to these questions, and whether the published opinions are based on sound scientific research.

The basic view of asymmetrical movement of the vertebral column is that taken by osteopaths, and described by Stoddard (1961), Lewit (1977), and Grieve (1981). Their interpretation, which is based in part on the original studies by Lovett (1916) and Freyette (1954), is as follows.

In the neutral position (symmetrical posture) and in the extension position of the lumbar and thoracic vertebral column, the vertebral bodies rotate during sidebending in the direction of the convexity of the vertebral column (contralateral rotation). In a predominantly flexion position of the lumbar and thoracic vertebral column, the vertebral bodies rotate during sidebending in the direction of the concavity of the vertebral column (ipsilateral rotation).

It may be noted that the upper part of the thoracic vertebral column (consisting of T1 to T4)—which is called the cervicothoracic transitional area—functions like the cervical spinal column. In the cervical region, in both ventral and extension, the sidebending and the rotation are in the same direction (ipsilateral rotation). These movement combinations are described as "three-dimensional physiological movements." Van der Bijl Sr. (1969) carried out studies of three-dimensional movement in the vertebral column, on the basis of which he formulated laws of movement. These laws incorporate a distinction between physiologic movement and physiologic fixation. They are in conflict with the osteopathic view, except for the laws that apply to the cervical vertebral column, where he is in agreement about the direction of the accompanying rotation during sidebending from an extension position.

In general, we can say that apart from this exception, the movement combinations that the osteopaths call physiologic movements are called physiologic fixations by Van der Bijl Sr. The movement combinations that the osteopaths use to arrive at their three-dimensional locking (fixation) are classed as physiologic movement by Van der Bijl Sr.

In an attempt to identify at a scientifically validated position, Seroo and Hulsbosch (1982) carried out a literature search. They compared the work of Lovett (1916) and Freyette (1954) with that of a number of more recent authors, such as Lijssel (1969), Schultz and Galante (1970), and White (1971). The conclusions of their comparative study are described in the next section.

Literature Review With Regard to the Coupling Between Sidebending and Rotation of the Human Spine

Few authors have described the three-dimensional movement pattern of the whole vertebral column. The best-known publications on the subject are those of Lovett and of Freyette.

When we compare the works of these two authors, the first thing we notice is the difference in definitions. Lovett calls a forward-bending movement flexion and a backward bend extension. Freyette on the other hand defines flexion according to the literal meaning of the word, as an increase in initial curvature, and extension as a decrease in initial curvature. Given the three basic curves in the spinal column in the sagittal plane, namely, the cervical lordosis, thoracic kyphosis, and lumbar lordosis, a forward bend, according to Freyette, consists in extension of the cervical vertebral column, flexion of the thoracic vertebral column, and extension of the lumbar vertebral column.

To describe three-dimensional patterns of movement vectors are used. Following the "corkscrew rule," the direction of the vector is linked to the direction of rotation. When the corkscrew is turned, the vector direction is the same as the direction in which the corkscrew is moving. During rotation to the right, it moves into the cork. In a sideways bend to the left, therefore, there will be a rotation vector in a dorsal direction (**Figure 4–8**).

This provides a simple way of indicating the position of all the vertebrae in relation to each other. A local system of axes is defined for each vertebra, consisting of an X axis, a Y axis, and a Z axis. The axes are perpendicular to each other (**Figure 4–9**). The Z axis is vertical and has a positive direction, toward the cranial end of the spinal column; the X axis is at a right angle to it and has a positive ventral direction;

the Y axis is at right angles to both and has a positive lateral direction to the left. All movements of the vertebral column can be described within this system of axes. Rotation about the X axis is a sidebending; in the positive X direction, it is sidebending to the right; in the negative X direction, it is a sidebending to the left. Rotation about the Y axis is ventral/extension; in the positive Y direction, it is flexion; in the negative Y direction, it is extension. Rotation round the Z axis is rotation; in the positive Z direction, it is rotation to the left; in the negative Z direction, it is rotation to the right.

Where possible, when vectors are given, the sequence of the movements is indicated. The basic curvature can also be specified because the system starts from a straight spine (**Figure 4–10**). When the experimental participant or the patient bends forward, or has a basic forward curvature, this is indicated by vector 1. He or she then performs a lateroflexion to the right, indicated by vector 2. This results in an axial rotation, indicated by vector 3. The whole movement is a rotation to the right.

Table 4–5 shows that the two authors differ only with regard to the lumbar part of the vertebral column. The difference is in the representation of axial rotation combined with extension in the lumbar region.

Following are shown additional comparisons of the work of a number of other authors. The latter only make incidental mention of a three-dimensional movement pattern. Where

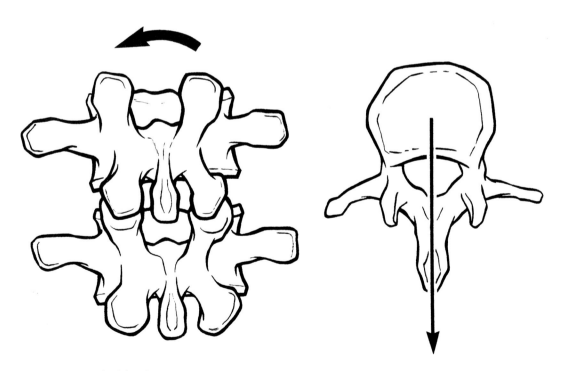

Figure 4–8   Vector rotation of sidebending.

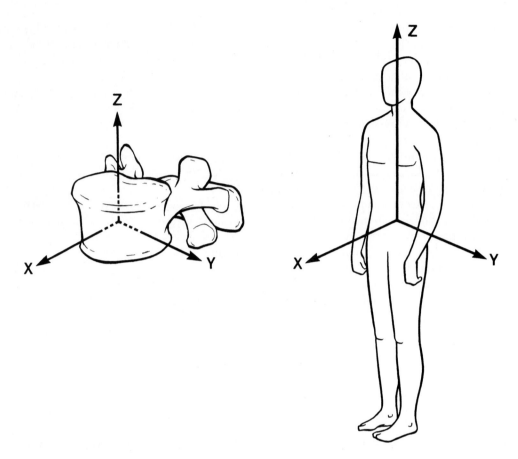

Figure 4–9   Schematic representation of orthogonal axes.

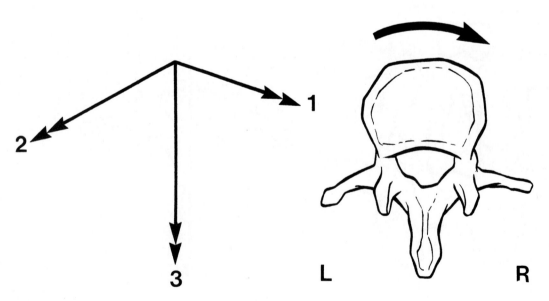

Figure 4–10   Movement sequence by means of vector rotation.

Table 4–5   Comparing the Systems of Lovett and Freyette

Region / Position (Researchers)	Position	Lovett	Freyette
Cervical	Flexion	x ↗ ↓z ↘ y	x ↗ ↓z ↘ y
Cervical	Extension	y↘ x↙ ↘z	y↘ x↙ ↘z
Thoracic	Flexion	z↑ x↙ ↘y	z↑ x↙ ↘y
Thoracic	Extension	Barely noticable rotation	y↘ x↙ ↘z
Lumbar	Flexion	x↙ ↓z ↘y	x↖ ↓z ↘y
Lumbar	Extension	y↘ x↙ ↘z	y↘ z↑ ↙x

researchers have worked with X-rays, a three-dimensional study is extremely complicated, if not impossible, because in X-rays the spinal column is projected onto a two-dimensional plane.

Table 4–6 offers an overview of data including the more recent researchers. It, too, is limited to the combination of sidebending with axial rotation; the authors included do not discuss ventral or extension. In general, the differences between authors are small and can probably be explained by the use of different research methods.

Overall, there are two main research methods, namely, the use of cadavers, and the use of X-rays of living persons. Given that movements are the result of forces, it makes a great deal of difference whether a spinal column is brought into a particular final position by the application of one force, as in the case of cadavers, or by an extremely complicated interplay among the muscles and connective tissues that affect the spinal column directly or indirectly, as in X-ray studies. The difference is that between a passive and an active pattern. Patterns of movement can be discussed meaningfully only when the type of force applied is taken into account.

With regard to the discrepancies between the laws of movement developed by Van der Bijl Sr. and those used by osteopaths, we might conclude, cautiously, that Van der Bijl Sr. developed his laws in the context of active movement. The osteopaths, on the other hand—among whom Freyette made the most detailed analysis of the subject—arrived at their laws by studying passive movements in a loaded condition (sitting position).

Summary

The literature search carried out by Seroo and Hulsbosch (1982) indicates that in the context of active movement in three dimensions, no firm conclusions can be drawn about the direction of the rotation component during sidebending. This is because there are many unknown factors, especially those connected with the influence of the muscles. With regard to passive movements, it seems likely that the passive biomechanical behavior of the spine as described previously can be aligned with the work of Freyette, who carried out his research on cadavers and who

Table 4–6   Comparing Approaches to the Combination of Sidebending and Rotation

Region \ Researchers	Lovett	Freyette	Lyssel	White	Schultz/Galante
Cervical	↗↘	↗↘	↗↘	↗↘	↗↘
Thoracic	↙↑	↙↑	—	↗↘ (upper thoracic) / ↙↖ | ↙↑ (mid and lower thoracic)	↗↘ (upper) / ↙↑ (mid and lower thoracic)
Lumbar	↗↘	↙↑	—	—	↗↘

applied transverse forces to the spine in the loaded condition. It must be emphasized that passive movements performed on living organisms differ greatly from those carried out on cadavers. In the living organism, the musculature always maintains a basic tone, which is present even during so-called passive movements.

Freyette's research is the most extensive. Although the research methods of the modern authors have greater validity, their work is not comprehensive because they concerned themselves only with the spinal column moving from the neutral position. Lovett and Freyette are the only researchers to present data on the vertebral column in various positions in the sagittal plane (flexion, neutral position, extension, and extreme extension). We may conclude that Freyette's research is the most reliable. However, it is based on passive movement in the loaded condition, so it offers no information about active movement and movement in the unloaded condition. Freyette's model can be used only as a biomechanical research model for passive movement examination in the loaded condition.

In summary, we have to state that even Freyette's research has produced insufficient data for constructing a practical model upon which we can base the clinical examination. This means that in an evidence-based physical examination process all three-dimensional movements need to be performed in an active-assisted format.

Three-Dimensional Movement Analysis of the Human Spine According to Freyette

Freyette describes asymmetrical movements in terms of a clear sequence according to position in the sagittal plane and region of the spinal column. From a biomechanical point of view, however, his explanation of the sequences is summary and most unsatisfactory. An attempt will be made here to give a hypothetical explanation, as far as possible, of Freyette's sequence of movements in the different spinal regions. With regard to the direction of movement, the basic biomechanical principle is assumed that all movements are caused by the application of forces, and that the direction of the movement is determined by the direction of the resulting forces and moments.

The Lumbar Spine

Studies of the kinesiology of the lumbar spine (T10 to L5 inclusive) show that in flexion and extreme extension, bony apposition occurs in the intervertebral joints. In the neutral position and in less extreme extension positions, there is no bone-to-bone contact (Putz, 1977b).

In asymmetrical movements, when there is bony apposition of the intervertebral joints, the position of those joints determines how the movement pattern will proceed. When there is no bone-to-bone contact, the subsequent movement pattern is determined by the center of rotation (located in the dorsal intervertebral disk).

The consequence of this for the movement sequence is that in those positions of the spinal column in the sagittal plane in which the intervertebral joints make bone-to-bone contact, sidebending can take place only if there has been a previous rotation. The direction of this rotation is governed by the orientation of the intervertebral joints. In the lumbar spine, the intervertebral joints consist of a frontally and a sagittally oriented demifacet (Putz, 1981). Sagittally, the intervertebral joints tend to converge in an anterior direction, which means that the sagittal demifacet converges less than the frontal demifacet. In the caudocranial direction, the frontally oriented demifacet has a slight ventral inclination. The sagittally orientated demifacet converges toward the caudal end.

The movement sequence from the different positions in the sagittal plane is as follows:

1. In the flexion position, rotation and sidebending occur in the same direction.

2. In sidebending in the neutral position and in incomplete extension positions, the rotation is in the opposite direction until there is bone contact in intervertebral joints. After that, sidebending can be increased only if movement takes place in the sagittal plane (flexion–extension), combined with rotation in the same direction.

3. In the complete extension position, rotation and sidebending occur in the same direction.

Further, regarding item 1 in the preceding list, in the flexion position, the contact in the intervertebral joint is of a focal nature. The inferior articular processes of the cranial vertebra make contact with the cranial edges of the articular surfaces of the superior articular processes of the caudal vertebra (**Figure 4–11**). The orientation of the articular surfaces of the superior articular processes of the caudal vertebra plays the dominant role. The situation is depicted from above in **Figure 4–12**.

When a right sidebending is initiated, the right inferior articular process of the cranial vertebra tries to move in a lateral and caudal direction. The lateral movement, indicated by A in Figure 4–12, is hindered by the interlocking bone contact occurring between the articular processes of the two vertebrae. The vertebra above must first rotate to create the necessary room for movement. As a result of the orientation of the intervertebral joints, only a dorsal movement component is possible in the right intervertebral joint; this is marked B. In the left intervertebral joint, the move-

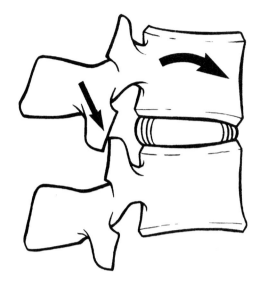

Figure 4–11   Focal bony contact in flexion.

ment needed for right sidebending does not take place in the direction of the bony contact, so the bones present no resistance. The situation is the same in a right rotation combined with right sidebending. The spatial movement of the vertebrae in relation to each other during sidebending is shown in different planes in **Figure 4–13**.

Further, in regard to item 2 in the preceding list, in the neutral position and in the nonendrange extension position, there is no bone-to-bone contact in the intervertebral joints. The movement is, therefore, determined by the active forces that are applied to the vertebra from outside. These are muscle power, the force of gravity, and the forces exerted by an external load. In the resting state, the passive reaction forces in the spinal column control mechanical balance.

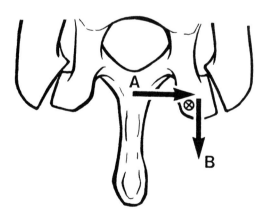

Figure 4–12   Movement components in the intervertebral joint.

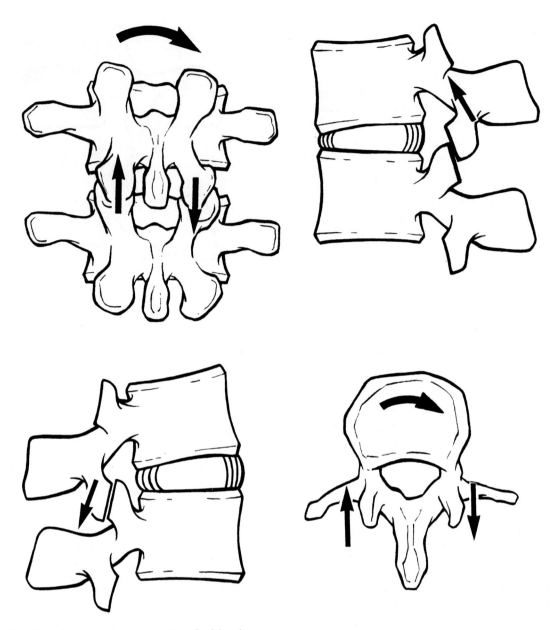

Figure 4–13   Three-dimensional representation of sidebending.

These passive forces are exerted by connective tissues, ligaments, capsule, pressures in the nucleus pulposus, and basic muscle tone. During a sidebending movement, the forces causing the movement will consist of external frontal plane forces and moments, the effects of which are increased by the movement of the center of gravity of the trunk in the direction of the sidebending.

In addition, in the spinal column and in the body, muscles become active to bring about the movement. In the motion segment, the sum of the moments of the forces reaches a point where the part of the body located cranial to it performs a pure sidebending. When indicating the vectors, for a right sidebending, the moment can be represented by a horizontal vector that is directed ventrally (**Figure 4–14**).

This vector can be broken down into two components. For the lower lumbar part of the spinal column, one component runs in the direction of the vertebral body and determines the direction of its sidebending. The second component runs in the axial direction of the vertebral body and is directed cranioventrally (**Figure 4–15A**).

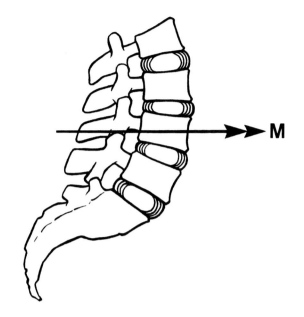

For the individual vertebra, this means a moment of rotation with a direction opposite to that of the sidebending. In the example given, this is a left rotation with a right sidebending. This breakdown of vectors applies only to the vertebrae within the lordotic curve, which have a dorsal-ventral slope in the caudal direction.

The vertebrae above the deepest point of the lordosis show a dorsal-ventral slope in the caudal direction. The breakdown of vectors here leads to a rotation in the opposite direction, that is, a right rotation in right sidebending (**Figure 4–15B**).

This account implies that when lateral forces are applied to the spinal column, in the absence of resistance caused by bone contact, the direction of rotation in the spinal column depends on whether in the sagittal plane the vertebra slopes toward the cranial or the caudal end of the spine. This principle applies to the whole of the vertebral column. The consequence is that if a sidebending can take place without bone-to-bone contact, the direction of the accompanying rotation always reverses at the top of the curve (**Figure 4–16**).

Figure 4–14   Moment causing sidebending right.

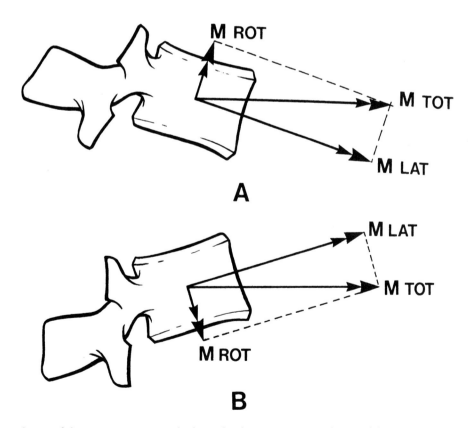

Figure 4–15   A. Dissolution of the moment vector in the lower lumbar spine. B. Dissolution of the moment vector in the upper lumbar spine.

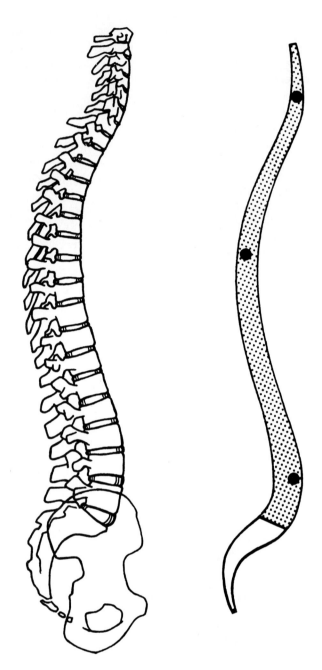

Figure 4–16   Reversal points of the rotation vector.

In clinical practice, the occurrence of sidebending without bony apposition seems to be extremely limited. Following even a small sidebending, with a rotation component that can barely be registered, bone-to-bone contact occurs in the intervertebral joints. From that point on, the rest of the movement sequence will not be purely dynamic, but will be of a kinematic nature, determined by the geometry of the intervertebral joints. It is obvious that in the case of the lumbar spine, which has a natural lordosis, the expected

pattern of movement is consistent with that described below in relation to sidebending in the extreme extension position. The rotation sequence is thus in the same direction as the sidebending.

Further, in regard to item 3 in the preceding list, in the extreme extension position, there is also bilateral focal bony apposition in the intervertebral joints (**Figure 4–17**).

Compared with the flexion position, the contact area is located more caudally. It is formed by the caudal extremities of the inferior articular processes of the cranial vertebra and the caudal edges of the articulating surfaces of the superior articular processes of the caudal vertebra. Whenever a sidebending is initiated from this extreme extension position, the bony geometry determines the movement sequence, as in the flexion position. The sagittally oriented articulating surfaces, which diverge in the dorsal direction and converge in the caudal direction, will hinder the movement of the inferior articular process of the cranial vertebra on the side of the sidebending.

Freedom of movement can be created only if the inferior articular process of the cranial vertebra moves in a dorsal direction on the ipsilateral side. On the contralateral side, the bone-to-bone contact between the articular surfaces presents no obstacle, so the inferior articular process can move freely in a medioventrocranial direction. For the whole vertebra, this means a rotation in the same direction as that of the sidebending, as described in flexion.

Thoracic Vertebral Column

The movement sequence that Freyette describes for different positions of the thoracic vertebral column in the sagittal plane is difficult to explain. This is because, from a biomechanical point of view, the geometrical relationships

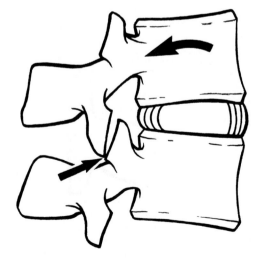

Figure 4–17   Focal bony contact with extension.

arising from the rib–vertebra connections are extremely complicated (**Figure 4–18**).

The disk, vertebral body, intervertebral joints, transverse process, rib, and sternum together form a kinematic chain. The movement pattern of this chain is closely determined by the interactions among the nine joints that are part of it in each segment. During sidebending, an additional biomechanical component is involved because of the bone contact that is possible between the rib arches. Because of individual differences in the measurements of joints that can function as centers of rotation, and the positions of the muscles and ligaments that are responsible for exerting pressure, there can be no single and definitive description of the kinematic behavior of the thoracic spinal column. It is similarly impossible to give a balanced biomechanical explanation of the movement patterns described in the literature. We cannot, therefore, make an unambiguous statement, based on a reasoned position, about direction of movement and movement sequence in the thoracic region.

The upper thoracic region (consisting of T1 to T4) seems to follow the movement pattern of the cervical vertebral column. There are no differences of opinion on this in the literature.

Cervical Vertebral Column

Freyette's description of the movement sequence in the cervical vertebral column (C2–T5) is also difficult to under-

stand because of the geometry of the connections between the vertebrae. Here, too, conclusions are hypothetical.

There is no discussion in the literature of the direction of rotation that accompanies sidebending. As noted earlier, independently of the position of the vertebral column, in the sagittal plane it always takes place in the direction of the concavity of the lateroflexion. The following is a possible explanation for Freyette's movement sequence.

In the ventral flexed position, the lower articular surfaces of the upper vertebra make focal bone-to-bone contact with the cranioventral extremities of the upper articular surfaces of the caudal vertebra. When a lateral force is applied, there will initially be no bony obstruction. The contact point with the concave part of the joint will act as a tipping point. This means that limited sidebending can take place, followed directly by the rotation.

In the ventral flexed position, there is no initial bone resistance during sidebending. One might, therefore, expect that the rotation component would change direction at the top of the curve. Because the lordosis of the cervical vertebral column disappears in the ventral flexed position, the pattern of reversal should not take place, so the rotation would continue in the same direction.

If a lateral force is applied in the dorsal flexed position, the bones of the uncovertebral and intervertebral joints will hinder the sidebending at the concavity of the bend. Sidebending can continue only if there is a rotation that,

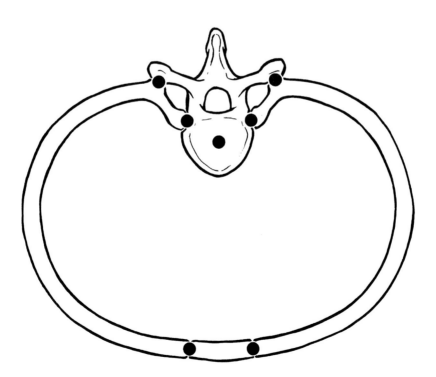

Figure 4–18 Joints of the thoracic kinematic chain.

given the geometric relationships in the motion segment, can be broken down into a sidebending component and a pure axial rotation. Depending on the geometry and condition of the articular surfaces of the upper cervical vertebrae (C2–C3–C4) and the lower cervical vertebrae (C4–C5–C6), relatively more sidebending should take place in the upper cervical region and relatively more rotation in the lower cervical region.

Segments C0–C1 and C1–C2 have a special function in the cervical region. The functional mechanism of these segments, and their behavior in motion, are explained in Chapter 17 "Examination of the Upper Cervical Spine."

Diagram Showing Direction of Movement and Movement Sequence

In **Table 4–7**, vector labeling is used to show which rotational movement occurs in response to a sidebending impulse at different positions in the sagittal plane. It also shows the sequence in which the movements will occur relative to the geometry of the motion segment. With regard to the area consisting of T5 to T9 inclusive, many authors—including Freyette—argue that different combinations and sequences are possible. This is indicated in the diagram by a dotted line and the bracketing of sequences.

Table 4–7　Rotation Direction Coupled to a Primary Movement of Sidebending in the Various Spinal Regions

Key to the diagram

Ipsilateral rotation = Rotation in the direction of the concave part of the lateral curve

Contralateral rotation = Rotation in the direction of the convex part of the lateral curve

Lumbar vertebral column (T10 to L5 inclusive)

Ventral flexed position
Direction of rotation: ipsilateral
Movement sequence: rotation, sidebending

Neutral position or extension, nonendrange position
Direction of rotation: contralateral
Movement sequence: sidebending, rotation

Extension, endrange position
Direction of rotation: ipsilateral
Movement sequence: rotation, sidebending

Thoracic vertebral column (T5 to T9 inclusive)

Neutral position and ventral flexed position
Direction of rotation: ipsilateral
Movement sequence: sidebending, rotation
(other directions of rotation and movement sequences are possible here)

Dorsal flexed position
Direction of rotation: ipsilateral
Movement sequence: rotation, sidebending
(other directions of rotation and movement sequences are possible here)

Cervical vertebral column (C2 to T4 inclusive)

Ventral flexed position
Direction of rotation: ipsilateral
Movement sequence: sidebending, rotation

Dorsal flexed position
Direction of rotation: ipsilateral
Movement sequence: rotation, sidebending

THREE-DIMENSIONAL EXAMINATION OF THE SPINE

The description given previously of three-dimensional movement in the vertebral column gives some idea of the complexity of spinal movement. Numerous authors have studied the three-dimensional movement of the different spinal regions using cadavers. Further data to be found in the literature (Grieve, 1981), and research carried out by the Manual Therapy Training Foundation (Stichting Opleiding Manuele Therapie) at the Free University of Amsterdam (Van Zoest, 1985) has shown considerable individual differences in the orientation and shape of the facets in different regions and segments of the spine.

Movement in the individual is affected by congenital and acquired deviations, morphology developed in response to use, and variations in centers of gravity of different parts of the body. It should, therefore, be clear that comparisons involving quantitative measures of apparently identical movements, or combinations of movements, make little sense. Assuming symmetry of movement as a general rule does not offer appropriate criteria for assessing the functioning of the vertebral column. Comparison of mobility in neighboring segments within a region also fails to provide a reliable guide to overall function. Although one needs to know the general principles according to which the vertebral column works, functional examination of the vertebral column of the individual needs to be qualitative in nature.

The authors discussed earlier describe relationships among the components of particular movements and the sequence in which they take place. However, the human vertebral column seems able to respond to all the positions and movement combinations that occur. The fact that some combinations of movements can be performed more easily or efficiently than others can is an individual matter, determined by congenital characteristics and the development of preferred patterns during daily life (work, sports, hobbies). The movements that the vertebral column has to make in normal life are mostly three-dimensional in nature. Even a seemingly one-dimensional movement of the vertebral column results in movements in several planes.

Functional disturbances of the spinal column are thus likely to appear predominantly, or to a large extent, during three-dimensional movements. It is, therefore, evident that the qualitative examination of the functioning of the spinal column should be carried out primarily in three dimensions. The exception is examination of movement in the sagittal plane because this is a frequent part of normal activities. Sagittal plane motion, therefore, should be added to the active and active-assisted regional examination.

Although ventral/extension should not be regarded as a purely two-dimensional movement, it is performed during the examination as a movement that takes place about a instantaneous axis of rotation located in the frontal plane. This movement in the sagittal plane is added to the three-dimensional functional examination partly to gain extra information about the dynamic functioning of the spinal column, and partly to identify or rule out spinal cord, dural, or nerve root compression.

The vertebral column has a capacity for movement that forms a prerequisite to all human activities; this means, of course, that it is prone to dysfunction. Its mobility is based on eight main three-dimensional movements, to which the two others in the sagittal plane are added. In examinations of dysfunctions of the spinal column, certain movements must first be performed actively to find out which ones are dysfunctional. Once it is clear in which region the dysfunction is located, there should be an active-assisted regional examination, followed by a similar examination at the segmental level. This will allow a more precise localization of the problem.

To gain further information about the eight three-dimensional movements, a pilot study was carried out on 150 patients with spinal dysfunction. Those with rib fixations and radicular symptomatology were excluded. The research variables were pain and disturbances of endfeel. In 147 patients, the disturbance seemed to be present in one three-dimensional ipsilateral movement, or two or more three-dimensional ipsilateral and/or contralateral movements. In three patients, the disturbance showed only in one three-dimensional contralateral movement. In two of these three cases, the problem was localized in the thoracic vertebral column, and the third, in a highly mobile person, in the cervical vertebral column.

The findings of the pilot study were that in only 3 out of 150 cases of nonradicular disorders of the spinal column—that is, in 2%—only one three-dimensional contralateral movement was disturbed. In the 147 other cases—that is, in 98%—either just one three-dimensional ipsilateral movement seemed to be affected or several ipsilateral and contralateral movements.

Every movement is unique and imposes a specific load on tissue structures in the sense of tensile and compressive loads. Nevertheless, a general examination strategy was developed following the pilot study. The procedure is as follows:

For the examination of active function, eight three-dimensional movements are performed, plus ventral and extension. If these show that ipsilateral, or ipsilateral and contralateral, three-dimensional movements are affected only in a particular region, then during the active-assisted regional and segmental examinations, only the ipsilateral three-dimensional movements are examined initially so as to cause the patient as little discomfort as possible.

After the segmental ipsilateral three-dimensional dysfunctions have been dealt with, the contralateral movements that were shown dysfunctional during the examination of active function must also be checked. If the assessment of active function shows disturbance of only one or more contralateral functions, only these movements are checked during the active-assisted examination of regional and segmental function.

When the three-dimensional functioning of a segment is examined, the separate orthogonal movement components are loaded at the end of the movement to identify the one that is causing the most difficulty. The stressing of the endrange of the different orthogonal movement components should be carried out from the position adopted to avoid unlocking the three-dimensional endrange state. In treatment, attention should be paid to the component that caused the most difficulty during three-dimensional mobilization, whether loaded or unloaded, depending on the circumstances.

During evaluation of findings of the functional examination, the emphasis should be on quality of movement. With regard to the quantity of movement in a segment, the only important consideration is whether or not any movement is present. To shed more light on the examination procedure, some concepts and particular regions are described in greater detail in the following subsections.

Quantitative vs. Qualitative Examination

Quantitative judgments of segmental movement do not provide a meaningful criterion. Individual anomalies, scoliosis, and the development of different preferred movement patterns lead to asymmetries in the spinal column, which means that quantitative right-left comparisons within the same segment, or cranial-to-caudal comparisons between adjacent segments, are bound to give misleading information. Subtle differences in movement are also difficult to detect. The only useful quantitative criterion in assessing movement is not the number of degrees of movement, but whether movement is present or absent.

Qualitative assessment of movement in relation to the segmental symptoms offers a more efficient approach to identifying the affected segment and the nature of the dysfunction. In an examination of segmental function, the critical factors are, therefore, the quality of the movement and the nature of the associated symptoms.

In a segment that is free of dysfunction, movement is possible in all directions; the slack can be taken up; there is a normal endfeel related to bones, ligaments, capsules, and soft tissues limiting the respective movements; the movement is stable and pain-free; there are no pseudoradicular or radicular symptoms; and there are no specific pain points or *referred sensations* associated with the specific segment.

Pathologic Hypo-/Hypermobility

A qualitative approach to the assessment of movement entails a different interpretation of terms such as pathologic hypomobility and hypermobility. Changes in the quality of movement as a result of impairments in the bones, cartilage, capsules, ligaments, disks, and dura can be accompanied by decreased or increased mobility. A qualitative examination of segmental function should not exclude hypomobility and hypermobility as phenomena, but should not use them as evaluation criteria. Individual differences in movement can be caused by the morphology of the segment, but this need not mean that the movement is adversely affected or imply the existence of a pathologic state.

It seems reasonable to speak of pathologic hypo- or hypermobility in cases where a qualitative disturbance of movement is associated with very limited mobility or extreme mobility. However, the absence of quantitative norms for the mobility of individual segments makes concepts such as hypomobility and hypermobility impossible to use as diagnostic criteria. This does not mean that a therapeutic assessment, which is based among other things on the quality of the endfeel, should disregard the presence of increased or limited movement in the segment.

Other determining factors include previous history, injury or illness, and the phase of the movement in which the disturbance appears. Where internal or peripheral pathology is present, it is possible that the moving and vegetative segments involved by it are not yet affected from the point of view of movement, or are not yet perceptibly affected in this respect. From a neurophysiologic point of view, a segment of this kind, defined not on functional examination but by pathologic signs and symptoms, should be noted in the therapeutic assessment. From the biomechanical viewpoint also, all the joints and tissues associated with a segmental dysfunction should be included in the examination to help identify the etiologic factors.

Weight-Bearing and Non-Weight-Bearing Examination

Weight-Bearing

To the extent possible, both the assessment of active function and the examination of active-assisted regional and segmental function should be carried out under weight-bearing conditions. This is because of the following reasons:

- Ninety-nine percent of human activity takes place in the loaded condition.
- Functioning in the weight-bearing condition is responsible for most of the dysfunctions from which pathology can develop.

- Symptoms noted in the weight-bearing condition provide the most realistic picture of patient status.
- The patient can perform tasks naturally in this position.
- The therapist can examine the patient easily and efficiently in this position, though this applies to a lesser extent in the case of the lumbar region.

Non-Weight-Bearing

Although it is preferable to assess movement in the weight-bearing position, there are times when it is desirable or necessary to carry out the examination in a non-weight-bearing position. In some circumstances, a non-weight-bearing examination may be the only possibility, or it may be indicated as a supplementary assessment. From a practical point of view, it is possible to examine unloaded three-dimensional movement in the lumbar and cervical regions, but it can be problematic with regard to the thoracic region. Here it may be necessary to limit oneself to carrying out local provocation and oscillation tests with the patient lying prone.

Examination in the non-weight-bearing condition may be carried out in the following cases:

- Pathology resulting from compression
- Predominant defensive muscular tension
- Suspected passive instability
- Increase in problems during examination in the weight-bearing position, for example, the mushroom phenomenon
- Overwhelming pain
- Radicular symptomatology

If three-dimensional functioning cannot be examined in either the weight-bearing or the non-weight-bearing condition, one must make inferences from other aspects of the patient presentation. Other parts of the manual diagnostic procedure, such as the history and/or the neurologic examination, provide guiding input to the decisions that have to be made. Persisting with a three-dimensional examination of the segment under adverse circumstances is a mistake. The findings with regard to treatment posture, directional emphasis, and technique choice are the deciding factors in planning treatment.

Guided vs. Active-Assisted Examination

The passive functional examination is replaced by the guided and active-assisted functional examination. Observation of the body in action allows one to observe recipro-

cal inhibition. During therapist-guided activity, the movement pattern chosen by the patient can be observed; during the active-assisted movement part of the examination, the therapist can discover what is possible or impossible for the patient. During examinations of regional function, both guided and active-assisted movements are observed; during segmental examinations, only active-assisted movements are assessed. The assessment of active-assisted function ends with a passive examination to test the endfeel, and by way of tissue provocation elicit potential symptoms.

Tissue Loading and Unloading

In general, when the body moves in the sagittal plane, the tissues dorsal to the axis of movement is stretched during flexion, and those ventral to the axis are compressed, or relaxed. The reverse applies during extension. The exception is the interspinous ligament, which is stretched during extension. During combined movements, tissues on both sides, both concave and convex, are liable to be stretched and compressed. The compression factor is greatest on the concave side and the stretch factor on the convex side.

It is important to be able to distinguish which tissues are involved in segmental dysfunction. When planning therapy, it is equally important to be able to determine and interpret the extent of the symptoms. For this, knowledge of segmental and intersegmental relationships and of neurophysiologic processes is essential. Factors that can serve as criteria include sensory function of the skin; connective tissue adhesions; muscular hypertonicity; nerve root irritation; decreased muscle strength; capsular, ligamentous, and periostal pain; trigger points; and the endfeel of segmental movements.

The joints and tissue structures most directly affected by a segmental dysfunction and most likely to develop symptoms are intervertebral joints, uncovertebral joints, rib joints, intervertebral formina, intervertebral disk, spinal cord, dura mater, nerve root, the segmental muscles, ligaments, and capsules, and in the cervical region, the vertebral artery. For the purposes of planning appropriate therapy, it is important to establish whether the disturbance in the movement trajectory of a particular segment is caused by arthrogenic, capsuloligamentous, muscular, vascular, diskogenic, or neurogenic factors, and at what level of activity the sympathetic nervous system is functioning.

Specific Regions

C0–C3

The assessment of the functional unit of C0–C3 occupies a special place in the examination of three-dimensional function. In this region, exceptionally, the three-dimensional contralateral movements should be examined in the first instance because of the ligamentary restraints. The functional interdependency of the upper cervical segments raises a problem regarding the order of segmental examination. For various reasons (see the section titled "Examination Sequence C0 to C3" in Chapter 17), the preference is for the examination to proceed from caudal to cranial.

Pelvis

The functioning of the sacroiliac joints involves the eight three-dimensional movement combinations of the lumbar spine and the accompanying movements of the pelvis that are listed as follows. Combinations III, IV, V, and VI are based on the functional walking pattern (Marsman, 1981):

I. *Flexion, left sidebending, left rotation.*
   - Left half of pelvis higher than right
   - Backward tilt of sacrum relative to lumbar vertebral column
   - Forward rotation of right side of sacrum
   - Backward rotation of right innominate relative to right side of sacrum
   - Backward rotation of left side of sacrum
   - Forward rotation of left innominate relative to left side of sacrum
   - Pelvic shift to right side

II. *Flexion, right sidebending, right rotation.*
   - Right half of pelvis higher than left
   - Backward tilt of sacrum relative to lumbar spine
   - Forward rotation of left side of sacrum
   - Backward rotation of left innominate relative to left side of sacrum
   - Backward rotation of right side of sacrum
   - Forward rotation of right innominate relative to right side of sacrum
   - Pelvic shift to left side

III. *Extension, left sidebending, left rotation (push-off phase, left leg).*
   - Left half of pelvis higher than right
   - Forward tilt of sacrum relative to lumbar spine
   - Forward rotation of right side of sacrum
   - Backward rotation of right innominate relative to right side of sacrum

   - Backward rotation of left side of sacrum
   - Forward rotation of left innominate relative to left side of sacrum
   - Pelvic shift to right side

IV. *Extension, right sidebending, right rotation (push-off phase, right leg).*
   - Right half of pelvis higher than left
   - Forward tilt of sacrum relative to lumbar spine
   - Forward rotation of left side of sacrum
   - Backward rotation of left innominate relative to left side of sacrum
   - Backward rotation of right side of sacrum
   - Forward rotation of right innominate relative to right side of sacrum
   - Pelvic shift to left side

V. *Flexion, left sidebending, right rotation (swing phase, left leg).*
   - Left half of pelvis higher than right
   - Backward tilt of sacrum relative to lumbar vertebral column
   - Forward rotation of left side of sacrum
   - Backward rotation of left innominate relative to left side of sacrum
   - Backward rotation of right side of sacrum
   - Forward rotation of right innominate relative to right side of sacrum
   - Pelvic shift to right side

VI. *Flexion, right sidebending, left rotation (swing phase, right leg).*
   - Right half of pelvis higher than left
   - Backward tilt of sacrum relative to lumbar vertebral column
   - Forward rotation of right side of sacrum
   - Backward rotation of right innominate relative to right side of sacrum
   - Backward rotation of left side of sacrum
   - Forward rotation of left innominate relative to left side of sacrum
   - Pelvic shift to left side

VII. *Extension, left sidebending, right rotation.*
   - Left half of pelvis higher than right
   - Forward tilt of sacrum relative to lumbar spine
   - Forward rotation of left side of sacrum

- Backward rotation of left innominate relative to left side of sacrum
- Backward rotation of right side of sacrum
- Forward rotation of right innominate relative to right side of sacrum
- Pelvic shift to right side

VIII. *Extension, right sidebending, left rotation.*
- Right side of pelvis higher than left
- Forward tilt of sacrum relative to lumbar spine
- Forward rotation of right side of sacrum
- Backward rotation of right innominate relative to right side of sacrum
- Backward rotation of left side of sacrum
- Forward rotation of left innominate relative to left side of sacrum
- Pelvic shift to left side

Normal functioning of the pelvis, at the base of the spine, is important for the optimal functioning of the spinal column as a whole and of the lumbar region in particular. Dysfunction in one or both of the sacroiliac joints can consist of joint fixation in the neutral, posterior, or anterior position; pelvic torsion without fixation; ligamentous laxity; or instability. This can have a negative effect on the three-dimensional mobility of the lumbar spine.

Locking of the Spine

Spinal locking is the patient- or therapist-induced fixation of one or more segments of the vertebral column. It can be brought about either actively or passively. The aim is to create an adequate lever function so that forces applied to the spinal column can be processed as efficiently as possible. Locking can also serve to localize forces to the segment that is being examined or mobilized.

There are several ways of achieving spinal locking:

- By ligamentous locking
- By bony apposition locking
- By including both these components

Locking primarily by ligamentous fixation can occur only in symmetrical movements in which the ligaments are brought under tension. For the spinal column, this means flexion. Locking primarily by bony apposition occurs only in symmetrical movements where bony structures (facets, spinous processes) limit further movement. In the spinal

column, this happens in extension. A combination of ligamentous and bony apposition locking can occur only in asymmetrical movements where movement is obstructed both by ligaments under tension and by bony structures. Optimal locking by ligament and bony apposition occurs when the spinal column is in an endrange position in all three dimensions.

Three-Dimensional Locking (Osteopathic View)

Osteopaths regard three-dimensional locking as an absolute prerequisite for creating a good lever function in segments on which certain examinations and treatments are to be carried out. The locking is brought about by changing one component in a three-dimensional physiologic position. It is only functional in the endrange position.

Locking for the Purpose of Examination

Every endrange position of a joint, regardless of which movement or combination of movements is being performed, leads to fixation and can be regarded as locking. Three-dimensional endrange positions offer optimal locking.

Three-dimensional locking is used where necessary for active-assisted examinations in which only three-dimensional movements will be carried out. The locking is applied so that it matches the three-dimensional movement that is to be carried out. The only exception to this rule is examination of the upper cervical region, in which the middle and lower cervical region is locked in three dimensions. Here, locking in one of the planes (sagittal) differs from the movement combination to be examined.

TERMS USED IN DESCRIBING THE EXAMINATION STRATEGY

The following sections contain definitions of terms that are used to describe examinations and to list and interpret possible etiologic factors.

Load

Load can be defined as "the physical and psychological stress that an individual tolerates or undergoes." Load is determined by the extent, duration, and frequency of the stresses, and the circumstances under which they are (or must be) handled. Several types of stress may be distinguished, notably psychosocial, general, local, and regional.

(See also the section titled "Examination Strategy" in Chapter 10.)

Load-Bearing Capacity

Load-bearing capacity can be defined as "the maximum physical and psychosocial load that an individual can tolerate at a given time and in given circumstances." It is determined by the following factors:

- Morphologic structure
- Mental fitness
- The effectiveness of the physiologic adaptation mechanisms
- Age and gender

The limits on both physical and psychological load-bearing capacity can be changed by appropriate physical and mental training. There are several kinds of load-bearing capacity, namely, psychosocial, general, local, regional, and segmental. (See the section titled "Examination Strategy" in Chapter 10.)

CHAPTER 5

Introduction to Test Psychometric Properties

Peter A. Huijbregts

STANDARDIZATION

Standardization means carrying out a test in a strictly defined manner, according to written instructions or previous agreement.

RELIABILITY

Many tests used within orthopaedic manual therapy (OMT) diagnosis yield a nominal-level or dichotomous outcome. In this regard, we might think of pain provocation tests that can produce either a positive (pain present) or a negative (pain absent) response, but we can also grade segmental mobility tests based on presence or absence of a segmental dysfunction or fixation. Other tests yield ordinal-level outcomes: 3-point grading scales can be used to express the finding of increased, normal, or decreased mobility on segmental mobility tests. Various authors have suggested extended multipoint rating scales allowing for further, therapy-relevant gradation of mobility findings. Less relevant to the specific OMT tests described in this text but important when using, for example, the active and passive general or regional range of motion tests that usually precede more segment- or structure-specific tests in the OMT evaluative process are continuous data on an interval and ratio levels.

Within the evidence-informed paradigm, diagnostic tests preferably need to have demonstrated sufficient research-based reliability and validity before their findings can be considered for use in the diagnostic process. In the absence of a clear, consensus-based gold standard test as often oc-

curs with OMT diagnostic tests, it may be impossible to establish diagnostic test validity. In this scenario, per force sufficient reliability is considered the only and necessary prerequisite for construct validity. In the absence of sufficient reliability, we have to seriously doubt the true existence of the construct that the test is intended to measure.

Reliability can be defined as the extent to which a measurement obtained by doing a test or measure is consistent and free of error (Portney and Watkins, 2008). To indicate this psychometric property of a test or measure the terms *reliability*, *repeatability*, *retest reliability*, *consistency*, and *stability* are often used interchangeably in the literature (Batterham and George, 2003).

There are five forms of reliability relevant to diagnostic and prognostic tests and measures used in clinical practice. However, with parallel forms reliability and internal consistency reliability more related to questionnaire-type tests and outcome measures not discussed in this text and test-retest reliability more relevant with regard to instrumental tests and measures and not the manual tests described here, we limit our discussion to intra- and interrater reliability.

Intrarater reliability is used to determine the repeatability of a measurement by a single rater or observer. Here, multiple measurements of the same characteristics by one observer are compared. If reliability is good, then the variation between repeated measurements from that one observer for the same characteristics should be small.

Interrater reliability is used to determine the repeatability of measurements obtained from multiple raters or observers (Batterham and George, 2003; Portney and Watkins, 2008). If reliability is good, then the measurements taken are similar to each other. In other words, the measurements taken by different raters show little variation. Relevant to interrater reliability, especially within the context of OMT diagnosis, is that the different raters need to agree on what it is they are measuring. This may involve consensus meetings and training sessions using the established consensus on what in fact is being measured prior to the actual study of interrater reliability.

When evaluating the methodological quality of reliability research, we need to consider several internal validity threats. For one, the time between test and retest is critical. Maturation and history can threaten reliability findings because too large of a gap between measurements can cause the variable being measured to change, and the reliability determined may not necessarily be indicative of truly poor reliability but rather of maturation and history effects (Batterham and George, 2003). If the time interval between the measurements is small, history or maturation threats are diminished. However, too short of a time between tests might cause undesirable testing effects such as fatigue and unintended (non)therapeutic effects.

Perhaps more relevant to interrater reliability, we could also wonder if repeated testing of, say, an intervertebral segmental restriction would not result in the second tester not measuring the same restriction present for the first tester but rather the effect of the mobilizing force exerted by the first tester during the test on the now less hypomobile intervertebral articulation? Some OMT tests may also suffer from a learning effect where the subjects are better able to comply with the test's imposed movement after they have experienced it before. Finally, the threat of regression to the mean necessitates standardization of testing circumstances. Perhaps most relevant with regard to this internal validity threat is standardization of test instructions to the subjects.

The use of inappropriate statistical tests is a threat to research validity of a research study. Reliability studies quantitatively express the level of reliability by way of an index of agreement. Which index of agreement or statistical measure is used depends first and foremost on the type of measurement performed. For test and measures scored at the nominal or ordinal levels, researchers have used percentage agreement values, kappa (κ) statistics, Spearman rank correlation coefficients, phi coefficients, and tests of statistical significance (Huijbregts, 2002). If tests or measures are scored on an interval or ratio level of measurement, then statistical measures such as tests of statistical significance, standard error of the measurement, limits of agreement, generalizability coefficients, Pearson product-moment correlation coefficients, and intraclass correlation coefficients may be used. Additional considerations in the choice of statistical measure concern the number of raters used and the number of retests performed (Batterham and George, 2003; Portney and Watkins, 2008). Although the reader is encouraged to review the references provided in this section

for a more in-depth discussion of this topic, some statistical measures are commonly used in OMT test reliability research and need to be discussed to allow for interpretation of this research.

The simplest index of agreement is the percentage agreement (PA) value, which is defined as the ratio of the number of agreements to the total number of ratings made (Haas, 1991). It is most commonly used for nominal and ordinal scale data but can also be used with higher scale data. Because it does not correct for chance agreement, it may provide a misleadingly high estimate of reliability (Haas, 1991; Maher and Adams, 1994; Portney and Watkins, 2008). Consider the following example: Two therapists want to establish the interrater reliability of a palpatory test for identification of an active myofascial trigger point in a given muscle. They agree that a positive finding is defined as the presence of a taut band, a hypersensitive nodule in this band, and referral in a characteristic agreed-upon pattern upon palpation. The therapists collect data on 50 patients, with and without trigger points. The results can be found in **Table 5–1**. We can calculate the percentage agreement value by adding the number of agreements on positive and negative findings and dividing this number by the total number of ratings (Batterham and George, 2003). In this case, the PA value is $(20 + 15) / 50 = 35 / 50 = 0.7$ (70%). A value of 100% would, of course, indicate perfect agreement between these two raters.

As noted previously, the problem with the PA value as an index of agreement is that it does not take into account the occurrence of agreement based on chance alone. In the case of a dichotomous test as discussed earlier, we would expect a chance agreement of 50%. The κ statistic is a chance-corrected index of agreement for use with nominal and ordinal-level data (Haas, 1991; Portney and Watkins, 2008). In its simplest form, the formula used to calculate the κ statistic is: $\kappa = (PA - PC) / (1 - PC)$ (Batterham and George, 2003). In this formula, PC indicates the agreement based on chance alone. In the preceding example of a dichotomous test with a PA of 70%, the κ value would be $(0.7 - 0.5) / (1 - 0.5) = 0.2 / 0.5 = 0.40$. It should be noted that there are various types of κ statistics, with

Table 5–1   Example of Findings for Diagnostic Palpation of Myofascial Trigger Points

	Therapist 1	
Therapist 2	Positive	Negative
Positive	20	5
Negative	10	15

weighted and mean κ statistics used and reported most commonly in the research and throughout this textbook; Huijbregts (2002) provides information on conditions for their use.

All variations of the κ statistic are inappropriate for use as a reliability statistic when there is limited variation in the data set. Limited variation occurs when there is a large proportion of agreement or when most agreement is limited to one of the possible rating categories (Haas, 1991). This can be the result of a study population that is highly homogeneous on the variable of interest; it can also occur as a result of rater bias or when the raters use only a limited portion of a multipoint rating scale (Lantz, 1997; Portney and Watkins, 2008).

Theoretically, κ can be negative if agreement is worse than chance. Practically, in clinical reliability studies, κ usually varies between 0.00 and 1.00 (Portney and Watkins, 2008). For the interpretation of the obtained κ values, benchmark values have been established. **Table 5–2** contains these benchmark values.

Whereas PA and κ statistics provide a measure of absolute agreement, correlation coefficients such as the Spearman rank correlation coefficient and phi coefficient are used to express relative agreement when using ordinal and nominal data, respectively. Pearson product-moment correlation coefficients are used for higher-level data. Therefore, correlation coefficients are not really appropriate as an index of agreement because they do not reflect agreement but rather covariance: they express the degree to which two variables vary in similar patterns (Maher and Adams, 1994; Portney and Watkins, 2008). Despite low actual agreement, a consistent difference between ratings will produce a large value for the correlation coefficient used, giving the misleading impression of high reliability. Correlation coefficients vary from −1.00 indicating a perfect negative correlation to 1.00 indicating a perfect positive correlation; a value of 0.00 indicates total absence of correlation. Despite drawbacks mentioned, benchmark values have also been established for the interpretation of these statistics in reliability research (see **Table 5–3**).

Table 5–2   Benchmark Values for κ Statistic

<40%	Poor to fair agreement
40–60%	Moderate agreement
60–80%	Substantial agreement
>80%	Excellent agreement
100%	Perfect agreement

Table 5–3   Benchmark Values for Correlation Coefficients

0.00–0.25	Little or no relationship
0.25–0.50	Fair relationship
0.50–0.75	Moderate to good relationship
>0.75	Good to excellent relationship

Some studies have used the nonparametric chi-square (χ^2) test or parametric tests of significance with higher-level data to establish reliability. The χ^2 statistic cannot distinguish a significant relationship predominated by agreement from one predominated by disagreement: deviation from chance in either direction contributes to the magnitude of χ^2 (Haas, 1991). Looking at reliability by determining that a κ value obtained significantly differs from 0 is also of little value: large samples tend to produce small yet significant κ values, whereas small samples may cause even large κ values to be statistically insignificant (Haas, 1991). Sample size also affects significance of correlation coefficients: large samples produce statistical significance despite a low actual value for the correlation coefficient used (Portney and Watkins, 2008).

The statistic most commonly used in reliability research for interval- or ratio-level data is the intraclass correlation coefficient (ICC). The ICC is a reliability coefficient calculated with variance estimates obtained through an analysis of variance (ANOVA). This statistic can be used for two or more raters or ratings and it does not require the same number of raters per subject. Although designed for interval or ratio scale data, it can also be used for ordinal scale data, provided the intervals between the ratings are assumed to be equivalent (Portney and Watkins, 2008). Of note is that there are six different types of ICC to be used in different reliability research methodologies. Because the choice of ICC used affects the numerical value of ICC with the same data set used, the type of ICC used should be reported in research studies (Portney and Watkins, 2008). Limited variation within the data set also makes the ICC an unreliable indicator of reliability. In case of limited variation, ICC can exceed 1.00, but normally ICC varies between 0.00 and 1.00. Portney and Watkins (2008) provided benchmark values for using ICC in reliability studies (see **Table 5–4**).

Table 5–4   ICC Benchmark Values

<0.75	Poor to moderate agreement
>0.75	Good agreement
>0.90	Reasonable agreement for clinical measurements

Throughout the remainder of this text, research-based data on test reliability are provided where available.

VALIDITY

Perhaps confusing to some, research validity used to assess methodological quality of research studies is different from test validity. Test validity includes four different aspects: face validity, content validity, criterion-related validity, and construct validity.

The most basic and least rigorous way to establish validity of a test or measure is face validity, that is, does the test on face value seem to test what it purports to measure? Establishing face validity is easiest for concepts, that is, directly observable abstractions. Consider the high level of face validity one easily attributes to a goniometric evaluation of a joint to establish joint mobility or to a manual muscle test to establish muscle strength. Establishing face validity of constructs, which are nonobservable abstractions of reality (Portney and Watkins, 2008), may be less simple. Examples of constructs relevant to OMT diagnosis are outcome measures such as patient self-report measures of function (eg, Oswestry Disability Index, Neck Disability Index) and quality of life (eg, Short Form 36) questionnaires. A test or measure either has or does not have face validity: it is an all-or-none quality that it is not further quantifiable. It is important in that clinicians and researchers will likely not use or study a test that in their opinion has no face validity.

Many OMT constructs have a theoretical domain that describes the content of that construct. Most obvious are simple constructs such as activities of daily living and how they might be affected by low back or neck function; quality of life is an example of a more complex construct. More relevant to OMT diagnostic tests are, for example, the characteristics thought to represent a positive finding on a segmental mobility test. Think of range of motion, resistance during range, endfeel, pain, tissue response, and many other possible variables on which frequently no profession-wide consensus has been established. When constructing a test or measure intended to capture those complex constructs, which aspects do we need to include?

Content validity (also known as domain validity or intrinsic validity) is the adequacy or degree to which a theoretical domain or universe of content is represented by a specific test or measure. Content validity is an important characteristic of multi-item tests and measures such as questionnaires, comprehensive examination procedures, inventories, and interviews that try to capture a range of information relevant to a specific construct. Generally, a panel of experts who review the test or measure and determine whether the items within the test satisfy the content domain establish its content validity. Delphi analysis is another method used within current-day OMT research to establish content validity of a complex construct.

Construct validity is the most difficult to determine of all forms of test validity. A construct does not have "reality status" or construct validity until such time that it conforms to a host of scientific requirements. We discussed earlier in the chapter how reliability testing is the most basic way to address concerns with regard to construct validity. Without going into further detail, other avenues include concurrent, convergent, and discriminative validity testing.

Criterion-related validity is the most relevant aspect of test validity when it comes to clinical diagnostic decision making. The word *criterion* in criterion-related validity refers to the fact that we are comparing a test or measure to a test that is commonly considered the best test available. This best available test is called the criterion or gold standard test. Some examples of criterion tests are radiographs for establishing the presence of lumbar spondylolisthesis, magnetic resonance imaging for determining intervertebral disk disease staging, intra-articular infiltration, or arthroscopic findings. The test to which we compare this criterion test is usually a more clinical, less invasive, less dangerous, and/or less expensive test or measure. **Table 5–5** provides some examples of criterion tests and related clinical tests. It is obvious why we would want to replace some of these criterion tests with clinical tests. Of course, at times we could argue that the criterion tests might not in fact be the best tests available.

There are four different types of criterion-related validity. Conversion validity is the degree to which a test or measure is similar to other tests or measures that theoretically should be similar to each other. Think of comparing visual estimates of range of motion (ROM) to goniometric ROM scores or radiographic measurements from the same subject. Discriminative validity is the degree to which a test or measure is not similar to other tests or measures that theoretically should not be similar to each other. This type of

Table 5–5   Examples of Criterion and Clinical Tests

Criterion Test	Clinical Test
Radiographs	Step palpation test for spondylolisthesis
Magnetic resonance imaging	McKenzie repeated movement exam
Intra-articular infiltration	Sacroiliac pain provocation tests
Arthroscopy	McMurray tests

validity might be used to validate a test or measure for assessing local stabilizing system function with one that is used to evaluate global stabilizing system function. Predictive validity establishes the extent to which a test or measure can forecast or predict some future event or criterion. Most relevant to current OMT clinical practice is the recent research into the predictive validity of a test cluster to determine the chance of meaningful improvement with lumbosacral manipulation (Childs et al., 2004a). Concurrent validity is the degree to which the outcomes of one test or measure correlate with outcomes on a criterion test when both tests are given at about the same time (Portney and Watkins, 2008). We discuss the two clinically more relevant forms of criterion validity: concurrent and predictive criterion-related validity. Although the following discussion is tailored more to concurrent validity, the same information applies to predictive validity.

In contrast to face and content validity, concurrent and predictive criterion-related validity can be expressed in a quantitative manner. Diagnostic tests and measures frequently yield dichotomous results such that the person either has or does not have the disease or dysfunction. When comparing a dichotomous clinical test or measure to a dichotomous gold standard test, there are four possible outcomes (Huijbregts, et al., 2005):

- *True positive (TP)*. The test indicates that the person has the disease or dysfunction and this is confirmed by the gold standard test.
- *False positive (FP)*. The clinical test indicates that the disease or dysfunction is present, but this is not confirmed by the gold standard test.
- *False negative (FN)*. The clinical test indicates absence of the disorder, but the gold standard test shows that the disease or dysfunction is present.
- *True negative (TN)*. Both the clinical and the gold standard tests agree that a disease or dysfunction is absent.

These outcomes can be tabulated in a two-by-two or truth table (**Table 5–6**).

The values in the truth table are then used to calculate the statistical measures of accuracy, sensitivity, specificity, negative and positive predictive values, and negative and positive likelihood ratios (Davidson, 2002). (See **Table 5–7**.) These are all ways to statistically express concurrent and predictive criterion-related validity of tests and measures.

The statistical measure of accuracy provides a quantitative measure of the overall value of a diagnostic test but has minimal value in the diagnostic decisions because it does not differentiate between the diagnostic value of positive and negative test results. In clinical practice, we can, therefore, disregard this statistical measure altogether.

Interpretation of sensitivity and specificity values is easiest when their values are high. When a test has high sensitivity, negative test results will likely rule out the disease or dysfunction because there are very few false negatives when sensitivity is high. When a test has high specificity, a positive test result will rule in the disease or dysfunction with a high degree of confidence because there are very few false positives when specificity is high (Davidson, 2002; Huijbregts et al., 2005). Without providing specific quantitative cut-off points, Davidson (2002) used the following mnemonics:

- SnNOUT. With highly Sensitive tests, a Negative result will rule a disorder OUT.
- SpPIN. With highly Specific tests, a Positive result will rule a disorder IN.

For most diagnostic procedures, the statistical measures of sensitivity and specificity are inversely related: tests with high sensitivity often have lower specificity, and vice versa (Huijbregts et al., 2005). A diagnostic test can be 100% sensitive and 100% specific only if there is no overlap between the population that has the disease or dysfunction and the population that does not (Huijbregts et al., 2005). Davidson (2002) also noted that sensitivity and specificity tell us how often a test will be positive or negative in patients that we already know have or do not have the disease or dysfunction. Obviously, this does not correspond with the clinical situation, where it is not known whether the disease or dysfunction is present.

Table 5–6   Truth Table

	Positive Criterion Test	Negative Criterion Test	Totals
Positive Clinical Test	True Positive (TP)	False Positive (FP)	TP + FP
Negative Clinical Test	False Negative (FN)	True Negative (TN)	FN + TN
Totals	TP + FN	FP + TN	TP + FP + FN + TN

Table 5–7   Definition and Calculation of Statistical Measures of Concurrent Criterion-Related Validity

Statistical Measure	Definition	Calculation
Accuracy	The proportion of people who were correctly identified as either having or not having the disease or dysfunction	(TP + TN) / (TP + FP + FN + TN)
Sensitivity	The proportion of people who have the disease or dysfunction who test positive	TP / (TP + FN)
Specificity	The proportion of people who do not have the disease or dysfunction who test negative	TN / (FP + TN)
Positive predictive value	The proportion of people who test positive and who have the disease or dysfunction	TP / (TP + FP)
Negative predictive value	The proportion of people who test negative and who do not have the disease or dysfunction	TN / (FN + TN)
Positive likelihood ratio	How likely a positive test result is in people who have the disease or dysfunction as compared to how likely it is in those who do not have the disease or dysfunction	Sensitivity / (1 − Specificity)
Negative likelihood ratio	How likely a negative test result is in people who have the disease or dysfunction as compared to how likely it is in those who do not have the disease or dysfunction	(1 − Sensitivity) / Specificity

Note: TP, true positive; TN, true negative; FP, false positive; FN, false negative.

At first glance, the usefulness of positive and negative predictive values seems greater than that of sensitivity and specificity. However, their usefulness is limited by the fact that for predictive values to apply, the prevalence in the clinical population being examined has to be identical to the prevalence in the study population from which the predictive values were derived (Davidson, 2002; Huijbregts et al., 2005). Prevalence is defined as the number of cases of a disease or dysfunction at a given point in time expressed as a percentage of the total population at risk (Portney and Watkins, 2008). Clinically, we establish prevalence by gathering data from published research, but more frequently we will estimate prevalence based on our clinical experience. Davidson (2002) notes that because of the issue of different or unknown prevalence positive and negative predictive values should be virtually disregarded in the diagnostic process.

The most useful statistical measures to express concurrent and predictive criterion-related validity of a test or measure are, therefore, not accuracy, sensitivity, specificity, or positive and negative predictive values but rather a measure called a (positive or negative) likelihood ratio. Likelihood ratios (LR) summarize the data of sensitivity and specificity (Davidson, 2002; Huijbregts et al., 2005). Within evidence-informed OMT clinical practice—whenever available—diagnostic accuracy statistics such as LR should be used to calculate shifts from the pretest probability that a pa-

tient has or does not have a particular condition to the posttest probability of a specific diagnosis. Data on LR can be used to calculate posttest from pretest probabilities. Jaeschke et al. (1994) provide guidelines for the clinical interpretation of LR data (see **Table 5–8**).

Data on prevalence provide the clinician with information on pretest probability. Of course, frequently one has no data from epidemiologic studies that look at the incidence and prevalence of certain dysfunctions and diseases in certain populations to establish this prevalence. If the patient we see fits to an acceptable degree within a population studied, that is, if the epidemiologic study has sufficient external validity to allow for extrapolation to our particular clinical setting, we may assume that prevalence and incidence and thus pretest probability for this patient are similar to that reported in the literature for similar subjects. Another frequent—but perhaps more fallible—source for data on pretest probability is simply clinician expertise and familiarity with the clinical population with which the clinician works.

We can use LR to calculate the posttest probabilities in two ways. The more exact way involves calculating odds ratios:

- *Estimate pretest probability.* For this example, we use a prevalence of a disorder of 70%, or 0.70.
- Pretest odds are Probability / (1 − Probability), that is, 0.70 / (1 − 0.70) = 2.3.

Table 5–8 Effect of Positive and Negative Likelihood Ratios on Posttest Probability

LR+	Interpretation
>10	Large and often conclusive increase in the likelihood of disease
5–10	Moderate increase in the likelihood of disease
2–5	Small increase in the likelihood of disease
1–2	Minimal increase in the likelihood of disease
1	No change in the likelihood of disease

LR−	Interpretation
1	No change in the likelihood of disease
0.5–1.0	Minimal decrease in the likelihood of disease
0.2–0.5	Small decrease in the likelihood of disease
0.1–0.2	Moderate decrease in the likelihood of disease
<0.1	Large and often conclusive decrease in the likelihood of disease

- Multiply pretest odds by the LR to get posttest odds. If the positive LR = 10, then this produces $2.3 \times 10 = 23$.
- Convert posttest odds to posttest probability by using the following equation: Odds / (Odds + 1), that is, $23 / 24 = 0.96$.

One could also use a nomogram (**Figure 5–1**): draw a line from pretest probability through the LR to get the posttest probability. Although obviously easier, this method is less precise. Where available we have provided data throughout this text on predictive and concurrent criterion-related validity for the diagnostic tests described.

RESPONSIVENESS

Responsiveness is the sensitivity to change of a diagnostic test or outcome measure (Stratford, Binkley, and Riddle, 1996). Sensitivity used in the context of responsiveness should not be confused with the statistical measure of sensitivity discussed in the context of criterion-related validity. Using a test or measure that has sufficient responsiveness is very relevant for research purposes. A test or measure used to assess outcomes that lacks a sufficient degree of responsiveness reduces precision and necessitates an increase in sample size or effect of an intervention to still allow the researcher to pick up a statistically relevant difference (Scrimshaw and Maher, 2001). A responsive test also allows the clinician to establish with research-based confidence whether a true and/or meaningful change has

occurred over the course of treatment. There are two types of relevant change with regard to diagnostic tests or outcome measures:

- Minimal detectable change (MDC)
- Minimal clinically important change (MCID)

The MDC refers to a change in your measurement on a diagnostic test or the score on an outcome measure that indicates that—when exceeded—a true change has occurred. A test or measure with a high MDC is an unresponsive test: if, for example, the MDC on goniometric measurement of shoulder abduction is 20°, you could conclude only that a true change had occurred—whether resulting from natural history or intervention—if there is a 20° change or greater for the better on two consecutive measurements. The MDC is mathematically related to the standard error of measurement (SEM; mentioned briefly as an index of agreement earlier in this chapter): $MDC_{95} = (1.96) \times \sqrt{(2)} \times (SEM)$ (Eliasziw, Young, Woodbury, and Fryday-Field, 1994; Stratford, 2004). Further, relevant to clinicians interested in calculating the MDC is that the SEM can be calculated from ICC values also discussed as indices of agreement using the formula $SEM = SD \times \sqrt{(1 - ICC)}$ (Weir, 2005).

This MDC_{95} value comes with a bit of statistical uncertainty: using the preceding formula to calculate the MDC, we can be 95% confident that if a patient exceeds the MDC it is thus determined that a true change has occurred. Some MDC values come with a different degree of statistical uncertainty. This is indicated (or should be indicated) with a number after the MDC. An MDC_{90} is the amount of change

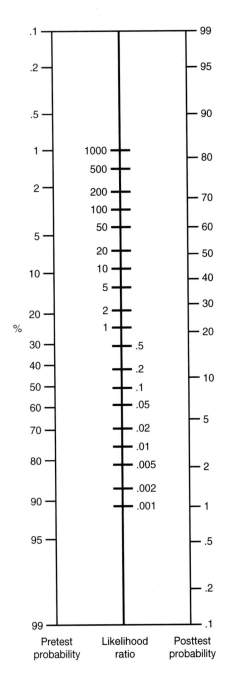

Pretest
probability

Likelihood
ratio

Posttest
probability

Figure 5–1 Nomogram.

value of change than the MDC. The MCID can be calculated by way of either distribution- or anchor-based calculation methods (Stratford et al., 1996). Coefficients commonly used in the distribution-based method include effect size, standardized response mean, and receiver operating characteristic curve area. For a more in-depth discussion of this method for determining the MCID, see Stratford and colleagues (1996). The anchor-based method of calculation is the preferred method: it compares changes in the health status measures under investigation with concurrent changes on a standard or criterion test indicating a change in health status. Frequently, this criterion standard is the global rating of change. This method is preferred mainly because it provides more clinically meaningful descriptions whereas the distribution-based method provides, at times, difficult to interpret indications of statistical significance of the change score (Stratford et al., 1996). From the preceding discussion, it is obvious that the psychometric property of responsiveness has little relevance to most tests used as part of OMT diagnosis; however, responsiveness can be relevant when using range of motion measures as impairment-level outcome measures or when interpreting standardized patient-report questionnaires on function or quality of life.

CONFIDENCE INTERVALS

It has been said, "Statistics is nothing but a means to never have to say you are certain." Throughout this text psychometric data on reliability, validity, and responsiveness are presented where such data are available with confidence intervals. The most commonly used form of the confidence interval in this text is the 95% confidence interval (abbreviated throughout this text as 95% CI). A 95% CI is a means of estimating—with 95% confidence—what the true findings would be in the clinical population and is presented as a range between a lower and a higher value (Bolton, 2007). An example of this is a discussion of interrater reliability reporting a κ value of 0.57 (95% CI: –0.20–0.89). Other psychometric data reported in this text with confidence intervals include percentage agreement, intraclass correlation coefficient, sensitivity, specificity, and likelihood, odds, and prevalence ratio values.

Relevant to the interpretation of confidence intervals is to see whether this interval includes a value that equates to "no effect" (Bolton, 2007). In the context of data on reliability, this no-effect value is usually determined by the benchmark values presented previously (Portney and Watkins, 2008). In the absence of benchmark values helpful in their interpretation, the no-effect value is less clear with regard to data on sensitivity and specificity. The benchmark values

in scores required to be 90% confident that a true change has in fact occurred.

The second aspect of responsiveness is MCID. The MCID is also known as minimal clinically significant difference (MCSD). When a patient exceeds the MCID on a test or measure, we can be confident that not only a true but also a clinically meaningful change has occurred for this patient. It should be obvious that the MCID is likely a greater proposed by Jaeschke et al. (1994) can help establish the no-effect value for likelihood ratios. However, it is obvious that clinician interpretation of what constitutes a no-effect value in these cases strongly affects interpretation of confidence intervals. In the case of ratio statistics, the interpretation is less ambivalent: a ratio statistic, whether likelihood, odds, or prevalence ratio, with a value of 1 included in the confidence interval equates to the possibility of no effect.

Another important aspect of interpretation of confidence intervals is related to how wide the interval is. A narrow confidence interval means that we can be fairly certain of the true population value, whereas a wide confidence interval means that we cannot be very precise about the population estimate. The main reason for wide confidence intervals is usually a small sample size, a situation all too common in the OMT research presented throughout this text (Bolton, 2007).

PART II

Examination

CHAPTER 6

History and Examination: General Structure and Special Considerations

A. History: Components of a comprehensive history taking are discussed in more detail later in this chapter.

B. Present patient status is determined during the physical examination in a structured format consisting of the following components:

   Observation by way of a visual assessment with attention to:

   - Activities of daily living (ADLs)
   - Posture and gait
   - Shape
   - Skin
   - Assistive devices used

   The physical examination consists of a general, a regional, and a segmental component:

   The general component includes:

   - Active range of motion examination
   - Active range of motion examination with specific instructions as to performance of the motions

   The regional component includes:

   - Active guided range of motion examination
   - Active assisted range of motion examination
   - Resistance tests
   - Differential diagnostic tests
   - Provocation tests

   The segmental component consists of:

   - Tissue-specific examination
   - Provocation tests
   - Active-assisted segmental range of motion tests

   The orientation and palpation portion of the examination focus on:

   - Body regions
   - Topographic orientation
   - Palpation of specific tissues and organs
   - Specific pain points

   The neurologic examination includes tests for:

   - Radicular syndrome
   - Thoracic outlet compression syndrome
   - Sensory examination
   - Segment
   - Pseudoradicular syndrome
   - Lesions of the plexi and peripheral nerves
   - Places predisposed to entrapment syndromes
   - Coordination
   - Motor function
   - Circulation

   Finally, a supplementary examination may include:

   - Radiography and other imaging studies
   - Electrodiagnostics
   - Biopsy, puncture
   - Laboratory tests
   - Other specialist medical examinations

C. Clinical impression

D. Kinesiologic diagnosis

E. Trial treatment

F. Definitive therapy (repeated diagnostic examination)

125

The preceding general protocol for examinations, as developed by Frisch (1977), is used—with some modifications and additions—as a model for examining the neuromusculoskeletal system. It is intended to provide guidelines for completing a maximally comprehensive assessment. In clinical practice, reasoned choices must be made according to circumstances with regard to the components to be included in the examination and the sequence in which they will be carried out. An efficient examination is one that takes a minimum of time, causes the patient minimal discomfort, and yields the best possible information. For more information about aspects of the examination that are not treated fully here, you may wish to consult the literature or appropriate medical specializations.

EXAMINATION

After indicating the general content of the history and examination process at the beginning of this chapter, we now proceed with a more in-depth discussion of the various components.

Patient History

Document the patient's personal details:

- *Administrative.* Name, address, telephone number, sex, age, family physician, referring physician, health-care insurance
- *Social.* Marital status, family details, home situation (past and present), occupation, working conditions, sports, hobbies

Document in the history specific information with regard to their present complaint:

- *Pain.* Where, when, type, onset, course, pattern, day or night, referral; aggravating factors and whether effects are immediate or delayed; easing factors
- *Disturbances of posture.* Forced posture; inability to assume a particular position
- *Disturbances of movement.* Difficulty, quality, course, coordination, associated noises, relapses, secondary movement dysfunctions
- *Disturbances of sensation.* Hyperesthesia, paresthesia, hypesthesia, anesthesia
- *Motor disturbances.* Reduced strength, paresis
- *Vegetative disturbances.* Hidrosis, trichosis, hyperesthesia, color, cramp

- *General well-being*
- *Previous therapies*
- *Patient's own beliefs about the cause of the symptoms*

Take down the supplementary history:

- *System-based history/screening examination*
- *Central nervous system.* Headache, balance
- *Sensory organs.* Double vision, seeing stars, visual complaints, deafness, tinnitus, dizziness
- *Respiratory organs.* Shortness of breath, cough, sputum
- *Circulatory system.* Palpitations, angina, dyspnea, edema
- *Gastrointestinal system.* Swallowing problems, appetite, thirst, stomach pain, heartburn, vomiting, abdominal pain, defecation
- *Urogenital system.* Micturition, frequency of urination, incontinence, menstruation, sexuality
- *Hormonal system*
- *Medication history*
- *Psyche*
- *Supplementary examinations.* Radiology, laboratory tests, other specialist medical examinations
- *Development.* Illnesses, hospital admissions, surgeries

Document the family history: hereditary history, anomalies, illnesses. After the history taking process the clinician formulates a list of likely provisional diagnoses.

Inspection

During inspection, attention is usually paid to the following:

- Body type
- General presentation
- Activities of daily living (ADLs)
- Posture and gait
- Abnormalities with regard to shape
- Skin color
- Scars
- Hair growth pattern and distribution
- Use of orthoses and prostheses

When evaluating static spinal posture, the lower extremities should be taken into account because of their effect on pelvic position.

A plumb line is used in assessing changes in posture in the vertebral column in the sagittal and frontal planes, or in a combination of the two planes. For assessment in the frontal plane, the plumb line is suspended from the external occipital protuberance; for assessment in the sagittal plane, it is suspended from the external auditory meatus (external ear canal). It is important to establish whether changes in the posture of the vertebral column are compensated, and whether this is happening inside or outside the vertebral column.

Examination

The Basic Planes, Axes, and Directions

In functional diagnosis, the concept of the zero position is used. It is also called the anatomic position. The zero position is the internationally accepted starting position for describing and measuring joint movements. The movements are described in three basic planes (as shown in **Figure 6–1**):

- Sagittal (A)
- Frontal (B)
- Transverse (C)

Movements in each of these planes are performed about the following axes:

- Frontal axis (a)
- Sagittal axis (b)
- Vertical axis (c)

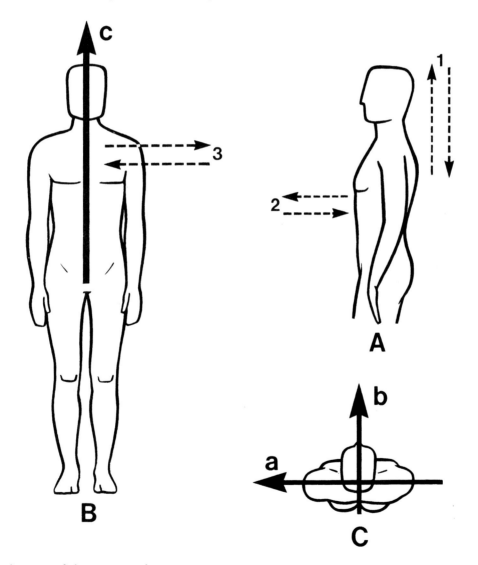

Figure 6–1   Basic directions of planes, axes, and movements.

To specify the direction of a movement, the following terms are used:

- Caudal–cranial (1)
- Ventral–dorsal (2)
- Medial–lateral (3)
- Combinations of the preceding

When describing the direction, it is assumed for all starting positions that the upper vertebra moves in relation to the one below it.

General Examination

Considerations Preceding Examination

It is only partly true to say that examinations of the neuromusculoskeletal system follow a particular sequence. An examination always begins with history taking. This is followed if possible by observation. The rest of the examination strategy is then planned in the light of the findings up to this point. If a specialist medical examination is indicated, should a neurologic assessment, for instance, precede or follow the functional assessment?

In every phase of the examination, there comes a moment of decision about what should come next. It would be unjustifiably dogmatic to stick to an arbitrarily imposed examination protocol. The examination should not be unnecessarily stressful for the patient and must in no circumstances aggravate the symptoms or cause them to spread. The place of the functional assessment, or its continuation, depends on the circumstances of the moment. In general, if central neurologic signs or radicular symptoms are present, the neurologic examination should precede the active examination. If, however, there are no reasons for referring to a medical specialist first, the limits of the patient's load-bearing capacity will not be exceeded, and there is a positive belief that the active examination will provide valuable further information, the therapist may decide to continue the assessment by carrying out a targeted functional examination. This involves the selection of appropriate diagnostic and manual examination tests from the range available. The therapist must also decide to what extent the examination should include, in addition to the specific problem area, the whole segment, its sphere of influence, and vegetatively related segments.

Active Examination

During the active examination, the movements that the patient is asked to make are initially performed freely. After that, he or she may be set tasks that will yield further information or will confirm the presence of dysfunctions that were noted in earlier parts of the examination. During the active examination, the examiner looks for pathologic signs and symptoms, and observes the way in which the patient makes the movements.

The movements that are included in the active examination are as follows:

Flexion	- Extension		
Flexion	- Sidebending	- Ipsilateral rotation	L + R
Extension	- Sidebending	- Ipsilateral rotation	L + R
Flexion	- Sidebending	- Contralateral rotation	L + R
Extension	- Sidebending	- Contralateral rotation	L + R

Regional Examination

Active-Guided Regional Examination

During active-guided examination of a region, no corrections are made if the patient does not perform the requested actions appropriately. The therapist follows the movement to look for possible deviations within a given movement pattern. In this part of the examination, the quality of the endfeel is of secondary importance.

Active-Assisted Regional Examination

During active-assisted examination of a region, the movements are controlled by the therapist. If a movement is problematic, the therapist will note the associated assistance. In this part of the examination, special attention is paid to the quality of the endfeel.

The regional active examination is carried out in the regions C0–T4, T4–T12, and T12–S1. The restraining hand is placed on the last vertebra of the region. The working hand/arm leads the movements by directing the patient's head, arms, and thorax. When assessing the ventral/extension component in the lumbar region, backward and forward tipping of the pelvis can be used.

The movements to be carried out during the active-assisted examination are as follows:

Flexion	- Extension		
Flexion	- Sidebending	- Ipsilateral rotation	L + R
Extension	- Sidebending	- Ipsilateral rotation	L + R

and depending on the active examination:

Flexion	- Sidebending	- Contralateral rotation	L + R
Extension	- Sidebending	- Contralateral rotation	L + R

THE ENDFEEL

The endfeel is the quality of the resistance at the end of the movement. The following distinctions are made according to the structure that is limiting the movement (Cyriax, 1947):
Normal:

- *Hard.* Bony resistance at the end of a physiologic movement
- *Firm.* Ligamentous resistance at the end of a physiologic movement
- *Elastic resilient.* Capsular resistance at the end of a physiologic movement
- *Soft.* Noneccentric resistance of soft tissues at the end of a physiologic movement

Pathological:

- *Hard.* Bony resistance at a point before the physiologic end of the movement
- *Firm.* Ligamentous resistance at a point before the physiologic end of the movement
- *Firm resilient.* Muscular spasm at every stage
- *Resilient.* Capsular resistance at some stage before the physiologic end of the movement
- *Rebound.* Jack-knife phenomenon, fixation of meniscus or segment
- *Empty.* No resistance, pain in serious disorders

Patla and Paris (1982) have provided a slightly different classification with regard to endfeel:
Normal:

- *Soft tissue approximation.* Soft and spongy. Examples: elbow or knee flexion
- *Muscle.* Elastic reflex resistance with discomfort. Examples: maximal hip flexion with stretched knee (SLR)
- *Ligament.* Firm arrest of movement with no perceptible give or creep. Example: abduction or extension of the knee
- *Cartilage.* Sudden stopping of the movement, without hard resistance. Example: extension of the elbow
- *Capsular.* Firm resistance to the movement, which can, however, be continued to a limited extent. Example: hyperextension of the elbow

Pathological:

- *Capsular.* Expressed in patterns specific to the joint: (a) chronic inflammation; (b) acute inflammation. Therapy: stretching

- *Adhesions and scars.* Sudden, sharp arrest in one direction. Therapy: tone inhibition
- *Bony block.* Sudden, hard stop before the end of the movement. Example: myositis ossificans
- *Bony grating (crepitation).* Caused by uneven, rough joint facets. Example: advanced chondromalacy
- *Springy rebound.* Example: luxated meniscus. Therapy: manual therapy
- *Pannus.* A slightly grinding, squelching endfeel. Example: generally in extension of the elbow
- *Loose, slack, too lax.* Expressed with laxity of the ligaments and general hypermobility. Therapy: stabilization
- *Empty.* Boggy and soft. Examples: synovitis, hemarthrosis
- *Painful.* Marked pain before the end of the movement. A distinction is made between an endfeel where the resistance is caused by pain and an endfeel caused by inflammation of the capsule, callus formation, or muscle spasms. Examples: "suspicious" disorders, including neoplasms

During the active-assisted examination of spinal regions, the therapist gains no more than an impression of the quality of endfeel throughout the whole chain of joints in the region. Localized pain and other signs of segmental dysfunction may point to specific segments within the region. Nevertheless, the active-assisted examination, in which the quality of endfeel in all the segments in the affected region should be examined, will identify the location of the dysfunction.

Manual Muscle Tests

During manual muscle tests, examples of which are illustrated in **Figures 6–2, 6–3, 6–4,** and **6–5,** the emphasis is on provocation of the musculotendinous system. The tests are carried out isometrically and should be repeated several times. They can yield information about the following factors:

- Willingness to move
- Strength
- Coordination
- Pain

A manual muscle test can yield information about strength and pain that will help to distinguish among the following possibilities:

Normal strength, no pain: No abnormalities

Normal strength, pain: Small lesion in musculotendinous system

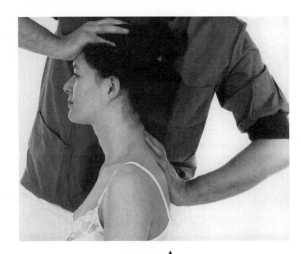

Figure 6–2   Manual muscle test. ↑

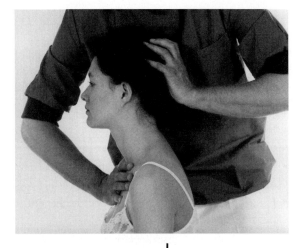

Figure 6–3   Manual muscle test. ↓

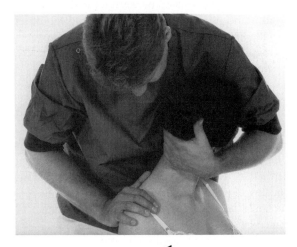

Figure 6–4   Manual muscle test.

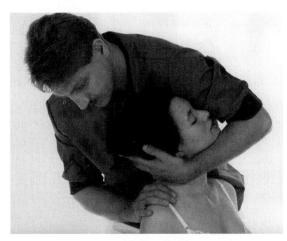

Figure 6–5   Manual muscle test.

Reduced strength, no pain: Neurogenic lesion, recently healed musculotendinous rupture

No strength, no pain: Neurogenic lesion, total musculotendinous rupture

Normal strength, pain on repetition: Arterial disorder

Normal strength, pain on all resistance tests: Acute lesion, serious disorder, psychogenic

The patient may experience so much pain that he or she is unwilling to engage in muscular activity. The examiner should be aware that under these circumstances, it is impossible to gain an accurate impression of muscular strength.

Selective Tissue Tension Examination

Unlike the active-assisted examination, this examination is described as "passive," which means that the active component should be switched off to the extent possible during the assisted movements. The clinical findings described by Cyriax (1947) are listed subsequently, together with possible interpretations.

Both active and passive movements are limited and painful in the same direction. Pain is felt at the endrange of the movement. The resistance test is not painful. A noncontractile structure is damaged, or a contractile structure is painfully shortened. Possible interpretations are:

- *Capsular pattern.* This is a set pattern of restricted movements, with or without pain, characteristic of a particular joint or of the joints in a particular region of the vertebral column. The capsular pattern indicates a dysfunction of the whole joint. The muscular adaptation is secondary. The degree of restriction on movement depends on the extent of the disorder.
  - *Cervical spine.* Extension, sidebending, and left and right rotation are the most limited and are limited to a similar degree. Flexion is the least limited.
  - *Thoracic spine.* Left and right rotation are the most restricted movements and are affected first.
  - *Lumbar spine.* Extension and right and left sidebending are the most limited. Flexion is the least restricted.

The capsular pattern is described here as described by Cyriax (1947). It has been the subject of a great deal of discussion because of the complicated structure of the vertebral column. However, there seems to be a fair measure of agreement about the fact that in all regions of the spine, flexion is the least limited and is affected last.

- *Noncapsular pattern.* This consists in restricted movement(s) in one or more directions, with or without pain, and not corresponding to the capsular pattern. Localization of the damage:

Intra-articular

Internal derangement
- Arthropathy
- Osteophytosis
- Ankylosis

Capsular
- Partial capsular adhesion

Extra-articular
- Osteogenic deformity
- Ligamentous adhesion
- Cyst
- Lymph blockage
- Hematoma
- Neuromuscular reflex contracture (Lasègue)
- Musculotendinous shortening (contracture, adhesions, calcifications, stenosis)

Intervertebral disk
- Pathology of the endplates
- Disk narrowing
- Protrusion
- Prolapse

No restriction of active or passive movement. Painful in the same direction. The resistance test is not painful:

Articular. Arthritis in the initial stages:
- Intervertebral joint
- Costovertebral joint
- Costotransverse joint
- Sternocostal joint

Extra-articular
- Ligamentous lesion

Intervertebral disk
- Small protrusion

No restriction of active or passive movement in the same direction. No change in basic pain level during active examination. Referred pain caused by pathology elsewhere in the body. The range of active and passive movements in the same direction is increased. Pain may or may not be present:
- Arthrogenic deformation
- Capsuloligamentous hypermobility
- Spondylolisthesis
- Fracture

Full passive range of movement, limited active range, in the same direction pain may or may not be present:
- Myogenic lesion
- Tendinous lesion
- Partial musculotendinous rupture
- Neurogenic lesion
- Psychogenic lesion

Passive movement is painful and may be restricted in one direction. Active movement is painful and may be restricted in the opposite direction:
- Musculotendinous lesion

REGIONAL PROVOCATION TESTS

Regional provocation tests are tests in which one or more movements is/are carried out for the purpose of loading particular tissues or organs in the region (**Figure 6–6**). Positive findings form a basis for some of the decisions involved in differential diagnosis.

Regional Springing Test

The regional springing test (A) gives a general idea of the elasticity of a region and of the pain present. If a particular

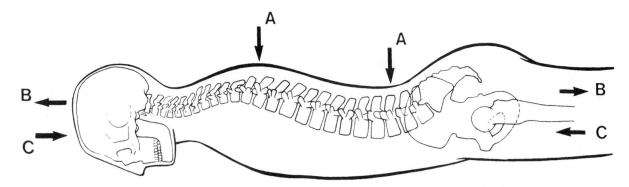

Figure 6–6　Regional springing, traction, and compression tests.

region is painful, or in some degree stiff relative to other regions, a more detailed specific examination is indicated.

Regional Traction Test

In the regional traction test (B), pressure on the intervertebral disks is reduced and a more or less translatory movement takes place in the intervertebral joints. The test yields information about the intersegmental structures at one or more levels. Some symptoms may appear under traction, and others may disappear.

Regional Compression Test

In the regional compression test (C), the intervertebral disks are compressed and a more or less translatory movement takes place in the intervertebral joints. This test can yield information about the intersegmental structures at one or more levels (for information on carrying out the test, see Chapter 14 and Chapter 15).

SEGMENTAL EXAMINATION

Segmental Tissue-Specific Examination

Where there is dysfunction in a particular segment, provocation tests will be carried out and the joints examined in that segment. However, the following tissue-specific tests are carried out first:

- Light touch test
- Kibler test
- Palpation for hypertonicity of intrinsic musculature
- Coordination test of segmental musculature
- Palpation of specific pain points

Segmental Provocation Tests

Segmental provocation tests are a number of tests aimed at assessing the function of the segmental joint mechanisms. These are carried out in addition to the active-assisted examination and the regional provocation tests.

Segmental Springing Test

The segmental springing test is only performed on the lumbar and thoracic regions. It is applied via the transverse or spinous processes in a posterior-to-anterior direction. The main function of this test is to provide information about the resilience of the segment (elastic behavior). The examiner also looks for any evidence of pain and any other symptomatology arising from the segment. The movements that take place in the intervertebral joints above and below the segment differ according to the region of the spine.

Figure 6–7 shows springing via the transverse processes.

Thoracic. Gapping at the caudal level (the joints open caudally and are compressed cranially). There is traction at the cranial aspect.

Lumbar. Translation: the inferior articular processes move in a dorsocranial direction, and the superior articular processes move in a ventrocranial direction.

Springing in a ventral direction via the spinous processes results in the following movements in different regions (**Figure 6–8**):

Thoracic. Compression in the caudal joints and gapping in the cranial ones.

Lumbar. In the caudal joints, the inferior articular processes slide in a ventral direction, which is associated with in-

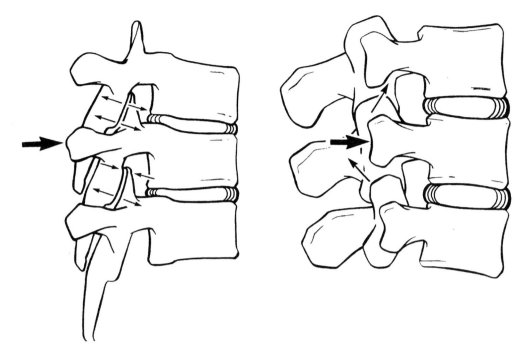

Figure 6–7 Segmental springing test via transverse processes.

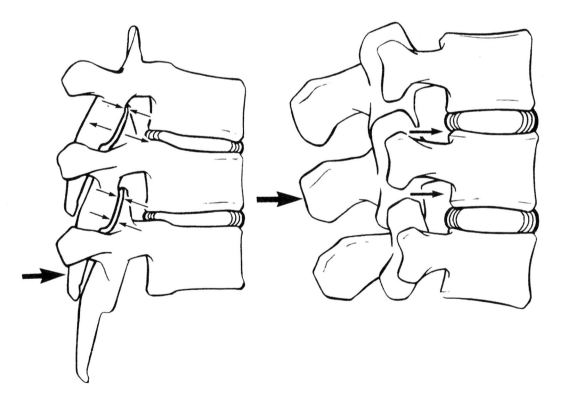

Figure 6–8 Segmental springing test via spinous processes.

creasing compression depending on how far forward the joint facets are. In the joints that lie above, the superior articular processes also slide in a ventral direction. This is accompanied by extension.

Finally, in the thorax, it is possible to carry out the spring test via the caudal aspect of the spinous process in a cranioventral direction. When this is done, the inferior and superior articular processes both slide in a cranioventral direction, which causes dorsal flexing in the segment above and ventral flexing in the segment below.

The segmental spring test technique is also suitable for examining the mobility of the sacroiliac joint.

Segmental Traction Test

The traction test described earlier can also be carried out at the segmental level, though in practice, it can be used only in the cervical region. The segments above the level to be worked on are locked. The working hand is placed above the segment to be moved and as close to it as possible. The other hand restrains the lower vertebra of the segment.

Segmental Rotation Test

This test is performed on the thoracic and lumbar segments of the spinal column (**Figure 6–9**). The movements that take place in the intervertebral joints above and below differ according to the region.

Thoracic. When left rotational pressure is applied, the contralateral inferior articular process of the joint to be moved slides in a ventral-lateral-cranial direction. The ipsilateral inferior articular process of the joint slides in a dorsal-medial-caudal direction.

Lumbar. When left rotational pressure is applied, there is compression in the contralateral joint, and the inferior articular process of the joint to be moved slides in a ventral-medial-cranial direction. In the ipsilateral joint, there is traction accompanied by sliding in a dorsal-lateral-cranial direction.

Active-Assisted Segmental Examination

A dysfunctional segment can have a biomechanical as well as a neuroreflexogenic effect on other segments in the spinal column. Where a segment is dysfunctional, therefore, the whole spinal column should be examined. The following will serve as a basic order of examination:

- The level indicated by the symptoms
- Neighboring levels
- Sympathetically related levels
- Transitional areas
- The rest of the segments, if the existing information about them is insufficient

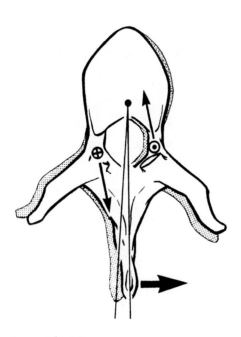
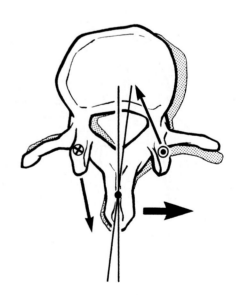

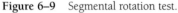

Figure 6–9   Segmental rotation test.

The following movements are carried out during the active-assisted examination:

Flexion   - Extension
Flexion   - Sidebending - Ipsilateral rotation   L + R
Extension - Sidebending - Ipsilateral rotation   L + R

and, depending on the results of the active examination:

Flexion   - Sidebending - Contralateral rotation L + R
Extension - Sidebending - Contralateral rotation L + R

Notation of Findings

The factors that can be noted simply in a diagram during a movement examination are disturbance of direction of movement in three dimensions, the structure responsible, the most disturbed component, and the pain factor. Other symptoms, such as skin and tissue reactions, hypertonicity, trigger points, and the degree of radicular referral, should be recorded separately (**Figure 6–10**).

ORIENTATION AND PALPATION

Palpation of Specific Tissues and Organs

The changes in organs and tissues that can be identified on observation as well as palpation, and which are measurable, are shown in **Table 6–1**.

Specific Palpatory Pain Points

Points that are painful under pressure have been described in different ways by a number of authors (Sell, 1969; Simons, 1976; Travell, 1976, 1981; Melzack, 1981; Reynolds, 1969; Dvorak and Dvorak, 1983). The range of terms that has been used (myogeloses, *Muskelhärte*, soft tissue rheumatism, muscular rheumatism, and fibrositis) suggests that the authors were striving to put their clinical findings into words. In the modern literature, we find the terms *tender point, myofascial trigger point,* and *tendomyosis* (Barker and Saito, 1981; Sutter, 1974; Oostendorp, 1984, 1985, 1988; Hagenaars, Dekker, van der Plaats, Bernards, and Oostendorp, 1985).

On the basis of clinical findings, three specific pain points are distinguished, though they have one feature in common, namely, they are spontaneously painful, or sensitive to pressure, by comparison with the surrounding tissues. In the muscles where pressure-sensitive points are found, additional signs are often encountered, for example, hypertonicity, stiffness, fatigue, shortening, pain with contraction, and an altered endfeel during passive stretching. These muscular changes indicate segmental muscle problems. Owing to trophic dysregulation, there may also be specific reactions in other tissues in the segment. The changes in cross-striated muscle are thought to result from the effects of the sympathetic nervous system on these muscles (Hagenaars et al., 1985). In segments C8–L2, the lateral horns contain both the preganglionic neurons of the local innervation and the peripheral innervation of the sympathetic nervous system. The peripheral sympathetic innervation of the head, arm, and leg is from segments C8–T3, T3–T9, and T10–L2.

The postganglionic sympathetic fibers may course along the blood vessels or with the spinal nerves. Nociceptive afferents enter the dorsal horn synapse via interneurons with (**Figures 6–11** and **6–12**):

- The motor neurons in the motor ventral horn
- The preganglionic neurons of the sympathetic nervous system in the motor lateral horn (Hagenaars, 1987)
- Neurons whose axons join the ascending conductive pathways

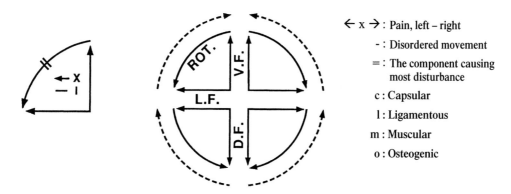

Figure 6–10   Notation graphic; LF = Sidebending, VF = Flexion, DF = Extension.

Table 6-1   Visible, Papable, and Measurable Findings

	Visible	Palpable	Measurable
Skin and subcutaneous connective tissue	Color Swelling Hair growth Pigmentation Moisture Scars Striae Dimpling	Temperature Moisture Edema Tissue resistance Tissue consistency Mobility/pliability Sensitivity Pain Point	Temperature Circumference Degree of sensitivity
Muscles, myotendinous junction, tendons, and tendon attachments	Shape Contour Volume	Tone Myogeloses Taut band formation Pain point	Circumference Myogeloses power Length when stretched
Tendon sheaths and bursae	Shape Swelling	Swelling Crepitus Pain point	Swelling
Synovial joint	Shape Contour Position Swelling	Endfeel Joint play Swelling Shape changes Crepitus Pain point	Range of motion Circumference Swelling
Bone/periosteum	Shape Thickening	Consistency Pain point	Vibration sense
Nerves		Pain on compression or tensile loading Pain point	Conduction
Blood vessels	Filling Pulsation	Pulsation Consistency	Frequency Blood pressure

Nociceptive afferent input that enters above C8 and below L2 can also pass to preganglionic neurons of the local innervation area of the sympathetic innervation and can influence the tissue structures that are linked with these segments. This is possible in the absence of selective blocking of the inhibitory descending pathways and a segmental imbalance between thick-fiber gnostic and thin-fiber nociceptive information.

Under normal circumstances, the nociceptive input is controlled by the interaction between the thick-fiber gnostic and thin-fiber nociceptive input and the endogenous pain control system. The inhibitory pathways that are active in this control process are the dorsolateral funiculus from the nucleus raphe magnus, the rubrospinal tract, and the lateral corticospinal tract.

In an alarm phase (Selye, 1978; Lurija, 1982; Bernards, 1991), with continuing increase in nociceptive input, the ac-

tivity of the sympathetic nervous system will increase. This stimulates the ergotrophic functions and increases activity in the interneuron population. According to the size principle (Henneman, 1980), there will be an increase in tonic activity in the smallest preganglionic neurons in the lateral horn and the smallest motor neurons in the ventral horn. The tonic activity is most marked in the vasoconstrictory neurons of the blood vessels in the cross-striated muscles and skin, and less so in the sudomotor neurons. Prolonged increase in sympathetic activity seems not only to affect the synovial joints and skin, but also to have a number of pathologic effects on the cross-striated muscles, which could explain the clinical signs. These effects are (Hagenaars et al., 1985) as follows:

- *Hypertonicity.* In the a-selective phase of the central nervous system, there is increased activity in the reticular formation, which leads to increased activity of

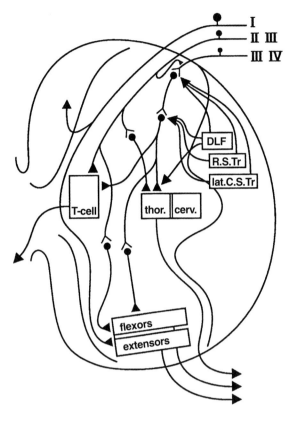

Figure 6–12 Afferent entrance, synaptic connections, and descending influences at the thoracic spinal cord level. *Source:* Reproduced from Hagenaars, 1987.

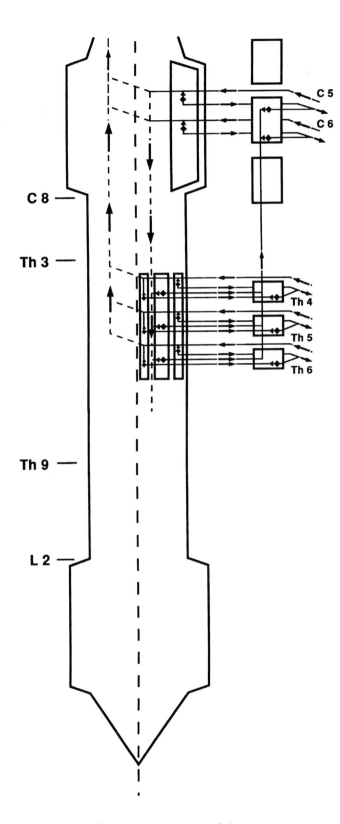

Figure 6–11 Schematic representation of the synaptic connections of the nociceptive afferents. *Source:* Reproduced from Hagenaars, 1987.

the spinal interneurons in lamina VII. These interneurons synapse on the motor neurons in lamina IX of the spinal cord. The motor neuron pools of the flexors are situated dorsally of the motor neuron pools of the extensors in the ventral horn (**Figure 6–13**).

As a result, when there is increased activity in the sympathetic nervous system, the hypertonicity shows primarily in the flexors. When there is segmental imbalance between thick-fibered gnostic afferents and thin-fibered nociceptive afferents, and no selective blocking of the inhibitory descending pathways, the activity of the interneuron population will also increase. Because the nociceptive afferents project on to the interneurons of lamina VII of the spinal cord, tone will increase in the segmentally related cross-striated muscles via synapses on the motor neurons in lamina IX. Moreover, because the nociceptive afferents are not blocked, their influence will cause the activity in the preganglionic neurons in the lateral horn of the spinal cord to increase. This may also lead to increased tone in the cross-striated segmental muscles.

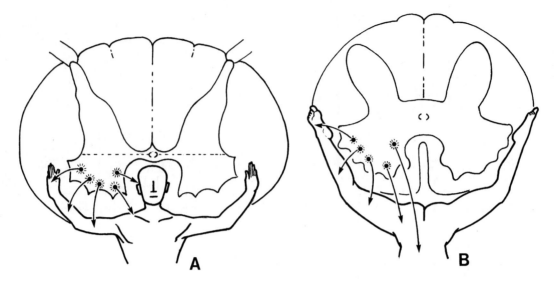

Figure 6–13   Localization of the motor neurons in the ventral horn of the spinal cord: A. cervical level; B. lumbar level.

• *Reduction in effective circulation.* When the activity of the preganglionic neurons is not selectively dampened by inhibitory descending pathways, the result is an overactive sympathetic nervous system. If in addition the balance between thick-fibered and thin-fibered afferents appears disturbed in certain segments, the tonic activity in the vasoconstrictive neurons of the blood vessels of the cross-striated muscles will increase even more. The resulting vasoconstriction affects the arterioles as well as the venules (Blumberg and Jänig, 1983) in the muscles whose blood vessels are innervated by the affected segment (**Figure 6–14**).

The vasoconstriction leads to an increase in vessel resistance in the affected muscles. Blood vessel resis-

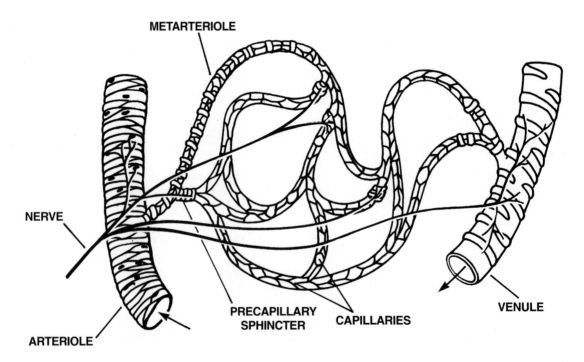

Figure 6–14   Sympathetic innervation of the blood vessels.

tance is not increased in the muscles of the unaffected segments. The blood therefore follows the path of least resistance. The volume of arterial blood that passes through the narrowed blood vessels per unit time therefore declines. The reduction in effective blood supply to the affected musculature may explain the earlier occurrence of fatigue in a particular muscle.

- *Changes in the muscular connective tissue.* The reduction in circulation affects the metabolism of the connective tissue. The quantity of matrix (ground substance) is reduced and its composition changes, which affects viscosity. The decrease in ground substance and the reduction in activity because of pain and the tendency to tire more easily lead to changes in the structure of the connective tissues. The three-dimensional pattern of the existing collagen fibers will be disturbed by the newly synthesized fibers (**Figure 6–15**).

These new fibers will bind themselves to the existing collagen fibers by means of cross-links, thus changing the behavior of the connective tissue in the muscles (Donatelli and Owens-Burkhart, 1981; Heerkens, 1987). This connective tissue will gain in mechanical resistance and will thus become stiffer and less able to cope with external forces. This may explain clinical signs such as stiffness, a tough passive endfeel, and reduced range of movement (Oostendorp, 1988). Although there is no scientific support for this, Sutter (1974) suggests that functional changes in the muscular connective tissue are reflexogenic in origin because the changes can disappear as soon as the nociceptive stimulation stops. Paravertebral tender points may also be seen in this light because they disappear spontaneously when the joint recovers its normal function.

- *Increased receptor sensitivity.* The threshold of the receptors in the cross-striated muscle is lower when the

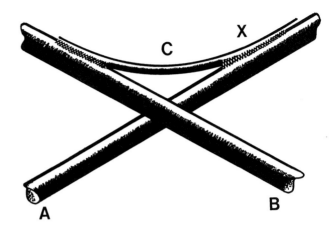

Figure 6–15 Cross-links (X) between existing collagen fibers (A, B) and a newly synthesized fiber (C).

activity of the segmental sympathetic nervous system is raised. When the generator potential increases, the Pacinian pressure receptors become more sensitive. In this state of increased sensitivity, even weak stimulation of the Pacini corpuscle produces a high discharge frequency, which, entering the nervous system in the alarm phase, is experienced as pain. Under these circumstances, even mild pressure on the muscle, or mild contraction, can cause pain (Nathan, 1983; Wiesenfeld-Hallin and Hallin, 1983). The concentration of Pacini corpuscles seems to be greatest in the tendon and around the motor endplate of the muscle. When the pressure receptors are in a state of increased sensitivity, these locations are especially sensitive to pressure and may be identified as specific pain points. If there is pain referral during pressure, this is called a *myofascial trigger point* (Travell and Simons, 1984) (**Figure 6–16**).

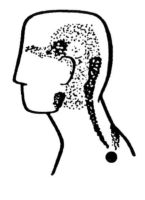 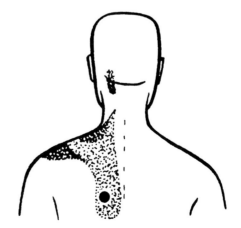

Figure 6–16 Myofascial trigger points in the trapezius muscle.

We may conclude from the preceding that the following factors can cause damage to the movement systems, including the cross-striated muscles:

- Absence of selective blocking by inhibitory descending pathways, and segmental imbalance between thick-fibered gnostic afferents and thin-fibered nociceptive afferents
- Increased activity in the sympathetic part of the vegetative nervous system
- Reduced dynamic activity as a result of pain and fatigue (Bernards and Oostendorp, 1988)

The consequences are most apparent in the areas innervated by the ramdorsal and meningeal rami of the spinal nerves at the C8–L2 levels.

TENDER POINT, MYOFASCIAL TRIGGER POINT, AND TENDOMYOSIS

Distinctions are made in the literature between tender point, myofascial trigger point, and tendomyosis. Given the circumstances under which these specific pain points develop, and the ways in which they do so, it is probably appropriate to consider them together. The differences among them may be caused by variations in the level and duration of increased activity in the sympathetic nervous system.

For both methodological and clinical reasons, the clinical signs of the three kinds of specific pain points are described separately.

Tender Point Clinical Signs

The following signs of tender points can usually be found:

- Usually in the vicinity of the affected joint.
- Mildly swollen and sensitive to pressure.
- Relatively small surface area, 0.5–1 cm².
- The muscles respond to mechanical stimulation with a local contraction (twitch).
- There is no referral with mechanical pressure.
- The patient is usually unaware of the tender point (Hoogland, 1987).
- In spondylogenic dysfunction, there are often a number of paravertebral tender points.
- With appropriate therapy, tender points become less acute.

- Inappropriate therapy causes them to become more sensitive.

The presence of tender points may indicate—through nociceptive afferent input—a slight increase in the local activity of the sympathetic nervous system, resulting in increased sensitivity of the alpha motor neurons at the level of the affected segment (Hoogland, 1987). This is possible when the nociceptive activity is relatively limited and the inhibitory descending pathways block the surrounding segments selectively (Azevedo and Soares da Silva, 1981; Basbaum and Fields, 1984). It is not clear what kinds of tissue are affected. Generally, it is likely to be richly innervated tissues such as muscle tissue, joint capsule, and branches of the dorsal ramus and the spinal nerve (Hoogland, 1987). There are no obvious structural changes in the tissue. With focused therapy, the pain point always disappears directly and completely.

The innervation of the paravertebral musculature is organized more or less according to segments. Tender points are therefore most prominent in the context of dysfunction within the Junghanns movement segment (Korr, 1978). The tender points of the spinal column, which are also diagnostically important, appear at the level of the intervertebral joints. Please see Chapter 11 for the locations of the other tender points.

Myofascial Trigger Point

The concept of the myofascial trigger point has been described by many authors (Simons, 1976; Travell, 1976, 1981; Melzack, 1981; Reynolds, 1969). According to Travell (1976), the clinical signs are as follows:

- Circumscript areas of deep sensitivity in the muscle, having an area of 1 cm².
- Exogenous stimulation by pressing or needling causes a local contraction (twitch) or fasciculation of the muscle.
- When pressure passes the threshold level, referral occurs.

Van Stralen (1985) adds the following signs:

- The patient is usually unaware of the point.
- It may or may not be part of the reported symptoms.
- Stimulation of the point may be felt at the spot or elsewhere.
- The point is not associated with a specific disorder.

The literature affords little information about how trigger points arise. Hagenaars et al. (1985) and Oostendorp (1988) maintain that insufficient selective blocking of nociceptive transmission by the endogenous pain control system, and imbalance between thick-fibered and thin-fibered afferent nerves, lead to increased activity in the sympathetic nervous system. This in turn causes the sensitivity of receptors, including the Pacinian pressure receptors, to increase. The Pacini corpuscles seem to occur in great concentration around the motor endplate of the muscle and in the tendon. When there is a marked increase in sensitivity, these locations are extra sensitive, and a pain point may develop. If pain referral occurs when sufficient pressure is applied, the point may be considered a myofascial trigger point (Hagenaars et al., 1985). Van Stralen (1985) states that the afferents from the myofascial trigger point reach the level of the preganglionic sympathetic neurons via the spinal cord, and that treatment of the point will normalize the raised sympathetic activity.

In summary, the most important signs of a myofascial trigger point are the following:

- The occurrence of referral when sufficient pressure is applied
- The link with sympathetic innervation

Tendomyosis

Clinical signs of tendomyosis are the following (Brügger, 1965):

- The muscle tires relatively quickly.
- Rigor-like tone in the muscle (stiffness).
- Increased sensitivity to pressure, both exogenous and endogenous (contraction). The sensation, which may be reported as piercing, prickly, burning, or dull, can be localized in the muscle, the myotendinous region, the tendon, or the tenoperiosteal region.
- Tendency to fasciculation.
- Muscle shortening.
- Changed endfeel during passive elongation.
- Specific pain points.

The influence of increased activity of the sympathetic nervous system on the cross-striated muscle (Hagenaars et al., 1985; Oostendorp, 1988) is described in the introduc-

tion. The effects of this on the cross-striated muscle—such as hypertonicity, reduction in effective circulation, changes in the functional characteristics of the muscle connective tissue, and raised receptor sensitivity—appear to offer a satisfactory explanation of the clinical signs of tendomyosis.

The fact that the tendomyotic changes are segment-related has implications for therapy (Hagenaars, 1987). An inhibitory influence can be exercised on nociceptive transmission to the preganglionic neurons and in the dorsal horn through type II or fast type III receptors, such that afferent nerve fibers belonging to the same segment are stimulated. To promote continuing recovery, efforts must also be made to ensure that the phase of a-selective ergotrophic activity of the nervous system moves into a phase of selective tropotrophic activity. In the phase of renewed selective activity, the endogenous pain control system can be activated during recovery by graded stimulation of the nociceptive thin-fiber afferents.

This has a positive effect on the control of activity in the lateral horn. If the tonic preganglionic neurons of the associated local segment appear to be in a state of increased activity, this segment should be included initially in the treatment.

Therapy may lead to one of three clinically observable patterns (Hoogland, 1987):

- The phenomena disappear quickly and completely. In this case, it is probable that the reflexogenic component, for example, hypertonicity, was dominant, and that there are no structural changes in the affected tissues.
- The phenomena reduce, but do not disappear completely. This suggests that limited structural change has taken place.
- The signs only disappear after a long time. If it takes the signs weeks or months to reduce or disappear, it is likely that serious structural changes have taken place.

Nerve Pressure Points

Nerve pressure points can also be regarded as trigger points. They are in locations where peripheral nerves can be provoked for diagnostic or therapeutic purposes.

CHAPTER 7

Neurologic and Neurovascular Examination

In this book, only those aspects of neurologic examination are described that are most relevant to the examination of the spinal column. The reader is referred to the literature for a more extensive description of neurologic examination procedures.

Before we discuss the neurologic tests, some of which are shown in the illustrations, it is useful to provide a more detailed definition of the term *radicular syndrome*.

RADICULAR SYNDROME

The term *radicular syndrome* is used to indicate damage to a single root as a result of compression or tension (Brüegger, 1969).

The symptoms are as follows:

- Pain in the area innervated by the respective nerve root. According to Urban (1981), pressure on a nerve, or stretching, does not necessarily cause pain. Pain does always occur, however, when there is an inflammatory reaction with fibrosis in the nerve. Because the lymphatic system is poorly developed, the exudate from the inflammation cannot easily be carried away, which may be the cause of fibrosis after an inflammatory reaction. MacRae (Krämer, 1978) states that pain is experienced whenever chemical changes take place that cause the acidity level (pH) to fall below 7.

- Sensory abnormalities, especially affecting pain sense or algesia. An anesthetic zone appears only if more roots are damaged. In regard to the algesia, each segment has a specific area of innervation. There is much

less segmental overlapping of the pain sense than with other aspects of sensation.

With regard to aesthesia, hyperesthesia usually occurs initially and may be followed by hypesthesia, paresthesiae, or anesthesia. The loss of sensation is associated with a dermatomal distribution.

- Motor function loss corresponding to the radicular innervation of specific muscles that derive innervation exclusively from a particular segment. Failure of deep tendon or myotatic reflexes associated with the damaged root. Initially, this may cause hyperreflexia followed by hyporeflexia or areflexia. This must be differentiated from reflex loss resulting from a damaged peripheral nerve.

- Disturbance of paravertebral sensation; this happens when the root is damaged before the dorsal ramus branches away from the spinal nerve in the lateral aspect of the intervertebral foramen.

- Sympathetic phenomena such as piloerection and effects on secretion of sweat, vasomotor responses, and the musculoskeletal system can occur in acute root lesions. In certain circumstances, pronounced Sudeck's dystrophy can even be a consequence.

Neural Tension and Compression Tests

Neuromechanosensitivity is generally part of the clinical presentation of radicular syndrome. The clinician can test for the increased sensitivity of neural structures to mechanical stimuli by way of nerve tension and compression tests.

Tension Tests

Neural tension tests include various tests for the neural structures of both upper and lower quadrant.

Lasègue's Test, or Straight Leg Raise Test   With the patient supine, the straight leg at the involved side is flexed at the hip. (See **Figure 7–1**.) If pressure from a dorsolateral prolapse is obstructing the movement of the dural sleeve of the nerve root, or of the root itself, this hip flexion will be limited by pain and/or a sensory referral. The extent to which flexion is limited varies with the severity of the compressive factor or of any adhesions that may be present. If the restrictions of hip flexion occur at more than 60° to 70°, the test result is not considered positive. If a painful arc occurs in the course of the movement, this can indicate a small protrusion causing temporary compression of the nerve root or the spinal nerve. The test provides positive findings if the nerve roots of L4 to S2 are compressed.

Bertilson et al. (2006) rated the straight leg raise test as positive if pain radiated below the knee and if pain increased when the neck was flexed or the ankle dorsiflexed. This study established a percentage agreement of 98% and a κ value of 0.92 (95% CI: 0.65–1.00) for interrater agreement. Deville et al. (2000) compiled the results of 15 studies that looked at the diagnostic accuracy of the straight leg raise test for the clinical diagnosis of herniated lumbar disks. They calculated a sensitivity of 0.91 (95% CI: 0.82–0.94) and a specificity of 0.26 (95% CI: 0.16–0.38). This provided a positive likelihood ratio of 1.2 and a negative likelihood ratio of 3.5.

Pseudo Lasègue   If symptoms suggestive of compression occur, the amount of hip flexion is reduced until these disappear. The patient is then asked to contract the hamstring muscles hard against resistance. When after this contraction it is possible to bring the hip into the position in which previously symptoms suggestive of compression were reported without these symptoms recurring, this test finding is called a pseudo Lasègue (shortened hamstring muscles).

If symptoms of compression occur, the flexion of the hip is reduced until they disappear. The piriformis muscle is then tensed by internal rotation and adduction of the hip joint. If the symptoms of compression then reappear, this is probably caused by the M. piriformis compressing the sciatic nerve.

Bragard's Test   If the result of Lasègue's test is positive, the flexion of the hip is reduced until the symptoms of compression disappear. The foot is then moved passively and forcefully into dorsiflexion. If the symptoms of nerve root compression reappear, the Bragard's test is considered positive. (See **Figure 7–2**.)

Neck Flexion Test (Neri)   The neck is flexed, which stretches the dura mater (**Figure 7–3**). The symptoms may be provoked, depending on the level and location at which the root is stimulated.

Other possibilities are the following:

- An electrical sensation in the midline and occasionally pins and needles in hands and feet (L'Hermitte's sign, indicative of a central neurologic lesion)
- Pain in head and foot (Brudzinski I, indicative of meningitis)

This test is usually carried out in combination with Lasègue's test. For purposes of differential diagnosis, the

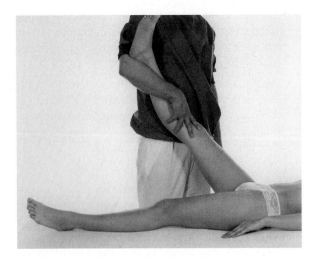

Figure 7–1

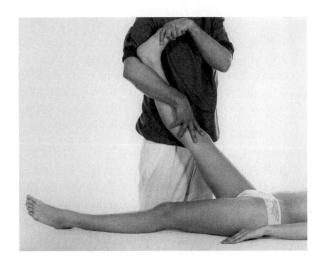

Figure 7–2

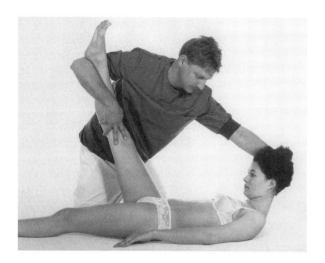

Figure 7–3

symptoms that are revealed by each of the three tests (Neri, Lasègue, and Bragard) must be carefully distinguished.

Uchihara et al. (1994) reported a sensitivity of 0.03 and a specificity of 0.97 for the L'Hermitte's sign in the diagnosis of focal myelopathic lesions, multiple sclerosis, or stenotic myelopathy.

Reverse Lasègue, or Prone Knee Bend Test The patient lies prone. The leg on the involved side is flexed at the knee joint and extended at the hip joint. (See **Figure 7–4**). If the compressive factor is limiting the mobility of the dural sleeve of the L3 nerve root, or the nerve root itself, this test will provoke the symptoms.

Porchet et al. (1994) reported a sensitivity of 0.84 for the prone knee bend test in the diagnosis of far lateral disk herniations at L3–S1. Kobayashi et al. (2003) reported a

92.8–100% reduction in intraoperative intraradicular blood flow and decrease of nerve root mobility to mere millimeters with the prone knee bend test in four patients with L3–L4 disk herniation.

Cross-Over Lasègue The patient lies supine and the leg on the uninvolved side is flexed at the hip, which pulls the dura in a caudal direction. This can bring about indirect compression of the nerve root on the involved side, causing a shooting pain in the nonflexed leg.

Alternatively, the flexion of the hip may cause the ilium on the ipsilateral side to tilt posteriorly, which also delivers a backward impulse on that side to the lower lumbar vertebrae. This brings about a small rotation, which may influence the structure that is compressing the contralateral root.

According to Zizina (1910), a positive Lasègue indicates that the lesion is in the spinal canal. According to Cyriax (1947), the compression occurs between the dura mater and the nerve root. A positive cross-over Lasègue would be most prevalent in the case of an axillary prolapse and at the level of the L4 nerve root.

Deville et al. (2000) compiled the results of eight studies that looked at the diagnostic accuracy of the cross-over straight leg raise test for the clinical diagnosis of herniated lumbar disks. They calculated a sensitivity of 0.29 (95% CI: 0.24–0.34) and a specificity of 0.88 (95% CI: 0.86–0.90). This provided a positive likelihood ratio of 2.4 and a negative likelihood ratio of 0.80.

Forward Bending Test The patient bends forward from a sitting or standing position, with the legs extended. (See **Figure 7–5**.) This stretches the dura and bilateral nerve roots. The test will be positive if there is compression of the

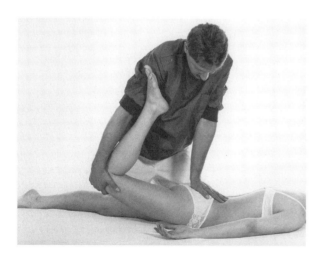

Figure 7–4

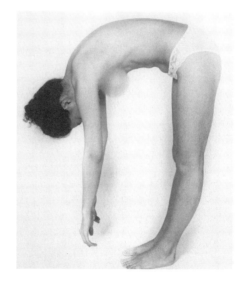

Figure 7–5

nerve roots of L4 to S2. Because it puts a greater load on the intervertebral disk, this test can give a positive result when Lasègue's test is negative.

Scapular Adduction Test   The test involves adduction of both scapulae, which stretches the first and second thoracic nerves and the dura in a cranial direction. (See **Figure 7–6**.) This can cause provocation at the level where irritation of the root or dura is suspected.

Brachial Plexus Tension Test   Following scientific studies, Elvey (1979) devised a procedure for placing the brachial plexus under tension. (See **Figures 7–7, 7–8, 7–9,** and **7–10**.) The patient lies supine and the following movements are carried out:

- Depression of shoulder girdle
- Abduction of upper arm to 90°
- External rotation of upper arm, hand behind shoulder
- Extension of elbow
- Dorsiflexion of wrist and fingers
- Supination of forearm
- Contralateral sidebending of cervical spine

This last movement is added if there is low irritability or to differentiate from other upper extremity pathology.

The test puts the following nerve tissues under maximum tension:

- Cervical nerve roots with their dural sleeve
- The dura that is anatomically related to said roots
- The brachial plexus and peripheral nerves

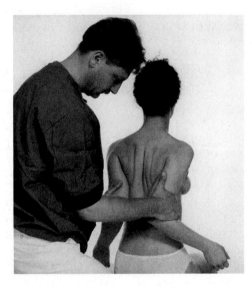

Figure 7–6

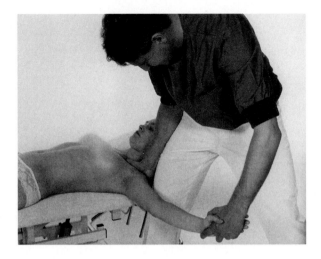

Figure 7–7

Biomechanically, the tension is brought about as follows: the median nerve, which lies anterior to the axis of extension of the elbow, is put under tension by extending the elbow and the wrist. The ulnar nerve, which runs along the medial aspect of the lower arm, is twisted and tensioned during supination. As a variation on the preceding test, the radial nerve–which lies posterior to the flexion axis of the elbow–can be stretched by bending the elbow.

The musculocutaneous nerve, which runs along the medial aspect of the upper arm, is twisted around the humerus and tensioned during external rotation of the upper arm. The same applies to a lesser degree to the median nerve. The brachial plexus is located inferior to the abduction axis of the upper arm and is stretched during abduction.

Finally, the nerve roots are put under extra tension by inducing contralateral sidebending of the cervical spine and by depressing the shoulder girdle.

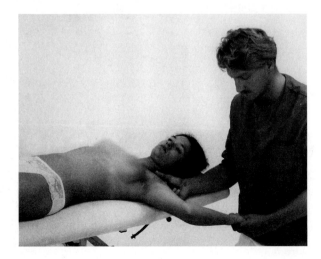

Figure 7–8

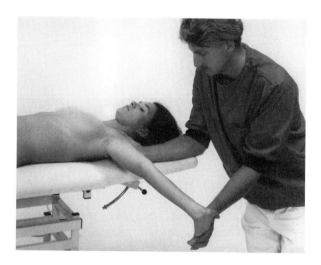

Figure 7–9

As with the straight leg raise test, this test allows quantification of the degree of dysfunction. The same starting position is used, but with the elbow bent. The point at which the symptoms occur as the elbow is extended is taken as an indicator of the degree of dysfunction.

The following sensitizing movements can be added to the test:

- Abduction and external rotation of the contralateral arm.
- Full flexion of the cervical spine. The cranial movement of the dura increases the tension on the intradural and extradural roots.
- Traction to the cervical spine.

An additional movement that may cause the symptoms to decrease is the 90° bilateral straight leg raise. This results

in some caudal movement of the dura, which reduces the load imposed during the test.

The provocation induced during the brachial plexus tension test has the greatest effect on the C5 and C6 nerve roots. It affects the C7 root to a lesser extent. Subjectively, the effects are experienced in the referral area in the arm and may also sometimes be felt at the medial edge of the scapula, the whole of the scapula, or in the pectoral area.

Wainner et al. (2003) established a κ value of 0.76 (95% CI: 0.51–1.0) for the interrater reliability of this test in the diagnosis of cervical radiculopathy. A positive test was defined as reproduction of the patient-reported symptoms, discrepancy in side-to-side elbow extension of >10°, or decrease in symptoms with ipsilateral cervical sidebending or increase with contralateral sidebending with regard to the symptomatic limb. Compared to a gold standard test of electrodiagnostic test findings, these authors also established a sensitivity of 0.97 (95% CI: 0.90–1.0) and a specificity of 0.22 (95% CI: 0.12–0.33). These values yielded a positive likelihood ratio of 0.12 (95% CI: 0.01–1.9) and a negative likelihood ratio of 1.3 (95% CI: 1.1–1.5).

Contralateral Cervical Sidebending Test If contralateral sidebending of the cervical spine is painful while all other cervical movements are free and painless, the possibility arises of a superior sulcus tumor (Cyriax, 1947). (See **Figure 7–11**.) If the result of the test is positive, elevation of the shoulder girdle and arm on the ipsilateral side should also be tried. If these movements are painful too, the patient should be referred to a medical specialist.

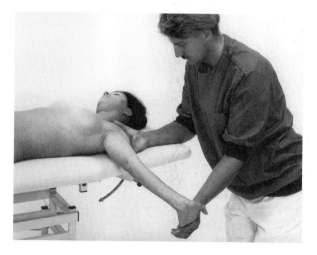

Figure 7–10

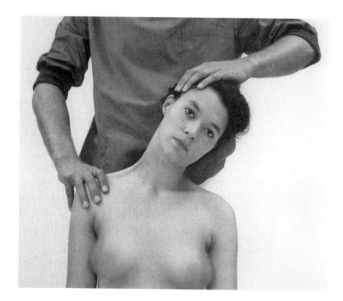

Figure 7–11

Compression Tests

Naffziger's Test   The jugular vein is compressed on both sides, which increases cerebrospinal fluid pressure. (See **Figure 7–12**.) This causes the pain to increase if there is a compressive pathology in the spinal canal.

Heel drop Test   The patient stands on tiptoes, and then drops onto his or her heels (**Figure 7–13**). This compresses the intervertebral disks, and the damaged disk may transfer the pressure to neighboring structures located dorsally or dorsolaterally.

Nerve Root Compression Test (Kemp)   The spinal column is extended dorsally and laterally, and rotated ipsilaterally in an extension quadrant position. (See **Figure 7–14**.) This test is intended to increase the compression on the ipsilateral side, thus provoking the symptoms. However, depending upon the position of the compressive pathology, the test can also produce a positive result on the contralateral side.

Extension Test   This test consists in extension from a standing position (**Figure 7–15**). If radicular pathology is present, and the movement provokes symptoms, whereas flexion of the trunk produces no symptoms, a disturbance at the level of L4–L5 is very probable.

Valsalva Maneuver   Coughing, sneezing, and straining cause an increase in intra-abdominal and intrathoracic pressure. The intravenous pressure and the cerebrospinal fluid pressure also increase. If a compressive pathology is present, these increases can compress dorsal or dorsolateral structures.

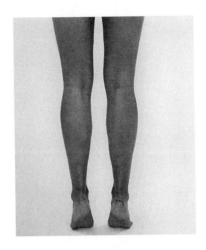

Figure 7–13

Wainner et al. (2003) established a κ value of 0.69 (95% CI: 0.36–1.0) for the interrater reliability of this test in the diagnosis of cervical radiculopathy. A positive test was defined as reproduction of the patient-reported symptoms. Compared to a gold standard test of electrodiagnostic test findings, these authors also established a sensitivity of 0.22 (95% CI: 0.03–0.41) and a specificity of 0.94 (95% CI: 0.88–1.0). These values yielded a positive likelihood ratio of 0.83 (95% CI: 0.64–1.1) and a negative likelihood ratio of 3.5 (95% CI: 0.97–12.6).

Piriformis Test   The patient lies supine. While the pelvis is held in contact with the surface below, the thigh is passively flexed through about 90° and brought into inter-

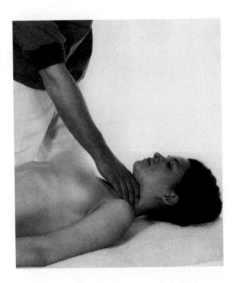

Figure 7–12

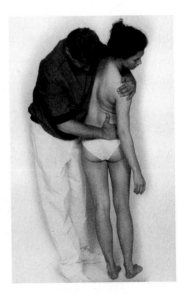

Figure 7–14

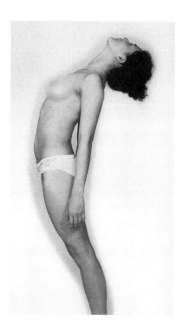

Figure 7–15

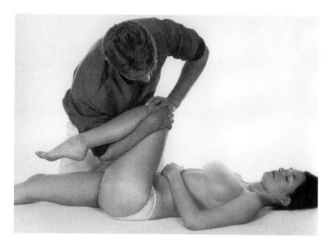

Figure 7–16

nal rotation and adduction. (See **Figure 7–16**.) The lower leg is flexed. This test is carried out when there are indications that symptoms may be caused by the piriformis muscle pressing on the sciatic nerve (See the section titled "Pseudo Lasègue" earlier in this chapter).

THORACIC OUTLET COMPRESSION SYNDROME

The structures that are involved in thoracic outlet compression syndrome are the cervical and upper thoracic spinal column, the cervical rib if present, the first rib, the collar bone, the shoulder blade, the scalenes, the subclavius, the sternocleidomastoid, the pectoralis minor, the subclavian artery, the subclavian vein, and the brachial plexus. The following definitions of the costoclavicular space, the anterior scalene port, the dorsal scalene port, and the coracopectoral port may be helpful (Van Meerwijk, 1979, 1984, 1986):

The *costoclavicular space* is the space between the first rib and the clavicle through which the neurovascular bundle courses.

The *anterior scalene port* is the space between the clavicular part of the sternocleidomastoid and the anterior scalene. Through this port run the subclavian vein, small arteries, the phrenic nerve, the omohyoideus muscle, and the large lymphatic vessels.

The *posterior scalene port* is the space between the anterior and middle scalenes. Through this port run the subclavian artery and the brachial plexus.

The *coracopectoral port* is the space between the attachments of the pectoralis minor to the coracoid process and the upper ribs. The neurovascular bundle courses through this space.

If compressive forces arise in these passages because of structural, congenital, or acquired abnormalities, and if these cause disorders, this is called a "pure" thoracic outlet compression syndrome.

Possible symptoms include the following:

- Pain in the neck, which may radiate to the back of the head
- Pain in the shoulder girdle
- Pain in the arm, sometimes radiating as far as the little finger
- A dull feeling and paresthesia in the area of the supraspinatus and the upper trapezius
- A feeling of loss of power in the arm and hand
- Difficulty in carrying heavy loads
- Inability to perform activities with the arms in a raised position for any length of time
- Shoulder–arm problems (heavy feeling, paresthesia) during sleep, particularly when the patient sleeps with his or her arms above the head

Neurovascular Tests

Adson Test

For this test, the patient stands or sits with the arms at the sides. (See **Figure 7–17**.) The head is held in maximum

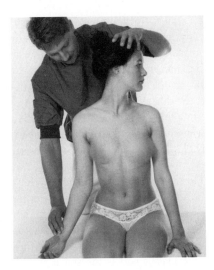

Figure 7–17

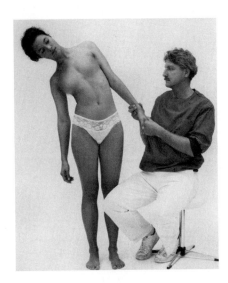

Figure 7–18

extension and ipsilateral rotation (in this position, the ipsilateral scalenes scissor each other) or contralateral rotation (the ipsilateral scalenes are thereby placed under tension). In this position, the patient breathes in deeply, which causes the scalenes to thicken (the first rib also rises). The position is held for 20 to 30 seconds. During the test, the quality of pulsations in the radial artery is examined. The therapist also looks for complaints that were noted in the history and the occurrence of a supraclavicular *souffle* (stethoscope) or, if the *souffle* was already present, the examiner checks whether it is now louder. This test is used if a compression is suspected in the dorsal scalene port, causing pressure on the neurovascular bundle.

Gillard et al. (2001) calculated a sensitivity of 0.79 and a specificity of 0.76 for the Adson test with the test scored positive if the radial pulse was abolished and/or the patient-reported symptoms were reproduced. Gold standard was a varied combination of findings on electrodiagnostic, computed tomography, and ultrasound studies.

Costoclavicular Test

During this test, the examiner sits on a stool. The patient stands with his or her back to the examiner and leans against the examiner's knee. (See **Figure 7–18.**) The patient's shoulder (clavicle) is moved downward and backward. The examiner asks the patient to bend his or her trunk over to the opposite side a little and to breathe in deeply, which causes the first rib to rise. This position is held for 20 to 30 seconds. During this test, the quality of pulsations in the radial artery is checked. The examiner also

watches for any complaints that were noted in the history and for the occurrence of a supraclavicular *souffle* (stethoscope), or an increase in the volume of a *souffle* already noted. This test is used if compression of the neurovascular bundle in the costoclavicular space is suspected. This pressure may be exerted by a cervical rib, the first rib, the clavicle, the subclavius muscle, and the costocoracoid ligament. According to Cyriax (1947), when the load is taken off the shoulder girdle, particularly at night, pins and needles are experienced in the hands.

The results of the Adson test and the costoclavicular test are always assessed in combination.

Plewa and Delinger (1998) reported a specificity of 0.89 for the costoclavicular test if vascular changes were considered a positive finding. When pain was considered a positive finding the specificity was 1.00 and with paresthesiae as a positive test, specificity was 0.85.

Hyperabduction Test

For this test, that patient's arm is guided slowly into an elevated hyperabduction position. This brings about a pulley action of the pectoralis minor around the coracoid process. The clavicle rotates around its longitudinal axis in a posterior direction. (See **Figures 7–19** and **7–20.**) During this test the quality of the pulsations in the radial artery is observed, and the occurrence of symptoms noted in the history. The examiner also watches whether the hands become white, and whether the capillaries fill after termination of the test. This test is used if compression of the neurovascular bundle in the coracopectoral port is suspected.

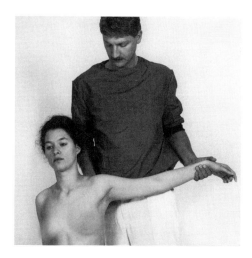

Figure 7–19

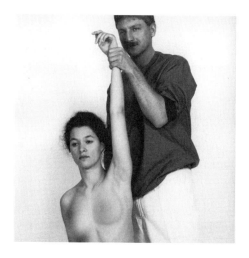

Figure 7–20

Sensitivity was established as 0.52 and 0.84 if a positive finding was defined as pulse abolition or symptom reproduction, respectively. Specificity was 0.90 and 0.40, respectively (Gillard et al., 2001).

Roos Test

During this test, the lower arms are bent at an angle of 90°, both upper arms are brought into 90° abduction/external rotation, and the shoulder girdle into depression/retraction. In this position, the hands are slowly clenched into fists and opened again for 3 minutes. (See **Figures 7–21** and **7–22**.) The criteria for this test are the quality of the radial pulse, the occurrence of signs and symptoms, the occurrence of a supraclavicular *souffle,* the hands turning white, and the filling of the capillaries after test termination.

Because these tests can also produce symptoms in people who have no complaints, they must be interpreted together. They must evoke or aggravate the complaints noted in the history. An asymmetrical pattern of complaints is the most likely clinical presentation.

Gillard et al. (2001) reported a sensitivity of 0.84 and a specificity of 0.30 for the Roos test with a positive test defined as reproduction of patient-reported symptoms.

Sensory Tests

Sensory tests form part of a full examination of sensorimotor function. Exteroception, proprioception, and enteroception are separate aspects of sensory function.

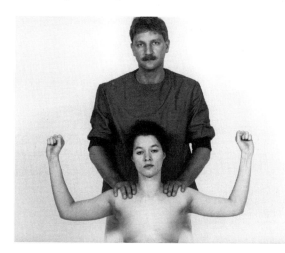

Figure 7–21

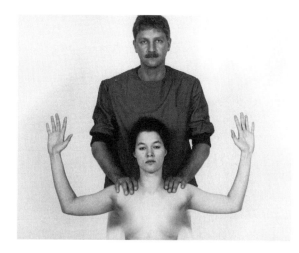

Figure 7–22

Exteroception

Exteroception is tested by examining the sensory function of the surface of the skin. First, the multisegmental peripheral nerve distribution (peripheral innervation) must be differentiated from the monosegmental radicular skin innervation (radicular innervation, dermatome). The boundaries are established with the aid of a small pinwheel. For purposes of differential diagnosis, changes in sensory function arising from pseudoradicular syndromes, nociceptive somatosympathetic syndromes, and entrapment neuropathies must also be included in the examination.

With regard to skin sensory function, the following can be distinguished:

- Surface tactile sensitivity to light touch, examined with a cotton wool ball or a brush (**Figure 7–23**) or quantified by using Semmes–Weinstein monofilaments (Peeters et al., 1998)
- Thermal sensitivity, examined with the aid of two tubes, one filled with cold water and one with warm (**Figure 7–24**)
- Surface sensitivity to pain, tested with an esthesiometer allowing for adjustable pressure, with a wheel, or by way of pinprick (**Figure 7–25**)

Qualitative distinctions are made using the following terms:

an	-	aesthesia	an	-	algesia
hypo	-	aesthesia	hyp	-	algesia
norm	-	aesthesia	norm	-	algesia
hyper	-	aesthesia	hyper	-	algesia
par	-	aesthesia	par	-	algesia
dys	-	aesthesia	dys	-	algesia

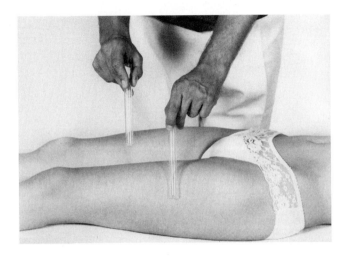

Figure 7–24

Proprioception

Proprioception is tested via deep sensitivity. The proprioceptive sensors can be grouped into capsular receptors, muscle receptors, tendon receptors, periosteal receptors, pressure receptors, and pain receptors.

Capsular Receptors   Wyke (1966) distinguishes four types of mechanoreceptors (see **Table 7–1**). There are mechanoreceptors that inform the nervous system about position and changes in position; these are type I and type II receptors. Type III receptors, situated in the ligaments, provide protection against excessive tension, analogous to that provided by the Golgi system in tendons. Finally, Wyke describes type IV receptors, which signal joint pain.

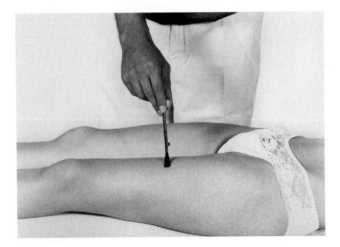

Figure 7–23

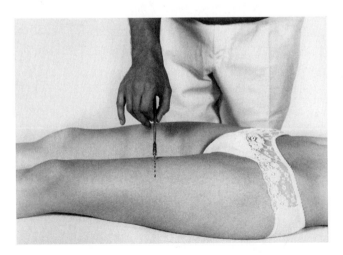

Figure 7–25

Table 7-1 Classification of Joint Receptors

Type	Structure	Location	Nerve fibers	Characteristics	Function
I	Thin capsule Round or ovoid corpuscles (100-40 micrometers) Units of 3-6 corpuscles	Fibrous joint capsule Mainly superficially located • Extremity joints (greater density proximal as compared to distal) • Zygapophyseal joint (highest density in cervical spine) • Temporomandibular joint	Thinly myelinated 6-9 micrometers (Type II)	Static and dynamic Low threshold Slow adaptation	• Tonic reflex effects on neck, jaw, extremities, and ocular muscles • Postural kinaesthetic sensation • Suppression of nociception
II	Thick capsule Conoid corpuscles (280-140 micrometers) Units of 2-4 corpuscles	Fibrous joint capsule Mainly in deeper locations and in joint capsule fat deposits • Extremity joints (greater density distal as compared to proximal) • Zygapophyseal joint • Temporomandibular joint • Intercartilaginous laryngeal connections (high density)	Moderately myelinated 9-12 micrometers (Type II)	Dynamic Low threshold Rapid adaptation	• Phasic reflex effects on neck, jaw, extremities, and ocular muscles • Suppression of nociception
III	Thin capsule Spindle-shaped corpuscles (600-100 micrometers) (large quantity of nerve endings almost identical to Golgi tendon organs)	Ligaments (extrinsic, intrinsic, usually near bony insertion) • Intrinsic, e.g., cruciate ligaments of the knee and round ligament of the hip • Extrinsic, e.g., collateral ligaments of the knee Not in longitudinal and interspinous ligaments of the vertebral column	Thickly myelinated 13-17 micrometers (Type I)	Dynamic (endrange positions) High threshold Very slow adaptation	
IV	Lattice-like organization of unmyelinated nerve fibers or free nerve endings	Fibrous joint capsule Adjacent to the periosteum Joint capsule fat deposits Ligaments Blood vessel walls • Extremity joints • Zygapophyseal joint • Temporomandibular joints Not in: • Synovial membrane • Menisci of the knee • Intervertebral disks	Very thinly myelinated 2-5 micrometers (Type III) Unmyelinated < 2 micrometers (Type IV)	Rapid nociceptive system (vasomotor reaction) Acute pain High threshold Adaptation Slow nociceptive fibers Chronic pain High threshold No adaptation	• Phasic reflex effects on neck, jaw, extremities, and ocular muscles • Nociception • Respiratory and cardiovascular reflex effects

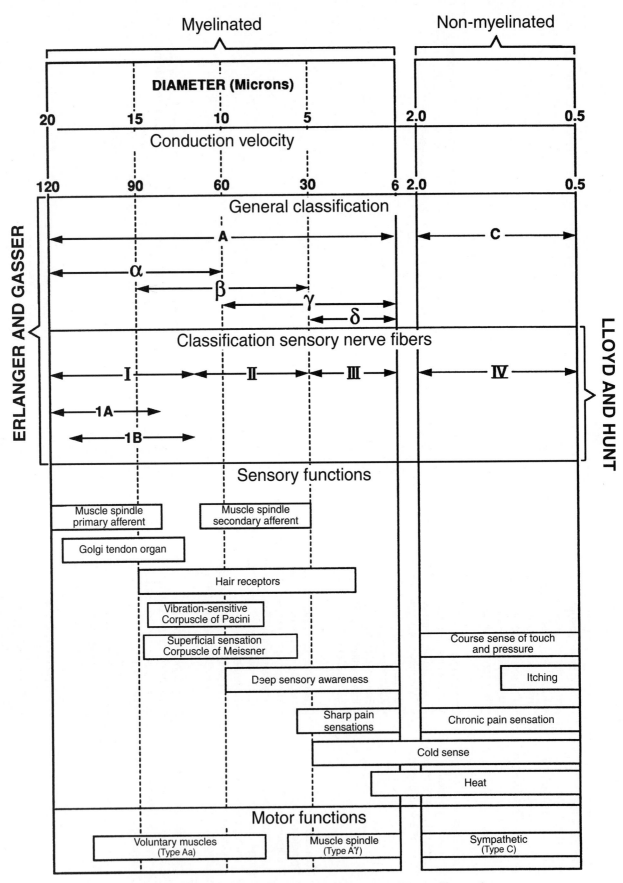

Physiologic classification of Nerve Fiber Function
(Adapted from Guyton AC, 1986).

Type I are static/dynamic mechanoreceptors and type II are dynamic mechanoreceptors. Both have a low threshold to depolarization. Goldscheider's test and Hautant's test, the latter test described later in this chapter, offer some insight into capsular sensory function. Goldscheider's test provides data on the dynamic component and Hautant's test on the static component. These tests are only meaningful if the influence of the central nervous system has been examined and found normal. Among the large joints, the proximal joints have greater proprioceptive sensitivity than the distal joints because the number of receptors is related to the surface area of the capsule. Greater demands are placed on the larger joints.

There are more type I receptors in the intervertebral joints of the cervical spine than in the joints of the more caudal parts of the vertebral column. There are more type II receptors in the intervertebral joints of the caudal parts of the spine.

Goldscheider's Test

It is difficult to test proprioception in the separate vertebral joints. The capsular receptors in the peripheral joints are tested via the small joints. If a change in movement of 3° per second and the position of the joint can be reported, it is assumed that capsular information is intact. If the change in movement within the set unit of time is not perceived, the time can be shortened or the extent of the movement increased. Proprioceptive sensitivity is expressed on a scale from 1 to 5. On this scale, time is always halved, or the extent of the movement is multiplied by a factor of 3. (See **Figure 7–26**.)

Type III receptors cannot be tested. Disturbance in the system is identified by indirect means and from the clinical

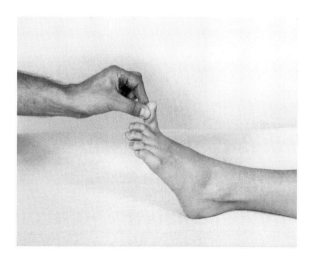

Figure 7–26

presentation. The functioning of type IV receptors is manifested as pain during movements in which the capsule comes under tension, and sometimes as pain in the resting state, which increases with tension on the capsule. Because this kind of receptor does not adapt to any great extent, pain will be present during tension and will ease only slowly or not at all.

Muscle Spindle Receptors

The muscle spindles can normally be tested via the response during myotatic reflexes:

- Increase during tension and (light) contraction
- Decrease through reciprocal innervation

The muscle spindle receptors can also be tested by slow passive extension of the muscle. This should bring about adaptation of the tension-sensitive muscle spindle, so there will be little or no increase in muscle tone. If the sensitivity to stimulation of the muscle spindle is raised because of lack of inhibition from the central nervous system, muscle tone will increase unevenly as the muscle is lengthened.

If tone increases during both lengthening and shortening of the muscle, the cause may be rigidity.

Tone is regulated primarily by the following structures:

- Reticular formation (static component)
- Basal ganglia (dynamic component)

In clinical practice, spasticity and rigidity almost always are found to occur together because the dystonia that occurs is a consequence of the imbalance between the gamma and the alpha motor system. Spasticity occurs when the gamma system is more sensitive to stimulation. In rigidity, the gamma system does not respond to stimulation. Both these situations cause imbalance between the alpha and gamma systems. Depending on whether the disturbance of the balance, and hence the observed abnormalities, are caused by the gamma system or the alpha system, we can distinguish between the following:

- Gamma spasticity
- Alpha rigidity

Gamma Spasticity

The characteristic sign of gamma spasticity is the clasp-knife phenomenon. Because the gamma system is persistently overstimulated or underinhibited, muscle tension increases so much during extension that the Golgi receptors are stimulated. This causes inhibition of the extended muscle. This form of spasticity occurs only if the spinal neurons are intact.

Alpha Rigidity

Alpha rigidity causes continual changes in resistance during passive movement. There is increased activity in the alpha neurons. Cogwheel phenomenon can occur if the tone-leveling function of the basal ganglia is faulty during passive shortening of the muscle.

Tendon Receptors

Testing the proprioceptive functioning of the tendon receptors is particularly difficult. These receptors discharge during tensile forces equal to or exceeding level 2 on the 0–5 manual muscle testing scale. The blocking of the A alpha neurons occurs when muscle exertion exceeds level 5 of this scale. When this happens, they function as a protective mechanism.

This is only one of the functions of the tendon receptors. Whereas an increase in muscle tension leads to inhibition of the homonymous motor neurons via the tendon receptors, a reduction in muscle tension leads to a reduction in discharge frequency in the Ib fibers, and thus to disinhibition of the homonymous motor neurons, so the tension tends to increase again. In other words, the tendon organ reflex circuit works so as to keep the muscle tension constant.

In every muscle there are two feedback systems:

- A length control system with the muscle spindle as receptor
- A tension control system with the Golgi tendon organ as receptor

The interplay between the tendon system and the muscle spindle system is best seen in the coordination of active movements, which should occur smoothly.

Periosteal Receptors

The periosteal receptors are tested via the vibration sense. The test is carried out with a tuning fork (**Figure 7–27**). The amplitude of the vibration is noted at the moment when it is no longer perceived. The vibration sense is generally tested at bony prominences, for example, the medial malleolus. The periosteal receptors can also evoke a sensation of deep pressure or a dull pain, especially if pathology is present.

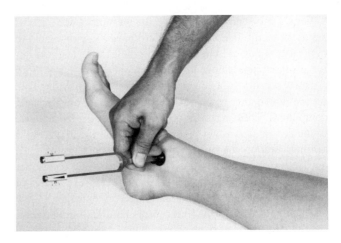

Figure 7–27

SEGMENT

The segment is named after the nerve root by which it is supplied (C1 to S5). Embryologically, it specifies interrelationships among the skin, the muscular system, the skeleton, organs, blood vessels, and nervous system. In this context, we speak of the dermatome, myotome, sclerotome, viscerotome, angiotome, and neurotome. A disturbance in a structure within one segment can cause disturbance in other structures in the same segment. Because most structures are organized multisegmentally, the disturbance spreads over several segments. The sympathetic innervation of the tissues originates from spinal segments C8 to L2, unlike the voluntary innervation of the movement systems, which is based on spinal segments C1 to S5 (Cocc.1).

Skin

The area innervated by a single spinal nerve, together with the gray communicating rami, is called a segment. The area of skin that is innervated by the sensory fibers of the spinal nerve is called a dermatome. The individual dermatomes vary. In the literature, the center of the dermatome is generally specified. The locations of the dermatome and myotome belonging to a particular segment do not coincide.

Dermatomes (**Figure 7–28**):

C2:   Temporal and occipital region

C3:   Neck, throat, jaw, and posterior half of the ear

C4:   Inferior aspect of throat and neck

C5:   Area of deltoid muscle and ventroradial aspect of arm to base of the hand

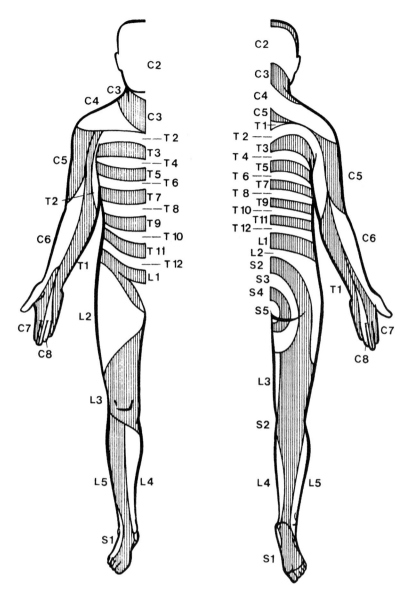

Figure 7–28   Dermatomes.

C6:   Radial aspect of arm up to and including thumb and index finger

C7:   Distal dorsal aspect of forearm, dorsal and ventral side of middle part of hand, second, third, and fourth fingers

C8:   Distal dorsolateral aspect of forearm, ulnar side of hand, fourth and fifth fingers

T1:   Dorsal aspect of upper arm, ulnar aspect of forearm to base of hand

T2:   Level T2, dorsomedial and ventromedial aspect of upper arm

T3:   Axillary region

T4:   Dorsally, approximately evenly spread from T4 to S1; ventrally, approximately evenly spread from the inferior aspect of sternal manubrium to top of symphysis

L1:   Back, top of ilium, groin

L2:   Back-ilium, ventral aspect of thigh, central-medial aspect of thigh, scrotum

L3:   Dorsolateral aspect of hip, ventromedial side of thigh-patella, and medial tibia condyle

L4:   Dorsolateral aspect of gluteal area, lateral side of thigh, ventromedial side of lower leg, medial side of foot, base of big toe

L5:   Ventrolateral aspect of lower leg, dorsal and plantar side of foot, first and second toes

S1:   Dorsolateral aspect of thigh, dorsal aspect of lower leg and heel, lateral plantar and dorsal aspect of foot, third, fourth, and fifth toes

S2:   Gluteal area, dorsomedial aspect of thigh and lower leg, penis

S3:   Dorsomedial aspect of gluteal area, proximal dorso-medial side of thigh and scrotum

S4:   Area around anus

S5:   Anus

Jepsen et al. (2006) reported on interrater reliability for peripheral nerve sensation testing of the upper extremity using a 3-point rating scale of normal, mild, and marked deviation. **Table 7–2** provides κ values and 95% confidence intervals.

Wainner et al. (2003) reported on interrater reliability and diagnostic accuracy of pinprick dermatomal sensation testing using a dichotomous rating scale of normal or de-creased. **Table 7–3** provides interrater κ values with a 95% confidence interval and data on sensitivity, specificity, and likelihood ratios (LR), also with a 95% confidence interval.

Bertilson et al. (2006) studied interrater reliability of pin-wheel dermatomal testing for pain sensation. Abnormal or asymmetric responses were deemed not normal. These au-thors reported κ values of 0.50 (95% CI: 0.26–0.74) for the L4, 0.71 (95% CI: 0.44–0.97) for the L5, and 0.68 (95% CI: 0.42–0.94) for the S1 dermatome.

Peeters et al. (1998) reported on diagnostic accuracy for dermatomal testing using Semmes–Weinstein monofila-ments; data are presented in **Table 7–4**.

Muscular System

Although the cross-striated musculature is in general multisegmentally innervated, a number of muscles are in-nervated more or less segmentally. These are called the *my-otomal muscles*. If there is a clear difference in strength or visible atrophy between a myotomal muscle and the same muscle on the other side, this can indicate dysfunction in the corresponding segment. Electromyography will provide objective information about this.

Myotomes

C1:   Rectus capitis anterior and lateralis muscles (**Figure 7–29**).

C2:   Obliquus capitis superior, rectus capitis poste-rior minor/major muscles (**Figure 7–30**).

C2:   Sternocleidomastoid muscle (**Figure 7–31**).

C3:   Upper trapezius, levator scapulae muscles (**Figure 7–32**).

Table 7–2   Interrater Agreement Upper Extremity Peripheral Nerve Sensation Testing

Sensory Nerve	Innervated Area	Light Touch	Pinprick
Axillary	Deltoid region	0.69 (0.45–0.93)	0.54 (0.33–0.75)
Medial cutaneous brachial	Medial upper arm	0.90 (0.71–1.00)	0.42 (0.14–0.69)
Medial cutaneous antebrachial	Medial forearm	0.75 (0.47–0.98)	0.69 (0.48–0.91)
Musculocutaneous	Lateral forearm	0.67 (0.40–0.95)	0.48 (0.25–0.71)
Radial	1st dorsal web space	0.31 (0.00–0.64)	0.48 (0.25–0.71)
Median	Palmar tip index finger	0.73 (0.50–0.96)	0.43 (0.20–0.66)
Ulnar	Palmar tip little finger	0.59 (0.29–0.89)	0.48 (0.23–0.74)

Table 7–3   Interrater Agreement and Diagnostic Accuracy Upper Extremity Dermatomal Pinprick Testing

Dermatome	Reliability	Sensitivity	Specificity	−LR	+LR
C5	0.67 (0.33–1.00)	0.29 (0.08–0.51)	0.86 (0.77–0.94)	0.82 (0.60–1.1)	2.1 (0.79–5.3)
C6	0.28 (0.00–0.58)	0.24 (0.03–0.44)	0.66 (0.54–0.78)	1.16 (0.84–1.6)	0.69 (0.28–1.8)
C7	0.40 (0.06–0.74)	0.18 (0.0–0.36)	0.77 (0.66–0.87)	1.07 (0.83–1.4)	0.76 (0.25–2.3)
C8	0.16 (0.00–0.50)	0.12 (0.0–0.27)	0.81 (0.71–0.90)	1.09 (0.88–1.4)	0.61 (0.15–2.5)
T1	0.46 (0.04–0.88)	0.18 (0.0–0.36)	0.79 (0.68–0.89)	1.05 (0.81–1.4)	0.83 (0.27–2.6)

Table 7–4 Diagnostic Accuracy Data for Lower Extremity Dermatomal Light Touch Sensation Testing

	Sensitivity	Specificity	+LR	−LR
L4 (L3–L4 disk herniation)	0.50	0.875	4	0.6
L5 (L3–L4 disk herniation)	0.50	1.0	NA	NA
S1 (L3–L4 disk herniation)	0.0	0.875	0	0
L4 (L4–L5 disk herniation)	0.59	0.875	4.7	0.5
L5 (L4–L5 disk herniation)	0.50	1.0	NA	NA
S1 (L4–L5 disk herniation)	0.23	0.875	1.8	0.9
L4 (L5–S1 disk herniation)	0.16	0.875	1.3	0.96
L5 (L5–S1 disk herniation)	0.42	1.0	NA	NA
S1 (L5–S1 disk herniation)	0.74	0.875	5.9	0.3

C4: Diaphragm, trapezius, rhomboid muscles (**Figure 7–33**).

C5: Deltoid, supraspinatus muscles (**Figure 7–34**).

C6: Biceps brachii, extensor carpi radialis muscles (**Figure 7–35**).

C7: Long head of the triceps brachii, flexor carpi radialis, opponens pollicis muscles (**Figure 7–36**).

C8: Adductor pollicis, abductor digiti minimi, extensor pollicis, flexor and extensor carpi ulnaris muscles (**Figures 7–37** and **7–38**).

T1: Interossei palmares/dorsales, adductor digiti minimi muscles (**Figures 7–39** and **7–40**).

T2 to T12: External and internal intercostals. No illustrations are given for these muscles because loss of power in them cannot be measured manually.

L1: Iliopsoas muscle (**Figure 7–41**).

L2: Adductor, rectus femoris, vastus medialis muscles (**Figure 7–42**).

L3: Quadriceps femoris muscle (**Figure 7–43**).

L4: Tibialis anterior muscle (**Figure 7–44**).

L5: Extensor hallucis longus, extensor digitorum brevis muscles (**Figure 7–45**).

S1: Triceps surae, peroneal muscles (**Figure 7–46**).

S1: Peroneus tertius muscle (**Figure 7–47**).

S2: Gluteus maximus muscle (**Figure 7–48**).

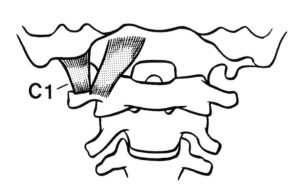
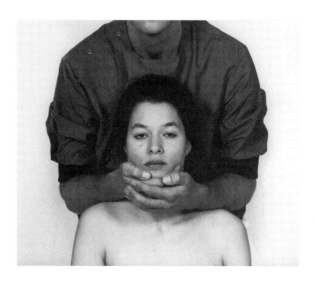

Figure 7–29 Myotome C1.

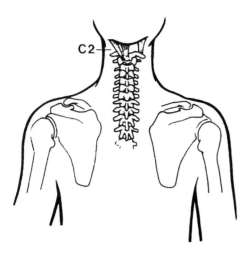

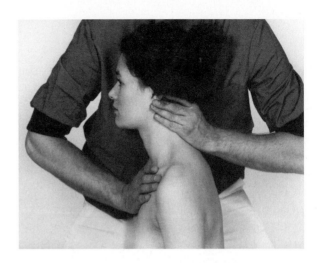

Figure 7–30 Myotome C2.

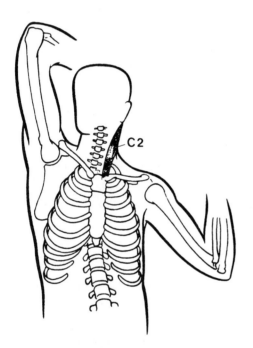

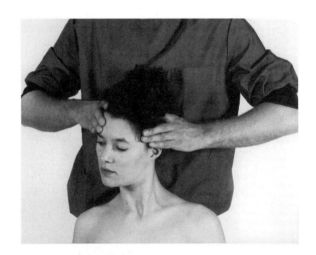

Figure 7–31 Myotome C2.

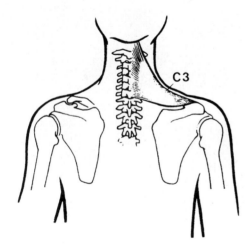

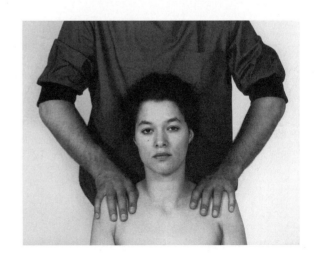

Figure 7–32 Myotome C3.

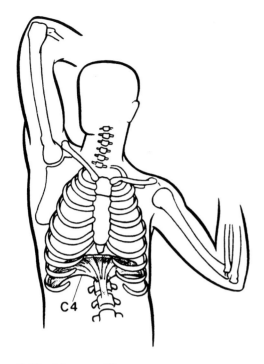

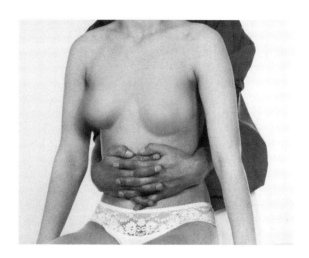

Figure 7–33   Myotome C4.

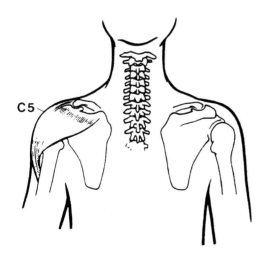

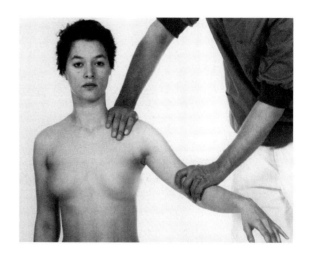

Figure 7–34   Myotome C5.

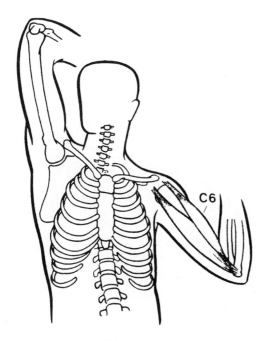

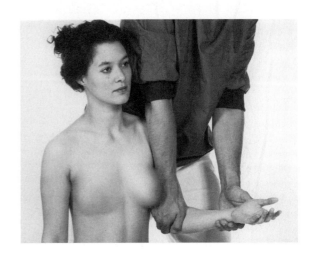

Figure 7–35   Myotome C6.

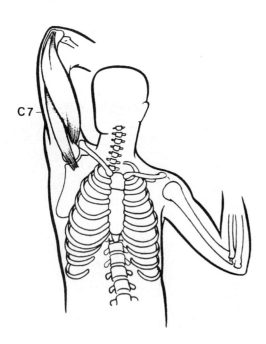

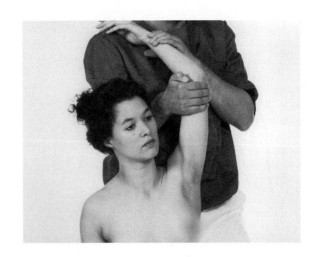

Figure 7–36   Myotome C7.

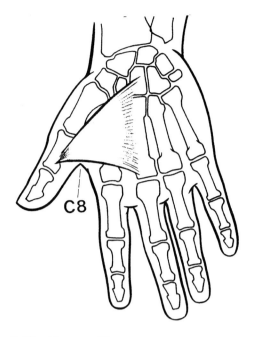
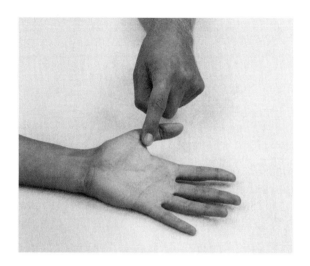

Figure 7–37 Myotome C8.

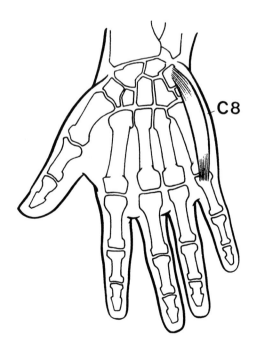
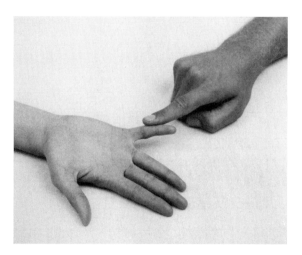

Figure 7–38 Myotome C8.

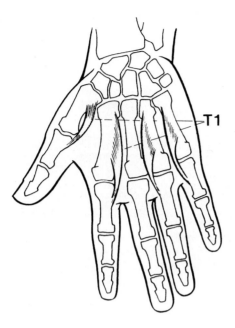

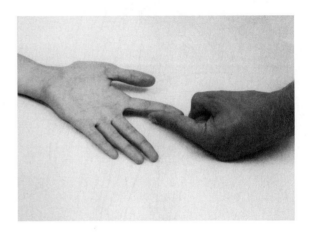

Figure 7–39   Myotome T1.

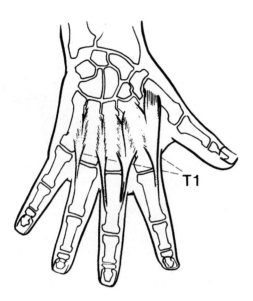

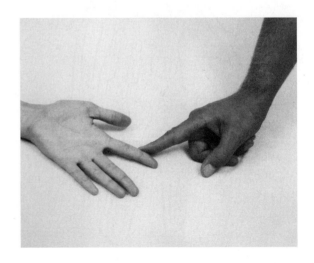

Figure 7–40   Myotome T1.

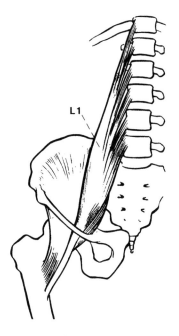

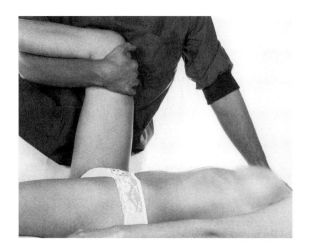

Figure 7–41   Myotome L1.

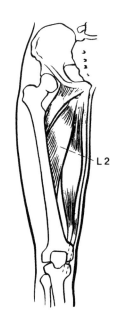

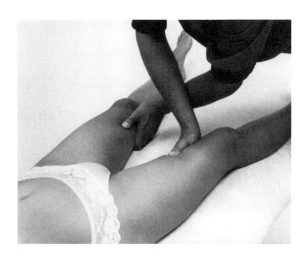

Figure 7–42   Myotome L2.

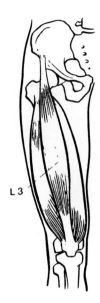

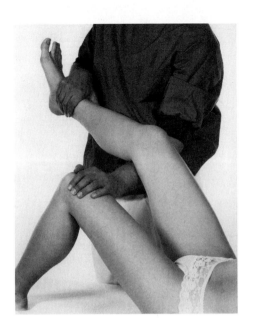

Figure 7–43   Myotome L3.

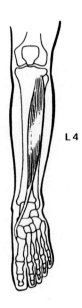

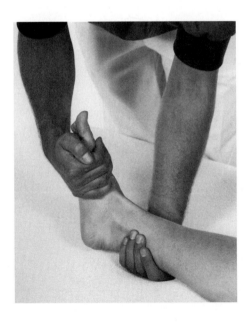

Figure 7–44   Myotome L4.

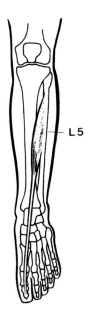 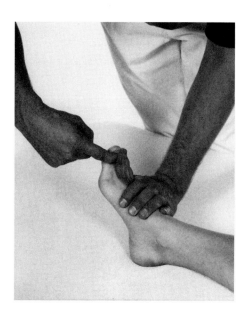

Figure 7–45   Myotome L5.

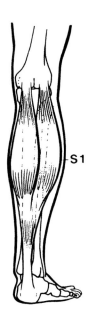 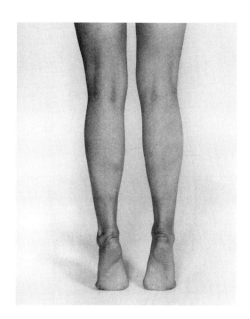

Figure 7–46   Myotome S1.

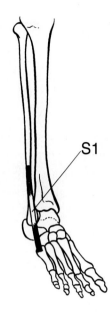

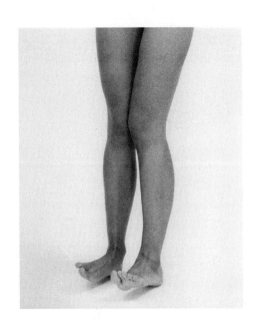

Figure 7–47   Myotome S1.

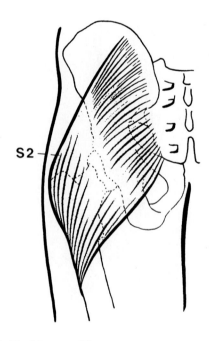

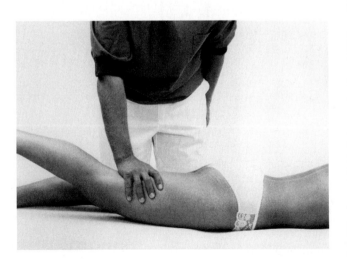

Figure 7–48   Myotome S2.

Wainner et al. (2003) reported interrater reliability and diagnostic accuracy of upper extremity myotomal muscle testing for the diagnosis of cervical radiculopathy compared to a gold standard of electrodiagnostic findings. **Table 7–5** provides interrater κ values with a 95% confidence interval and data on sensitivity, specificity, and likelihood ratios (LR), also with a 95% confidence interval.

Knuttson (1961) studied the diagnostic accuracy of great toe weakness in the diagnosis of lumbar nerve root compression and noted sensitivity of 0.48, 0.74, and 1.0 for the diagnosis of L5, L4, and L3 root compression; specificity was 0.50, 0.50, and 0.50, respectively.

Kerr et al. (1988) studied the diagnostic accuracy of hip extension weakness for the diagnosis of L4–L5 and L5–S1 disk protrusion: sensitivity was 0.12 and 0.09 and specificity 0.96 and 0.89, respectively. Ankle dorsiflexion weakness had a sensitivity of 0.33, 0.66, and 0.49 for L3–L4, L4–L5, and L5–S1 disk protrusion, respectively; specificity values were 0.89 for all levels. Ankle plantar-flexion weakness had 0.0, 0.0, and 0.28 sensitivity for the diagnosis of L3–L4, L4–L5, and L5–S1 disk protrusion, respectively; specificity values were 1.0 for all levels.

Skeleton

Relatively little is known about the segmental structure of the skeleton (sclerotome). Only the sclerotomes described by Inman and Saunders (Chusid, 1982) and de Palma and Rothman (1970), and shown in **Figures 7–49** and **7–50**, are discussed here. The sclerotomes that often coincide peripherally with the attachments of the myotomal muscles are of little extra significance in examinations.

C4: Ventral and dorsolateral aspect of clavicle, medial aspect of scapula

C5: Acromion, ventral aspect of humerus, lateral aspect of scapula

C6: Humeral head, distal ventral aspect of humerus, radius, first metacarpal

C7: Ventral/dorsocaudal aspect of scapula; proximal two thirds of dorsomedial aspect of humerus; olecranon; medial/lateral epicondyle; dorsal aspect of half of second, third, and fourth ray; ventral aspect of head of the radius; ventral side of first radius and half of second radius

C8: Distal-dorsal one third of humerus, distal dorsal two thirds of ulna, aspect of first ray, dorsal aspect of first and fifth ray, and radial half of second ray

L2: Iliac crest, mediocranial part of femur

L3: Ventrocranial edge of ilium, superior pubic ramus femur from collum femoris, patella, and medial tibial condyl

L4: Middle part of inner surface of the ilium, femoral neck, inferior pubic ramus, ventromedial aspect of tibia and medial aspect of talus, calcaneus, navicular and first cuneiform

L5: Body of the ischium, ischial tuberosity, greater trochanter, ventrolateral aspect of tibia, top two thirds of ventral part of fibula and ventral aspect of talus, calcaneus, navicular, first ray, distal interphalangeal (DIP), and proximal interphalangeal (PIP)

S1: Ventromedial aspect of ilium, caudal one third of fibula, cuboid, second and third cuneiform

S2: Second, third, fourth, and fifth ray

Enteroception

The visceral receptors are situated in or on the epithelium of the organs. Stimulation passes through the viscerosensory fibers (afferent C-fibers).

Organ

Organs are allocated to segments according to their autonomic innervation; segmentation is thus limited to the segments C8 to L2. The autonomic lateral horn cells of these

Table 7–5 Interrater Agreement and Diagnostic Accuracy Data Upper Extremity Myotomal Strength Testing

Myotomal Muscle	Reliability	Sensitivity	Specificity	−LR	+LR
Deltoid	0.62 (0.28–0.96)	0.24 (0.03–0.44)	0.89 (0.81–0.97)	0.86 (0.65–1.1)	2.1 (0.70–6.4)
Biceps brachii	0.69 (0.36–1.0)	0.24 (0.03–0.44)	0.94 (0.88–1.0)	0.82 (0.62–1.1)	3.7 (1.0–13.3)
Extensor carpi radial brevis/longus	0.63 (0.26–1.0)	0.12 (0.0–0.27)	0.90 (0.83–0.98)	0.98 (0.81–1.2)	1.2 (0.27–5.6)
Triceps brachii	0.29 (0.0–0.79)	0.12 (0.0–0.27)	0.94 (0.88–1.0)	0.94 (0.78–1.1)	1.9 (0.37–9.3)
Flexor carpi radialis	0.23 (0.0–0.69)	0.06 (0.0–0.17)	0.89 (0.82–0.97)	1.05 (0.91–1.2)	0.55 (0.07–4.2)
Abductor pollicis brevis	0.39 (0.0–0.8)	0.06 (0.0–0.17)	0.84 (0.75–0.93)	1.12 (0.95–1.3)	0.37 (0.05–2.7)
First dorsal interosseus	0.37 (0.0–0.8)	0.03 (0.0–0.1)	0.93 (0.87–0.99)	1.05 (0.94–1.2)	0.40 (0.02–7.0)

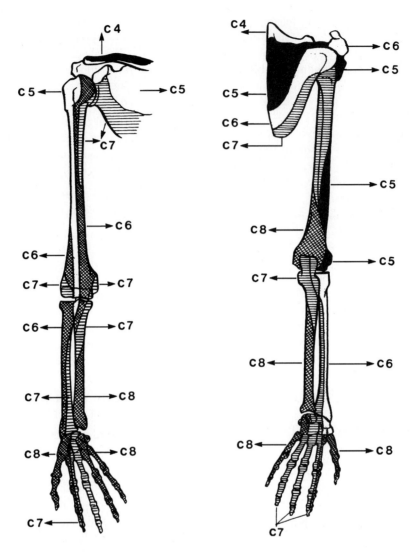

Figure 7–49   Sclerotomes, upper extremity.

segments are functionally linked with sympathetic ganglionic cord, which runs the entire length of the spinal column. Very little of the original parasympathetic segmentation remains except for the segmental structure in sacral segments S2 to S5. In the course of human evolution, the segmental structure in the area innervated by the vagus nerve has completely disappeared.

When the term *organ* is understood in its broadest sense, then an overall segmental division can be made with regard to the sympathetic autonomic innervation of the locomotor apparatus:

Head/throat: C8–T3
Arms: T3–T9

Trunk: T10–T12
Legs: T10–L2

with some overlap in both cranial and caudal directions.

Sweat Secretion   Secretion of sweat is segmentally organized, as follows (see **Figure 7–51**):

Head/throat/tops of shoulders: T1–T4
Trunk/arms: T5–T7
Lower body/legs: T8–L3

The frequent involvement of segments C3 and C4 may be resulting from the fact that a proportion of afferent input

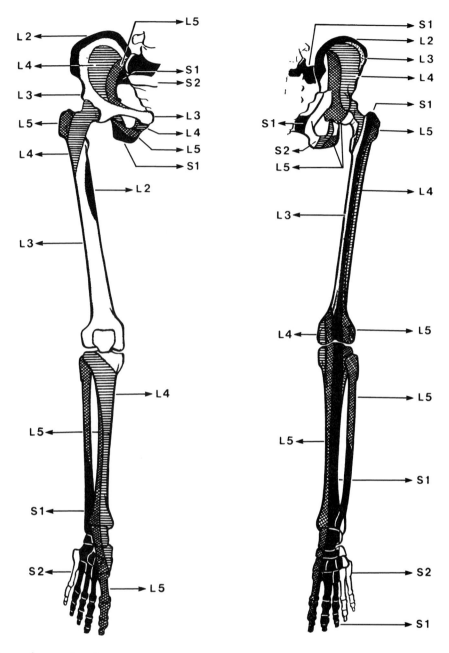

Figure 7–50   Sclerotomes, lower extremity.

from the diaphragm and the deeper abdominal structures passes through the afferent fibers of the phrenic nerve.

Symptoms of Pathologically Raised Sympathetic Activity
The primary symptoms are the following:

Sensory: Hyperesthesia and hyperalgesia *(referred sensation)*

Motor: Hypertonia, *défense musculaire* (pressure defense tension)

Eye: Mydriasis (widening of pupil)

Hair: Goose bumps

Sweat glands: Hyperhidrosis (increased secretion of sweat)

Blood vessels: Pallor, coldness

Lymphatic system: Swelling

Internal organs: Disturbance of function

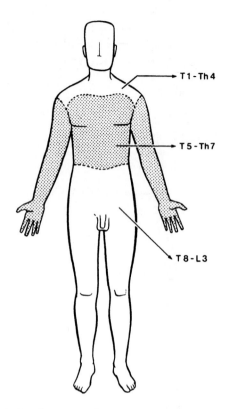

Figure 7–51   Sweat secretion.

Secondary symptoms are as follows:

Skin: Changes in elasticity, flaking, connective tissue zones

Connective tissue: Changes in elasticity, changes in consistency

Musculature: Tender points, myofascial trigger points, tendomyoses

Joint capsule: Changes in elasticity/limitations on movement

Periosteum: Swelling (Vögler points)

Internal organs: Disturbance of function, possible structural changes

A prolonged increase in the activity of the sympathetic autonomic nervous system, associated with inactivity, can be damaging to the movement apparatus. The consequences are seen most clearly in the areas innervated by the rami dorsales and meninges of the spinal nerves that leave the spinal canal between C7 and L2. Changes that may take place in the skin, the cross-striated muscle, and the synovial joint, and the consequences of those changes are described next.

The Skin

- Changes in the elasticity of the connective tissue
- Increased sensitivity of the nociceptors: Hyperalgesic zones associated with visceral pathology are described in **Table 7–6**
- Increased tone in the erector pili muscles
- Increased secretion of sweat

Panniculosis and skin connective tissue zones may develop as a result.

The Cross-Striated Muscle

- Hypertonicity
- Changes in the elasticity of the connective tissue in the muscle
- Reduced effective circulation in the muscle
- Increased sensitivity of the muscle receptors

As a result, tender points, myofascial trigger points, or tendomyoses may develop.

The Synovial Joint

- Qualitative and quantitative changes in the production of synovia
- Changes in the elasticity of the connective tissue in the membrana fibrosa capsula synovialis
- Increased sensitivity of the nociceptors
- Tendomyotic changes in the periarticular musculature

These may lead to disturbance of function, pain, and restriction of movement.

Blood Vessels

Blood vessels are doubly innervated by the autonomic nervous system, once via the dorsal root and peripheral nerves, and again via the perivasal pathways, the long spinal rami, and the sympathetic chain (Lazorthes, 1949) (**Figure 7–52**).

Foerster (1922), Fleisch (1956), and Lériche (1949, 1958) researched the innervation and pain transmission of the blood vessels. They found that irritation of the blood vessels gives rise initially to a sharp pain, giving way after a short time to a dull, glowing, burning traumatic and psychological component.

Table 7–6 Hyperalgesic Zones Resulting From Internal Organ Dysfunction

Viscerotomes (HANSEN and SCHLIAK, 1962)

Hyperalgesic zones resulting from internal organ dysfunction

	Ipsilateral pupal dilation	C3	C4	C5	C6	C7	C8	T1	T2	T3	T4	T5	T6	T7	T8	T9	T10	T11	T12	L1	L2	L3	
Heart, pericardium	left	+	+				+	+	+	+	+	+	+	+	+								left
Lung and bronchi	right/left	+	+							+	+	+	+	+	+	+							right/left
Pleura	right/left	+	?						(+)	+	+	+	+	+	+	+	+	(+)	(+)				right/left
Esophagus stomach	?	?	?																				left
Stomach (Corpus, Fundus)	left	+	+									+	•	+	+	+							right or left
Pyloris	right/left	+	+									+	•	+	+	+							right
Duodenum	right	(+)											+	+	+	+	+	+					right
Jejunum	left	+	+											+	+	+	+	+					left
Ilium	right ?	?	?											(+)	(+)	+	+	+					right
Pancreas	left	+	+											+	+	+							left
Liver, gallbladder	right	+	+										+	+	+	•	+	+					right
Spleen	left	+	+										+	+	+	+	•						left
Cecum, Appendix	right	+	+													+	•	•	•	•			right
Ascending colon																(+)	+	+	+				
Colon transvers./prox.	right	+													(+)	+	+	+					right
Colon transvers./dist.																+	+	+					
Colon desc., Sygmoid, Rectum	left	+	+												+	(+) (+)				+	(+)	(•)	left
Kidney	right/left	+	+												+	(+)	+	+	+	(+)	(+)		right/left
Urethra	right/left	+	+												+	+	+	+	+	+	•	(•)	right/left
Genitalia	right/left	+	+												+	+	+	+	+	+	•		right/left
Peritoneum	?	+									+	+	+	+	+	+	+	+	+				?

Right or left refers to the organ located on that side

• **Refers to the innervation area as determined by anesthesiologic testing**

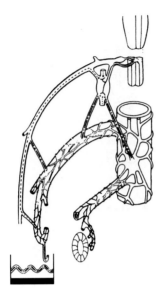

Figure 7–52   Innervation of the blood vessels.
Source: Lazorthes, 1949.

In addition to the radicular innervation area and the peripheral nerve innervation area, there is also a vascular innervation area. There is some confusion around the meaning of the term *vascular innervation area*:

- It is sometimes used to mean the area served by the sympathetic nervous system of the blood vessels; this defines it in terms of an efferent function.
- It is also used to refer to the area served by the blood vessels from which pathologic stimulation can originate; this defines it in terms of an afferent function.

Afferent input from the blood vessels themselves, or from the area served by the blood vessels, for example, as a result of ischemia, gives rise to pain and an increase in sympathetic activity. This creates a vicious circle. A disturbance in the periarterial autonomic nervous supply is characterized by abnormal topography. The vascular innervation area is defined as the area of skin that is vascularized by one artery.

Angiotomes (vascular innervation area) (**Figure 7–53**):

Common carotid artery (a): Ipsilateral side of head upper quadrant

Subclavian artery (b): Neck, arm, shoulder, cervical trunk

Aorta (c): Waist area

Internal iliac artery (d): Gluteal strip, lumbosacral trunk

External iliac artery (e): Leg (femoral artery)

In terms of innervation, neighboring vascular areas are linked by perivasal pathways and the sympathetic chain.

The carotid artery and the subclavian artery, for example, together form the upper quadrant. From the point of view of sympathetic innervation, this belongs to the cervical trunk. Vascular zones and quadrants have the same significance for autonomic innervation as the segment has in identifying disturbances of the spinal cord and its roots. It is clinically important to know all aspects of the innervation and vascularization of the skin to be able to distinguish the following conditions:

- Radicular and pseudoradicular syndrome
- Disorders of the peripheral nerves (entrapment syndrome, other neuropathies, lesions in peripheral nerves)
- Vascular quadrant syndrome, Sudeck's dystrophy

Reflexes
Aad van der El and Peter A. Huijbregts

The following kinds of reflexes can be distinguished: the intrinsic reflex (physiologic reflex), which can be monosynaptic, but probably has a central component; the extrinsic reflex (pathologic reflex), which is always multisynaptic; and the autonomic reflex, which is associated with the autonomic nervous system.

Intrinsic Reflex

The myotatic, periosteal, bone, joint, and tonic reflexes are intrinsic reflexes. They represent one neurologic segmental level. Central disturbance and absence of the inhibitory effect of the descending pathways almost always causes hyperreflexia. Partial breakdown of the primary reflex circuit, resulting from, for example, compression of the peripheral or spinal nerve, causes hyporeflexia in the later stages.

Extrinsic Reflex

A disturbance of the descending pathways causes hyporeflexia or areflexia. The corticospinal pathways must be intact for the extrinsic reflex to function. If there is a disturbance in the corticospinal pathways, the effects on the intrinsic reflex and the extrinsic reflex can be opposite: spastic hemiplegia on the right causes hyperreflexia in the intrinsic reflexes on the right and hyporeflexia of the extrinsic reflexes on the right.

Within the context of Orthopaedic Manual Therapy (OMT) diagnosis, pathologic reflexes play an important role in picking up on contraindications to OMT management and the need for medical-surgical referral. Positive findings

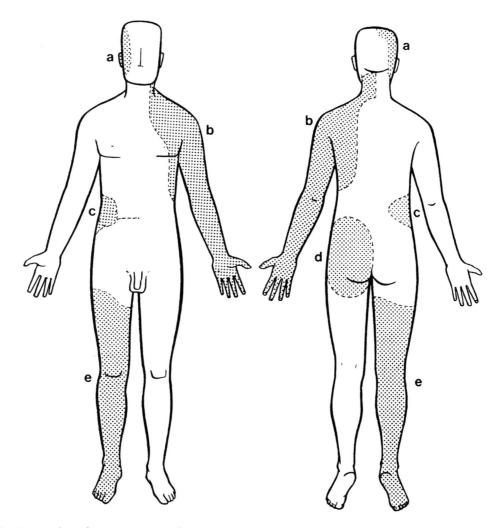

Figure 7–53   Angiotomes (vascular innervation area).

on pathologic reflexes may indicate central neurologic pathologies including global and supraspinal degenerative conditions such as Parkinson's disease, amyotrophic lateral sclerosis, multiple sclerosis, and other neurologic conditions but also spinal conditions, most notably myelopathy.

Reflexes clinically helpful in implicating supraspinal pathology but also spinal cord pathology include the jaw jerk or masseter reflex and the palmomental reflex. These reflexes are not present in patients with solely spinal cord pathology. Although not a reflex, the L'Hermitte sign discussed earlier in this chapter also serves this purpose. As noted, Uchihara et al. (1994) established a sensitivity of 0.03 and a specificity of 0.97 for this test in the diagnosis of spinal cord pathology and multiple sclerosis; it should be noted that this low sensitivity value makes this test poorly suited as a screening test. For the masseter reflex, the examiner taps his or her own finger placed centrally on the slightly opened mandible of the patient. Hyperreflexia is considered a positive finding and indicative of supraspinal nervous system pathology (McCormick et al., 2003). However, data on psychometric properties of this test are not available. With the palmomental reflex, stroking either the thenar or the hypothenar eminence in proximal to distal direction causing wrinkling of the skin of the chin and slight jaw retraction that does not diminish on repeated testing is considered indicative of Parkinson disease and other neurologic diseases. August and Miller (1952) calculated sensitivity of 0.95 and specificity of 0.98 for this reflex; positive and negative likelihood ratios were 38 and 0.21, respectively. However, Isakov et al. (1984) reported sensitivity of 0.78, specificity of 0.58, and positive and negative likelihood ratios of 1.8 and 0.22, respectively. Of specific relevance to OMT diagnosis is that a decreased corneal reflex has been implicated in cervical artery dissection as a sign of ischemic or nonischemic cranial nerve involvement (Kerry and Taylor, 2006).

With the Hoffman sign the examiner stabilizes the middle finger proximal to the distal interphalangeal joint, cradling the patient's hand with the forearm pronated and supported. Nipping the fingernail or flicking the middle finger may cause a positive response in the sense of adduction-opposition of the thumb and mild finger flexion. Sung and Wang (2001) in a sample of asymptomatic patients with positive tests reported only sensitivity of 0.94 for this test in the diagnosis of cervical pathology with cord compression due to a herniated disc. Wong et al. (2004) in a sample of patients with cervical myelopathy noted a sensitivity of 0.82. Glaser et al. (2001) reported a specificity of 0.58 and a specificity of 0.74 if the rater was not blinded to other findings, but a sensitivity of only 0.28 and a specificity of 0.71 if the rater was blinded.

The Babinski sign is positive when upgoing, meaning extension of the big toe and abduction of the other toes. Miller and Johnston (2005) reported a κ value of 0.73 for interrater agreement and sensitivity of 0.35 and specificity of 0.77 for the Babinski sign in the diagnosis of upper motor neuron pathology.

The radial periosteal reflex can be indicative in the form of an inverted supinator sign: finger flexion and slight elbow extension rather than the normal response of elbow flexion as with tapping the brachioradialis muscle more proximally is likely related to increased alpha motor neuron activity below the level of the myelopathic lesion. No data are available on psychometric properties of this pathologic reflex (Cook and Hegedus, 2008).

Autonomic Reflex

In the autonomic reflex, the proprioceptive and exteroceptive contributions of the precipitating stimulations cannot always be distinguished. The autonomic reflexes include the pupil reflex, the reflexes of the sweat glands and vascular nerves, the piloerection reflex (somatosympathetic reflexes), and the bladder, bowel, and sexual reflexes (somatoparasympathetic reflexes).

Reflexes of the Head Area and Tonic Reflexes

Head Area
Pupil reflex
Corneal reflex
Pain reflex
Masseter reflex
Choking reflex

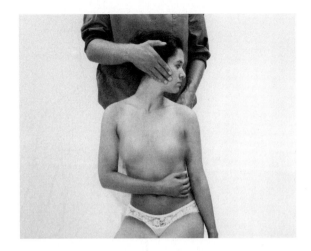

Figure 7–54   Postural reflex (tonic, neck, and labyrinthine reflex).

Eating and sucking reflexes
Palmomental reflex
Pouting reflex
Head retraction reflex
Chvostek phenomenon

Tonic Reflexes
Postural reflex (**Figure 7–54**) (tonic, neck, and labyrinthine reflex)
Adaptation reflex
Fixation reflex
Stretch reflex
Support reflex (**Figure 7–55**)
Rising reflex

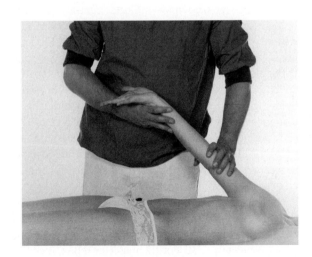

Figure 7–55   Support reflex.

*Reflexes of the Shoulder, Arm, and Trunk Areas and the
  Lower Extremity*

Reflexes of the shoulder, arm, and trunk areas and the
lower extremity are shown in the following grid.

Shoulder–Arm Area		*Trunk Area (External Reflexes)*		*Lower Extremity*	
Scapulohumeral reflex	C4–C5	Epigastric reflex	T5–T6	Adductor reflex (**Figure 7–64**)	L2–L4
Biceps reflex (**Figure 7–56**)	C5–C6	Upper abdominal skin reflex, motor: sensory:	T7 T9	Quadriceps femoris reflex (**Figure 6–65**)	(L2) L3–L4
Brachioradialis reflex (**Figure 7–57**)	C5–C6	Middle abdominal skin reflex, motor: sensory:	T8–T10 T8–T10	Gluteus reflex (External reflex)	L4–S1
Radius-periosteal reflex (**Figure 7–58**)	C5–C6	Lower abdominal skin reflex, motor: (**Figure 7–63**) sensory:	(T9) T10 T12(L1)	Tibialis posterior reflex (**Figure 7–66**)	L5
Triceps reflex (**Figure 7–59**)	C6–C7	Cremaster reflex	L1–L2	Peroneus longus reflex	L5–S1
Mayer's MCP joint reflex	C6–T1	Bulbocavernosus reflex	S3	Semimembranosus semitendinosus reflex	S1
Thenar reflex (**Figure 7–60**)	C6–C8	Anal reflex	S5	Biceps-femoris reflex	S1–S2
Hand bending reflex	C7–T1			Triceps surae reflex (**Figures 7–67** and **7–68**)	L5–S2
Trömmer reflex (**Figures 7–61** and **7–62**)	C7–C8			Back of foot reflex (**Figure 7–69**)	L5–S1
Wrist reflex	C6–C8			Sole of foot reflex (I.R.) Strumpell (**Figure 7–70**) Babinski (Extrinsic reflex)	(Exrinsic reflex)
Hoffman sign				Jendrassik's hand grip (**Figure 7–71**)	

For interpretation of these reflexes, please see Mumenthaler (1973) and Bronisch (1973).

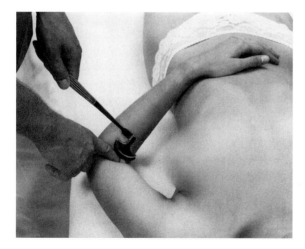

Figure 7–56 Biceps reflex.

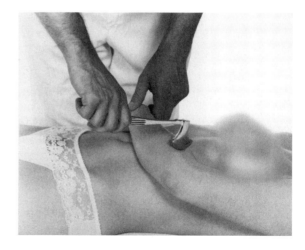

Figure 7–57 Brachioradialis reflex.

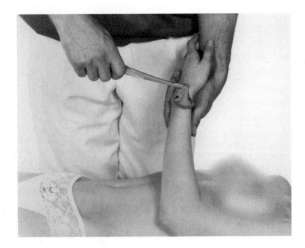

Figure 7–58   Radius-periosteal reflex.

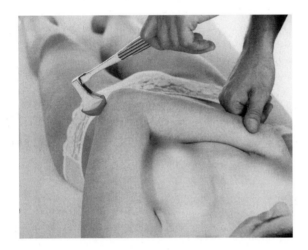

Figure 7–59   Triceps reflex.

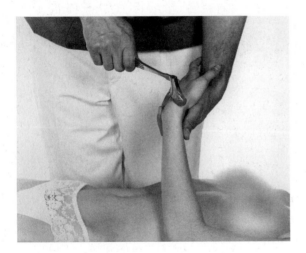

Figure 7–60   Thenar reflex.

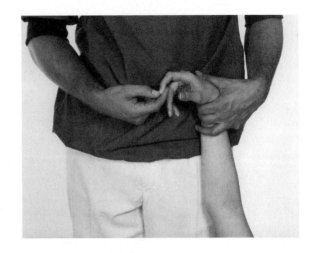

Figure 7–61   Trömmer reflex.

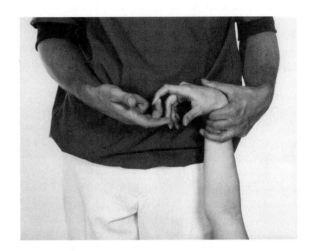

Figure 7–62   Trömmer reflex.

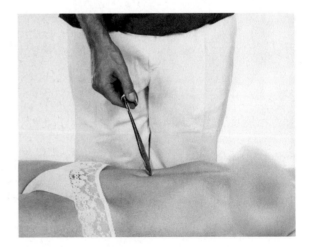

Figure 7–63   Lower abdominal skin reflex, motor.

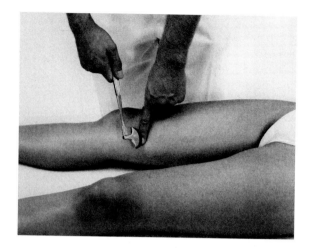

Figure 7–64 Adductor reflex.

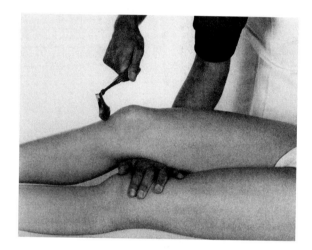

Figure 7–65 Quadriceps femoris reflex.

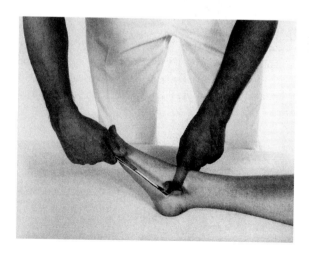

Figure 7–66 Tibialis posterior reflex.

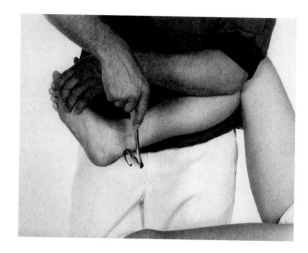

Figure 7–67 Triceps surae reflex.

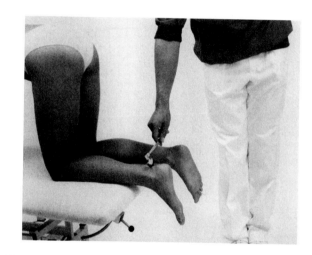

Figure 7–68 Triceps surae reflex.

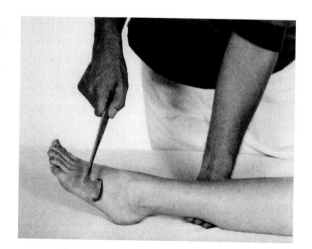

Figure 7–69 Back of foot reflex.

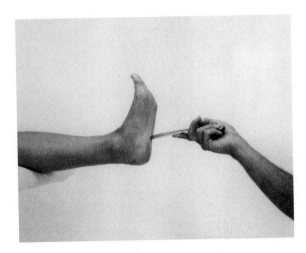

Figure 7–70   Strumpell.

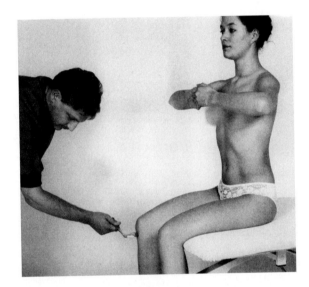

Figure 7–71   Jendrassik's hand grip.

Using a 3-point grading scale of reduced/absent, normal, or increased, Wainner et al. (2003) established a κ value of 0.73 (95% CI: 0.38–1.0) for the interrater reliability of the biceps brachii myotatic reflex test. With asym-

metry or either weak or strong response noted a positive in a 2-point grading system, Bertilson et al. (2003) reported 94%, 98%, 94%, and 90% agreement for the supraspinatus, biceps, brachioradialis, and triceps myotatic reflex tests, respectively. Wainner et al. (2003) also reported diagnostic accuracy statistics (with 95% confidence intervals) for the upper extremity myotatic reflexes in the diagnosis of cervical radiculopathy. Data are provided in **Table 7–7**.

Knuttson (1961) reported a sensitivity of 0.12 and a specificity of 0.65 for the quadriceps myotatic reflex in the diagnosis of L4 nerve root compression; sensitivity and specificity were 1.0 and 0.65, respectively, for L3 nerve root compression and 0.14 and 0.65 for L5 nerve root compression. Kerr et al. (1988) reported sensitivity of 0.87 and specificity of 0.89 for the Achilles tendon reflex in the diagnosis of L5–S1 disk herniation and sensitivity of 0.12 and specificity of 0.89 for the diagnosis of L4–L5 disk herniation. Marin et al. (1995) reported sensitivity of 0.18 and specificity of 0.91 for the diagnosis of L5 radiculopathy and sensitivity of 0.11 with specificity at 0.91 for the diagnosis of S1 radiculopathy for the back of the foot or extensor digitorum brevis myotatic reflex.

PSEUDORADICULAR SYNDROME

The pseudoradicular syndrome is characterized by referred pain sensations, not caused by stimulation of one or more nerve roots (Brügger, 1969). These painful sensations may result from a disturbance in the functional relationship between the joints and the muscles that move the joints either directly or indirectly. Note that the thoracic outlet compression syndrome, blood vessels, and so forth can also cause pseudoradicular symptoms.

A muscular limitation of movement caused by pain is mainly found where there is a painful capsule. The muscle tone changes; it may be slack, cramped by spasticity, or increased to the point of rigor. Tendomyoses (myogeloses, myotendinoses, tendinoses, tenoperiostoses) may also occur (**Figure 7–72**).

Table 7–7   Diagnostic Accuracy Statistics for Upper Extremity Myotatic Reflexes in the Diagnosis of Cervical Radiculopathy

Reflex	Sensitivity	Specificity	+LR	−LR
Biceps brachii	0.24 (0.3–0.44)	0.95 (0.90–1.0)	0.80 (0.61–1.1)	4.9 (1.2–20)
Brachioradialis	0.06 (0.0–0.17)	0.95 (0.90–1.0)	0.99 (0.87–1.1)	1.2 (0.14–11.1)
Triceps	0.03 (0.0–0.1)	0.93 (0.87–0.99)	1.05 (0.94–1.2)	0.40 (0.02–7.0)

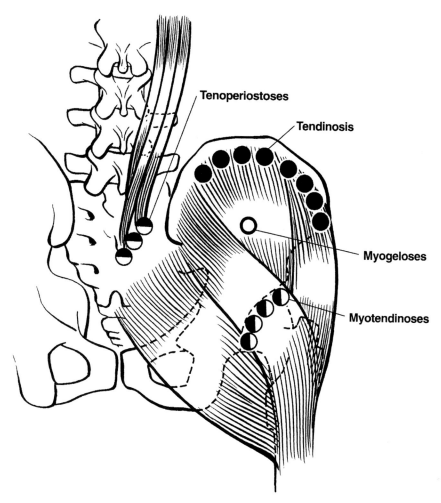

Figure 7–72   Tendomyoses.

Joints can also influence each other via nervous connections. Every joint has a typical peripheral representation area. The pseudoradicular syndromes are described extensively by Brügger and Rhonheimer (1965); we shall limit ourselves here to describing a few examples.

Cervical Intervertebral Joints

Primary symptoms: chronic or shooting headaches (frontal, parietal, temporal, and occipital). Secondary symptoms: possibly cervical brachialgias, overloading of the sternoclavicular joint, referred pain in the upper quadrant, dizziness, and acroparesthesias.

Findings: painful cervical intervertebral joints; tendomyoses in the muscles of the neck, frontalis, and possibly temporalis, trapezius, serratus anterior, and the arm muscles; possibly pressure paresthesias from the intercosto-brachial nerves; limitation of movement in the cervical spine.

Dwyer et al. (1990) established pain referral patterns emanating from cervical intervertebral joints by way of facet joint infiltration in normal subjects (**Figure 7–73**).

Sternoclavicular Joint

Primary symptoms: pain that can radiate from the neck to the forehead; pain in the face and ear on one or both sides; prearticular pains on one or both sides. (See **Figures 7–74 and 7–75**.) Secondary symptoms: secondary overloading of the cervical intervertebral joints, the jaw joint, and the acromioclavicular joint, with consequences such as cervicobrachialgia and acroparesthesias, possible dizziness, ringing in the ears, overstimulation of the sternocostal joints and the costocartilagenous attachments, with precardial pains.

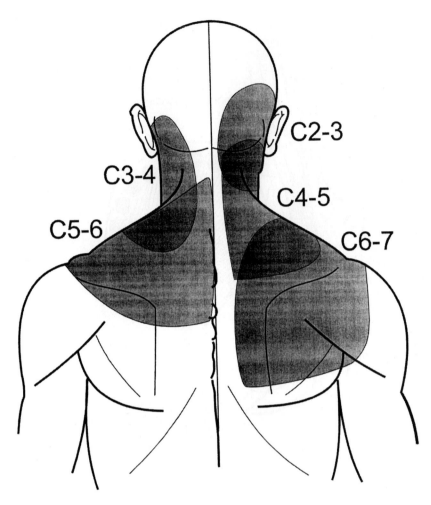

Figure 7–73   Referral patterns cervical facet joints.
Source: Reproduced from Fernández-de-las-Peñas C., Arendt-Nielsen L., Gerwin R. Diagnosis and Management of Tension-Type and Cerviocengenic Headache. Sudbury, MA: Jones and Bartlett Publishers, 2009.

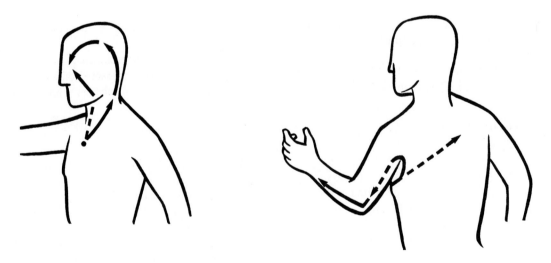

Figure 7–74   Pain referral of sternoclavicular joint. *Source:* Brügger, 1977.

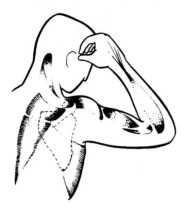

Figure 7–75   Tendomyoses of sternoclavicular joint.
Source: Brügger, 1977.

Findings: painful sternoclavicular joint, usually combined with painful cervical intervertebral joints, possibly painful temporomandibular joint and painful sternocostal joints; tendomyoses in the neck musculature and sternocleidomastoid with painful mastoid bones, shortening of the sternocleidomastoid and the neck musculature, possible symptoms arising from the cervical intervertebral joints, dizziness on extension or rotation of the cervical spine, limited movement in the cervical spine, painful symphysis.

Acromioclavicular Joint

Primary symptoms: cervicobrachialgias and pain in the neck and back of the head. Secondary symptoms: possible secondary overloading of the sternoclavicular joint, the shoulder joint, and the cervical intervertebral joints, with symptoms such as dizziness and acroparesthesias.

Findings: acromioclavicular joint painful on pressure; painful internal rotation of the upper arm; referred pain in the lateral aspect of the upper arm to the elbow, sometimes in the forearm, occasionally in the area of the serratus anterior muscle; tendomyoses in the trapezius, serratus anterior, serratus lateralis, biceps brachii, coracobrachialis, and hand and finger extensors.

Sternocostal Joint and Costocartilaginous Connection

Primary symptoms: referred pain in the area of the thoracic spine, between the shoulder blades, precardial pains, and cervicobrachialgias. (See **Figures 7–76** and **7–77**.) Secondary symptoms: secondary overloading of the sternoclavicular joint and the cervical intervertebral joints, with the associated symptomatology.

Findings: pain on pressure in the sternocostal joints, the costocartilaginous connections, and possibly in the

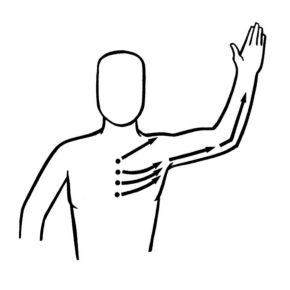

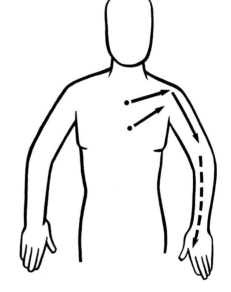

Figure 7–76   Pain referral sternocostal joints. *Source:* Brügger, 1977.

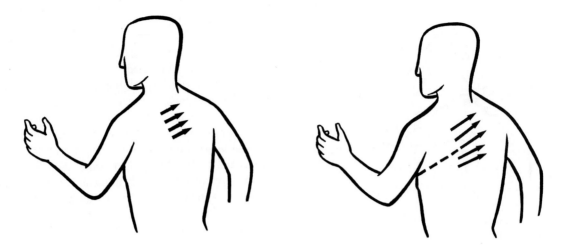

Figure 7–77   Pain referral sternocostal connections. *Source:* Brügger, 1977.

sternoclavicular joint; tendomyoses of the pectoral and the abdominal musculature.

Costovertebral and Costotransverse Joints

Primary symptoms: pain radiating toward the front wall of the thorax; precardial pains. Secondary symptoms: Possible secondary overloading of the costocartilaginous connections, the sternocostal connections and the sternoclavicular joint; sometimes radiating pain in the arm via the intercostobrachial nerve.

Findings: Pain on pressure in the costotransverse and costosternal joints and in the costocartilaginous connections; possible pressure paresthesias of the intercostobrachial nerves.

Pubic Symphysis

Primary symptoms: pain radiating toward the lumbar spine and from there to the waist, often also in the abdomen or in the groin area, sometimes as far as the knee. (See **Figures 7–78** and **7–79**.) Secondary symptoms: in rare cases, overloading of the sternocostal and sternoclavicular joints and the cervical intervertebral joints.

Findings: symphysis painful on pressure, tendomyoses in the abdominal musculature, lumbar spinal erector, gluteus maximus, adductors, hamstring muscles, triceps surae; spasms of the adductors; can sometimes lead to pressure paresthesias of the lateral and anterior femoral cutaneous nerves.

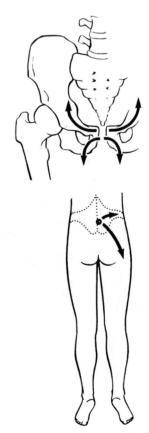

Figure 7–78   Pain referral of pubic symphysis. *Source:* Brügger, 1977.

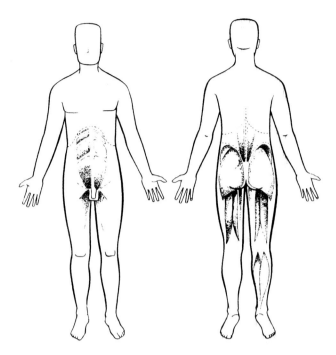

Figure 7–79 Tendomyoses of pubic symphysis. *Source:* Brügger, 1977.

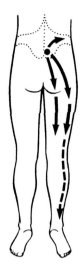

Figure 7–80 Pain referral of the lower lumbar intervertebral joints. *Source:* Brügger, 1977.

Lower Lumbar Intervertebral Joints

Primary symptoms: pain is possible that radiates to the flank, iliac crest, gluteal region, and the whole leg to the big toe. (See **Figures 7–80** and **7–81**.) Secondary symptoms: Possible secondary overloading of the sacroiliac, hip, and knee joints.

Findings: iliac crest painful on pressure, tendomyoses in the spinal erector trunci, gluteus maximus, hamstring muscles, and sometimes in the triceps surae, oblique abdominals, quadratus lumborum, gluteus medius, tensor fasciae latae, and peroneals.

Schwarzer et al. (1994) established the prevalence of pain patterns in 176 patients with lumbar facet joint pain confirmed by diagnostic blocks:

- Left groin 15%, right groin 3%
- Left buttock 42%; right buttock 15%
- Left thigh 38%; right thigh 38%
- Left calf 27%; right calf 15%
- Left foot 31%; right foot 8%

Sacroiliac Joint

Primary symptoms: pain at the level of the sacroiliac joint, especially when climbing stairs, referring to the pelvic rim, along the dorsolateral side of the thigh, sometimes as far as the knee. Secondary symptoms: Possible secondary overloading of the hip joint and the lower lumbar intervertebral joints.

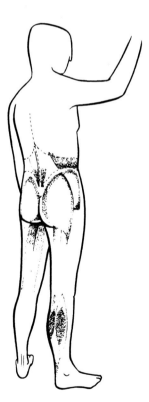

Figure 7–81 Tendomyoses of the lower lumbar intervertebral joints. *Source:* Brügger, 1977.

Findings: Pain on pressure on the sacroiliac joint and the inner top corner of the iliac crest; tendomyoses in the multifidi, gluteus maximus, piriformis, and pain on pressure in the iliacus, iliopsoas muscles, and the iliolumbar ligament.

Fortin et al. (1994b) established an area of sensory changes, approximately 3 cm wide and 10 cm long, just inferior to the PSIS in 10 asymptomatic subjects with fluoroscopically guided provocation arthrography to the right SIJ (Fortin et al., 1994b). Using the criterion of the patient indicating a predominantly unilateral pain in this area for the diagnosis of sacroiliac joint dysfunction, Fortin et al. (1994a) established a κ of 0.96 for the interrater reliability of this diagnostic test. Pointing to the area of pain referral established in these studies has since been introduced in the literature as the Fortin finger test.

Schwarzer et al. (1995) used a fluoroscopically guided SIJ block with at least a 75% reduction of pain over the SIJ and buttock as a gold standard test in patients with chronic low back pain; L4–S1 facet joint infiltrations for all and discography for some patients served as control procedures. The only statistically significant characteristic pain pattern in patients with sacroiliac pain was the presence of groin pain ($P < .001$). The prevalence of buttock, thigh, calf, and foot pain was not statistically different between sacroiliac and nonsacroiliac patients.

Table 7–8 Sacroiliac Pain Referral Patterns in Study by Slipman et al. (2000)

Anatomic Region	Percentage	
Upper lumbar	06	
Lower lumbar	72	
Buttock	94	
Groin	14	
Abdomen	02	
Thigh	48	
• Posterior		• 30
• Lateral		• 20
• Anterior		• 10
• Medial		• 00
Lower leg	28	
• Posterior		• 18
• Lateral		• 12
• Anterior		• 10
• Medial		• 00
Ankle	14	
Foot	12	
• Lateral		• 08
• Plantar		• 04
• Dorsal		• 04
• Medial		• 00

Dreyfuss et al. (1996) used a gold standard test of 90–100% reduction in pain after a fluoroscopically guided SIJ block. They reported 81% interrater agreement (κ = 0.60), a sensitivity of 0.76, and a specificity of 0.47 for the Fortin finger test. Sensitivity for a pain drawing indicating sacroiliac joint, groin, or buttock pain was 0.85, 0.19, and 0.80, respectively. Specificity was 0.08, 0.63, and 0.14, respectively.

Using a gold standard test of 80% or greater reduction in pain after a fluoroscopically guided sacroiliac joint block, Slipman et al. (2000) reported the frequency of pain referral patterns noted (see **Table 7–8**).

LESIONS OF THE PLEXUS AND PERIPHERAL NERVES

This topic is important to create a better understanding of central and segmental pathology. The reader is recommended to look at the existing literature (Mumenthaler and Schliack, 1973).

LOCATIONS WHERE NERVE ENTRAPMENT MAY OCCUR

For the purpose of differential diagnosis, the practitioner needs to have an understanding of the kinds of compression lesions that can affect the peripheral nerves and what the practical skills are to elicit them. Some additional information on this topic may be found under the heading "Nerve Pressure Points" in Chapter 11, page 289; for further discussion, the reader is recommended to look at the literature (Kopell and Thompson, 1976).

COORDINATION

To have coordinated movement there needs to be a fine balance between the sensory and motor functions within the sensorimotor loop. This balance can be disturbed by central and peripheral neurologic disorders.

Central Neurologic Disorders

Central neurologic disorders can include proprioceptive disturbance, cerebellar disturbance, and vestibular disturbance. These disturbances can have the following consequences:

- Extreme increase in motor restlessness, possibly with the inability to maintain a standing position. This can be a sign of disturbance in central or peripheral nerve conduction.
- A limited increase in motor restlessness. This can be caused by dysfunction of the cerebellar system.
- A fall tendency to the same side. This may be caused by a dysfunction of the vestibular system.

In addition to the proprioceptive, cerebellar, and vestibular ataxias, the following may also be distinguished:

Extrapyramidal ataxia

Cerebral ataxia

Psychogenic ataxia

Extrapyramidal system

This includes:

- The corpus striatum:

     Neostriatum—nucleus caudatum, putamen

     Paleostriatum—globus pallidus
- The mesencephalic nuclei: Nucleus ruber, substantia nigra, nucleus subthalamicus
- The medulla oblongata: Nucleus olivarius inferior, substantia reticularis
- The cortical areas outside the primary motor zone

Extrapyramidal disturbances can be divided into the following categories:

Hypokinetic rigid syndromes, which are characterized by decreased movement patterns and increased muscle tone, such as Parkinson disease and the juvenile form of Huntington's disease

Hyperkinetic syndromes, which are characterized by excessive movement patterns, such as Huntington's disease and chorea minor

The symptomatology is as follows:

- Disturbances in muscle tone, usually hypertonia, occasionally hypotonia. This is characterized by the "lead pipe" and the "cogwheel" phenomena.
- The occurrence of involuntary movements:

     Slow tremors

     Choreatic movements

     Athetosis

     Hemiballistic movements

     Myoclonias, tics
- Disturbances in motor tempo and automatic functions:

     Hypokinesis

     Hypomimia, mask face

     Absence of trunk rotation

     Walking with small steps

     Flexed posture, tendency to fall

     Inability to start or stop

     Monotonous dysarthric speech

     Micrography

Note that the patient's emotional life is usually unaffected.

Cortical motor functions are generally intact, so complex movements can be performed without difficulty.

Cerebral Ataxia

This form of ataxia involves a tendency to fall backward, without attempts to correct this tendency.

Psychogenic Ataxia

In this condition, "clownish" movements can often be seen. Difficult tasks may be performed better than simple ones.

Peripheral Neurologic Disorders

When making a differential diagnosis in cases where the center of gravity is displaced, the therapist must consider the possibility of peripheral neurologic disorders. Difficulties in regulating posture can be caused by lesions of the tibial and the peroneal nerves, and to radicular symptomatology from the L5–S1 (myotomal muscles) segment. If there is a syndrome affecting L5–S1, the flexor digitorum brevis muscle may not function normally; this can be seen by a displacement of the center of gravity in a forward direction.

STATIC AND DYNAMIC COORDINATION

Coordination can be divided into static and dynamic coordination. Static coordination is about regulation of posture, whereas dynamic coordination concerns regulation of coordinated movements. In the text below several tests are described. Their purpose is to exclude central and peripheral neurologic disorders as underlying causes of the coordination issues. The result in most cases is either positive or negative depending on whether an impairment of static or dynamic coordination is present.

Static Coordination

Standing

Standing is a dynamic state of balance. It is a continuous process of subtle movement, as a result of which the center of gravity moves slightly within the base of support. The small displacements of the center of gravity are corrected and coordinated by the musculature of the lower leg. By challenging the individual through movements causing a displacement of the center of gravity in all directions, the therapist can discover how and to what extent the corrections are taking place. Postural corrections should normally occur within the base of support.

The base can also be made smaller, for example, by asking the patient to stand on one leg. The capsular receptors in the peripheral joints and the mechanoreceptors in the intervertebral joints play a primary role in maintaining this position. These receptors have a low discharge threshold, which plays a vital part in the ability to make the necessary corrections to stay balanced.

Romberg Test

The person being tested stands with feet close together but not touching. The test is performed with eyes open and with eyes closed (**Figure 7–82**). The patient's ability to maintain the position for 30 seconds is observed. This test can be modified, making it more sensitive, by having the subject stand with one foot in front of the other (**Figure 7–83**).

Other modifications include standing on one leg and the addition of flexion and extension of the cervical spine. Cervical extension causes a challenge of the vestibular system without reducing blood flow in the vertebral arteries. These modifications to the Romberg test can help to confirm symptoms noted during the "standard" test—such as motor overactivity or muscular overcorrection—because they may elicit them more clearly.

Hautant's Test

The subject sits upright with both eyes closed, the back supported, with the feet on the ground and arms out-

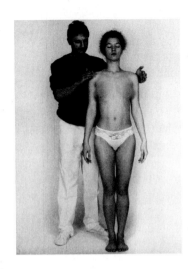

Figure 7–82

stretched in front. The forearms are pronated (palms down). The therapist stands in front and places his or her thumbs in front of the subject's middle fingers. The thumbs will be used to judge whether the patient's arms are deviating sideways (**Figure 7–84**). The patient initially holds his or her head still and the therapist looks for sideways movement of the arm(s) consistent with any tendency to fall when standing with eyes closed (Romberg test), or the deviation from a straight line when walking. If sideways movement of the arms should occur, this would be another possible symptom of vestibular dysfunction.

To explore the effects of upper cervical movements on the ability to maintain the arm position, the subject is asked

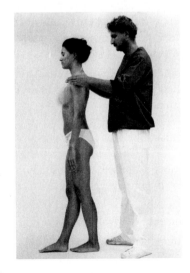

Figure 7–83

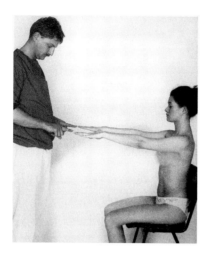

Figure 7–84

to make an extension movement of the cervical spine while rotating his or her head (**Figure 7–85**). During this maneuver, the therapist holds the subject's arms firmly in a neutral position, to prevent physiologic synkinetic arm movement; however, after this the thumbs of the therapist are again placed in front of the subject's middle fingers. The end position of the head movement must be held for a short time (20–30 seconds) because there is a latent period before the sideways movement of the arms begins.

Oostendorp (1984) performed an extensive literature search on the many interpretations of Hautant's test. His review indicates that the most relevant findings are those reported by Lewit and Berger (1985). These authors performed the test on 85 patients who suffered from vertiginous dizziness. They found three kinds of reaction to the test:

- *Reaction typical of cervical joint fixation.* During extension and rotation of the upper cervical spine in the direction of the cervical fixation, the sideways movement of the contralateral arm is opposite to that of the head. During flexion of the cervical spine and rotation of the head in the opposite (unloading) direction of the fixation, the deviation of the contralateral arm corrects itself.
- *Reaction partially typical of cervical fixation.* Also in this situation the sideways movement of the contralateral arm is in the direction opposite to that of the head movement. However, the movement of the upper cervical spine is not in the same direction as the direction of fixation.
- *Reaction not typical of cervical fixation.* In this situation, the result of Hautant's test is considered negative or the sideways deviation of the arm is in the same direction as the head movement.

Ninety percent of the patients who took part in the study of Lewit and Berger showed a reaction typical of a cervical joint fixation.

Hautant's test resembles a functional test of the vestibular system (Romberg test, Unterberger, Babinsky–Weil); however, differences become evident if there are symptoms in the direction of the nondominant vestibular organ (*harmonie vestibulaire*). In this case, the typical reaction to Hautant's test is not consistent with the direction of the tendency to fall or the pointing past the nose, which can be the result of a disturbance of the vestibular system. Hautant's test is clearly aimed at testing a different organ. Lewit and Berger (1985) attach great importance to disturbances of proprioceptive functioning as a result of dysfunctions in the upper cervical joints.

We may conclude that when the patient complains of dizziness, and when Hautant's test elicits the reaction typical of cervical spine fixation (as described earlier), the dizziness is most probably a consequence of upper cervical dysfunction. The symptoms of upper cervical fixation are largely identical to those of vertebrobasilar insufficiency.

Lewit (1986) states that proprioceptive vertebrogenic dizziness can be distinguished from dizziness caused by circulatory problems. Proprioceptive vertebrogenic dizziness occurs immediately and then decreases, whereas the dizziness as a result of circulatory problems has a latency period and then increases. Nevertheless, one must exercise extreme caution in evaluating and diagnosing dizziness.

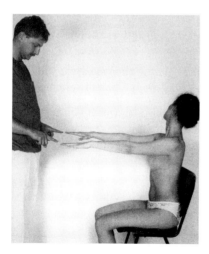

Figure 7–85

When deciding whether or not manual therapy is indicated, a detailed neurologic medical examination is often essential. Changes in afferent input associated with functional disturbances of the upper cervical area are not the only cause that could result in dysbalance in levels of stimulation of the left and right vestibular nuclei. Others are the following:

- Otitis media
- Arteriosclerosis (labyrinthine arteries)
- Vertebrobasilar insufficiency resulting from mechanical obstructions such as osteophytes, uncovertebral degenerative changes, prolapsed disk, hypertonic neck muscles, and raised sympathetic tone

Barré Test

In this test, which can be carried out either standing or sitting, the arms are extended horizontally, palms face upward, and the eyes are closed (**Figure 7–86**). If one of the arms lowers slowly, with a simultaneous pronation of the forearm, this could indicate a mild paresis of central neurologic origin.

To evaluate the lower extremities, the test is carried out in the prone position (**Figure 7–87**). The knees are bent at an angle of 45° so that the lower legs make an angle of 45° with the examination table. If one of the lower legs lowers (often jerkily), this can also indicate a mild paresis of central origin.

Dynamic Coordination

Ambulation

When ambulation is being examined, it is essential that there is enough space for the patient to walk a reasonable distance. Additional tasks can be imposed that determine

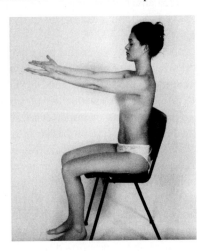

Figure 7–86

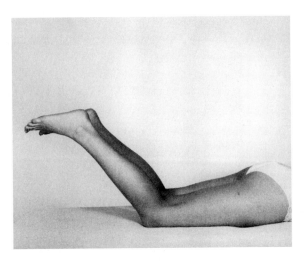

Figure 7–87

how the patient walks, for example, walking along a line while placing the feet in front of each other or next to each other, or walking with eyes closed.

There are two main kinds of abnormal gait patterns:

- The *spastic gait*, in which the flexion-extension mechanism is disturbed because dissociation between flexion and extension is not possible.
- The *ataxic gait*, in which the steps are uneven in length and direction. Continual corrections are necessary.

These atypical gait patterns may be caused by the following conditions:

- Central neurologic disorders
- Peripheral neurologic disorders
- Disorders of the lower limbs and pelvis

Central Neurologic Disorders

Disturbances during the gait cycle with the eyes closed can indicate disorders in different systems:

- A clearly visible abnormality of gait can indicate a disturbance of the proprioceptive system, although this is not necessarily the result of a central neurologic disorder. Dysmetria can also be a result of proprioceptive disturbances.
- A wide stance ambulation pattern with a less obvious disturbance of the gait cycle can indicate a disturbance of the cerebrovestibular system.
- An abnormality of the gait cycle that is always in the same direction can point to a disturbance of the vestibular system.

Peripheral Neurologic Disorders

Peripheral nerve lesions and radicular and pseudoradicular symptomatology can all be associated with abnormal gait patterns. Steppage gait and staggering can be both caused by peripheral as well as central neurologic disturbance.

Disorders of the Legs and Pelvis

If the patient's gait cycle is abnormal, the condition of the foot, ankle, knee, hip, and sacroiliac joints must be taken into account, as well as the possible presence of any leg length difference or congenital deformities.

Unterberger's Test

The subject is asked to walk on the spot, eyes closed, while flexing the hips and knees to an angle of 90°. (See **Figure 7–88**.) A turn of the body by about 45° for every 50 steps is considered normal. If the subject turns more than 45°, the test result is considered positive, and the number of degrees in excess of 45° is noted.

The direction of the turn is also recorded. Turning direction indicates an ipsilateral vestibular disturbance. Turning in various directions indicates a cerebellar disturbance. The test should be carried out in a quiet room with low lighting.

Babinski and Weil Test

The subject is asked to close his or her eyes and take five steps forward and five steps backward and repeat this a few times. If there is a disturbance in the balance system, the subject will make a star shape (*marche en étoile*) pattern. The direction of deviation in this case will be the same as that shown in Unterberger's test. This test too should be carried out in a quiet room with low lighting.

Upper Limb

The following tests can be used: fingertip-to-nose test, finger-to-ear test, tip-to-tip test, and the dysdiadochokinesia test.

Fingertip-to-Nose Test   In this test, the subject's eyes are closed and the subject is asked to touch his or her nose with a fingertip. (See **Figure 7–89**.) This is done with both the right hand and the left hand. If there is a disturbance of the vestibular system, the subject will miss and point to the side of the nondominant vestibular system. Mild cerebellar ataxia results in an intention tremor near beginning and end of the movement with possible overshooting of the target. This test has poor test-retest and interrater reliability for dysmetria and tremor, but excellent reliability for time of execution (Vidal and Huijbregts, 2005). Swaine et al. (2005a, 2005b) reported mean test-retest reliability coefficients of 0.77–0.82 for time of execution of five repetitions of the fingertip-to-nose test indicating clinically sufficient test-retest reliability in healthy adults and also established norms for healthy subjects aged 15 to 34 years.

Dysdiadochokinesia Test   In this test, opposing movements are performed quickly, for example, opposing pronation and supination movements with the lower arms, which are bent at an angle of 90°. (See **Figures 7–90** and **7–91**.) Other possible tests include rapid alternating finger or foot tapping (Vidal and Huijbregts, 2005).

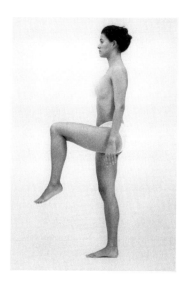

Figure 7–88

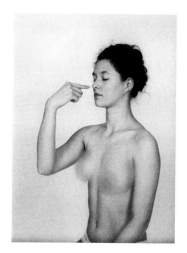

Figure 7–89

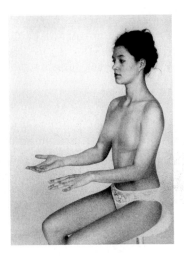

Figure 7–90

Lower limb

Knee-Heel Test   The subject is asked to bring the heel of one foot to the knee of the other leg, while having the eyes closed. (See **Figure 7–92**.)

Heel-Lower Leg Test   The patient is asked to move the heel from one foot over the dorsal aspect of the opposite foot over the shin toward the knee, while maintaining a constant distance above the lower leg with the foot. (See **Figure 7–93**.)

The De Kleyn–Nieuwenhuyse Test

In 1927, on the basis of their research on cadavers, De Kleyn and Nieuwenhuyse stated that cervical extension

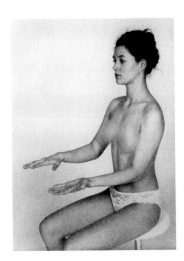

Figure 7–91

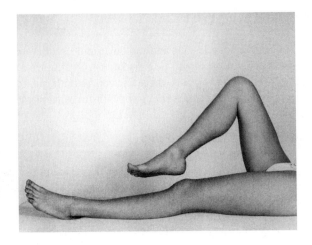

Figure 7–92

in combination with rotation of the head causes a decrease in blood flow in the contralateral vertebral artery. Many subsequent authors have cited this maneuver, sometimes describing it with small modifications, as a way of testing the functioning of the vertebrobasilar system. The modified tests that are presented in the literature do not differ much on the essentials of the maneuver; however, there is no consensus on the signs and symptoms that are considered positive indication of vertebrobasilar insufficiency (Oostendorp, 1988).

One of the most important symptoms generally included in the list, and which could be established objectively, is dizziness. From both a neuroanatomic and a neurophysiologic point of view, there are functional links between the vestibular-vertebral, oculomotor-vertebral, and cervicovertebral systems down to the segment C3–C4. Hülse (1983a, 1983b) speaks in this context of cervico-vestibulo-ocular reflexes. It seems logical that disorders in this sensory orien-

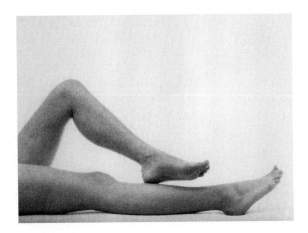

Figure 7–93

tation system and its central representation could lead to dizziness. Oosterveld (1984) describes dizziness as a sensation of undergoing nonexistent patterns of posture and movement.

The aim of the De Kleyn and Nieuwenhuyse procedure is to test the flow of blood in the vertebral arteries during the endrange of specific movements of the cervical spine, including the C0–C1 segment. Blood flow in one vertebral artery is tested by decreasing the flow in the other as much as possible. Reducing or blocking the blood flow in one vertebral artery can, if there is insufficient compensation through the opposite side or through the anterior internal carotid system, lead to disturbances and decreased perfusion in the area supplied by the vertebrobasilar system (see later in this chapter).

The Modified De Kleyn–Nieuwenhuyse Test

The patient is supine on the examination table in such a manner that the head is free to move to endrange in all directions. The eyes are kept open. (See **Figure 7–94**.) The practitioner sits at the short end of the table behind the patient's head and slowly places the cervical spine through the different movements. The endrange of each movement is held until the patient reports identifiable symptoms (to a maximum of 2 minutes per movement). The head is then brought back to the neutral position. The practitioner waits a minimum of 1 minute before carrying out the next movement, or longer until the symptoms disappear. The patient is asked to report when the symptoms appear (latency) and when they disappear (recovery time) (Oostendorp, 1988).

The test is positive—which would be an indication of a functional vertebrobasilar insufficiency—when, in the absence of an identifiable organic cause, the symptoms and complaints increase during or after the cervical provocation tests, and this is confirmed by the patient.

Order of Cervical Movements　Mechanical loads are applied to the vertebral artery by means of cervical movements that are made in the following order:

- Flexion
- Extension
- Bilateral sidebending
- Bilateral rotation
- Flexion in combination with bilateral rotation
- Extension in combination with bilateral rotation

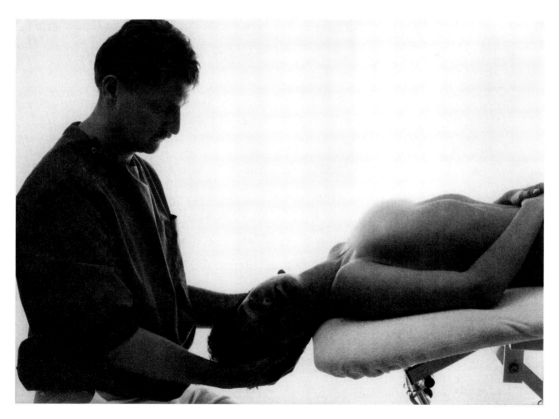

Figure 7–94

- Extension, sidebending, and bilateral ipsilateral rotation
- Flexion, sidebending, and bilateral contralateral rotation

Oostendorp (1988) states in his doctoral thesis that the following cervical movements are the most likely to elicit symptoms in cases of vertebrobasilar insufficiency:

- Extension, probably based on a neurogenic mechanism
- Left and right rotation
- Extension in combination with right and left rotation

The clinician may, therefore, want to utilize only these movements when using the De Kleyn–Nieuwenhuyse test.

The limitation of the De Kleyn–Nieuwenhuyse test lies in the fact that if movement is limited, especially in the upper cervical spine, the vertebral artery cannot be fully elongated. The clinician should keep in mind that the reduction of movement may be the result of a natural protective mechanism. If this is the case, it is called a *Schutzblockierung* ("protective fixation").

Signs and Symptoms   Later in this chapter we discuss signs and symptoms of cervical artery dysfunction including both the vertebrobasilar and internal carotid systems. However, based on what is still the most extensive study in this area, Oostendorp (1988) mentions the following symptoms, when performing the modified De Kleyn–Nieuwenhuyse test, as being the most likely to reveal vertebrobasilar insufficiency:

- Dizziness on rotation, without or without other symptoms such as ringing in the ears, vomiting, and other autonomic symptoms
- Headache
- Neck pain
- Nystagmus
- Lowering of consciousness, syncopic attacks
- Disturbances of the visual field
- Paresthesias in the face, and/or arms, and/or legs
- Drop attacks

For the result of the De Kleyn–Nieuwenhuyse test to be considered positive, it is not necessary for all of these symptoms to appear together. The three symptoms that are conclusive for vertebrobasilar insufficiency include headache, neck pain, and dizziness on rotation.

Frenzel glasses are useful in checking eye movements for nystagmus (see the section titled "Nystagmus" later in this chapter) because the surroundings appear blurred to the patient, making optokinetic fixation practically impossible.

If the modified De Kleyn–Nieuwenhuyse test reveals the presence of a nystagmus, dizziness on rotation, lowering of consciousness, disturbances of the visual field, drop attacks, and paresthesias in the arms/legs either separately or together, a medical consultation will be necessary to obtain a differential diagnosis. Manual therapy is contraindicated.

In the section titled "Movements of the Cervical Spine and Their Effect on Cervical Artery Perfusion" later in this chapter, we discuss research into the effect of cervical motions on vertebrobasilar and internal carotid system hemodynamics and the equivocal results this research has produced. Richter and Reinking (2005) have calculated diagnostic accuracy statistics for the De Kleyn–Nieuwenhuyse test based on studies by Côté et al. (1996) and Sakaguchi et al. (2003) by comparing ultrasound flow study findings to clinical symptoms thought indicative of vertebral artery compression. Sensitivity for both vertebral arteries in the Côté et al. (1996) study was 0% and specificity for the right vertebral artery was 86%, whereas the left artery scored 67%. Note that a positive test was defined as the occurrence on a 30-second hold of vertigo, nausea, tinnitus, lightheadedness, visual problems, numbness of the face or on one side of the body, nystagmus, vomiting, or loss of consciousness. Diagnostic accuracy data calculated from the Sakaguchi et al. (2003) study included sensitivity of 9.3% (95% CI: 4–19.9%), specificity of 97.8% (95% CI: 96.7–98.5%), a positive likelihood ratio of 4.243 (95% CI: 1.678–10.729), and a negative likelihood ratio of 0.928 (95% CI: 0.851–1.011). It is clear that with such sensitivity values the De Kleyn–Nieuwenhuyse test is without any research-based value in its common clinical use as a screening test. In contrast, it may have value as a diagnostic test because of its high specificity. However, with an established incidence of cervical artery dissection in the general population of 2.6 per 100,000 as the pretest probability, we have to question the effect of a positive test finding on posttest probability despite a moderately high positive likelihood ratio of 4.243 (Graziano et al., 2007).

In addition, Thiel and Rix (2005) rightfully question the ability of positional testing in a still patent vessel to produce clinically useful information with regard to the risk of adverse effects with manipulative intervention. These authors also noted that the test itself may put the patient at risk in case of a pathologically weakened vessel, especially because cadaver studies have shown greater strain values with the test as compared to manipulation. Haldeman et al. (2002) also questioned the predictive validity of the test: in their retrospective review of 64 medicolegal cases where manipulation was associated with stroke, in 27 patients the test was documented with negative results in all cases.

Visual Field Test

The patient is asked to look straight ahead while the clinician holds the index fingers of both hands about 40 inches in front of the patient's nose. (See **Figure 7–95.**) The clinician then moves his or her fingers away from each other. The patient indicates when he or she can no longer see them. It is considered normal for the fingers to be visible to the width of the shoulders. This test is important because it can indicate disturbance of the optical nerve. Visual field confrontation testing had low sensitivity but high specificity (0.97) and positive predictive value (0.9) when compared to automated perimetry (Shahinfar et al., 1995), indicating that a confrontation-method visual field test may have diagnostic value only if positive.

Visual Fixation Test

Before performing this test, the eyes are checked for nystagmus with the patient looking straight ahead. The clinician then holds the index finger of one hand at the height of the patient's nose and about 40 inches in front of it. (See **Figure 7–96.**) The patient is asked to focus on the finger with both eyes; the practitioner observes the patient's eyes for the presence of a nystagmus.

Visual Tracking Test

The practitioner moves the index finger of one hand, at the patient's eye level and 40 inches away, at an angle of 45°

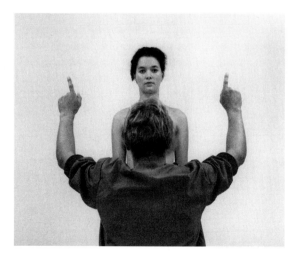

Figure 7–95

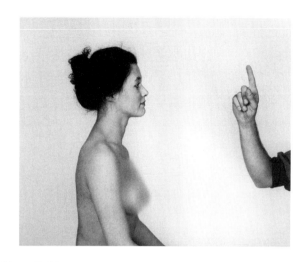

Figure 7–96

equally to the left and to the right, and at an angle of 30° upward and downward. (See **Figures 7–97** and **7–98.**) The patient is asked to follow the finger with his or her eyes. To exclude the cervico-ocular and spino-ocular reflexes, the patient may not move his or her head or cervical spine. The clinician watches the eyes for signs of nystagmus.

Saccadic Eye Movement Test

The examiner holds the index fingers of both hands at the patient's eye level and 40 inches away, at an angle of 30° to the patient's nose. (See **Figure 7–99.**) The patient is asked to look with both eyes first to the one finger and then the other, without moving his or her head. The clinician watches the *saccades* to see whether the eye movements overshoot the target.

Hearing Test

Rinne's tuning fork test is used to screen hearing. The tuning fork, sounding C at 128 Hz, is placed on the patient's mastoid process. (See **Figure 7–100.**) As soon as the patient no longer can hear the sound, the tuning fork is held in front of the ear; in the normal situation the patient should hear the sound again.

Rotation Stop Test

The patient sits on a rotating stool, with or without van Frenzel glasses. He or she is spun around for 20 seconds and then suddenly stopped. (See **Figure 7–101.**) During this test, the patient is dependent on the vestibular system

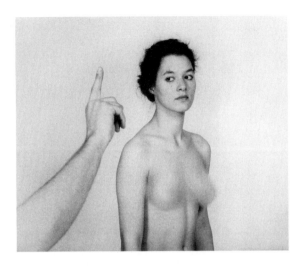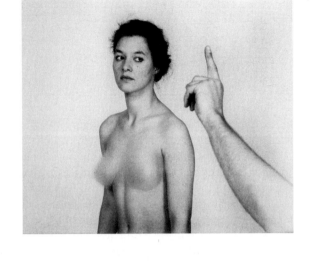

Figure 7–97

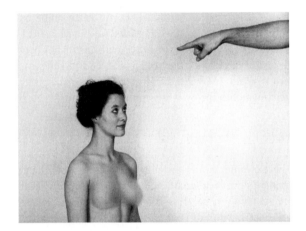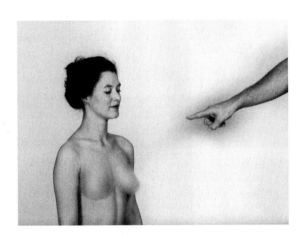

Figure 7–98

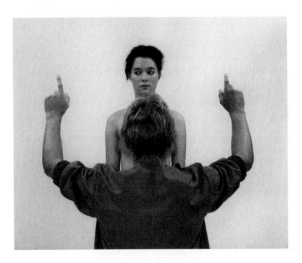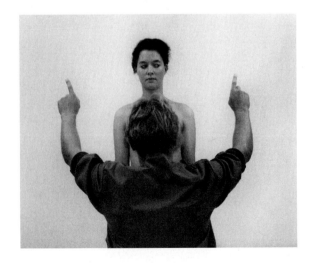

Figure 7–99

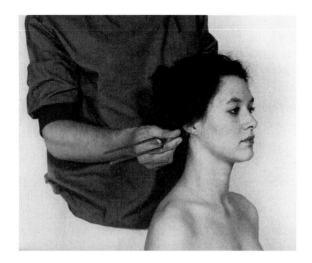

Figure 7–100

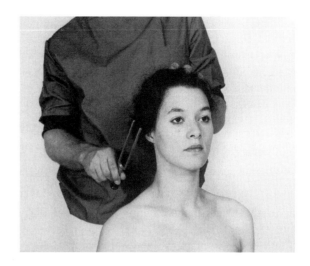

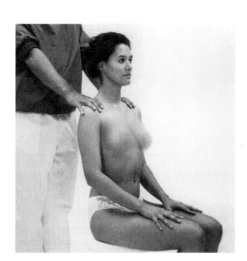

Figure 7–101

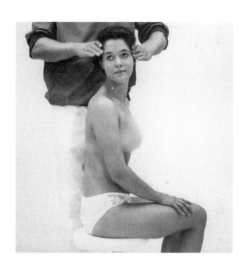

Figure 7–102

and to a lesser extent on the proprioceptive system. The criterion for this test is based on the fact that the physiologically occurring nystagmus should disappear within 30 seconds. Nausea and dizziness may occur as additional symptoms during the period that the nystagmus is present.

Sinusoidal Rotation Test

The patient sits on a rotating stool, with or without van Frenzel glasses. The clinician holds the patient's head immobile and rotates the stool through about 60° alternately to the right and left. (See **Figure 7–102**.) As a result of this manual fixation of the head the vestibular system is not di-

rectly stimulated, although it is possible that it could be indirectly stimulated through the cervical spine.

Normally, there should be no nystagmus. If a nystagmus does occur, it is probably of cervical origin, and further differential diagnosis is needed to rule out a vascular nystagmus.

NYSTAGMUS

In a number of the tests described earlier, the criterion for a positive result was the occurrence of a nystagmus. Recent work (Oostendorp et al., 1990) has shown that the methods used in manual diagnostics for observing eye movements, namely, Frenzel glasses and visual judgments of eye movements, are only of limited value. In the literature on vertebrobasilar insufficiency, much attention is paid to positional nystagmus; therefore, this is now discussed in greater detail.

Two forms of positional nystagmus of cervical origin should be distinguished:

- Vascular form
- Proprioceptive form

The Vascular Positional Nystagmus of Cervical Origin

The vascular form of positional nystagmus of cervical origin is a result of unilateral malfunction in the vestibular nuclei and the vestibular organ, caused by temporary disturbance of blood flow in the vertebrobasilar supply area during movement of the cervical spine. Oostendorp (1988) lists the following characteristics of the vascular form:

- A latency period lasting seconds to minutes during maximal rotation of the cervical spine.
- A *crescendo* pattern.
- Usually present only on one side; however, it can also be absent in patients with vertebrobasilar insufficiency.
- Third-degree nystagmus according to Moser's (1974) classification.

The presence of vascular positional nystagmus of cervical origin is an absolute contraindication for manual therapy.

Proprioceptive Positional Nystagmus of Cervical Origin

The proprioceptive form of positional nystagmus in the cervical spine is thought to be pathognomonic for fixation in segments C0 through C4 (Oostendorp et al., 1990). Eye movements are regulated not only by visual signals, but also by proprioceptive signals from the vestibular system and the posture and movement systems, which are dependent on the cervical region. The optokinetic reflex (OKR), the vestibulo-ocular reflex (VOR), and the cervico-ocular reflex (COR) are distinguished according to their origin.

In adults, the cervico-ocular reflex can be elicited only if pathology is present, such as lesions of the vestibular system. We may conclude from this that the VOR dominates the COR; the OKR and the VOR must, therefore, be suppressed if the COR is to be assessed. This can be done by carrying out the examination in a dark room or asking the patient to wear Frenzel glasses, and making the cervical movements by moving the trunk while the head is kept

still. The rotational movements are the easiest to carry out. Rotating the trunk while the head is immobilized in a static position causes adequate stimulation of the static mechanoreceptors in the soft tissues and joints of the upper cervical region. Under these conditions, a positional nystagmus of cervical origin could be elicited if present. It is also possible to carry out a sinusoidal rotation of the trunk with the head in a fixed position. This stimulates the dynamic mechanoreceptors of the tissues and joints of the upper cervical region.

Propriosensory cervical positional nystagmus is often thought to be associated with joint fixation of spinal segments C0 through C4, but the mechanism by which it arises is still unknown. One hypothesis is that hypomobility of the upper cervical intervertebral joints reduces the discharging of the static and dynamic mechanoreceptors. This reduction in proprioceptive input from the upper cervical segments would cause dysregulation of the systems in the vestibular nuclei and the nuclei of the oculomotor nerves that control eye movements. A second hypothesis is that cartilaginous changes in the upper cervical spine cause mechanical stimulation of the cervical dorsal roots and/or dorsal ganglia. The resulting pathologically induced afferent stimulation would cause direct stimulation of the vestibular nuclei.

Hülse (1983a) describes the following as indicators of the proprioceptive positional nystagmus of cervical origin:

- No latency period
- A *decrescendo* pattern because of the rapid adaptation of the dynamic mechanoreceptors
- Usually present if there is fixation of the upper cervical segments and it can be elicited in different movement directions (horizontal, vertical, and rotational nystagmus)
- A first-degree nystagmus according to Moser's (1974) classification

In a study by Oostendorp et al. (1990) of 101 patients with one or more hypomobile upper cervical segments, visual detection of a proprioceptive positional nystagmus was possible in 10 patients. These patients had fixations at several levels in the upper cervical region (C0 to C4). In other studies reported in the literature using more or less identical assessment criteria for selecting the patient population, the frequency of the proprioceptive induced positional nystagmus is generally higher. In the study by Oostendorp et al. (1990), eye movements were observed while the patients were wearing Frenzel glasses, and the movements were judged visually. In the studies that showed higher frequencies, electronystagmography was used. This suggests that the methods normally used in manual diagnostics for assessing eye movements are inadequate. It is probable that the proprioceptively induced positional nystagmus can be detected visually only when several upper cervical movement segments are blocked and proprioceptive input from the upper cervical joints to the vestibular nuclei is consequently much reduced.

MOTOR FUNCTION

Examination of motor function includes assessment of sensorimotor activities in patients with central neurologic disorders. They are asked to adopt postures and carry out movements that appear sequentially during normal motor development. The practitioner needs to have knowledge of central neurologic disorders to interpret motor symptoms.

Complaints relating to the movement apparatus, especially the vertebral column, require a different approach to interpretation. When assessing motor function in these cases, more emphasis is placed on the way in which the vertebral column behaves during basic activities, such as standing up, sitting down, bending, lifting, raising, carrying, pulling, pushing, throwing, and catching. This part of the examination, which is normally carried out during the patient inspection, can be repeated when the pain is reduced or has disappeared. It can then be regarded as therapy for functional recovery; this is also called sensorimotor training.

CIRCULATION
Aad van der El and Peter A. Huijbregts

To allow for a comprehensive examination, the practitioner needs to have good working knowledge of the entire vascular system that supplies the brain and spinal cord. However, there are particular blood vessels that have special relevance to examination of spinal movement.

Spinal Arteries

The direct blood supply to the spinal cord is through the posterior and anterior spinal arteries. (See **Figure 7–103**.) Both these arteries originate from the radicular arteries, which enter the spinal canal through the intervertebral foramen. Narrowing of the intervertebral foramen can cause radicular and pseudoradicular symptoms and can cause a disturbance in the perfusion of the spinal cord, which in extreme cases can lead to ischemia of the spinal cord.

Vertebral Arteries and Basilar Artery

The vertebral arteries coursing through the cervical region join together intracranially to form the basilar artery and are responsible for about 20% of the cervical and intracranial blood supply (Graziano et al., 2007; Kerry and Taylor, 2006). (See **Figure 7–104**.) Considering the course of the vertebral arteries through the cervical spine, they play an important role in manual diagnosis of this spinal region.

The vertebral artery normally courses through the intertransverse foramina of the cervical vertebrae. However, there are reports of atypical cases in which this is not the case, or only partly so. In the individual foramina, the vertebral artery has essentially fixed attachments, resulting in tension on it during movements around the vertical and sagittal axes. According to Penning (1978), the axis of flexion–extension of the cervical segments lies at the level of the vertebral artery, so movement around this axis does not lengthen it (**Figure 7–105**). It is subject to most tensile force during rotation of the cervical spine. The functional

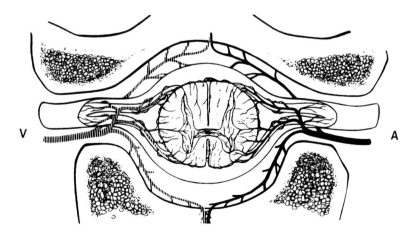

Figure 7–103 Vascular supply of the spinal cord.

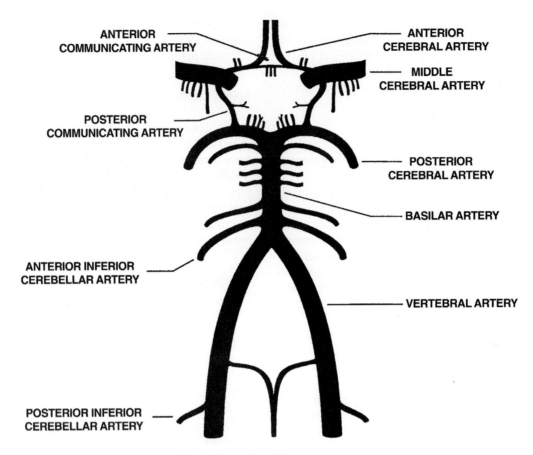

Figure 7–104   Vertebral and basilar arteries and their respective branches.

loop between C1 and C2 will be stretched when C1 is fully rotated in respect to C2 (**Figure 7–106**). The loop between C0 and C1, which is not stretched during movement, probably serves as a dampening mechanism for excessively strong pulsation (comparable to the carotid siphon, described by Dörfer and Spatz, 1935, in Penning, 1978).

Internal Carotid Arteries

The internal carotid artery branches off from the common carotid artery and runs cranially anterior to the transverse processes of C1–C3. It then enters the carotid canal in the petrous portion of the temporal bone (Clemente, 1985). Fixed to the anterior aspect of the vertebral body as well as in the carotid canal and traversing the sternocleidomastoid, longus capitis, stylohyoid, omohyoid, and digastric muscles it may experience tensile stress during cervical motions, especially contralateral rotation and extension-contralateral rotation, and the clinical tests for the vertebral arteries have also been proposed as tests for the internal carotid arteries (Haneline and Triano, 2005; Kerry and Taylor, 2006; Licht

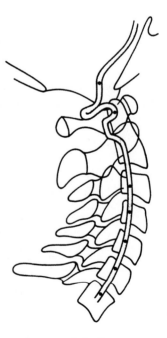

Figure 7–105   Localization of the flexion–extension axis in relation to the vertebral artery.

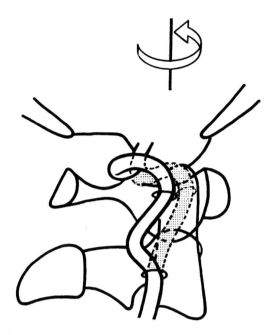

Figure 7–106 Elongation possibility of the upper cervical loop of the vertebral artery during rotation.

et al., 2002). Add to this the fact that 80% of the cerebral circulation is supplied by the internal carotid arteries and that, therefore, tests proposed in the past to examine the vertebrobasilar system could more reasonably be seen to test the ability of the internal carotid arteries to compensate for a physiologic and/or pathologic loss of posterior circulation, and the reemphasis in recent years from the posterior system to include also the anterior circulatory system and speak of cervical artery dysfunction becomes more understandable (Kerry and Taylor, 2006; Kerry et al., 2008). However, we need to still put this reemphasis in perspective by pointing out that Terrett (2000) in his review of 185 cases of manipulation-associated cervical artery injuries only found 5 cases (2.7%) that reported injuries to the internal carotid artery.

Structures Supplied by the Vertebrobasilar System

The area supplied by the vertebral arteries and the basilar artery, with their branches and anastosmoses with other arteries, include a cervical area and an intracranial area. (See **Figure 7–107**.)

The Cervical Supply Area

The branches of the vertebral artery that originate from it in the cervical region are the following:

- *Spinal arteries.* These divide into the anterior and the posterior radicular arteries that vascularize the anterior and posterior nerve root and the spinal ganglion. The anterior central artery and the anterior and posterior vertebral canal artery also branch from the vertebral artery.
- *The muscular, joint, and cutaneous rami.* These vascularize the intrinsic cervical musculature of the segments C2–C7, the interspinal ligament, the flaval ligament, the joint capsules of the intervertebral and uncovertebral joints, and the area of skin supplied by the dorsal ramus.
- *Ascending arteries of the axis.* These vascularize the body and dens of C2, the transverse ligament, and the cruciform atlantal ligament.

The branches of the vertebral artery that originate from it subforaminally (below the foramen magnum) are the anterior, posterior, and lateral spinal arteries. These arteries, which run longitudinally, with their transverse branches and anastosmotic connections with the radicular arteries, vascularize the cervical spinal cord. In most cases, the anterior spinal artery receives anastosmoses from the ventral radicular arteries only below C4. This means that the upper cervical spinal cord is more vulnerable with regard to its blood supply. In ischemia of the cervical cord, a number of clinical phenomena will occur that are consistent with a vertebrobasilar insufficiency (VBI) picture. The encephalic (or brain-related) symptoms indicative of other ischemic syndromes, however, are absent.

The Intracranial Supply Area

The vertebral arteries join together to form the basilar artery. Just before they join, the posterior inferior cerebellar artery branches off. This artery vascularizes the dorsolateral part of the medulla oblongata, a large part of the posterior lobe of the cerebellum, the cerebellar vermis, and a number of cerebellar nuclei.

The basilar artery with its branches vascularizes the medulla oblongata, the pons, the mesencephalon, and parts of the cerebellum. The reticular formation and the vestibular system with its nuclei also depend on the basilar artery and its branches for their blood supply. In fact, the labyrinthine arteries branch off early from the basilar artery or the anterior inferior cerebellar arteries to supply the vestibular nucleus and inner ears making these structures very susceptible to ischemia and explaining the symptom of dizziness as an early presentation of ischemic syndromes affecting the posterior circulation (Oostendorp, 1988).

The posterior cerebral arteries that originate from the basilar artery at the level of the clivus vascularize parts of

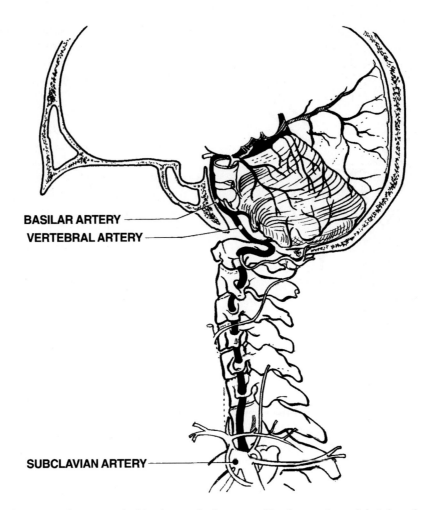

BASILAR ARTERY

VERTEBRAL ARTERY

SUBCLAVIAN ARTERY

Figure 7–107   Extra- and intracranial areas supplied by the vertebral artery and basilar arteries and their branches.

the thalamus and hypothalamus, the occipital lobe, the basal part of the temporal lobe, the dorsal part of the capsula interna, and the lateral corpus geniculatum.

The posterior cerebral arteries and the posterior communicating arteries join together to form the circle of Willis.

Segments of the vertebral artery

As shown in **Figure 7–108** the segments of the vertebral artery are the following:

V_1: In 89% of cases, the *extravertebral part* runs from its origin from the subclavian artery to the transverse foramen of C6. It enters at C7 in 3%, at C5 in 6%, and at C4 in 1% of the population (Thiel, 1991). In this area, the vertebral artery runs ventrally of the transverse process of

T1 and C7, and the first rib, and dorsally of the longus colli muscle and the anterior scalene muscle.

V_2: The *intravertebral part*, which in most cases runs anteromedially from C6 to C2 through the transverse foramina, is surrounded in between the foramina by ligament and muscle tissue. The uncovertebral joints form the anteromedial boundary. The cervical nerve roots and cervical spinal nerves lie dorsal to the vertebral artery.

V_3: The *atlantoaxial part* runs from C2 to C0. In this section, the vertebral artery forms a dorsolateral loop. From the transverse foramen of the atlas, which lies more laterally, the vertebral artery follows a medial path via the vertebral artery sulcus and behind the lateralis masses of the atlas. The ventral boundary is formed by the capsule of the atlanto-occipital joint and the dorsal boundary by the obliquus capitis superior muscle and the rectus capi-

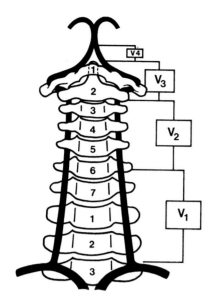

Figure 7–108 Segments of the vertebral artery.

tus posterior major muscle. In some patients, a bony bridge is present called the ponticulus posterior where the artery crosses over the posterior arch of the atlas: the added fixation is hypothesized to make the artery even more prone to tensile lesions at this level (Triano and Kawchuk, 2006).

V_4: The *subforaminal and intracranial part*. The subforaminal part of the vertebral artery passes through the posterior atlanto-occipital membrane, the dura mater, the pia mater, and the arachnoid, and continues its way intracranially.

Segments of the Internal Carotid Artery

As does the vertebral artery, the internal carotid artery also has four separate portions (Clemente, 1985): the cervical, petrous, cavernous, and cerebral portions.

The cervical portion is formed at the bifurcation of the common carotid into the external and internal carotid arteries at the upper border of the thyroid cartilage. The internal carotid artery is located here posterior and lateral to its external counterpart, overlapped by the sternocleidomastoid muscle and covered by the deep anterior cervical fascia, platysma, and the skin. Superiorly to this bifurcation the hypoglossal nerve (12th cranial nerve), the posterior belly of the digastric muscle, the stylohyoid muscle, and the occipital and posterior auricular branches of the external carotid artery traverse the internal carotid artery. Even more superior the artery is bordered by the glossopharyngeal nerve (9th cranial nerve), the pharyngeal branch of the va-

gus nerve (10th cranial nerve), the longus capitis muscle, the superior cervical sympathetic ganglion, and the superior laryngeal branch of the vagus nerve. At the skull base level, the artery borders the glossopharyngeal, vagus, accessory, and hypoglossal nerves (9th–12th cranial nerves). This close anatomic connection to the various cranial nerves will serve later to explain some of the nonischemic signs and symptoms of internal carotid artery dissection.

The petrous portion starts where the internal carotid artery enters the carotid canal in the petrous portion of the temporal bone. Relevant to the clinical presentation of internal carotid artery dissection is its close anatomic connection to the cochlea and tympanic cavity and also to the trigeminal ganglion (ganglion of the 5th cranial nerve).

The cavernous portion of the internal carotid artery is named after the close anatomic connection the artery has in this aspect of its course, with the layers of the dura forming the cavernous sinus. Most relevant to clinical presentation of a dissection is its close proximity to the abducens nerve (6th cranial nerve).

After perforating the dura mater the internal carotid artery passes between the optic and oculomotor nerves (2nd and 3rd cranial nerves) and then divides into its cerebral branches.

Structures Supplied by the Internal Carotid Artery

The cervical portion of the internal carotid artery gives off no branches (Clemente, 1985). The petrous portion mainly provides the caroticotympanic artery that supplies the tympanic membrane together with branches from the posterior auricular and maxillary arteries. The cavernous portion gives off the cavernous branches, hypophyseal branches, ganglionic branches, and the anterior meningeal branch, which provide the arterial supply to the hypophysis, the trigeminal ganglion, and the anterior cranial dura mater. The cerebral portion of the internal carotid artery provides the ophthalmic artery supplying the optic nerve, the orbital structures including the extraocular muscles, and the eyeball. After joining the circle of Willis by way of the posterior communicating arteries thereby establishing the major anastosmosis for a deficient posterior circulation, the cavernous portion of the internal carotid artery divides into the anterior and medial cerebral arteries that supply the major portions of both hemispheres (Clemente, 1985).

Movements of the Cervical Spine and Their Effect on Cervical Artery Perfusion

In 1927, De Kleyn and Nieuwenhuyse reported decreased and absent vertebral artery blood flow based on cadaver perfusion studies in various head and neck positions. Based on these early perfusion studies and on the anatomic considerations with regard to the cervical arteries discussed earlier, the sustained extension–rotation and sustained rotation tests have been proposed and widely instructed and clinically used as tests to determine the presence of vertebrobasilar artery dysfunction.

Chrost (Gutmann and Biedermann, 1984) and Hillen and Fonville (1980) discussed the effects of physiologic movements on blood flow in the vertebral artery. In line with the work by De Kleyn and Nieuwenhuyse (1927), their work is an example of the earlier work on this topic that has dominated clinical reasoning within OMT for decades, with changes occurring in this area only recently. These authors concluded that there is a reduction in blood flow in the vertebral artery during physiologic movement of the cervical spine even in the absence of any anomaly or pathology. Rotation of the cervical spine seems to have a particularly marked effect in reducing blood flow in the contralateral vertebral artery.

Hillen and Fonville (1980) report that the reduced vascular resistance in the vertebral artery during rotation of the cervical spine is the greatest in the ipsilateral vertebral artery at the atlantoaxial segment. They believe that this is because of the relatively long distance from the transverse foramen of the atlas to the centrally located axis of rotation of the cervical spine, and to the compression at the level of the transverse foramen of the atlas (**Figure 7–109**).

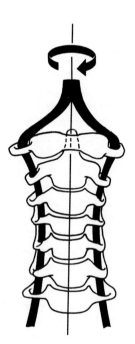

Figure 7–109   Distance of the vertebral artery to the axis of rotation of the cervical vertebrae.

Sidebending seems to have no effect on blood flow in the vertebral artery on the contralateral side, and only a limited influence (10%) ipsilaterally. Penning (1978) states that the position of the facet joints in the segments of C2–C7 during sidebending does not differ much from their position during rotation. He argues that the difference in osteokinematic trajectory between cervical rotation and sidebending must, therefore, be caused by the rotation of C1–C2 being added to the sidebending. This argument, and the relatively small reduction in blood flow during sidebending, supports the position of Hillen and Fonville (1980), namely, that during rotation in the atlantoaxial segment, the reduction in vascular resistance is greater on the ipsilateral side.

During flexion and extension of the cervical spine, there is no reduction in blood flow. This is also consistent with Penning's theory (Penning, 1978) (Figure 7–105). Although under normal circumstances extension does not lead to any reduction in blood flow in the vertebral artery, it seems capable of causing symptoms of functional vertebrobasilar insufficiency. This might be the result of a reflexogenic reaction to mechanical irritation of the smooth muscle tissue of the vertebral artery wall or mechanical stimulation of nociceptive units.

Chrost, referenced by Gutmann and Biedermann (1984), investigated the blood flow in both vertebral arteries during different movements of the cervical spine and produced a chart of the results (**Figure 7–110**). Expressed in percentages, these reductions are approximately as follows:

Flexion and Extension: 0%

Sidebending: Ipsilateral, 10%; contralateral, 0%

Rotation: Ipsilateral, 20%; contralateral, 75%

Flexion, rotation: Ipsilateral and contralateral, 55%

Extension, rotation: Ipsilateral, 50%; contralateral, 75%

Flexion, sidebending, contralateral rotation: Ipsilateral (with regard to the rotational component), 30%; contralateral, 95%

Although there is little or no difference in total blood flow between the two final movement combinations, the last one gives more information about the functioning of the less affected ipsilateral vertebral artery. The reduction of flow in the contralateral vertebral artery to 5% means that the body is almost completely dependent on the blood supply via the ipsilateral vertebral artery and the internal carotid arteries by way of the anastosmotic connection through the circle of Willis. It is not clear why Chrost (referenced by Gutmann and Biedermann, 1984) did not study the combinations of flexion with sidebending and ipsilateral rotation, or of extension with sidebending and ipsilateral and contralateral rotation. He also provides no explanation

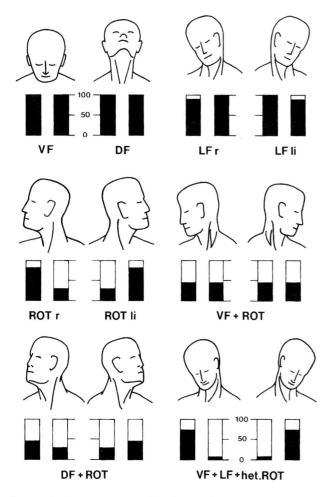

Figure 7–110 Percentage of perfusion of both vertebral arteries with uniplanar and multiplanar physiological motions of the cervical spine.

with regard to the fact that flexion and extension—unlike the combined movements—have no effect on blood flow in the vertebral arteries.

More recent studies have provided much less unequivocal findings than the older studies discussed earlier and have forced OMT clinicians to reevaluate the near-certainty with which in times past they approached the topic of cervical artery dysfunction based solely on history and physical examination data.

Extension–rotation as a clinical test—discussed in more detail in the section titled "Dynamic Coordination" earlier in this chapter—has been extensively studied with equivocal results. Some authors have reported significant decreases in blood flow (Rivett et al., 1999; Yi-Kai et al., 1999), whereas other studies have found no changes (Arnold et al., 2004; Licht et al., 2000). Case reports have noted false-negative results (Rivett et al., 1998; Westaway

et al., 2003), and case series have reported 75–100% false-positive results (Arnold et al., 2004; Haynes, 2002). Research findings for the sustained cervical rotation test are equally equivocal with significant decreases (Arnold et al., 2004; Mitchell, 2003; Nakamura et al., 1998; Rivett et al., 1999; Yi-Kai et al., 1999) or no effect noted on vertebral artery blood flow or volume (Haynes et al., 2002; Licht et al., 1999). We discussed data on concurrent criterion-related validity and clinical implications in the section titled "Dynamic Coordination" earlier.

Earlier studies concentrated solely on the effect of physiologic movements on perfusion in the vertebral arteries, but more recent studies have also studied the effects on perfusion in the internal carotid artery. Refshauge (1994) noted an increase in right internal carotid artery blood flow velocity with sustained contralateral rotation in healthy volunteers. In contrast, Licht et al. (2002) found no change in peak flow or time-averaged mean flow velocity in the ICA during sustained extension–rotation test. Clinically relevant is that the patients in that study nonetheless experienced symptoms (vertigo, visual blurring, nausea, hemicranial paresthesiae) classically considered a positive response on this test. Rivett et al. (1999) reported an increase in internal carotid artery blood flow velocity with cervical extension and attributed this to narrowing in the internal carotid artery. In contrast to the other two studies, they noted a decrease in peak systolic and end diastolic blood flow velocity in both ICA during sustained rotation. Again relevant with regard to the clinical interpretation is the fact that these authors found no between-group differences for subjects that were positive or negative on this test.

With all these studies, we have to of course acknowledge the chance of type II error (not finding a between-group difference where in reality one does exist) because of the small sample sizes used; for some studies, we must consider the effect of using asymptomatic subjects on external validity. In summary, research on the hemodynamic effect of the sustained rotation and the sustained extension rotation tests produces equivocal results, thereby calling into question our previously held assumptions with regard to the effect of physiologic movements of the cervical spine on cervical artery perfusion.

VERTEBROBASILAR INSUFFICIENCY

Both vertebral arteries and the internal carotid arteries form a functional unit. Under normal circumstances, reduction of the blood flow in one of the two vertebral arteries is completely compensated by an increase in blood flow in the other vertebral artery and the anterior system. If one vertebral artery is not able to compensate the partial or complete loss of flow in the other one, this may reduce perfusion of the area supplied by the vertebrobasilar system, especially in the case where the anterior system is insufficiently capable of compensating. The use of provocative movement of the cervical spine has been suggested as a way of testing this compensatory mechanism. Disturbance of blood flow in the vertebrobasilar system is called vertebrobasilar insufficiency. Ausman et al. (1985) define the term as follows:

> Vertebrobasilar insufficiency is the term used to denote recurrent periods of relative ischemia in the area supplied by the vertebrobasilar arterial system, consequent upon a temporary reduction or blocking of blood flow in the vertebral artery and the basilar artery together with their branches.

Oostendorp (1988) distinguishes between vertebrobasilar insufficiency and functional vertebrobasilar insufficiency. The former can be a consequence of organic abnormalities, physiologic movements of the cervical spine combined with increased sympathetic activity in the cervicothoracic transitional area, and or a combination of the two. Distinctions can, therefore, be made between structural, functional, and combined vertebrobasilar insufficiency.

Structural Vertebrobasilar Insufficiency

Structural vertebrobasilar insufficiency is the form of vertebrobasilar insufficiency in which identifiable symptoms occur as a consequence of an organic abnormality of the vertebral arteries, or changes in its lumen as a result of structural abnormalities in the cervical spine or the musculature that lies directly ventral to the vertebral artery.

Functional Vertebrobasilar Insufficiency

Functional vertebrobasilar insufficiency is the form of vertebrobasilar insufficiency that occurs in the absence of structural abnormality and in which complaints and symptoms are provoked by movements of the cervical spine, especially rotation (Oostendorp, 1988).

Temporary reduction in blood flow in the vertebral arteries as a result of physiologic movements of the cervical spine, in which there is an absence of structural abnormalities, is hypothesized to be caused by increased sympathetic activity in the cervicothoracic transitional area.

Combined Vertebrobasilar Insufficiency

Combined vertebrobasilar insufficiency is the form of vertebrobasilar insufficiency in which the occurrence of identifiable complaints and symptoms is the result of the combined factors responsible for structural and functional vertebrobasilar insufficiency.

It is clear from these definitions that the identifiable symptoms of vertebrobasilar insufficiency are caused by different mechanisms, which may be present separately or in combination. The abnormalities and changes that can play a part in structural or combined vertebrobasilar insufficiency are described in the section titled "Structures That Can Compress the Vertebral Artery," which follows.

Movements of the cervical spine generally cause changes in the length of the vertebral artery. The extent to which the vertebral artery, which is anchored in the transverse foramina, can be stretched without damage to its walls depends on the amount of surplus length present and the number of elastic fibers in the tunica media of the artery. If the elongation capacity of the vertebral artery is exceeded, there is a danger that its walls may be damaged.

Vulnerable locations are the following:

- The transverse process of the axis
- The transverse process of the atlas
- The lateral mass of the atlas
- The place where the vertebral artery passes through the dura mater

Structures That Can Compress the Vertebral Artery

The *extravertebral part* of the vertebral artery (segment V_1) has as its ventral boundary the longus colli and anterior scalene muscles, and as its dorsal boundary the transverse processes T1 and C7 and the first rib. Three-dimensional combined movement of extension, ipsilateral lateral flexion and rotation of the cervical spine lengthens these muscles as well as the vertebral artery. If the muscles are hypertonic and shortened, they will press the vertebral artery against the first rib and the transverse processes of T1 and C7. If the resulting reduction in blood flow is not fully compensated, it may result in symptoms and complaints typical of vertebrobasilar insufficiency.

The *intravertebral part* of the vertebral artery (segment V_2) has as its anteromedial boundary the uncovertebral joints. If as a result of osteoarthritic changes of the uncovertebral joint there is lateral osteophyte growth in the direction of the transverse foramen, this may cause compression of the vertebral artery, especially during sidebending and rotation of the cervical spine (**Figure 7–111**). Processes such as spondylosis or spondylarthrosis can also cause temporary compression of the vertebral artery in this segment during movement of the cervical spine. However, a prolapsed disk is more likely to compress the dural sleeve and the nerve root than the vertebral artery.

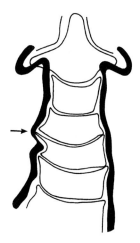

Figure 7–111 Compression of the vertebral artery as result of osteoarthritic changes of the uncovertebral joint.

In the *atlantoaxial part* of the vertebral artery (segment V_3), the changes in blood vessel resistance during rotation and extension of the cervical spine are the greatest in the contralateral vertebral artery. Normally, these changes in resistance do not cause problems; however, additional compressive factors such as congenital blood vessel abnormalities, or anomalies and abnormal positions of the segments of C1 and C2, can have a negative effect on blood flow. Other predisposing factors for vertebrobasilar insufficiency include congenital blood vessel abnormalities such as unilateral or bilateral hypoplasia or unilateral aplasia of the vertebral artery; anomalies of the circle of Willis; and anomalies, acquired structural changes, and positional deviations in the upper cervical spine including a ponticulus posterior (Triano and Kawchuk, 2006).

In the *intracranial part* of the vertebral artery (segment V_4), the only location where it is vulnerable from a biomechanical perspective is where it passes through the dura mater, the pia mater, and the arachnoid.

To study the commonly held assumption that the cervical artery seems most mechanically vulnerable in its V_3 segment, Kawchuk et al. (2008) studied two populations of patients with established cervical artery dissection. One group consisted of a 5-year retrospective cohort of 25 patients admitted to a hospital for vertebral artery dissection not related to major trauma or associated with cervical manipulation. The second group consisted of 26 of 64 cases on which Haldeman et al. (2002) reported in a retrospective review of medicolegal cases where manipulation was suggested as a causative factor for vertebral artery dissection. All cases included had diagnostic imaging or reports available to determine the level of the dissection. Kawchuk et al. (2008) noted that the V_3 segment was most affected with a prevalence ratio expressing prevalence in V_3 as compared to baseline prevalence in V_1 in the manipulation group of 8.46

(95% CI: 3.53–20.24). The prevalence ratio in the nonmanipulation group was 4.00 (95% CI: 1.43–11.15). The authors noted that there was a higher prevalence in the V_3 segment irrespective of exposure to cervical manipulation showing the inherent increased mechanical vulnerability of the V_3 segment.

Tonic Spasm of the Vertebral Artery

Another proposed important causal factor in vertebrobasilar insufficiency is vascular spasm (Gutmann, 1985). The pathophysiologic mechanism that causes vascular spasm is not fully understood, but it causes the smooth muscle fibers of the arterial wall to contract. The contraction may be of short or long duration. According to Lechtape-Grutter and Zülch (1971), a vascular spasm is a reversible contraction of the smooth muscle tissue of the arterial wall that may last minutes, hours, days, or weeks. This occurs in response to mechanical, and/or chemical, and/or neurogenic stimulation. Spasm of the vertebral artery, spreading to the basilar artery and its branches, causes temporary disturbances in perfusion of the area supplied by the vertebrobasilar arterial system. Gutmann (1985) distinguishes three kinds of factors that may cause vascular spasm. They are often present in combination.

Mechanical Stimulation

Rotation and movements that include rotation cause mechanical compression that may affect the blood flow in the vertebral artery. The mechanical effect on the vertebral artery, the nerve fibers of the perivascular plexus, and the vertebral nerve does not seem to be a direct cause of the vascular spasm; however, when mechanical stimulation causes local damage of the blood vessel wall causing the release of chemical substances, these might cause the vascular spasm indirectly.

Mechanically caused spasm of the vertebral artery without tissue damage has a short latency and generally lasts only a short time (seconds, minutes, hours); this means that the symptoms are often reversible. Mechanically caused spasm of the vertebral artery with tissue damage has a relatively longer latency and generally lasts longer (hours, days); the symptoms are becoming irreversible (Oostendorp, 1988).

Chemical Stimulation

When the wall of the blood vessel is damaged, substances such as prostaglandin E2 and serotonin are released. These substances increase the sensitivity to stimulation of the arterial wall and the free nerve endings of the perivascular plexus of the vertebral artery (Gutmann, 1985). This increased sensitivity is a predisposing factor for the vascular spasm. It means that a mechanical stimulation that under normal circumstances would not cross the threshold of the free nerve endings will now result in depolarization of these nerves. The increase in discharge frequency of the unmyelinated fibers causes an increase in the release of substance P at the peripheral and central endings of the primary nociceptive neurons. This sensitizes the peripheral and central receptive fields of these neurons. This nociceptive activity can lead to a short-term or long-term increase in the activity of the sympathetic system (Oostendorp, 1988).

Neurogenic Stimulation

Stressors can increase tonic activity within the sympathetic system even in the absence of a peripheral source of nociceptive stimulation. When the activity of the sympathetic system is chronically raised by stress (discussed in Chapter 8) a minor mechanical stimulus can cause an angiospasm. The evidence that the raised activity in the sympathetic nervous system is a causal factor in angiospasms lies in the fact that injecting substances that block alpha-receptors can end these spasms. The reaction of norepinephrin is blocked through blocking alpha-receptors; this removes the sympathetic effect on the muscles in the wall of the blood vessel.

A long-lasting increase in the activity of the vasoconstricting subsystems of the sympathetic system leads to hyperreactivity of the smooth muscle cells of the vertebral artery and dysregulation of the blood flow to the vertebral artery and its branches via the vasa vasorum (Oostendorp, 1988). The resulting trophic disturbance may lead to an ischemic or vascular inflammatory reaction. This increases the sensitivity of the vessel wall and of the perivascular nerve fibers. An inflammatory reaction with chronic trophic disturbance of the vessel wall leads to fibrosis of the wall and fibrotic attachments to the surrounding tissues. This reduces the viscoelasticity of the blood vessel wall and the mobility of the vertebral artery during movements of the cervical spine. Both these factors increase the likelihood of damage to the arterial wall. Therefore, from a diagnostic perspective, it is important to determine the reactivity of the autonomic system in general and of the wall of the vertebral artery in particular before carrying out cervical provocation tests and assessing and interpreting the results of these tests.

CERVICAL MANIPULATION AND THE RISK OF STROKE

In the context of the OMT assessment of circulatory function of the cervical region as a precursor to potential manipulative intervention in this region, we cannot ignore the association made between cervical manipulation and stroke, more specifically, cervical artery dissection. Although overall population incidence at 2.6 per 100,000 is extremely low, cervical artery dissections account for approximately 20% of strokes in young versus 2.5% of strokes in older patients (Graziano et al., 2007). As Terrett (2000) noted: "The temporal relationship between young healthy patients without osseous or vascular disease who attend a spinal manipulative therapy practitioner and then suffer these rare strokes is so well documented as to be beyond reasonable doubt indicating a possible causal relationship."

There are two types of vertebral artery–related strokes (Terrett, 2000). In Wallenberg syndrome or dorsolateral medullary syndrome of Wallenberg occlusion of the posterior inferior cerebellar artery, frequently resulting from distal extension of a vertebral artery dissection, leads to destruction of the nuclei and pathways in the dorsolateral medulla oblongata. Another cause may be the occlusion of the parent vertebral artery, in which case the syndrome is called syndrome of Babinski–Nageotte. Ischemia of the inferior cerebellar peduncle leads to ipsilateral ataxia and hypotonia. Destruction of the descending spinal tract and the trigeminal nucleus causes a loss of pain and temperature sensation on the ipsilateral face in addition to loss of the ipsilateral corneal reflex. Destruction of the ascending lateral spinothalamic tract causes loss of pain and temperature sensation in the contralateral trunk, which together with the sensory loss in the ipsilateral face results in a pathognomonic presentation of alternating analgesia. Ischemia of the descending sympathetic tract causes Horner's syndrome; damage to the lower vestibular nuclei causes nystagmus, vertigo, nausea, and vomiting; and ischemia in the nucleus ambiguous of the glossopharyngeal nerve can cause hoarseness, dysphagia, or intractable hiccups.

Locked-in syndrome or cerebromedullospinal disconnection syndrome occurs as a result of occlusion of the midbasilar artery. This effectively transects the brain stem at the midpons level. Because the reticular formation and the ventral pons are unaffected, the patient retains consciousness but decerebrate rigidity develops as a result of the cerebrospinal tracts having been destroyed. The nuclei for the 5th through 12th cranial nerves are destroyed, but the 4th cranial nerve is spared leaving only eye convergence and upward gaze for the patient to communicate with his environment. Skin sensation remains grossly intact because the lateral spinothalamic tract is usually spared and the patient can still hear because the auditory nerves ascend in the brainstem lateral to the infarction area.

Evidence linking manipulation to stroke has included multiple narrative reviews of case reports found in the literature (Di Fabio, 1999; Ernst, 2002; Terrett, 2000; Triano and Kawchuk, 2006). Hurwitz et al. (1996) acknowledged the likely high underreporting bias and noted an estimated risk adjusted for an only 10% reporting rate in the literature of 5–10 per 10 million for all complications, 6 in 10 million for serious complications, and 3 in 10 million for the risk of death.

Rothwell et al. (2001) compared 582 patients with vertebrobasilar accidents over the period 1993 to 1998 with age- and sex-matched controls from the provincial insurance database in Ontario, Canada. They also determined exposure to chiropractic using this same database. These authors found that subjects younger than 45 years were five times more likely (95% CI: 1.31–43.87) to have visited a chiropractor in the month preceding the stroke. This same age group was also five times (95% CI: 1.34–18.57) more likely to have had three or more chiropractic visits with a cervical diagnosis in the month prior to the stroke. No significant association was noted for subjects older than 45.

Cassidy et al. (2008) used a very similar study design comparing 818 patients with vertebrobasilar accidents to age- and sex-matched controls from a provincial insurance database and also found an odds ratio (OR) of 3.13 (95% CI: 0.52–1.32) for having visited a chiropractor in the month before the stroke in those younger than 45 years, whereas the OR was 0.83 (95% CI: 0.52–1.32) for those older than 45. However, these researchers also looked at visits to general medical practitioners preceding the stroke and found an OR of 3.57 (95% CI: 2.17–5.86) for those under 45 and 2.67 (95% CI: 2.25–3.17) for patients having visited their medical doctor in the month preceding the vertebrobasilar accident. These authors suggested that the similar association between chiropractic and medical visits might indicate that patients with an undiagnosed vertebral artery dissection seek clinical care for headache and neck pain before having a stroke.

Signs and Symptoms of Cervical Artery Dysfunction

Previously, we have discussed structural, functional, and mixed vertebrobasilar insufficiency. Within the context of structural insufficiency we have to address the possibility of vertebral artery dissection and subsequent thrombosis and embolization leading to both nonischemic and ischemic presentations. Despite the fact that clinical evidence indicates that cervical artery dysfunction predominantly affects the posterior circulation (Terrett, 2000), OMT clinicians also need to be familiar with the presentation of internal carotid artery dissection. This becomes all the more relevant considering the possibility that patients may seek out an OMT clinician with a stroke in progress mistakenly assuming that the initially mild symptoms may be helped with OMT intervention.

Clinicians are likely most familiar with the classic cardinal signs and symptoms (**Table 7–9**) of vertebrobasilar compromise. We should note that diagnostic utility of these symptoms has yet to be established. With regard to raising the clinical suspicion of cervical artery dissection, it is important to realize that ischemic symptoms are not the only symptoms that occur with cervical artery dissection. Nonischemic symptoms usually develop first and are likely the result of deformation of nerve endings in the tunica adventitia of the affected artery and direct compression on local somatic structures (Kerry and Taylor, 2006). In fact, these nonischemic symptoms occur hours to days and even a few weeks prior to the ischemic findings (Blunt and Galton, 1997). In the case of internal carotid artery dissection, this delay has even been reported to possibly be as much as years (Haneline and Lewkovich, 2004). Ischemic findings develop in 30–80% of all dissections. Up to 20% of patients progress to a full cerebrovascular accident (Blunt and Galton, 1997). Nonischemic symptoms are unique to the pathology of dissection but ischemic symptoms can, of course, be expected to be similar for all underlying causes of cervical artery dysfunction.

Although the classic cardinal signs and symptoms for vertebral artery compromise as discussed in Table 7–9 can be part of the presentation, additional symptoms have been described for cervical artery dysfunction. **Table 7–10** provides ischemic and nonischemic signs and symptoms associated with cervical artery dissection (Blunt and Galton, 1997; Haneline and Lewkovich, 2004; Kerry and Taylor, 2006). Relevant to the physical examination are the cranial nerve palsies that may occur with cervical artery dissection. In the section titled "Segments of the Internal Carotid Artery" earlier in the chapter, we discussed the close anatomic association of the internal carotid artery with multiple cranial nerves and their nuclei. It is easy to imagine how a dissecting artery with its increasing diameter may compress surrounding somatic structures including adjacent cranial nerve structures. Dissection of the internal

Table 7–9 Classic Cardinal Signs of Vertebrobasilar Compromise: Five Ds and Three Ns

Dizziness
Drop attacks
Diplopia (including amaurosis fugax and corneal reflux)
Dysarthria
Dysphagia (including hoarseness and hiccups)
Ataxia of gait
Nausea
Numbness (in ipsilateral face and/or contralateral body)
Nystagmus

Table 7–10   Nonischemic and Ischemic Signs and Symptoms of Cervical Artery Dysfunction

	Vertebrobasilar System	Internal Carotid Artery
Non-ischemic	Ipsilateral posterior neck pain Ipsilateral occipital headache Sudden onset and severe Described as stabbing, pulsating, aching, "thunderclap," sharp, or of an unusual character: "a headache unlike any experienced before" Very rarely C5–C6 nerve root impairment (due to local neural ischemia)	Ipsilateral upper and midcervical spine pain Ipsilateral frontal-temporal or periorbital headache Sudden onset, severe, and of an uncommon character Horner's syndrome Pulsatile tinnitus Cranial nerve palsies Ipsilateral carotid bruit Neck swelling Scalp tenderness Anhydrosis face
Ischemic	Five **D**s and three **N**s (see Table 7–9) Vomiting Loss of short-term memory Vagueness Hypotonia and limb weakness affecting arm or leg Anhydrosis: lack of facial sweating Hearing disturbances Malaise Perioral dysesthesia Photophobia Clumsiness Agitation Cranial nerve palsies Hindbrain stroke: Wallenberg or locked-in syndrome	Transient ischemic attack Middle cerebral artery distribution stroke Retinal infarction Amaurosis fugax: temporary blindness Localized patchy blurring of vision: scintillating scotomata Weakness of extraocular muscles Protrusion of the eye Swelling of the eye or conjunctiva

carotid artery mainly causes dysfunction of the 9th through 12th cranial nerves with the hypoglossal nerve initially affected and then the other three nerves; eventually all cranial nerves except the olfactory can be affected. Whereas cranial nerve dysfunction has a nonischemic etiology in internal carotid artery dissection, it is part of the ischemic presentation of a vertebral artery dissection. As noted earlier, ischemic signs and symptoms of cervical artery compromise can logically be expected to be similar irrespective of underlying pathology.

DIAGNOSIS

See the section titled "Examination Strategy" in Chapter 10, page 235 for more information.

History

When taking the history, the practitioner lists the patient's complaints and symptoms. Where cervical artery

dysfunction is suspected, there are three complaints that are of primary diagnostic significance. These are the following:

- Headache
- Neck pain
- Vertigo

Terrett (2000) provided data on the presenting complaints of 137 chiropractic patients who subsequently had a manipulation-associated stroke:

- 47.4% noted neck pain and stiffness
- 19.7% noted neck pain, stiffness, and headache
- 16.8% had torticollis

Additional presenting complaints included low back pain (2.2%), abdominal complaints (2.2%), (kypho)scoliosis (1.5%), head cold (1.5%), upper thoracic pain (1.5%), upper limb numbness (0.7%), and hay fever (0.7%). Keeping in mind the distinct differences between indications proposed for chiropractic manipulation and OMT intervention, we still have to note the nonspecific nature of these presenting complaints and, therefore, their limited value in identifying patients at risk for cervical artery dysfunction.

Whether cervical artery dysfunction is related to patients presenting with a stroke in progress or whether manipulation in fact causes these serious adverse events remains unclear, but it does seem plausible that in the case of a pathologically weakened artery mechanical forces such as those induced during OMT intervention may cause damage to the cervical arteries. In addition to the nonischemic and ischemic signs and symptoms of cervical artery dissection and other forms of insufficiency outlined previously, the OMT clinician also needs to identify possible risk factors predisposing the artery to dysfunction whether iatrogenic, caused by mechanical events other than manipulation, or spontaneous. **Table 7–11** provides risk factors as identified in the literature.

With regard to the role of iatrogenic causes and direct vessel trauma, we discussed the increased odds ratio of cervical artery dysfunction and cervical manipulation earlier but should note that association, of course, does not imply causation. Although no specific data are available relevant to OMT clinical practice, Beaudry and Spence (2003) attributed 70 of 80 traumatically induced cases of vertebrobasilar

Table 7–11 Proposed Risk Factors of Cervical Artery Dysfunction

Atherosclerosis
Hypertension
Hypercholesterolemia
Hyperlipidemia
Hyperhomocysteinemia
Diabetes mellitus
Genetic clotting disorders
Infections
Smoking
Free radicals
Upper cervical instability
Migraine
Direct vessel trauma
Iatrogenic causes
Endothelial inflammatory disease (eg, temporal arteriitis)
Arteriopathies
Age 30–45 years
Female gender
Thyroid disease
Oral contraceptive use

ischemia to motor vehicle accidents. From a differential diagnostic perspective it should be noted that many patients after whiplash trauma note dizziness and meet criteria for inner ear pathology (Grimm, 2002; Oostendorp et al., 1999; Wrisley et al., 2000).

Although age of 30 to 45 years and female gender have been proposed as risk factors, Terrett (2000) indicated that the overall distribution of patients with regard to gender and age attending for chiropractic care closely matches the gender and age distribution of those with serious adverse events, thereby somewhat discounting these proposed risk factors. Kawchuk et al. (2008) also found no association for age and gender and the incidence of cervical artery dissection.

Arteriopathies predisposing the artery to dysfunction as a result of pathologic weakening of the vessel wall include Marfan syndrome, Ehlers–Danlos syndrome, fibromuscular dysplasia, cystic medial necrosis, osteogenesis imperfecta, and autosomal dominant polycystic kidney disease. Alpha-1-antitrypsin deficiency initially showed highly elevated odds ratios, but this association currently finds little support in the literature. In all, these risk factors can at best be suspected based on physical examination but would seem relevant if noted in the medical history. Research evidence for these arteriopathies in the etiology of cervical artery dysfunction, however, is limited.

Cardiovascular risk factors proposed include hypertension, tobacco use, hypercholesterolemia, hyperlipidemia, diabetes, and atherosclerosis. Most research into this area has compared patients with cervical artery dysfunction to patients with ischemic strokes. Perhaps as a result of this underlying difference in pathophysiology most cardiovascular risk factors actually show an odds ratio below 1, indicating a "protective" function. Of course, this is likely because of the methodology of the research. Hypertension with an odds ratio of 1.94 (95% CI: 1.01–3.70) was the only significant risk factor. Although seemingly plausible, the evidence for atherosclerosis as a risk factor is based solely on cadaver studies and the finding that blood flow is proportional to the fourth power of vessel diameter (Mitchell, 2002).

There is a noted seasonal variation in the incidence of cervical artery dissection with significantly more cases occurring in winter as compared to other seasons (Paciaroni et al., 2006). Indeed, one study showed an adjusted odds ratio of 3.1 (95% CI: 1.1–9.2) for an acute infection in the 4 weeks preceding a cervical artery incident (Guillon et al., 2003).

Rubinstein et al. (2005), in a systematic review noted additional clinically relevant risk factors for migraine (OR = 3.6; 95% CI: 1.5–8.6); recent infection (OR = 1.6; 95% CI: 0.67–3.80), and trivial trauma including cervical manipulation (OR = 3.8; 95% CI: 1.3–11). Triano and Kawchuk (2006) reported an OR of 1.6 (95% CI: 0.67–3.80) for coughing, sneezing, or vomiting; vascular risk factors and a current smoking habit had odds ratios of 0.14 (95% CI: 0.34–0.65) and 0.49 (95% CI: 0.18–1.05). Although earlier research implicated oral contraceptive use as a risk factor, Haneline and Lewkovich (2004) indicated that currently no consensus exists on relevance of this proposed risk factor.

Physical Examination

When the history has been taken and the data analyzed, the aims of the subsequent examination are formulated. At this stage, the following questions must be answered:

- Is examination by a manual therapist indicated or contraindicated?
- Is imaging needed to rule out possible contraindications?
- If examination by a manual therapist is indicated, what tests should be carried out?
- In what order should they be carried out?

If the history does reveal any central neurologic symptoms that would suggest structural vertebrobasilar insufficiency, targeted neurologic and other tests are carried out that do not put the patient at risk. In this context, we should think of cranial nerve examination, especially considering the place cranial nerve palsies have in the nonischemic presentation of internal carotid dissection and the ischemic presentation of vertebral artery dissection. Observation of the miosis (inability to dilate a pupil), ptosis (droopy upper eye lid), enophthalmus (deeper seated eye), and anhydrosis (decreased sweating ipsilateral head and shoulders) consis-

tent with Horner's syndrome also should serve as a red flag in this regard. Auscultation for a carotid bruit may be indicated: Magyar et al. (2002) noted 56% sensitivity and 91% specificity for detection of a 70–99% carotid stenosis when compared to Doppler duplex ultrasound. In the absence of findings indicative of relevant pathology, the OMT clinician can continue with a careful progressive examination noting the very limited diagnostic utility of and potential dangers associated with the cervical extension and extension–rotation tests in the section titled "Dynamic Coordination." Any findings indicative of the nonischemic and ischemic presentation of cervical artery dysfunction require immediate referral for medical management.

For differential diagnosis of the headache complaint that may be part of the presentation of cervical artery dysfunction, it will be helpful to be familiar with the location and pain referral patterns of myofascial trigger points as described elsewhere in this text. Myofascial trigger points have been implicated in the etiology of tension-type headaches. Although less likely to be confused with cervical artery–related thunderclap headache, the clinician should be familiar with the International Headache Society diagnostic criteria of cervicogenic headache as well (Olesen, 2004). The headache most likely to be confused with thunderclap headache due to its intensity, location, and associated neurologic symptoms is migraine headache. The following clinical prediction rule for the diagnosis of migraine may be helpful in the differential diagnosis (Detsky et al., 2006). The rule consists of the following five questions:

1. Is it a pulsating headache?
2. Does it last between 4 and 72 hours without medication?

Table 7–12 Differential Diagnostic Characteristics for Cervicogenic Dizziness, Benign Paroxysmal Positional Vertigo (BPPV), and Cervical Artery Dysfunction

	Dizziness Type	Nystagmus and Dizziness Characteristics	Associated Signs and Symptoms
Cervicogenic dizziness	Positioning-type	No latency period Brief duration Fatigable with repeated motion	Nystagmus Neck pain Suboccipital headaches Cervical motion abnormality on examination
BPPV	Positioning-type	Short latency: 1–5 seconds Brief duration: < 30 seconds Fatigable with repeated motion	Nystagmus
Cervical artery dysfunction	Positional-type	Long latency: 55 ± 18 seconds (Oostendorp, 1988) Increasing symptoms and signs with maintained head position Not fatigable with repeated motion	Ischemic and (depending on etiology) possibly nonischemic signs and symptoms as described in Table 7–10

3. Is it unilateral?

4. Is there nausea?

5. Is the headache disabling (with disabling headaches defined as headaches that disrupt a patient's daily activities)?

When the patient answers yes to four or more of these five questions, the positive likelihood ratio (LR) for a diagnosis of migraine headache is 24 (95% CI: 1.5–388). With a yes answer to three questions, the positive LR is 3.5 (95% CI: 1.3–9.2). For a yes answer to one or two of these criteria, the positive LR is 0.41 (95% CI: 0.32–0.52). The mnemonic POUNDing (Pulsating, Duration of 4–72 hours, Unilateral, Nausea, Disabling) may be helpful for clinicians when using this clinical prediction rule.

For differential diagnosis of a main complaint of dizziness the spin-stop test may be helpful for implicating the vestibular system provided that tests for more serious pathology have all been negative. A Hallpike–Dix maneuver can also be helpful to implicate benign paroxysmal positional vertigo (BPPV): positional nystagmus has been shown to identify patients with posterior semicircular canal BPPV with 78% sensitivity, and specificity as high as 88% has been reported. The sinusoidal rotation test (discussed earlier in the section titled "Static and Dynamic Coordination") can be used to help in the differential diagnosis of cervicogenic dizziness. **Table 7–12** provides details helpful for the differential diagnosis of the more common forms of dizziness. Vidal and Huijbregts (2005) have provided an extensive template for the diagnostic process in patients with a main complaint of dizziness.

If cervicogenic dizziness is implicated, the next stages in the examination are functional examination of the cervical spine and examination for possible changes in particular organs and tissues. The results of these examinations will show whether the patient is likely to have any of the following conditions:

- A structural or a functional vertebrobasilar insufficiency/cervical artery dysfunction
- A vestibular disturbance caused by a local problem
- Functional disturbances of the spine
- Tonically raised sympathetic activity

CHAPTER 8

Psychological Aspects

STRESS

Selye (1976a,b) regards *stress* as a situation from which illness can develop. Van Wijk (1988) describes it as a process that occupies a central position between humans and the environment, and that is expressed in biochemical, physiologic, behavioral, and psychological changes. It follows from this description that stress exists both at the level of the physical organism, that is, the organs and cells, and at the psychological level. Any attempt at subdivision of the stress phenomenon is artificial and must, therefore, be in some respects incomplete. Nevertheless, for purposes of discussion, we look first at the effects of stress on the physical organism, and second at its effects at the psychological level.

Biological Aspects of Stress

We may adopt as a basic principle that stress is the nonspecific response of the body to every demand placed upon it. Although the body responds in different specific ways to different agents and stimuli (food, temperature), the general response is an increasing nonspecific attempt at the restoration of homeostasis. The result is adaptation (van Wijk, 1988). The intensity of the stimulus is more important than its nature or whether it is pleasurable or painful. A state of stress could be a response to news of a large and unexpected inheritance just as well as to the news that one is incurably ill. From this point of view, stress is common to all living organisms; it will arise if the extent of physiologic deviation from the normal state is sufficient (**Figure 8–1**). The range within which the organism is able to cope with differ-

ent situations without stress is called the neutral range; the body is attuned to this neutral range in which a certain set of fluctuations normally occur. If circumstances arise that overstep the limits of the neutral range and exceed the body's ability to adapt, stress develops. Selye (1976a,b) defines stress as "a process of adaptation to events in the environment that challenge the wellbeing of the organism." In a state of stress, the organism moves via exposure to threatening stressors to which it is not attuned to a state directed at nonspecific adaptation.

According to Selye (1976a,b), the process of adaptation involves a number of interrelated physiologic processes. He described a constant pattern of physiologic responses that is independent of the particular stimulus or stressor,

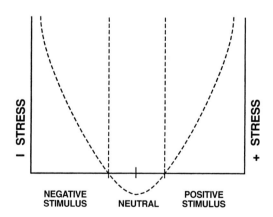

Figure 8–1   Degree of stress.

and that consists of three kinds of change that take place simultaneously:

- Enlargement of the adrenal cortex
- Atrophy of the thymus, spleen, and other lymphatic structures
- Stomach and duodenal ulcers

He distinguishes three phases in the response (see **Figure 8–2**):

- The *alarm phase* (A), during which the sympathetic nervous system is activated.
- The *adaptation phase* (B), in which the organism tolerates a higher level of threat before dying, or tolerates a higher level of the stimulus before particular responses are elicited.
- The *exhaustion phase* (C), which occurs if the organism is exposed for a long period to threat or noxious stimulation. The organism reacts to this as in the alarm phase.

The nonspecific response in its entirety is called the General Adaptation Syndrome (GAS). In addition to the changes already described, it is characterized by loss of body weight, loss of regulation of body temperature, the disappearance of certain cells from the circulating blood, and a number of chemical changes in the composition of body fluids and tissues. Short-term changes include changes in blood pressure, respiration, transpiration, skin resistance, digestion, blood glucose levels, white and red blood cell content, levels of free fatty acids and cholesterol in the blood, clotting factor in the blood, and excretion of adrenal cortex hormones. Davis (1957) found that when different sensory stimuli were applied, skin resistance and muscle tension changed in response to all of them, but that heart rate, peripheral circulation, and respiration were stimulus-dependent. Every condition seems to produce a different pattern.

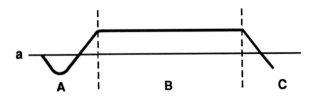

Figure 8–2   Normal level of stimulus response (a) and the three phases of stress (A, B, C).

The response pattern also differs between individuals exposed to the same stimulus; there is a great deal of variation in specific responses. The general character of the response can be explained by the fact that it is based on one general system consisting of two subsystems, namely:

- The endocrine system
- The autonomic nervous system

The hypothalamus (in its role as the main ganglion of the autonomic nervous system) serves an important function in the neural control of stress responses, as do the reticular formation and the limbic system. Stimuli and stressors recognized by the brain lead to activation of the autonomic nervous system, which stimulates the production of neurotransmitters such as epinephrine and acetylcholine at the nerve endings. These have a local influence in many areas on the physiologic processes that are characteristic of GAS. The autonomic nerve fibers that connect with the adrenal nerves produce epinephrine that is released into the blood, and thereby has more than a local effect.

A second important route by which stressors evoke responses is via the interaction of the hypothalamus with the pituitary gland, which secretes hormones that can activate other glands: the thyrotropic hormone affects the thyroid, and the adrenocorticotropic hormone affects the adrenal cortex. The adrenal cortex produces glucocorticoids and mineralocorticoids. The glucocorticoids raise blood glucose levels and have other functions that include an anti-inflammatory effect on connective tissues.

This is especially interesting because the inflammatory process is one of the stimuli that evoke the GAS, and the GAS prompts the production of the anti-inflammatory glucocorticoids, so there is a feedback loop. The glucocorticoids also have a dampening effect on lymphatic organs and certain white blood cells. The mineralocorticoids affect the regulation of mineral levels and promote the inflammatory process.

All the endocrine glands have a specific function, and they affect each other. The liver, which has many functions, plays an especially important part in biochemical regulation during stress, together with the kidneys and the thyroid.

In reality, every organ is drawn into the general stress reaction; there is a complex pattern of interactions among the various tissues and organs (**Figure 8–3**). Stress also changes the adjustment of the whole system: some activities increase, while others decrease. The relative priority of physiologic processes alters, and some physiologic changes take precedence over others.

GAS can be a response to both internal and external stressors. An internal stressor might, for instance, be overactivity in an organ, resulting in an inflammatory reaction.

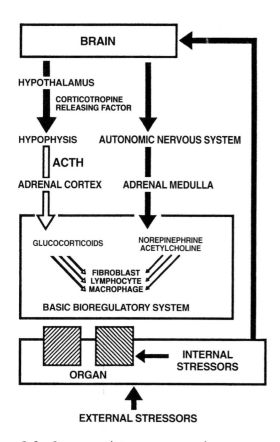

BRAIN

HYPOTHALAMUS

CORTICOTROPINE
RELEASING FACTOR

HYPOPHYSIS   AUTONOMIC NERVOUS SYSTEM

ACTH

ADRENAL CORTEX   ADRENAL MEDULLA

GLUCOCORTICOIDS   NOREPINEPHRINE
ACETYLCHOLINE

FIBROBLAST
LYMPHOCYTE
MACROPHAGE

BASIC BIOREGULATORY SYSTEM

ORGAN   INTERNAL
STRESSORS

EXTERNAL STRESSORS

Figure 8–3 Stressors and stress response pathways.

External stressors include ambient temperatures that are too high or too low, wounds, toxic substances with which the body comes into contact, and microbes. The presence of these stressors stimulates a local inflammatory reaction, which can be regarded as local adaptation. An active defense process begins, in which blood and connective tissues play an important part. The pattern of responses shows a high level of uniformity across individuals and different parts of the body and a large measure of nonspecificity with regard to the stimulus. The existence of a *local adaptation syndrome* (LAS) has, therefore, been suggested (van Wijk, 1988).

Interactions take place among cells, organs, and the organism. A threat to cells, which are the primary functional living units, causes a change in the functioning of those cells. It is, therefore, understandable that alarm signals should originate at cellular level. When the organism is confronted by stressors from the internal or external milieu, a general principle comes into action: at cellular level, groups of cells share a particular area. They make use of components from their surroundings to produce other components in their environment. Disturbance leads to

changes in the gradients of heat, nutrients, acidity, and oxygen. It is not clear, however, whether these changes in gradients are experienced by individual cells as stimuli for a nonspecific response pattern, whether the different changes lead to the same response pattern, and to which degree each individual cell has its own response pattern.

Cell death is regarded as an appropriate criterion for determining cell damage when investigating how different conditions cause such damage. The work of Loesberg et al. (1982a,b) has yielded information on the effects of heat. Individual cells produce heat as part of the metabolic process, but cell death occurs when cells are exposed to a temperature increase of a few degrees above body temperature. The effects of heat appear to be closely related to the acidity level of the cells. Hypothermia has a more damaging effect when pH levels are low, whereas an increase in cell metabolism, accompanied by higher levels of heat and acidity, increases the threat to cells and leads eventually to cell death. Hypoxic cells seem more sensitive to rises in temperature (Gerweck, Gillette, and Dewey, 1974). The amount of oxygen present depends on the available nutrients. All the gradients—temperature, nutrients, acidity, and oxygen—are interdependent. The threat arising from change in one of the gradients is limited in part by the other gradients. Freeman et al. (1980) believe that changes in acidity level pose a greater threat than do changes in oxygen level; however, little is known as yet about which factor is more likely to lead to cell death.

Normal gradients are vitally important to cellular processes. However, the normal gradients for temperature, nutrients, acidity, and oxygen within the cell can be disturbed by a number of stimuli or stressors.

Tissières, Mitchell, and Tracy (1974) maintain that when the cell is exposed to a temporary increase in temperature, levels of a particular group of proteins, which they call heat shock proteins (HSPs), increase within it. All cell types in different organisms show fundamentally the same reaction. Many other stressors—chiefly substances that influence energy metabolism—cause a response pattern identical to that which follows a rise in temperature. The heat shock proteins thus increase in quantity in circumstances other than heat shock. The increased production of HSPs seems to be a consequence of rapid change in the structural organization of genetic information stored in the DNA. This information can become available when changes occur in the relationship between the DNA molecule and certain other cell components. The complex consisting of DNA and some other molecules is known as chromatin. Changes in the structure of chromatin are basic to the cellular adaptation syndrome.

Stressors bring about other cellular changes in addition to the effects on DNA activity and the formation of HSPs. Researchers began to look for one primary initiator for the stress response. Their work produced a number of hypotheses, but no well-founded arguments have yet been put forward to support the basic assumption. Most of the research findings seem to point to a complete readjustment of the cell to changes in the speed at which several reactions proceed (van Wijk, 1988). In the cell and its immediate surroundings—as in the organism as a whole—a state of balanced adjustment normally prevails among all the ongoing reactions. If there is a change in the speed of one or more reactions, this will prompt a new adjustment or new priorities.

According to van Wijk (1988), there are indications of individual response patterns at cell level. Other writers argue that cellular adaptation proceeds through three phases (Li and Hahn, 1980):

- The early alarm phase, in which the stress process is initiated
- The adaptation phase, in which the cell becomes less sensitive to the stressor
- The exhaustion phase, in which the continuing stress leads to cell death

If the changes are small or proceed very slowly, an optimal readjustment of gradients may come about through rearrangement of cellular reactions. Every cell is capable of reacting in greater or lesser measure to specific changes, using its own range of molecular reaction capabilities. This means that when a particular gradient changes, not all cells will react directly or to the same extent. If the change in gradient is relatively marked, more cells will react. If there is a change in circumstances that affects all the cells in a population, some will have a better chance of survival than others will. This depends on which reactions the cell is capable of making based on its internal arrangement. Cells are multifunctional, but their structures differ. They complement each other and can meet a range of demands. They are capable of developing a new state of balance, not only within individual cells but also among themselves. If balance is not restored following a disturbance, this affects the milieu and every type of cell that interacts with it. This is also true of the dendrites of the sensory nerve cells in the connective tissue, which interact continuously with their environment. When they are not in a state of balance with their surroundings, they automatically register the loss of homeostasis.

Although there are many substances that occur locally in higher or lower concentrations at different times, there is no one specific substance that produces an alarm signal. The important factors are balance and organization. A cell as a living unit is characterized by a high degree of organization;

disturbance of the cell is expressed in its whole organizational structure and in neighboring structures. Changes in organization are transmitted to the nerve endings; disturbance of the intracellular organization in nerve cells, caused by instability in particular locations in the body, can ultimately be transmitted to areas of the brain that in turn are brought into a state of disorganization.

Where there is a local disturbance of gradients, cells will take on a regulating function by making internal adjustments to local levels. Their internal order will be registered and passed on. The local disturbance is, therefore, managed by two systems, namely, the organism as system and the cell as subsystem. During stress, both systems show changes in level of organization according to a more or less general response pattern that is specific to the (sub)system. The individual nature of the response may be associated with the function of the subsystem within the greater system (van Wijk, 1988).

Psychological Aspects of Stress

By analogy with the biological model, stress can be regarded as a state of psychological overload that threatens normal functioning. The situations that can result in overload may be related to marriage, family, work, and society.

Stress can arise as a result of a perceived imbalance between external demands and one's own capacity to meet them. Important factors affecting capacity are previous experience and the structure of the personality. In the interactions between the individual and his or her environment, previous experience may constitute a threat to which no adjustment is possible. The organism reacts to this with a pathologic defense mechanism.

During normal functioning, a state of continuous tension exists between the organism and the environment. On the one hand, the organism strives to maintain its freedom, identity, and balance; on the other hand, the environment often presents obstacles. The ways in which the individual is able to adapt to changing circumstances are of great importance. So long as the situations that arise fall within the individual's adaptive capability, all processes continue normally. If, however, that capability is not equal to the situation, the neuroendocrine system jumps into action and at the biological level, pathologic changes can occur. More highly developed organisms have a greater degree of freedom with regard to the environment; but the opportunities for tension with the environment are also more diverse, and the defense mechanisms are more extensive.

Humans develop patterns of behavior to meet changing circumstances. Situations have an affective coloring: they are named and recognized in terms of emotions such as fear, anxiety, anger, and pain. The need to avoid such emotions can result in a behavioral response. The body responds to danger with activation of the sympathetic system, including the adrenal cortex; this reflex reaction mobilizes defensive resources to deal with emergencies (Cannon, 1935). As in the biological model, a stressful stimulus activates both neurologic and endocrinological components, which then interact. The initial alarm phase is marked by activation of the sympathetic nervous system, including the adrenal cortex. The activation of the sympathetic nervous system is prompt, and it has immediate effects such as tachycardia, piloerection, pallor, and so forth, followed by rapid metabolic changes such as the breakdown of glycogen and fats (Smelik, 1982). The body is brought into a state of readiness for fight or flight.

In the second phase, the system based on the frontal lobe of the pituitary and the adrenal cortex is activated. In a sense, this can be seen as counteracting the original stress reaction. The coordination of the sympathetic-adrenomedullary system, which reacts first, and the pituitary-adrenocortical system, which reacts second, takes place in the hypothalamus, from which both systems are regulated. The affective behavior patterns linked with the neuroendocrine response are also anchored in the neural substrate of the hypothalamic circuits (Smelik, 1982). The stress-inducing stimuli are processed and the neuroendocrinological and behavioral outputs are produced via the hypothalamus.

Previously, the physical and chemical factors that contribute to stress input were described. The emotions also play an important part. It is the psychological component rather than the somatic stress-inducing stimuli that seems to be responsible for powerful stress reactions. The adrenal system is activated not only by the damaging stimulus, but also by the anticipation of threat implied by the stimulus. The individual's evaluation of the threat plays a key role. From a psychological point of view, experiencing and assessing the situation are important in relation to stress-inducing stimuli.

Psychologists refer to levels of alertness as *arousal*. A state of heightened arousal is associated with raised cortisol levels, which indicates that the organism is under attack. Aspecific arousal comes about through the reticular formation in the brain stem, where the ascending reticular activating system (ARAS) is located (Smelik, 1982). This system receives extensive collateral input from sensory systems and fans out in a diffuse manner to the cerebral cortex. If this system fails, the result is unconsciousness; if it stimulated, the result is a state of heightened alertness. Unexpected and powerful sensory stimuli can cause strong arousal, together with the associated neuroendocrine response.

In many cases, sensory stimuli seem to have an activating effect only when they have a certain emotional significance.

Arousal only takes place after the situation has been evaluated, by comparing it with previous experiences. Arousal can also be weaker, or absent, if memory (stored or recalled) indicates that adaptation to the situation is a possibility. The situation then corresponds to an expected pattern.

The stored patterns of expectation are important because they enable the individual to anticipate what might happen. Depending on expectation, anticipation can have an emotional component. When the organism recognizes the stimuli and evaluates them as nonthreatening, arousal is suppressed: the arousal system is not activated unconditionally by all sensory stimuli (**Figure 8–4**). It is not the stimuli themselves, but the individual perception of them that determines whether arousal takes place. This constitutes a filter system, which is difficult to locate anatomically, but it is clear that the limbic system is implicated.

The limbic system consists of a number of structures located inside the cerebral cortex and in the front part of the brain stem (Voorhoeve, 1978). The emotions and affective processes have their substrate here. It may be assumed that the emotional component of a situation is taken into account in these structures during the evaluation process. The limbic structures that are involved in feelings such as pleasure and displeasure have been charted during experiments based on (self-)stimulation. The following systems were identified:

- The system that leads to approach behavior (feelings of pleasure)
- The system that leads to avoidance behavior (feelings of displeasure)
- The system that leads to a powerful self-defense reaction (fight–flight, anger–fear)

Uncertainty and the absence of clear expectations play a part in activating the last of these systems. It involves a strong neuroendocrine reaction.

The arousal system (ARAS) and the evaluation system (limbic system) appear to be closely linked. Both can be seen as parts of a larger system (Smelik, 1982). The results of the processing of stimuli by these two systems are integrated at the level of the hypothalamus, which is the source of the signal for the integrated behavioral and neuroendocrine reaction.

Fear plays an important part in the avoidance behavior that is characterized by feelings of displeasure. Repetition of a threatening situation can lead to efficient adaptation in one individual and to a self-perpetuating progressive loss of adjustment in another. Weiss (in Smelik, 1982) performed experiments on rats in an attempt to identify the underlying factors.

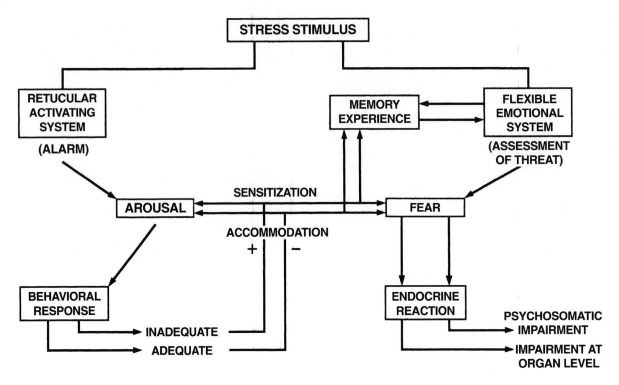

Figure 8–4   Processes during stress reaction.

Two rats received completely identical noxious stimuli. One rat was warned by a signal 5 seconds before the stimulus was applied; the other rat received no warning. After a few days, the second rat had developed gastric troubles, while the first rat, which received the warning, showed little sign of disturbance. Weiss concluded that it was not the threatening stimulus in itself that caused the pathologic symptoms, but the anticipation of fear. Fear and uncertainty about what will happen seem to intensify the stress reaction; the neuroendocrine reaction appears to be proportional to the level of nervous tension caused by fear. People use a number of techniques for reducing anxiety; these include action, verbalization, denial, and prayer.

When suffering from psychological stress, it is important for the individual to find ways of reducing the levels of fear and despair. Effective ways of protecting oneself can lead to successful adaptation: accurate anticipation, for instance, suppresses the physiologic stress reaction to the maximum extent possible. If the individual is not capable of adaptation and cannot find an effective way of anticipating, psychosomatic symptoms will occur. On the other hand, as feelings of self-efficacy grow, the anxiety decreases, and with it the somatic reaction. The most important thing is for the individual to feel defended and safe as an organism in relation to the environment. This subjective feeling is closely related both to personality and to experience.

Various factors can have a positive or negative influence on the state of mind. Negative factors such as feelings of powerlessness, being unable to do anything, loneliness, and feelings of abandonment increase the fear and tension. Positive factors that reduce fear include feelings of safety, of security within the group, of being able to tackle the situation, and of being able to act. If a way cannot be found of mastering the situation or adapting to it successfully, the individual is drawn into a downward spiral that can lead ultimately to breakdown. The spiral effect is a result of the presence of a constant threat against which there is no protection. The situation is experienced as increasingly threatening and unpleasant, and anxiety and tension increase. The somatic symptoms also become more serious and intense. Fear itself reinforces certain behaviors. Psychological conditions such as apathy, depression, and aggression are increasingly occurring because of "breakdown inadaptation."

From a diagnostic point of view, it is especially important to identify a parameter by means of which the level of anxiety can be measured. Therapeutically, a multidisciplinary approach is needed in many cases. Treatment by manual therapy of identifiable tissue-specific changes that have a psychological cause or a psychological component is no more than symptomatic treatment. It is only when the factors that precipitated the illness and those that now maintain it are identified that manual therapy can play a part in the curative process.

If a physical problem is the primary cause of the stress reaction, this should be treated in the first instance by manual therapy, with psychological input in a supporting role.

CHRONIC PAIN SYNDROME

Studies have shown that 86% of people are troubled by low back pain at some time in their lives, 5% of them every year. Of these, 19% have back pain that follows an atypical course, and they are referred to a manual therapist with chronic nonspecific low back pain. The manual therapist is regarded as competent to devise a behavioral approach in addition to offering the specific manual therapy skills.

Pain

Chronic pain syndrome is diagnosed in cases where a dysfunction accompanied by pain has lasted more than 12 weeks. Nociception is the signaling process that informs the central nervous system of tissue damage or threat of damage leading to a subjective experience of pain.

Pain is a subjective signal that can be described as a sensory and emotional experience associated with actual or potential tissue damage, or that is described by the sufferer in terms of such damage.

Every individual learns the meaning of the word *pain* through experiences related to a mishap earlier in life. Pain has both an organic and psychogenic component; these cannot be separated or distinguished. According to the gate theory of pain (Melzack and Wall, 1965), two different nerve conduction systems are involved: a pathway consisting of thick nerve fibers with a high depolarization threshold, and a pathway consisting of thin nerve fibers with a low depolarization threshold. Activity of the thick fibers obstructs signal transmission to the brain (closes the gate). Activity of the thin nerve fibers facilitates signal transmission to the brain (opens the gate). It is also known that information descending from the central nervous system can open the gate by stimulating transmission, and that it can close the gate by inhibiting transmission. The information thus obtained from the periphery and from higher centers determines whether, and to what extent, the pain signal is transmitted to the thalamus, the limbic system, and the cerebral cortex. Tension, grief, irritation, worrying about pain, fear, and inaccurate interpretations of the pain all seem to stimulate pain transmission; this causes the gate to open, and there is increasing pain awareness. An exciting sporting event or film, enjoyable music, and movement within the limits imposed by the pain seem to have an inhibitory effect on pain transmission; this causes the gate to close and stops awareness of pain.

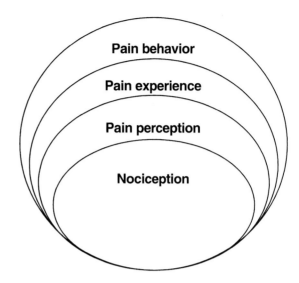

Figure 8–5   Loeser's Egg.

In "Loeser's egg" (Loeser, 1980), pain and its effects are represented as consequences of interactions among physical, emotional, and environmental factors (**Figure 8–5**).

Nociception is neurophysiologic transmission of the damage signal to the brain. *Pain perception* is the registration of the signal by the brain. *Pain experience* is the meaning that the individual attaches to the pain perception. *Pain behavior* is the individual's communication about the pain within his or her environment.

In patients with chronic pain, the pain experience and the pain behavior seem to be central. This suggests that the patient himself or herself may be able to do something about the pain by exercising various forms of control.

Classification of Dysfunctions

Complaints involving persistent pain in the movement system can be grouped as follows, according to their duration and to the objective somatic findings:

- Acute *dysfunction*, 0 to 6 weeks
- Subacute *dysfunction*, 7 to 12 weeks
- Chronic *dysfunction*, longer than 12 weeks

One of the most important features of the development of chronicity is the atypical course of the patient's recovery. Recovery is considered atypical when there is no reduction in pain, no lessening of the restrictions on movement and activities, and no change in participation levels within 3 weeks of onset. An atypical course of this kind indicates that the disorder needs a more comprehensive approach than the basic biomedical one. Psychosocial factors could be influencing the course of recovery and must be taken into account.

The atypical course of recovery and/or the persistence of the complaint may be caused by any of the following factors:

- Biomedical factors such as decreases in mobility, muscle strength, stability, and coordination (deconditioning)
- Psychological factors such as fear of movement (kinesiophobia), unrealistic thoughts about the pain, lack of confidence in the help provided, and increasing dramatization of the condition, leading to catastrophizing
- Social factors such as the work situation, lack of support and/or acceptance, reinforcement by the environment

The Guidelines on Manual Therapy for Low Back Pain issued by the Royal Dutch Society for Physical Therapy offer the following classification of recovery profiles:

Acute phase (0 to 6 weeks)
- Profile 1a: Normal course
- Profile 1b: Atypical course

Subacute phase (7 to 12 weeks)
- Profile 2a: Atypical course without social factors
- Profile 2b: Atypical course with social factors (yellow flags)

Chronic phase (up to 12 weeks)
- Profile 3a: Managing the complaint adequately
  High degree of self-efficacy
  Coping adequately (see the definition of coping with pain in the terminology section later in this chapter)
  Load adjusted to load-bearing capacity
  Appropriate participation
  Episodes of increased pain complaints
- Profile 3b: Inadequate management of the complaint
  Little or no self-efficacy
  Not coping adequately
  Load not adjusted to load-bearing capacity
  Reduced participation

Profile 2b does not belong in the chronic phase but has the potential to develop into a chronic state. The therapeutic approach is, therefore, the same as that for profile 3b, which does form part of the chronic phase.

Models of Development of Chronic Pain

The following three models can all contribute to an understanding of the etiology of the chronic pain syndrome:

- *Biomechanical model*: The basic assumption is that faulty patterns of muscle activity can lead to pain.
- *Reflex–spasm model*: Pain is regarded as a consequence of protective muscular hypertonicity following injury.
- *Psychosocial stress model*: Here, too, the pain is attributed to muscular tension, which is a consequence of inability to find solutions to emotional problems.

The chronic pain syndrome provides an illustration of the multimodal nature of long-standing problems. For some years now, approaches to diagnosis and treatment have taken into account psychological as well as biomedical factors.

The chemical processes that take place at the supraspinal level are not yet fully understood from a biomedical point of view and are, therefore, difficult to influence. This is probably the reason why behavioral therapists have become interested in the problem and have developed a behavioral approach consistent with the biopsychosocial view of humans (Vlaeyen, Kole-Snijders, and van Eek, 1996). This approach is based on the view that complex interactions among biological, psychological, and social variables can cause and/or maintain pain behavior.

The general characteristics of the chronic pain syndrome are as follows:

- Long-standing complaints of pain where no causal connection can be found with active physical pathology
- A history of a series of unsuccessful medical interventions
- Disturbed psychosocial functioning (Vlaeyen et al., 1996)

Special features of the chronic pain syndrome are as follows:

- Excessive use of medications, possibly with adverse effects
- Multiple surgical and pharmacologic treatments, with adverse effects
- Increasing physical restriction because of fear of pain and injury

- Growing feelings of hopelessness, powerlessness, and depression, despite the new treatments
- Conflicts with therapists and dissatisfaction with the treatments or with health care in general
- Interpersonal conflicts with partner and family members
- Negative affective disturbances
- Decrease in feelings of self-worth and self-confidence
- Increasing social isolation and loss of interest in social contact
- Decreasing ability to derive reinforcement from daily activities

Psychosocial factors that may indicate increased risk of chronicity (yellow flags) are discussed in the following lists (Waddell and Waddell, 2000; Vlaeyen et al., 1996):

Perceptions About Pain
- Back pain is a damaging disorder.
- Pain is uncontrollable.
- Rest is the best thing; activity aggravates the pain.
- Pain is a serious threat (catastrophizing).

Behavior
- Control of health is handed over to others (external locus of control)
- Use of orthoses and ambulatory aids, medication, and painkillers
- Much time devoted to bed rest; avoidance of daily activities
- Sleeping worse since pain started

Financial Consequences
- No financial motivation to resume work
- Problems over pay and benefits relating to previous prolonged absence because of the pain

Diagnosis and Treatment
- Confusion about the diagnosis
- Dependence on earlier treatments
- Passive forms of treatment
- Past experience of a series of ineffective treatments

Emotions
- Fearful of resuming work
- Depressive and more irritable than previously
- Fearful and more attentive to bodily feelings
- Decrease in self-worth and self-confidence

Family
- An overprotective partner who stresses the danger of damage and injury
- Insufficient support in resuming activities

Work/Sport
- Negative expectations with regard to resuming work and/or sport
- Conviction that work and/or sport is/are damaging
- Problems in present work setting
- Previous negative experiences when resuming work and taking up sport after an episode of pain

Terminology

Before discussing the behavioral examination, it will be useful to define some of the terms that are used.

Pain cognition: The subjective experience and interpretation of perceptual stimuli. The concepts of attribution and expectation are important in this context.

Attribution: The search for a cause to which the pain can be attributed. The cause is analyzed in terms of its relevance and its potential danger. It is the search for an answer to the question "why?" The consequences of pain are often seriously overestimated; this can lead to catastrophizing.

Expectations: The pain may be underestimated or overestimated. Acting as though one were stronger than one is can lead to overloading and unintended maintenance of the pain. The patient may also have expectations about the extent to which the pain can be controlled. This often results in avoidance of a range of activities. In the best case, the pain is less troublesome than expected during certain activities, and these can then be extended. This raises the patient's expectation of being able to manage the pain better, provided that he or she attributes the improvement to his or her own efforts (self-efficacy).

Pain coping: Pain coping is the cognitive and behavioral effort that the individual expends in trying to master, reduce, and tolerate the internal and external demands imposed by a stressor (Folkman and Lazarus, 1980). *Positive* coping means that the patient takes action to make the pain manageable. This self-initiated action might be cognitive, for instance, thinking of something else, or motoric, for example, relaxing or undertaking an activity. *Negative* coping is a tendency on the part of the patient to use passive methods of pain control, such as bed rest and medications. The patient regards himself or herself as dependent on others and restricts activities.

Stress: Stressors that have personal relevance can induce psycho/physiologic reactivity. Examples of such stressors are experiences of failure, stressful life events, unsatisfactory work, or being out of work. There is a high risk of stress if one is frequently confronted with problems that one cannot solve.

Family: Encouraging and rewarding partners and family members have a positive effect on the activity levels of patients suffering with chronic pain, whereas overanxious partners and family members have a negative effect.

Depression: Chronic pain and depression are often closely connected. This may be because of the loss of essential reinforcers such as work, sports, hobbies, and social contact. Chronic pain sufferers who are also depressed report more negative thoughts and are less able to self-manage the pain.

Kinesiophobia: The fear that activity might cause pain or new injury is not justified in terms of the reality of the tissue damage and can lead to kinesiophobia. Patients can be divided into "avoiders" of activities and "confronters." The avoiders may develop physical complications through long-term avoidance of physical and social activities; this may result in the disuse syndrome. Atrophy of the muscles reduces stability, which causes more pain and further avoidance. Psychologically, it can lead, among other things, to lower feelings of self-worth and to depression, which in turn lowers the pain threshold.

Diagnosis in Cases of Chronicity

The diagnostic process described here is appropriate for patients who are in the subacute phase and in whom the course of recovery is atypical; it is also for patients who are in the chronic phase and who are not managing their complaints adequately.

In the case of subacute patients showing an atypical course, it is important to discover what factors are causing or maintaining the complaints. Special attention is paid to the possibility of serious disorders (red flags) and/or psychosocial disturbances (yellow flags), the consistency of the findings from the physical examination, and the consistency of the links between impairments, limited activity, and participation problems.

History

When the history is taken, the topics that are explored include how the complaint arose, its nature, seriousness, and course; the patient's previous medical history (red flags); psychosocial factors (yellow flags); and the patient's work situation, family, personal lifestyle, and habits. These are all factors that may explain how the complaint started and why it persists. It is also important to know what significance the patient attaches to the complaints, whether there are any irrational thoughts, and whether the patient is able to control the complaint and/or has a fear of movement.

Special attention should be paid to any of the following:

- Psychosocial problems
- Exceeding the normal recovery period
- Absence of clear causal relationship between the physical substrate and the level of complaint-related behavior
- Unclear description or presentation of the complaint
- Excessive use of medications; "medical shopping"
- Family and others excessively concerned
- Reluctance to talk about psychosocial problems
- Unhealthy living and working habits
- Increasing feelings of hopelessness, depression, and /or powerlessness
- Decreasing feelings of self-worth
- Lack of coping skills

Obtain answers to the following questions about the history of the pain (Vlaeyen et al., 1996):

- When did the patient start to complain of pain?
- How did the patient cope with it?
- What treatments have been performed?
- What does the patient think is causing the pain?
- What makes the pain worse?
- What relieves the pain? (rest, medications)
- What does the patient no longer do because of the pain?
- How does the patient spend the day? (hobbies, leisure-time activities)
- What is the diurnal pattern of the pain?
- How does the patient sleep at night?
- How do the family members know when the patient is in pain?
- How do the family members react to it?
- What are the consequences of the pain for the patient's partner?
- How does the pain affect the relationship?

- How does the pain affect sexual behavior?
- Does the patient feel changed by the pain?
- From the patient's point of view, what is the aim of the treatment?
- What would the patient do again if the pain were less, or if he or she could cope with it better?

Following are the types of reinforcement of pain behavior:

- *Positive reinforcement of pain behavior*. The patient lacks healthy social skills and seeks social contact through pain behavior.
- *Negative reinforcement of pain behavior*. Negative reinforcement includes avoidance of events and activities. Reduced participation in social and physical activities leads to reduced load-bearing capacity. The patient falls into a negative spiral and the deconditioning syndrome may develop.
- *Little or no reinforcement of healthy behavior*. Others discourage the resumption of activities.

Examination

Diagnostic Subdivision of Physical Examination

According to Waddell and Waddell (2000), there are three distinct categories of pathology that may be responsible for low back pain:

- *Nonspecific low back pain*. Nonspecific low back pain is most common between the ages of 20 and 55. It may be related to overloading or dysfunction, or it may arise spontaneously. The pain often spreads across the lower back and into one or both buttocks or thighs. With regard to the cause, there is little correlation between the anatomic localization of the pain, clinical syndromes, and current pathology.
- *Nerve root pain*. Nerve root pain may be caused by a prolapsed disk, spinal stenosis, or postoperative adhesion. Mostly it affects just one nerve root. The pain occurs in a near-dermatomal distribution in one leg, extending past the knee to the foot and toes. There may be tingling and loss of feeling in the same area. Straight leg raising reproduces the pain in the leg. Nerve compression can result in motor, sensory, and reflex changes associated with a nerve root.
- *Serious disorders of the spinal column*. Tumors and infections are present in less than 1% of cases of low back pain. The pain is caused by rheumatic inflammation in less than 1% of cases. Less than 5% are caused by real nerve root pain; of these, only a small

percentage need surgical intervention. If a serious disorder is suspected, the examination must be expanded upon with supplementary examinations carried out to rule in or rule out pathology.

Red flags

I. Serious spinal disorders:
   - Presentation at less than 20 or more than 55 years of age
   - Trauma (fall or road accident)
   - Constant, progressive, nonmechanical pain
   - History of carcinoma, systemic steroids, drug misuse, or HIV
   - Feeling persistently unwell; weight loss
   - Persistent noted restriction of lumbar flexion
   - Widespread neurologic abnormalities
   - Structural deformities
II. Cauda equina syndrome or widespread neurologic disorders:
   - Problems with micturition
   - Loss of anal sphincter tone or rectal incontinence
   - Saddle anesthesia around anus, perineum, or genitalia
   - Widespread neurologic involvement (more than one nerve root), or progressive motor loss in the legs, or disturbance of gait
   - Sensory loss following spinal cord levels
III. Inflammatory disorders (ankylosing spondylitis and related conditions):
   - Gradual onset before age 40
   - Marked stiffness in the mornings
   - Persistent restriction of movement in all directions
   - Involvement of peripheral joints
   - Iritis, psoriasis, colitis, urethral discharge
   - Positive family history

The presentation of the symptoms should be analyzed in terms of the following four questions:

1. *Is the pain coming from the back?* Is the cause of the pain situated in the back, or is the back complaint part of a disorder in an organ or system? Are the hips involved? Is there a circulatory problem?
2. *Is there a major spinal deformity or a widespread neurologic disorder?* Is there a possibility of structural scoliosis or of pain deviation because of unilateral muscular

spasm? The latter often disappears when the patient lies down. Widespread neurologic symptoms affect several myotomes or both legs.

The gait may be disturbed or unstable. There may be problems with urinary retention or overflow incontinence. In case of doubt, a more extensive neurologic examination should be made, consisting of the following:

- Sensory tests of arms, trunk, and saddle area
- Palpation of bladder
- Examination for upper motor neuron signs: increased muscle tone, accentuated reflexes, clonus, upgoing plantar reflexes, loss of position sense in the toes, and positive result on heel-shin test

3. *Is a nerve root involved?* Stimulation of the nerve root causes a sharp, localized pain, which affects the associated dermatomes, while somatic referred pain, which seldom extends beyond the knee, causes a piercing, usually poorly localized pain. Nerve root compression, linking additionally to radicular pain, often gives rise to tingling and numbness. The pain in the leg is often more severe than the pain in the back. Ninety-eight percent of prolapsed disks affect the L5 and S1 nerve roots. Stretching the irritated root reproduces the nerve pain. Pain in the leg when coughing is a positive sign. For further information on nerve root problems, please see Chapter 7 titled "Neurological and Neurovascular Examination."

4. *Is there serious spinal pathology?* Although serious spinal pathology is found in only 1% of cases, the possibility should be explored to reassure the patient. There is a greater chance of spondylolisthesis in patients younger than the age of 20 years. In patients presenting with a first episode of back pain after the age of 55, there is a greater chance of metastases or osteoporosis. It is important to remember that nonmechanical back pain is independent of posture. All the points mentioned under I, II, and III must be carefully considered to ensure as far as possible that serious pathology has not been missed. Varied data must be considered together when forming a clinical opinion.

Behavioral Examination (Yellow Flags)

In cases of idiopathic disturbance without a clear cause, that is, where the physiologic substrate is unknown, the decision whether to adopt a biomedical and/or a behavioral treatment approach is made on the basis of the biopsychosocial history and the biomedical examination. If these reveal "yellow flags," a detailed examination is needed of the patient's psychosocial circumstances to establish whether these could be wholly or partly responsible for the pattern of complaints. If this proves to be the case, therapy must be planned accordingly.

When assessing patients who are in the chronic phase, the practitioner needs to explore the following questions:

- Is the patient coping with the complaint adequately or inadequately?
- Is the patient coping by exercising personal control (internal locus of control) or exercising little or no personal control (external locus of control)?
- Is the patient's way of coping adequate or inadequate?
- Are load and load-bearing capacity balanced, or not?
- Is the patient's level of participation appropriate, or is participation reduced?

Behavioral therapy

Proactive Measures Aimed at Preventing Chronicity

These measures are intended for patients in the subacute pain phase whose recovery is following an abnormal course:

- Information and guidance
- Graduated increase in level of activity
- Stimulating improvement of problem-solving skills

Inclusion Criteria
- Discrepancy between reported pain and objective medical findings.
- Painful complaints that limit the performance of desired motor activities.
- Ability to formulate concrete, attainable goals that are consistent with the therapeutic possibilities. The aim of treatment is not to reduce pain, but to improve functioning.
- The patient's partner is ready and able to take part in the partner course.

Exclusion Criteria
- Serious psychopathology such as psychosis, sociopathy
- Addiction problems, such as alcohol or drugs
- Other problems that affect the pain and that cannot be treated or alleviated by supportive care
- An ongoing legal dispute about the payment or retention of benefits

Arguments in favor of the behavioral approach include the following (Vlaeyen et al., 1996):

- Pain has at least three forms of expression: stress, pain cognition, and pain behavior.
- The presence of underlying physical pathology does not mean that cognitive and environmental factors have no influence on the pain.
- The factors that maintain the pain are not necessarily the same as the factors that caused it to develop in the first place.
- The extent to which patients are limited by pain is the product of interactions among physical, cognitive, emotional, and environmental factors.

Information and Advice

It is important initially to convince the patient that his or her behavior influences the pain and that he or she can have some control over recovery and on whether the complaint recurs or spreads. Factors that are important in this context include the patient's *attitude*: how the patient sees the behavioral changes in terms of *social influence*; how others regard the behavioral changes in *self-efficacy*; expectations as to whether the program will be successful.

The model described by van den Burgt and Verhulst (2003) consists of a series of steps called "being open," "understanding," "wanting to do," "being able to do," "doing," and "continuing to do." The patient is given information about the nature and course of the complaint, the relationship between load and load-bearing capacity, and the importance of an active lifestyle. It is important to explain to the patient that pain is not necessarily associated with tissue damage.

Attainable goals must be agreed upon in discussion with the patient, and the patient must be prepared to maintain the agreed-upon behavior. All information must be given in a language that the patient understands and in an atmosphere of trust to optimize the chances that the patient will use the information and put the advice into practice.

Behavioral Principles

Behavior therapy is appropriate in cases where it seems clear that the pain and restricted movement are a result not only of somatic factors, but also of possible psychological factors and the sickness behavior of the patient. When planning therapy in such cases, and treating joint dysfunction, the clinician emphasizes the use of behavioral principles. The aim of behavioral therapy in these circumstances is to change the patient's behavior in relation to movement functions.

There are three types of behavioral treatment:

- Operant approach
- Respondent or relaxation approach
- Cognitive approach

Operant Treatment

The aim of this treatment is to raise activity levels and decrease the pain. The first step is to establish the baseline for the exercise programmed. The patient is asked to perform a particular activity, for example, cycling on a home trainer, until the pain can no longer be tolerated. Using this as a baseline, the starting level is set just below it. Therapist and patient then agree on a short-term attainable goal. The patient reaches the goal in a series of time-contingent steps (graded activity).

The therapist and patient then negotiate and sign a treatment contract; this contains a treatment plan in which every stage is specified in terms of a starting level, a series of steps of increasing difficulty, and an end goal. The patient should do no more and no less than is stated for each activity in the contract. The long-term goals are set in terms of meaningful uses of time, such as hobbies, work, sport, and family activities. Positive reinforcement is vital when the patient succeeds in mastering steps in the plan.

When phobias are involved, exposure techniques are an option. For fuller information on the aims of operant treatment, please see *Psychology of Unexplained Chronic Pain* by Passchier et al. (1998).

Respondent or Relaxation Treatment

The first requirement is that the patient must be able to recognize stress. The methods used to achieve this include progressive relaxation, autogenic training, transcendental meditation, and yoga. The most suitable method next to operant treatment is relaxation through muscular activity (Jacobson method). This is a concrete, graded approach that places no demands on imagination.

In practice, the method is to contract a particular muscle or muscle group, and then relax it. The patient then practices relaxing the muscles without contracting them beforehand. The next stages are cue-controlled relaxation, where, using abdominal breathing, the patient counts to 3 while breathing in and to 6 while breathing out; differential relaxation, where only those muscles are contracted that are needed for a particular activity, while the rest remain relaxed; accelerated relaxation, where the patient relaxes for 20 to 30 seconds, preceded by abdominal breathing. This should be practiced 10 to 15 times a day while sitting, standing, and walking. The final stage is generalization: using relaxation in stressful situations or in moments of serious pain.

Cognitive Treatment

The purpose of this treatment is to change pain attributions and the patient's expectations about his or her own ability to control the pain. The locus of intervention can be either pain or stress. The treatment can be combined if desired with relaxation exercises.

The program consists of three phases:

- *Reconceptualization*: The therapist tries to reinforce active participation in an atmosphere of cooperation. Because cognitive factors play a part in the way pain is experienced, the therapist tries to change the patient's idea that pain is entirely caused by underlying pathology. The work is based on a biopsychosocial model in which pain is regarded as an experience that can be modified by one's emotions and by exercising control over oneself. The patient needs to become convinced that he or she can do something about the pain and can exercise control.
- *Acquiring capabilities*: Capabilities are acquired through imaginative exercises. Transformatory imagination is used to focus the patient's attention on the perception of pain. Metaphors and suggestions are then used to try to alter its meaning.
- *Generalization*: Patients are encouraged to perform the most demanding exercises in their imagination and then in actual life. Exercises are also given for homework; these can be checked to see what progress is being made.

When we consider the three kinds of treatment, it is clear that the operant approach combines best with the kinds of activities involved in manual therapy. The goals of the operant approach are as follows:

- Increase knowledge and insight with regard to the complaint
- Promote adequate ways of managing the symptoms
- Disengage avoidance behavior
- Raise activity levels
- Improve the relevant functions
- Gradually build up a program of exercises (graded activity)

- Introduce time-contingent exercise, in which the limiting factor is not the pain but the length of time during which the patient will exercise
- Positive reinforcement of completion of performance of the exercises
- Extinction of the pain behavior (Passchier et al., 1998)

The Therapeutic Process

In discussion with the patient, functions and/or activities are chosen that can be built up step by step from a baseline using time-contingent exercise (graded activity). The activities to be practiced should be those that are most important to the patient. The baseline is chosen so as to allow the patient to carry out the chosen activities as long, as frequently, and as well as possible without overdoing it. For every activity, the therapist and the patient work together to decide on an attainable goal in relation to the baseline. The period of treatment, duration, frequency, and intensity are agreed upon and written into the treatment plan.

If the exercise program is designed cooperatively by the patient and the therapist, the patient becomes co-responsible for the following:

- The functional and behavioral result
- The learning and relearning of motor and cognitive skills
- The time scale for achieving activities and participation
- The creation of a realistic approach to pain and pain behavior, in which pain is not synonymous with past or ongoing damage to the tissues

The time-dependent activities may not exceed the patient's load-bearing capacity, and neither may pain influence the performance of the task. If exercising at home does not lead to sufficient progress, the frequency of the therapist-directed sessions must be increased. If the results of the home exercise program are positive, the period between monitoring sessions can be increased. The ultimate aim is that when the goal is reached, the patient should take responsibility for continuing the exercise program: this is the final step.

The following measuring instruments can be used:

- Screening Questionnaire for Psychosocial Risk Factors (SQPRF) (Waddell and Waddell, 2000; Linton and Haldén, 1998).
- Patient-Specific Complaints (PsC) (Beurskens, Vet, and Köke, 1996). This identifies three to five physical

activities and the degree to which they are restricted, each rated on a 0–10 scale.

- Visual Analog Scale (VAS) or numeric pain rating scale (NPRS) (Köke, Heuts, Vlaeyen, and Weber, 1999). This scale determines how much difficulty the patient is having with the three most restricted physical activities. Kelly (2001) reported an overall minimal clinically significant score of 12 mm (95% CI: 9–15 mm) for the VAS measure with no significant between-group differences based on pain severity. Childs, Piva, and Fritz (2005) reported a 2-point difference as the minimal clinically important difference for the NPRS in patients with low back pain.

- Quebec Back Pain Disability Scale (QBPDS) (Köke et al., 1999). This scale charts restrictions and participation problems. It lists 20 daily activities, which are assigned to six categories: no difficulty at all; very little difficulty; some difficulty; much difficulty; extreme difficulty; and unable to answer.

- Acute Low Back Pain Screening Questionnaire (ALBSQ) (Vlaeyen and Heuts, 2000). This questionnaire is used to predict a possible atypical course and possible chronicity.

- Coping Strategies Questionnaire (CSQ) (Vlaeyen et al., 1996). This questionnaire is used to assess whether the patient is using positive or negative coping strategies.

- Pain control question list (Vlaeyen et al., 1996). The purpose of this list of questions is to determine whether the locus of control is internal or external.

- Tampa Scale for Kinesiophobia (TSK) (Vlaeyen et al., 1996). The scale measures the patient's fear of movement. Swinkels-Meewisse et al. (2003) reported a Crohnback alpha ranging from 0.70–0.76 for the internal consistency of the TSK. Test-retest reliability yielded Pearson's $r = 0.78$.

- Fear Avoidance Beliefs Questionnaire (FABQ). The role of this questionnaire as a predictor variable in various clinical prediction rules relevant to OMT clinical practice has been discussed earlier (in Chapter 4). Swinkels-Meewisse et al. (2003) reported a Crohnback alpha ranging from 0.70–0.72 for the internal consistency of the Physical Activity subscale of the FABQ; α ranged from 0.82–0.83 for the Work subscale. Test-retest reliability for the Physical Activity and Work subscales yielded Pearson's $r = 0.64$ and 0.80, respectively. Cleland, Fritz, and Brennan (2008) noted high (> 29) initial scores on the FABQ Work subscale as indicative of poor outcome only in patients with low back pain receiving workers' compensation. Low concurrent validity with the TSK (Spearman's rho $= 0.33$–0.59) indicates that it may be useful to use both the FABQ and the TSK in assessment of patients with low back pain (Swinkels-Meewisse et al., 2003).

This list of tests and measures is intended primarily to help the serious researcher to locate the literature in which the instruments are described and their background discussed. The clinician should have a thorough knowledge of the available instruments, how they were developed, and how to interpret them to make the right choice in each situation. The ultimate reason for using a valid, reliable, and responsive measurement tool is to objectify to the greatest extent possible information that is gathered by subjective methods. This provides a scientific basis for action. The patient has a right to the most objective assessment possible and to the most effective treatment.

CHAPTER 9

Supplementary Data, Diagnosis, and Treatment Planning

RADIOGRAPHY AND OTHER IMAGING STUDIES

When making a manual diagnosis, it is important to be aware of any physical anomalies, morphologic changes, and fractures. However, the first two cannot be objectively established by physical examination, and the last cannot always be identified with sufficient diagnostic certainty. Radiographs are therefore needed to provide definite answers. They serve two purposes: they provide either a supplementary or a definitive contribution to the physical examination, and they explain its findings.

When requesting radiographs, it is important to be able to justify the request. When interpreting the radiographs, uniform criteria should be used to gain a valid result. This plus the fact that a great deal of experience is needed to interpret radiographs makes a good working relationship with the radiologist both desirable and necessary.

Finally, although CT and MRI scans are too expensive for routine use, they can provide definite answers as to whether or not manual therapy is indicated.

ELECTRODIAGNOSTIC STUDIES

Electrocardiograms, electroencephalograms, and electromyograms can be produced and interpreted only by the appropriate medical specialists. Electromyography and nerve conduction velocity studies can be an important adjunct to manual assessment and are sometimes necessary for differential diagnosis.

BIOPSY

The manual therapy examination may yield findings that suggest tissue biopsy would be advisable. Examination of tissues and tissue fluids is one of the ways of establishing whether or not manual therapy is indicated.

LABORATORY TESTS

In cases where relative or absolute counterindications for manual therapy are suspected, laboratory tests can often give a definitive answer. The results of any previous laboratory tests should be taken into account, together with any treatment that was prescribed at the time, for example, insulin, antihypertensives, or anticoagulants.

OTHER SPECIAL MEDICAL TESTS

An accurate diagnosis may not be possible without input from other medical specialties such as gynecology; rheumatology; urology; ear, nose, and throat (ENT); internal medicine; and psychiatry. In manual diagnosis, the relationship between the internal organs and the spinal segments with which they are associated is also important: dysfunction in an internal organ can result in a presenting predominant pain in another structure that is related to the same segment. It is important when examining the patient to identify which structure is the cause of the pathologic loop (pathogenetic sensitivity diagnosis; Gutmann, 1970). The therapist must also pay attention to any pathology in secondary structures that are related to the segment because these can continuously reactivate the vicious cycle. Internal medicine thus can contribute not only to diagnosis but also to therapy.

OVERALL ASSESSMENT

During this assessment, data from the maximally comprehensive examination are evaluated in relation to each other with the goal of deriving an appropriate kinesiologic diagnosis.

KINESIOLOGIC DIAGNOSIS

Once the kinesiologic diagnosis has been made, the treatment plan can be drawn up. This is followed by the first treatment session, which is regarded as a trial treatment.

TRIAL TREATMENT

The outcome of the trial treatment may be negative. Possible reasons for this include inaccurate diagnosis, failure to choose the right therapy, or failure to administer it properly; under these circumstances, it may be necessary to restart the diagnostic process, adjust the therapy, or improve on its delivery. On the other hand, the outcome of the trial may be successful, in which case the probable diagnosis becomes definite and the trial therapy becomes the chosen therapy.

DEFINITIVE TREATMENT

The definitive treatment will need continual adjustment during the patient's recovery to take into account his or her changing condition.

CHAPTER 10

History and Examination: Practical Considerations

TERMINOLOGY

Functional mechanism. Before describing in chapters 13-18 the various regions of the spine and the temporomandibular joints, as well as the practical clinical examination procedures used in testing three-dimensional movement, we must look at the functional mechanisms that enable movement in the sagittal, frontal, and transverse (cardinal) planes separately in the chapter section titled "Functional Aspects." The reason for doing so is that the literature offers little or no scientifically supported information about the complicated mechanisms that underlie three-dimensional movement and the stresses it places on tissues. The whole is more than the sum of the parts and is different from it. Nevertheless, separate analyses of the different cardinal plane movements and the stresses they place on different tissues can provide some insight—by extrapolation—into the mechanisms and stresses involved in three-dimensional spinal movement.

Order of examination. The general principle for regional and segmental active-assisted examination is that three-dimensional movements involving sidebending and ipsilateral rotation are described before three-dimensional movements involving sidebending and contralateral rotation.

Side being examined—side not being examined. These terms refer to the starting position of the therapist with regard to the side or the direction of movement to be examined. During examination of three-dimensional function, the side to be examined is determined by the axial rotation component.

Ipsilateral, contralateral. These terms refer to the positioning of the therapist's hands in relation to the side or direction of movement to be examined. In this context, *ipsilateral* means on the side or in the direction of movement to be examined, and *contralateral* means the other side. During the examination of three-dimensional function, the direction of movement to be examined is determined by the axial rotation component.

Position of the patient during examination. Weight-bearing examinations of the thoracic and lumbar spine are carried out in a slightly flexed position unless this is prevented by dysfunction of the lumbar spine.

Therapist starting position. During examination of weight-bearing three-dimensional function of the cervical, thoracic, and lumbar spine, the therapist stands at the side being examined; this is determined by the direction of rotation.

Performance of examination. During weight-bearing three-dimensional examination of the lumbar spine, the patient's center of gravity should remain as close as possible above the point of support.

MANUAL THERAPY DOCUMENTATION

Table 10–1 can be used as a guide to which items should be documented during the diagnosis and management process in orthopaedic manual therapy.

Table 10–1   Steps in the Orthopaedic Manual Therapy Diagnosis and Management Process

Steps	Data
Details of patient and referring physician	Patient personal information Patient insurance information Date referral received Details of referral and referral source • Diagnosis on referral • Purpose of referral • Proposed treatment Treating manual therapist
History taken by manual therapist Examination by manual therapist	Patient's reason for seeking out treatment Complaint: nature/cause/location/severity/course Patient expectations Patient activities: Occupation/education/sports/hobbies Relevant medical details Relevant psychosocial details Other care and support Assistive devices used by the patient Results of examinations: • Inspection • Palpation • Neurologic examination • Movement examination • Other measurements and tests
Conclusions	Conclusions, with explanation Decision whether or not to treat Details outside the scope of manual therapy
Treatment plan	Impairments amenable to treatment Treatment goals Frequency of treatment Number of treatments Length of treatment sessions Details of intervention: Type/form/dosage /location information Advice and lifestyle guidance Appointments with patient Assistive devices Multidisciplinary appointments and referrals
Treatment evaluation	Documentation Details of treatment process Treatment results Results of discussions with: referral source/colleagues/other disciplines
Final treatment session	Reason for termination of treatment Date of report to referral source Details of post-discharge care

EXAMINATION STRATEGY

A clear formulation of the general and specific goals of the manual therapy examination is basic to a methodical and systematic approach to treatment (Hagenaars, Bernards, and Oostendorp, 1996). The taking of the history and the subsequent physical examination are the crucial elements in meeting those aims.

General Objectives

The manual therapist can make reasoned statements about the following factors:

- The appropriateness of the manual therapy referral
- Appropriate manual therapy goals for the individual patient
- The strategy for attaining those goals
- Appropriate manual therapy methods
- The most appropriate manual therapist

Before a statement of general objectives can be made, the general second-order objectives must be known (see next section).

General Second-Order Objectives

The manual therapist can identify and make reasoned statements about the following factors:

- The disorder (disease) affecting the patient, or the tissue or organ that is damaged
- The factors that were responsible for the onset of the patient's disorder (disease), or the damage to the tissue or organ
- The factors responsible for the patient's complaint (request for help)
- Whether the disorder (disease) or the damage to the tissues or organ is following a normal or an atypical course; the nature of any abnormality in the course, and the factors that have influenced it

Disorders (Diseases): Lesions in Tissues or Organs

As already discussed in more detail in Chapter 4, disorders (diseases) and lesions of tissues or organs may be classified according to any of the following diagnostic classification systems:

- Anatomic classification
- Medical classification
- Manual therapy classification
- Psychological classification

Anatomic Classification The manual therapist identifies the following:

- The location of the disorder or lesion
- The affected tissue
- The nature of the lesion

It is important to identify the damaged tissue to assess the adaptive capability of the area. Three kinds of tissue may be distinguished:

- *Mitotic tissue.* Continued cell division (blood, including bone marrow, and endothelial tissue)
- *Postmitotic tissue.* No cell division (muscle and nerve tissue)
- *Recurrent mitotic tissue.* Intermittent cell division (collagenous connective tissue)

Medical Classification Medical classification is based on the International Classification of Diseases (ICD). The diagnostic methods used are as follows:

- History
- Physical examination
- Additional examinations (X-ray, CT scan, MRI, laboratory tests, etc.)

The results of the medical diagnosis can be important for the manual therapist in determining adaptive potential and whether there are any absolute or relative contraindications for manual therapy.

Manual Therapy Classification Dysfunctions are classified as *local* or *segmental*. Where the dysfunction is segmental, there will be a complex set of dysfunctions in the tissues and organs innervated by one spinal nerve together with the gray communicating ramus. These are most likely to be expressed as changes in the mechanical behavior of connective tissue (mobility, endfeel).

Psychological Classification The following factors are important in this context:

- Ability to learn and to modify behavior in the short or long term

- Relevant personal characteristics, such as the following:

  Internal/external locus of control

  Attribution

  Coping style (active/passive/avoiding)

  Anxiety

  Depression

  Aggression

  Stress

  Nonspecific arousal

  Intelligence

  Willpower/motivation

- Social interaction

Inventarization   When information has been obtained under the preceding four headings, the therapist can evaluate the following:

- Capacity for local adaptation:

  Cell death

  Tissue type

  Age

  Gender

  Condition

  Constitution

- Local impediments:

  Positioning (position of vertebrae and sacroiliac joint)

  Circulatory disturbances (rupture, constricted blood vessel, edema)

- General impediments:

  Medical disorders

  Systemic diseases

  Disorders of organs that must be functioning well to enable adaptation of the neuromusculoskeletal system

  Individual patterns of posture and movement, which must sometimes be modified in the interest of local adaptation

  Aspects of life, or any affective coloring by the patient that creates unfavorable conditions for change

- The manual therapist must be able to recognize the general symptoms of stress and of strong nonspecific arousal to identify these factors.

Causes

The factors that were/are responsible for the onset of the disorder, or for the lesions in organs and tissues, may be of two kinds:

- Trauma
- Imbalance between load and load-bearing capacity

Presenting Complaint

There are three ways in which the patient's sickness behavior (presenting complaint) may be related to the physical factors:

- Complaint is related to the dysfunction and its consequences.
- Complaint is not related to the dysfunction and its consequences.
- Complaint is related both to the disorder and its consequences and to other unrelated problems.

Course

The nature of the disorder and the damage to the tissues or organ must first be identified. It may then be possible to establish whether the dysfunction (disease) is following a normal or an atypical course, and to identify any atypical features and their possible causes. Tissues and organs vary in their capacity to recover and the length of time this takes (de Morree, 1993; Junqueira et al., 1995). The course of a disorder can be atypical in nature and/or duration; this is influenced by both local and general impediments.

The history and the results of the physical examination must be available before the second-level objectives can be decided.

Patient History

The history should contain the following sections:

- Inventory of the patient's health problems.
- The point in time when the first symptoms appeared.
- List of the factors that were responsible for the onset of the disorder and the symptoms. This involves analyzing load in relation to load-bearing capacity, both at the local level (tissues and organs) and at the global level (the whole person).

- Description of the course of the complaints and the dysfunction.
- Description of the present status.

Inventory of Health Problems

The following information is gathered:

- Specific complaints and symptoms
- Impairments, disabilities, and handicaps (World Health Organization, 2001)
- Presenting problem

Complaints and Symptoms

- Pain:

  Location, nature, referral pattern

  Times when the pain appears and disappears

  Continuous or intermittent, diurnal/nocturnal rhythm

  Aggravating and relieving factors

  Any other influences

- Dysfunction:

  Nature of dysfunction

  Times when dysfunction appears or disappears

  Aggravating and relieving factors

  Any other influences

- Sensory abnormalities:

  Nature of disturbances (anesthesia, hypesthesia, hyperesthesia, paresthesia)

  Times when the disturbances appear and disappear

  Aggravating and relieving factors

  Any other influences

- Sympathetic dysfunction:

  Changes in perspiration

  Changes in temperature

  Changes in skin sensitivity

  Changes in muscle tone

Impairment, Disability, and Handicap   It should become clear from the history whether the patient is suffering from an impairment, and if so how this contributes to a possible disability or a handicap.

Presenting Complaint   On the subject of the presenting complaint, please see the section titled "Presenting Complaint" earlier in this chapter.

Time Line

The first step is to establish the time when the first symptoms appeared. This will show whether the patient has suffered from the complaint previously and whether it has been recurrent. The therapist then tries to discover what the cause was and in what circumstances the complaint arose; what its course was previously; whether any treatments were carried out, and how they were chosen; how long the treatment lasted, and whether it was successful.

Causes

As stated previously, the causes may be of two kinds: trauma and imbalance between load and load-bearing capacity.

Trauma   If the patient has suffered trauma, the therapist needs to form a picture of the mechanism of injury to tissues or organs. The important factors are the speed and direction of the forces that caused the lesion and the location of the impact.

Load   List the factors that were responsible for the onset of the disorder and the complaint. This is produced by analyzing load in relation to load-bearing capacity at the level of tissues and organs (local) and at the level of the whole person (general).

For the purposes of the manual therapy examination, factors are classified as contributing to the physical load (general, local, or regional) or to the psychosocial load.

General Physical Load   To form an initial picture, the therapist will ask about the following items:

- Work-related stress, sports, hobbies
- Smoking, alcohol consumption
- Medications and stimulants
- Current illnesses

Local Physical Load   Local loads—whether mechanical, thermal, or chemical—that exceed the limits of the physical load-bearing capacity can lead to disturbance in a kinesiologic unit or joint with associated muscles. Depending on the level of selectivity of the central nervous system and the persistence of nociceptive input, the disturbance may result in specific tissue changes elsewhere within the affected segment. With regard to work, sports, and hobbies, information is needed on the following specifics:

- Working hours, working conditions, and working position
- Type of sport, number of hours, at what level and under what conditions the patient participates
- Type of hobby, number of hours devoted to hobby, and conditions in which this time is spent

Regional Physical Load   A regional load that exceeds the limits of physiologic load-bearing capacity can lead to disturbance in a biomechanical unit consisting of several kinesiologic units. Depending on the level of selectivity of the central nervous system and the persistence of nociceptive input, the disturbance can result in the spread of tissue-specific changes elsewhere in the neuroanatomically related segments. The questions the therapist asks about the course of the complaint should reveal what the primary disturbance was and in what order and under what circumstances it spread.

The limits on physiologic load-bearing capacity may be exceeded by the following:

- Trauma
- Sudden changes in posture and movement habits
- Persistent holding of one-sided positions, or performance of movements with one side of the body

Psychosocial Load   Psychosocial load has an interface with working and living conditions. Occupational, family, and social circumstances can be threatening to the extent that they exceed load-bearing capacity.

Information is needed about the following factors:

- Work situation
- Family situation
- Social well-being

Load-Bearing Capacity   The information about load-bearing capacity gathered during the manual therapy examination can be classified as general, local/segmental, regional/segmental, thoracic/segmental, and psychological.

General Physical Load-Bearing Capacity   General physical load-bearing capacity can be lowered by the following items:

- Previous illnesses

- Previous surgery
- Present systemic disorders

The present status and the medical history are both important. The following questions may be asked to elicit the history:

- Have you ever had surgery?
- Have you had any serious illnesses?
- Have you ever had a serious accident?
- Have you ever taken any medicines? Which ones?
- Have you ever had an X-ray? Why?
- Have you ever had laboratory tests? Why?
- Have you suffered in the past from the complaints that you have now?
- Are you suffering from general fatigue?

Factors that can lower load-bearing capacity may result as follows:

- Increased susceptibility to viral or bacterial infections
- Tendency to tire easily
- Reduced functional movement
- Increased susceptibility to injury

Local/Segmental Physical Load-Bearing Capacity   Local capacity is load-bearing capacity within a kinesiologic unit and the related segment. Local load-bearing capacity can be reduced by a number of factors; these are listed in the next subsection on regional load-bearing capacity.

Regional/Segmental Physical Load-Bearing Capacity   Regional capacity is the load-bearing capacity of one or more kinesiologic units within a biomechanical chain and the related segments. Both local and regional load-bearing capacity can be reduced by the following factors:

- Previous trauma, inflammatory processes, surgery, disturbances in the affected region that may have caused reduced circulation and lymphatic drainage
- Previous disturbances in organs (internal organs and neuromusculoskeletal systems) in the same segment or in neuroanatomically related segments
- Current disturbances in other organs (internal organs and neuromusculoskeletal systems) in the same segment or in neuroanatomically related segments
- Anomalies in the affected area
- Spondyloses, uncarthroses, or spondylarthroses in the affected region

Thoracic/Segmental Load-Bearing Capacity This is the load-bearing capacity of the autonomic segments and their innervation area. The load-bearing capacity of these segments can be lowered by the following factors:

- Previous or current complaints affecting the internal organs or neuromusculoskeletal systems in the same segments or in neuroanatomically related segments
- Threats that exceed psychological load-bearing capacity

Psychological Load-Bearing Capacity Psychological load-bearing capacity can be lowered by previous psychological disturbances or current threats to general well-being. Nonspecific arousal can elicit a nonspecific reaction in the central nervous system; this is called nonselectivity. Persistent nonspecific arousal can lower load-bearing capacity. When combined with persisting nociceptive input, this can cause a lasting rise in the tonic activity of the sympathetic autonomic nervous system. The recognizable symptoms of this are changes specific to organs and tissues. These conditions can be responsible both for the onset of the complaint and for its maintenance and/or spread. To establish whether the patient is in a state of nonspecific arousal, the therapist should ask whether the patient is suffering from any of the following:

- Difficulty in falling asleep, restless sleep, night terrors, night sweats
- Poor appetite, nausea
- Irritability, feeling harassed, feeling bloated
- Poor concentration, aimless activity
- Hyperventilation, palpitations, swings in blood pressure
- Hyperhydrosis, loss of interest, and general fatigue

Course

Recording the Course of the Patient's Complaints and the Illness
The course of a complaint or an illness can be atypical in physiologic and/or pathologic terms. The atypical features of the course may be qualitative or have to do with its progression over time. In cases where the course of recovery is atypical, this may be due to the following:

- Local impediments such as inappropriate loading of the tissues
- General impediments such as nonselectivity of the central nervous system

The following questions are useful for elucidating the course of the complaint:

- When did the current complaint begin?
- Where did the present complaint begin?
- Has there been any improvement since the onset of the complaint?
- When did the improvement begin?
- Has improvement been continuous since then?
- Have there been times when the complaint became worse again?
- When did it become worse?
- What might have caused the deterioration?
- Was the deterioration followed by improvement?
- At what point did the improvement begin?
- Have other complaints developed in addition to the primary one?
- What are these additional complaints?
- When did the additional complaints arise?

The answers to these questions will show the pattern of development over a given period. Three different patterns are possible:

- Progressive improvement
- Mixed picture
- Spread of the illness or the pattern of complaints

If either the second or the third pattern applies, the practitioner will need to explore whether the load placed on the damaged tissues is inappropriate, and whether there is a degree of nonselectivity in the central nervous system.

Present Status

To assess the patient's present condition, it is essential to supplement the history with information about the complaints at the time of presentation.

Interpretation All the data obtained in the history must be organized and interpreted before proceeding to inspection and physical examination. The following kinds of information are needed about the illness, or the damaged organ or tissue:

- Location
- Location of the original complaint
- Distribution

- Factors responsible for onset and development
- Factors that influence the pattern of complaints

The practitioner should be able to make an overall judgment and a provisional differential diagnosis based on interpretation of the information recorded. If the referral for manual therapy proves to have been inappropriate, this finding is reported to the referrer, together with an explanation. If, however, the referral appears at this stage to be appropriate, the therapist will proceed to observation and physical examination to check and refine the information contained in the history.

Observation

The purpose behind the observation strategy is to confirm or supplement the details in the history. In most cases, a general observation is followed by a regional/local observation focused on the reported dysfunction (see the following section titled "Observation").

Physical examination

It should be clear from the history which region should be examined and which segments are likely to be related to the disorder. For a description of examination procedures, please see the appropriate chapters.

The examination must perform the following functions:

- Check symptoms that were named or indicated by the patient during the taking of the history; list symptoms that were not named, but which on theoretical grounds could be present
- Provide additional support for the conclusions reached so far about illness or damage to tissues or organs

Checking the History

The reasons for checking the details in the history are these:

- Possible loss of information resulting from inadequate communication between therapist and patient
- Incomplete information because of differences in interpretation between therapist and patient

Additional Support for Conclusions

Two questions should be asked at this point:

- Does the suspected illness have a characteristic clinical presentation, and can a manual therapist identify such a picture with a high level of confidence?
- Is this clinical presentation specific to this illness?

If the answers to these questions are positive, the level of confidence can be increased even further by means of appropriate tests.

When the results of the examination have been recorded and interpreted, a general opinion is formed and a provisional diagnosis made. The diagnosis will determine whether manual therapy is indicated, whether it is absolutely or relatively contraindicated, or whether it is contraindicated on functional grounds.

If manual therapy is indicated, the therapist must assess what results can reasonably be expected. The next question is whether manual therapy alone will suffice, or whether a multidisciplinary approach should be considered. If the next step is to be manual therapy, the therapist proceeds to a trial treatment. The definitive treatment follows if the trial treatment yields positive results. If the outcome of the trial treatment is negative, either the diagnostic process must be started afresh or the therapeutic approach must be modified.

OBSERVATION

During the observation, any abnormalities in shape or position and any special characteristics should be noted. Observation covers the head, shoulder girdle, upper limbs, trunk, pelvic girdle, and lower limbs. It is particularly important to assess the relationships among the different parts of the neuromusculoskeletal system.

Cleland et al. (2006) established interrater reliability for visual assessment of posture as a component for the development of a clinical prediction rule on the indications for thoracic spine manipulation in patients with mechanical neck pain (Cleland et al., 2007). Using a dichotomous rating scale, they reported 81% agreement for the assessment of forward head posture but a κ value of -0.1 (95% CI: -0.2–0.0) as a result of limited variation, that is, 90% prevalence. Visual assessment of excessive shoulder protraction yielded 95% agreement and a κ of 0.83 (95% CI: 0.51–1.0). Observation for excessive C7–T2 kyphosis yielded 90% agreement ($\kappa = 0.79$, 95% CI: 0.51–1.0). Interrater agreement for observation for excessive or decreased kyphosis at T3–T5 was 90% and 82% with κ values of 0.69 (95% CI: 0.3–1.0) and 0.58 (95% CI: 0.22–0.95). For excessive and decreased kyphosis at T6–T10, these values were 95% and 95% with κ values of 0.9 (95% CI: 0.74–1.0) and 0.9 (95% CI: 0.73–1.0), respectively.

In contrast to these high interrater reliability values, Fedorak et al. (2003) reported fair mean intrarater reliability ($\kappa = 0.50$) and poor mean interrater reliability ($\kappa = 0.16$) for visual assessment of lordotic posture of the cervical and lumbar spine when using a 3-point rating scale (ie, normal, increased, decreased). Using changes in posture as indicators of diagnosis and outcome has been questioned by Dunk et al. (2004), who noted large coefficients of variance reflecting substantial intrasubject variation in upright standing posture in asymptomatic adults even with digitized postural assessment. In contrast, Saxon-Bullock (1993) noted consistent spinal postural alignment using inclinometers and an electrogoniometer on various occasions on one day in pregnant women, women with low back pain, and asymptomatic subjects; asymptomatic subjects maintained consistent postural alignment even over a period of 2 years.

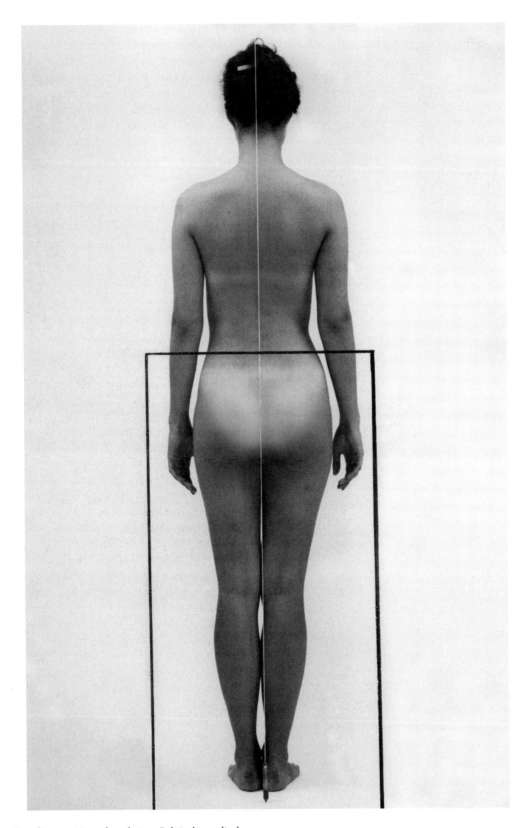

Figure 10–1   Standing position, dorsal view. Pelvis, lower limbs.

Pelvis and lower limbs	*Assessment*	*Criteria*
Pelvis	Position	Posterior superior iliac spines, iliac crests, trochanters, gluteal folds, gluteal cleft, lateral shift relative to shoulder girdle
	Musculature	Atrophy, hypertrophy, swelling
	Skin	Skin zones, swelling
Thighs	Position	Varus, valgus, rotation
	Musculature	Atrophy, hypertrophy, swelling
	Blood vessels	Varicose veins
	Knees	Varus or valgus position, popliteal folds
	Shape	Swelling
Lower legs	Position	Varus, valgus, rotation
	Shape	Varus, valgus
	Musculature	Atrophy, hypertrophy, swelling
	Blood vessels	Varicose veins
Ankles	Position	Asymmetry of medial malleoli
	Shape	Contours of Achilles tendons, swelling
Feet	Position	Calcaneus varus, valgus
	Shape	Swelling

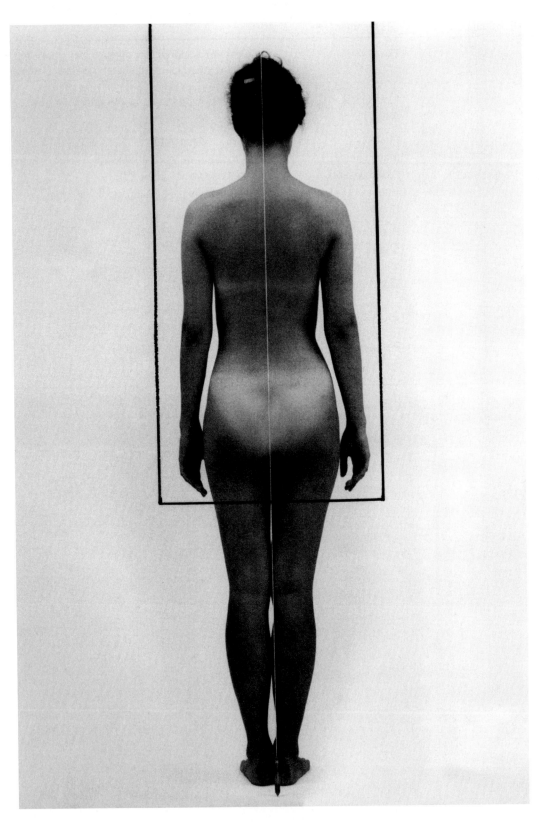

Figure 10–2   Standing position, dorsal. Spine, shoulder girdle, thorax, upper limbs.

	Assessment	Criteria
Cervical spine	Position	Sidebending, rotation, lateral shift
	Shape	Scoliosis
	Musculature	Atrophy, hypertrophy, swelling
Shoulder girdle	Position	Depression, elevation, asymmetric shoulder height
	Shape	Asymmetry of neck-shoulder angle
	Musculature	Atrophy, hypertrophy, swelling
Shoulder blades	Position	Scapula alata, protraction, retraction, rotation, difference in height, distance from spine
Thorax	Position	Asymmetrical rib arch, inspiration position, expiration position
	Shape	Gibbus (rib hump)
Thoracic/lumbar spine	Position	Scoliosis, torsion, shift, flank triangle
	Musculature	Atrophy, hypertrophy, swelling
	Skin	Skin zones, swelling, scars, hair growth
Upper arms	Position	Rotation
	Musculature	Atrophy, hypertrophy, swelling
Elbows	Shape	Swelling
	Skin	Color, folds
Forearms/hands	Position	Pronation, supination
	Musculature	Atrophy, hypertrophy, swelling
	Skin	Swelling, color

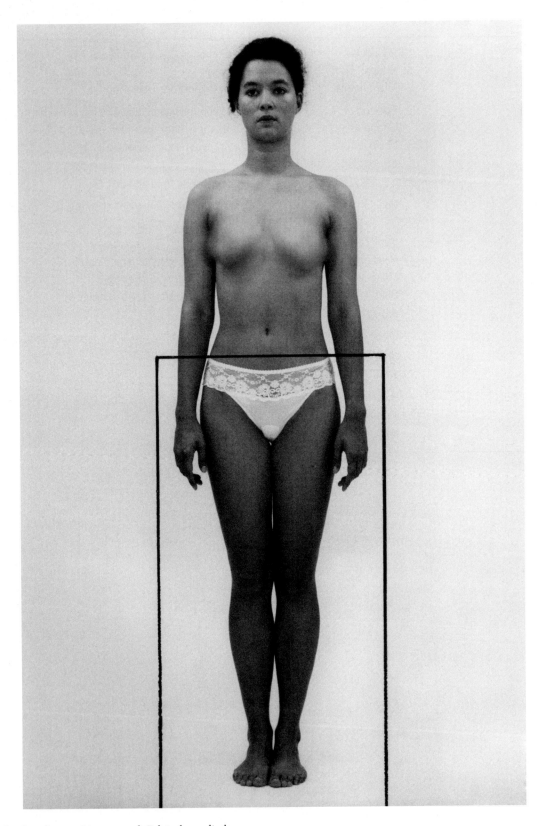

Figure 10–3   Standing position, ventral. Pelvis, lower limbs.

Pelvis and lower limbs	Assessment	Criteria
Pelvis	Position	Difference in height of anterior superior iliac spines
Thighs	Position	Varus, valgus, rotation
	Musculature	Atrophy, hypertrophy, swelling
	Blood vessels	Varicose veins
Knees	Position	Varus, valgus, position of patella
	Shape	Swelling
	Musculature	Atrophy, hypertrophy, swelling
Lower legs	Position	Varus, valgus
	Musculature	Atrophy, hypertrophy, swelling
	Blood vessels	Varicose veins
Ankles	Position	Asymmetry of medial malleoli
	Shape	Swelling
Feet	Position	Calcaneus varus, valgus, inversion, eversion
	Shape	Longitudinal arch, swelling
	Musculature	Atrophy, hypertrophy, swelling
	Skin	Swelling, color
Toes	Position	Abducted toes, hammer toes, claw toes, hallux valgus

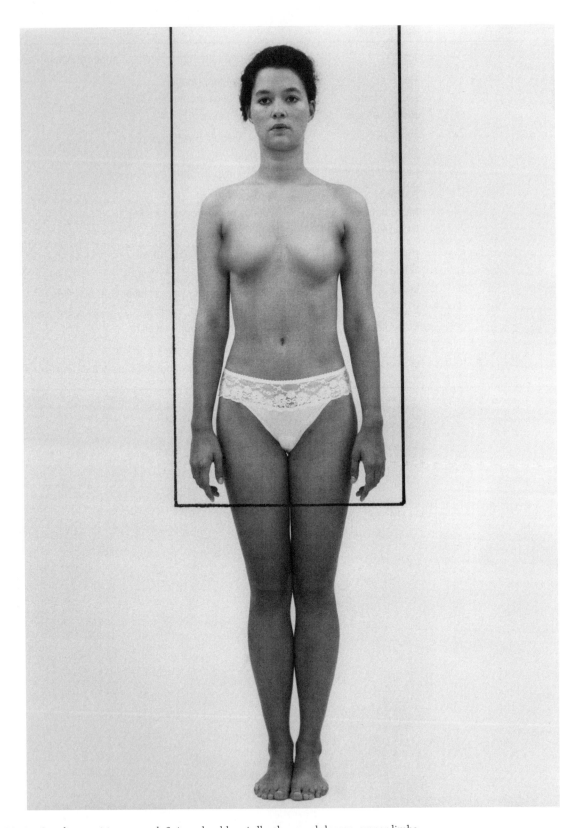

Figure 10–4   Standing position, ventral. Spine, shoulder girdle, thorax, abdomen, upper limbs.

Spine, shoulder girdle, thorax, abdomen, upper limbs	Assessment	Criteria
Head	Shape	Symmetry, swelling
	Musculature	Atrophy, hypertrophy, swelling
Cervical spine	Position	Sidebending, rotation, lateral shift
	Musculature	Atrophy, hypertrophy, swelling
	Skin	Scarring
Shoulder girdle	Position	Depression, elevation, protraction, retraction, asymmetric shoulder height
	Shape	Asymmetry of neck-shoulder angle, supraclavicular fossa, shoulder blades
	Musculature	Atrophy, hypertrophy, swelling
Thorax/abdomen	Position	Inspiration or expiration, position of sternum, navel
	Shape	Swelling, pectus excavatum ("sunken chest"), pectus carinatum ("pigeon chest"), asymmetry of rib bow, nipples, epigastric angle
	Musculature	Atrophy, hypertrophy, swelling
	Skin	Scars, striae
Upper arms	Position	Rotation
	Musculature	Atrophy, hypertrophy, swelling
Elbows	Position	Flexion
Forearms/hands	Position	Pronation/supination
	Musculature	Atrophy, hypertrophy, swelling
	Skin	Swelling, color

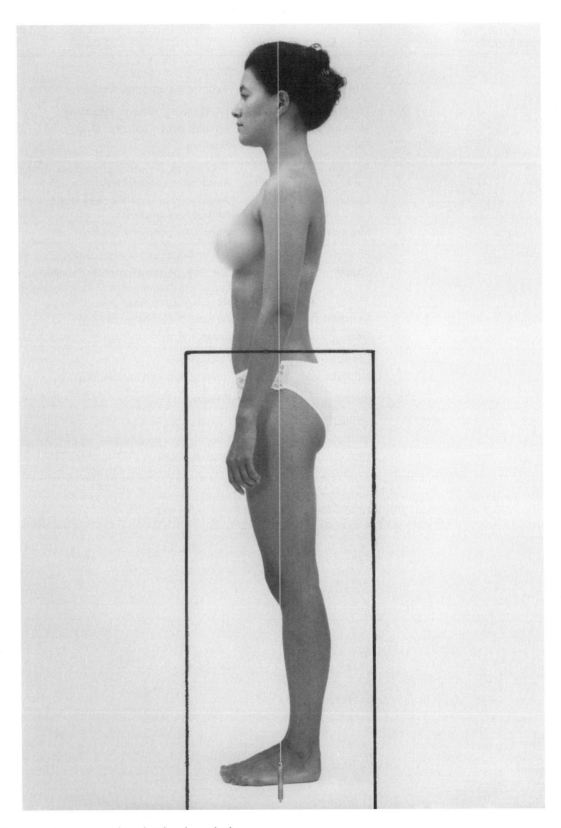

Figure 10–5   Standing position, lateral. Pelvis, lower limbs.

Pelvis and lower limbs	Assessment	Criteria
Pelvis	Position	Anterior and posterior superior iliac spines
	Musculature	Atrophy, hypertrophy, swelling
	Skin	Swelling, scarring
Thighs	Position	Hip flexion
	Musculature	Atrophy, hypertrophy, swelling
	Skin	Swelling, scarring
Knees	Position	Recurvatum, flexion (antecurvatum)
	Shape	Swelling
Lower legs	Shape	Saber-shaped shins
	Musculature	Atrophy, hypertrophy, swelling
Ankles	Position	Plantar- or dorsiflexion
Feet	Shape	Dorsal arch of the foot, swelling, other anomalies
Toes	Shape	Claw toes, hammer toes

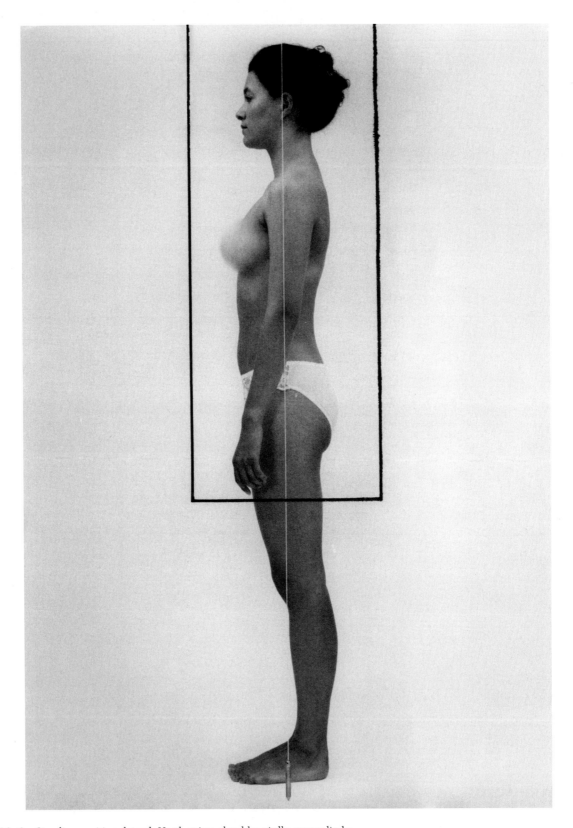

Figure 10–6   Standing position, lateral. Head, spine, shoulder girdle, upper limbs.

Head, spine, shoulder girdle, upper limbs	Assessment	Criteria
Head	Position	Protraction, retraction, flexion, or extension
Cervical spine	Position	Flexion and extension, ventral and dorsal shift
	Musculature	Atrophy, hypertrophy, swelling
	Skin	Scarring
Shoulder girdle	Position	Protraction, retraction
Scapulae	Position	Scapula alata
Thorax	Position	Torsion
	Shape	Gibbus (rib hump)
Thoracic/lumbar spine	Position	Kyphosis - lordosis, rotation, forward-backward carrying
Upper arms	Position	Rotation, position relative to trunk
	Musculature	Atrophy, hypertrophy, swelling
Elbows	Position	Flexion
	Shape	Swelling
	Skin	Color, folds
Forearms	Position	
	Musculature	Atrophy, hypertrophy, swelling
Hands	Shape	Swelling
	Musculature	Atrophy, hypertrophy, swelling
	Skin	Color
Fingers	Shape	Arthritic, rheumatic, traumatic abnormalities, hour glass deformity
	Skin	Color

Seated, dorsal

Following inspection in the standing position, the spine is inspected in a sitting position. The purpose of this is to exclude the effects of the lower limbs on the static position of the pelvis and the spinal column. It is important to note whether there are static changes in the spinal column in the frontal plane when compared with the standing position (**Figures 10–7** and **10–8**).

Changes in static position relative to the lower limbs can be caused by the following:

- Anatomic leg length difference
- Unilateral congenital abnormalities

- Unilateral pes varus or valgus
- Unilateral genua valga or vara
- Unilateral abduction or adduction of femur
- Unilateral abnormal rotation position of the femur
- Unilateral shortening of muscles
- Unilateral degenerative disorders of the joints
- Unilateral pain
- Asymmetries resulting from old fractures
- Surgeries

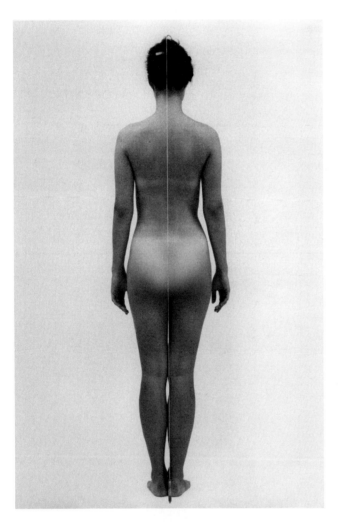

Figure 10–7   Inspection in standing position.

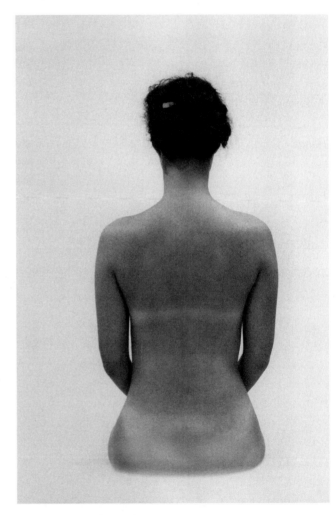

Figure 10–8   Inspection in sitting position.

CHAPTER 11

Palpatory Examination

REGIONS OF THE BODY SURFACE

The regions of the body that are not directly relevant with regard to examination by palpation are listed for information (see **Figure 11–1**).

1. Frontal region
2. Temporal region
3. Parietal region
4. Mastoid region
5. Occipital region
6. Parotid-masseter region
7. Zygomatic region
8. Supraorbital region
9. Orbital region
10. Nasal region
11. Infraorbital region
12. Oral region
13. Mental region
14. Buccal region
15. Midline superior anterior neck region
16. Midline inferior anterior neck region
17. Sternocleidomastoid region
18. Sternal region
19. Lateral anterior neck region
20. Clavicular region
21. Infraclavicular region
22. Nuchal region
23. Deltoid-pectoral trigonum (Mohrenheim fossa)
24. Acromial region
25. Deltoid region

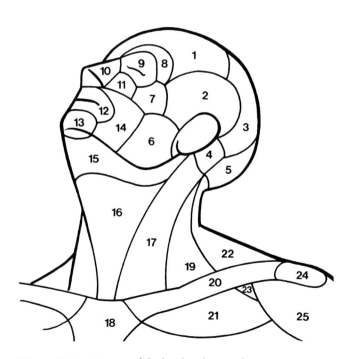

Figure 11–1   Regions of the head and cervical spine.

For the purpose of standardization of techniques, regions of the body that can be the topic of a palpatory examination are illustrated in **Figures 11–2** and **11–3**:

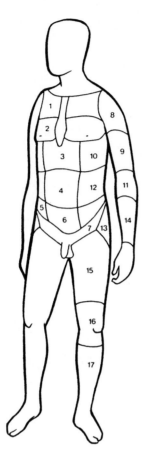

Figure 11–2   Regions of the body surface (ventral).

1. Infraclavicular region
2. Mammary region
3. Epigastric region
4. Umbilical region
5. Iliac fossa
6. Hypogastricum
7. Inguinal region
8. Deltoid region
9. Lateral humerus region
10. Hypochondrium
11. Lateral cubital region
12. Lateral abdominal region
13. Trochanteric region
14. Lateral antebrachial region
15. Anterior femoral region
16. Anterior knee region
17. Anterior crural region

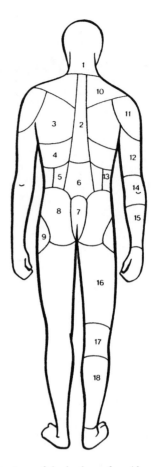

Figure 11–3   Regions of the body surface (dorsal).

1. Nuchal region
2. Superior spinal region
3. Scapular region
4. Infrascapular region
5. Lumbar region
6. Inferior spinal region
7. Sacral region
8. Gluteal region
9. Trochanteric region
10. Suprascapular region
11. Deltoid region
12. Posterior humerus region
13. Lateral region
14. Posterior cubital region
15. Posterior antebrachial region
16. Posterior femoral region
17. Popliteal region
18. Posterior crural region

TOPOGRAPHICAL GUIDE TO PALPATION OF BODY REGIONS

The orthopaedic manual therapist may use the following tables and figures as guides to palpation. (See **Figures 11–4** to **11–7**.)

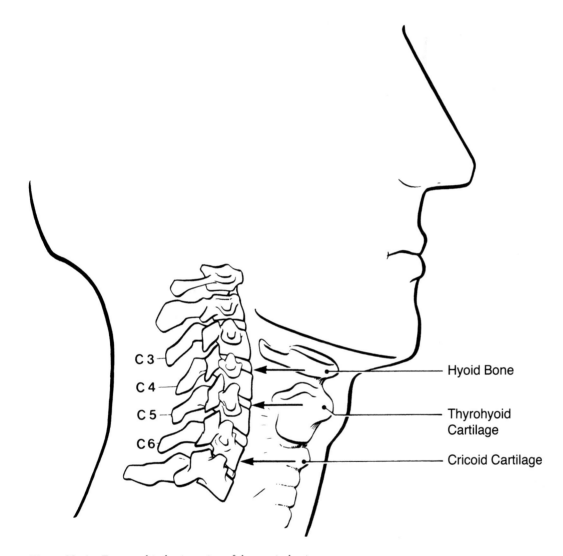

Figure 11–4   Topographical orientation of the cervical spine.

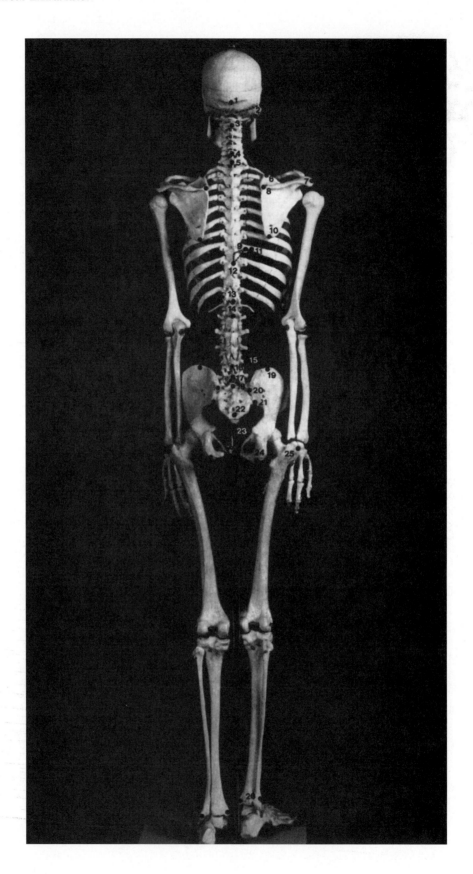

Figure 11-5

Table 11–1   Topographical Guide (Standing Position, Dorsal) **(Figure 11–5)**

Region	Location	Orientation
Head	1. External occipital protuberance	
	2. Mastoid process	Mandible/transverse process C1
	3. Spinous process C2	
Cervical Spine	4. Spinous process C6	
	5. Spinous process C7	Spinous process C6
Shoulder girdle	6. Superior scapular angle	2nd rib
and thoracic	7. Acromion	Acromioclavicular joint
spine	8. Trigonum or base scapular spine	3rd rib
	9. Transverse process T8	Spinous process T8
	10. Inferior scapular angle	7th rib
	11. Rib angle	
	12. Spinous process T8	Transverse process T8
	13. Spinous process T12	
Lumbar spine	14. Spinous process L1	
	15. Transverse process L4	
	16. Spinous process L4	Iliac crest
	17. Spinous process L5	
Pelvis	18. Spinous process S1	Posterior superior iliac spine
	19. Upper iliac crest	
	20. Posterior superior iliac spine	
	21. Posterior inferior iliac spine	
	22. Sacral hiatus	
	23. Coccyx	
	24. Ischial tuberosity	
Lower limb	25. Greater trochanter	
	26. Medial and lateral malleoli	

Haneline et al. (2008) report, based on a retrospective analysis of 50 radiographs, that the mean spinal level corresponding with the left inferior angle of the scapula was midway between the T8–T9 interspace and the upper T9 body (range: lower T7 to upper T10). The right inferior angle was slightly lower, located within the level of the T9 body (range: lower T7–lower T10). Despite considerable variability, most commonly the inferior angles of the scapulae corresponded with the level of the upper body of T9.

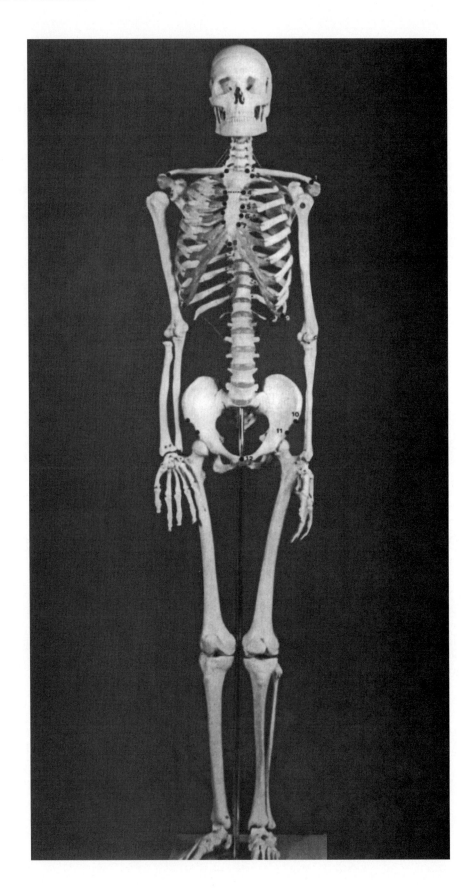

Figure 11–6

Table 11–2   Topographical Guide to Examination (Standing Position, Ventral) **(Figure 11–6)**

Region	Location	Orientation
Shoulder girdle and thoracic spine	1. Acromioclavicular joint	
	2. Sternoclavicular joint	
	3. Costosternal joint 1st rib	Just under sternoclavicular joint
	4. Costosternal joint 2nd rib	Transition between body and manubrium sterni
	5. Costosternal joint 3rd rib	
	6. Costosternal joint 4th rib	Nipple height
	7. Costosternal joint 5th rib	
	8. Xiphoid process	
	9. Lower thoracic aperture	
Pelvis	10. Anterior superior iliac spine	
	11. Anterior inferior iliac spine	
	12. Pubic symphysis	Greater trochanter

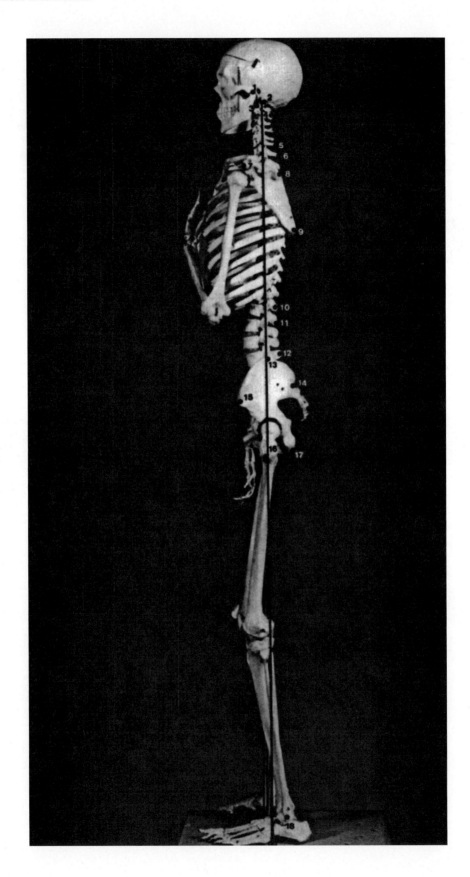

Figure 11–7

Table 11–3   Topographical Guide to Examination (Standing Position, Lateral) **(Figure 11–7)**

Region	Location	Orientation
Head and	1. Temporomandibular joint	External auditory meatus
cervical	2. Mastoid process	
spine	3. Transverse process C1	Mandible/mastoid process
Shoulder girdle	4. Spinous process C2	
and thoracic	5. Spinous process C6	
spine	6. Spinous process C7	Spinous process C6
	7. Acromion	
	8. Scapular spine	
	9. Inferior scapular angle	
	10. Spinous process T12	
Lumbar spine and pelvis	11. Spinous process L 1	
	12. Spinous process L4	Iliac crest
	13. Upper iliac crest	
	14. Superior posterior iliac crest	
	15. Superior anterior iliac crest	
	16. Greater trochanter	Ischial tuberosity
	17. Ischial tuberosity	
	18. Lateral malleolus	Plumb line

SPECIFIC PAIN POINTS

Palpatory examination of specific pain points includes palpation for:

1. Tender points
2. Specific segmental points as described by Sell (1969)
3. Myofascial trigger points as described by Travell and Rinzler (1952)
4. Tendomyoses as described by Dvorak and Dvorak (1983)
5. Nerve pressure points

Tender Points

Figure 11–8 shows tender points in the dorsal lumbopelvic region.

L: Tender points from the lumbar spine

S: Tender points from S1, S2, and the sacroiliac joint

Co: Tender points from sacrococcygeal joint

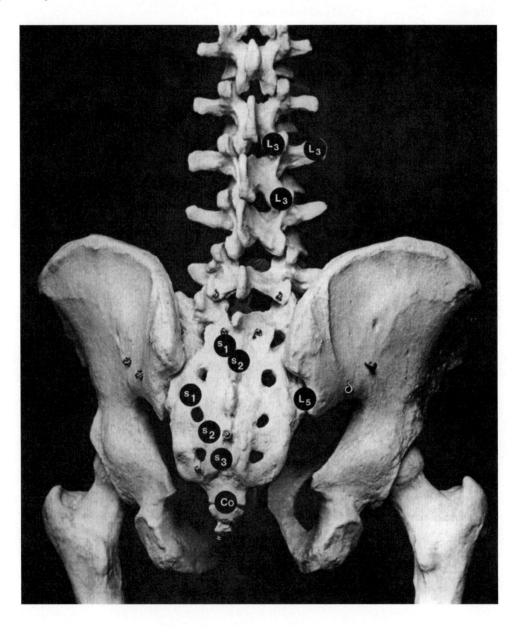

Figure 11–8

In **Figure 11–9**, tender points in the symphyseal and hip region are illustrated:

S: Tender points from the sacroiliac joint

Cx: Tender points from the hip joint

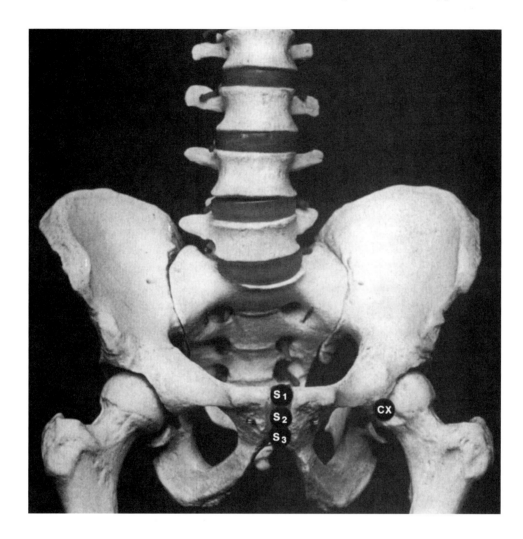

Figure 11–9

In **Figure 11–10** tender points in the dorsal cervicothoracic region are illustrated:

C: Tender points from the cervical spine

T: Tender points from the thoracic spine

CT: Tender points of the costotransverse joints

CO: Tender points of the ribs

L: Tender points from the lumbar spine

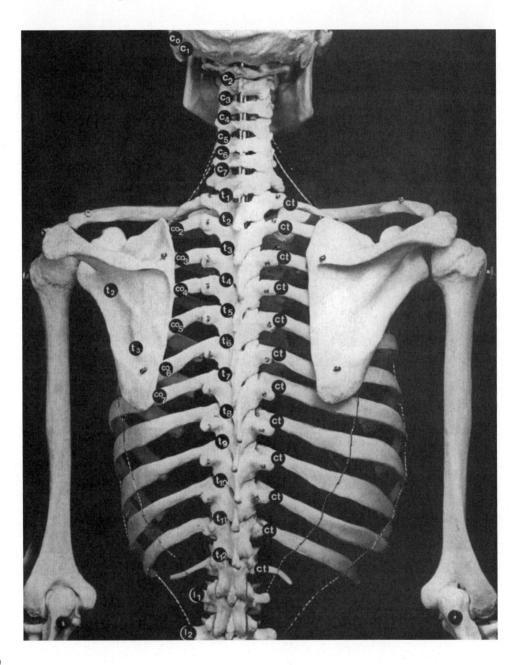

Figure 11–10

In **Figure 11–11** tender points in the ventral cervicothoracic region are illustrated:

AC: Tender points from the acromioclavicular joint

C7: Tender points from segment C7

SC: Tender points from the sternoclavicular joint

T: Tender points from segments T1 to T6

CO: Tender points from the sternocostal joints

Ich: Tender points from the interchondral attachments

Christensen et al. (2003) studied reliability of palpation for pain using a 3-point rating scale of no pain, tenderness, or severe tenderness when palpating the intercostal spaces II/III through VI/VII, that is, locations very similar to the sternocostal tender points noted here. They reported κ values ranging from –0.20 to 0.50 for hour-to-hour intrarater reliability, κ values ranging from –0.20 to 0.53 for day-to-day intrarater reliability, and κ values between 0.19 and 0.46 for interrater agreement.

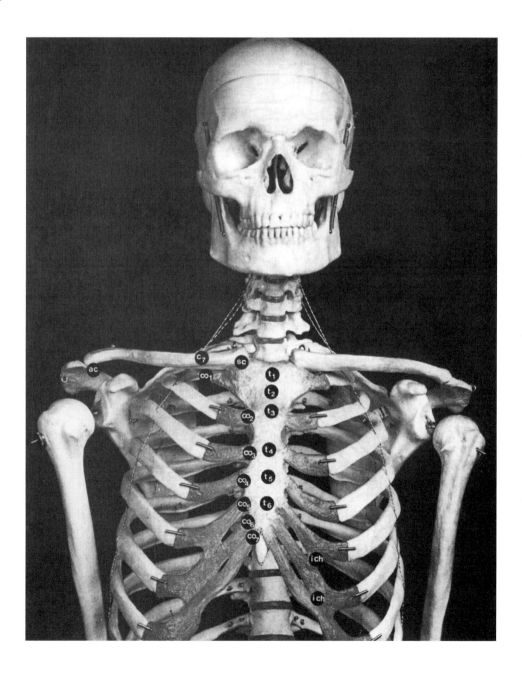

Figure 11–11

Sell's Specific Segmental Points

Sell (1969) described segment-specific pain points that he suggested would be helpful in establishing the level of segmental dysfunction. **Figure 11–12** shows these seg-ment-specific pain points for the cervical spine and **Figure 11–13** shows the pain points proposed to have diagnostic value in determining the level of dysfunction for L1-S1.

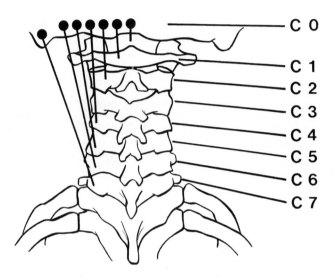

Figure 11–12   Cervical segmental points as described by Sell (1969).

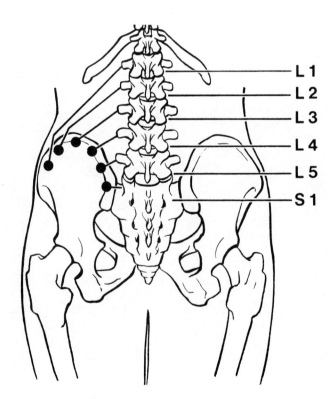

Figure 11–13   Lumbar segmental points as described by Sell (1969).

Myofascial Trigger Points

Travell and Rinzler (1952) established pain patterns indicative of myofascial trigger points in various muscles by way of intramuscular injections in normal subjects. Trigger points and referral zones are depicted in **Figures 11–14**

through **11–50**. The solid circles represent trigger points. Referral zones are darkly or lightly dotted indicating common and less common referral patterns.

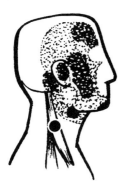

Figure 11–14   Sternocleidomastoid.

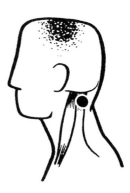

Figure 11–15   Splenius capitis.

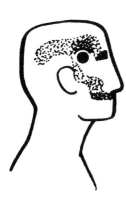

Figure 11–16   Temporalis.

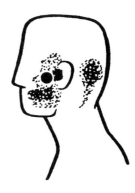

Figure 11–17   Masseter.

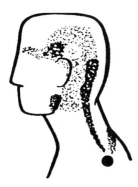

Figure 11–18   Trapezius.

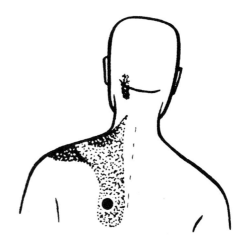

Figure 11–19   Trapezius.

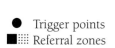
● Trigger points
■ Referral zones

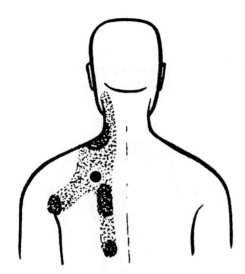

Figure 11–20   Levator scapulae.

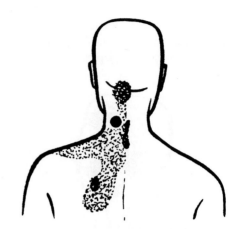

Figure 11–21   Rectus capitus posterior major.

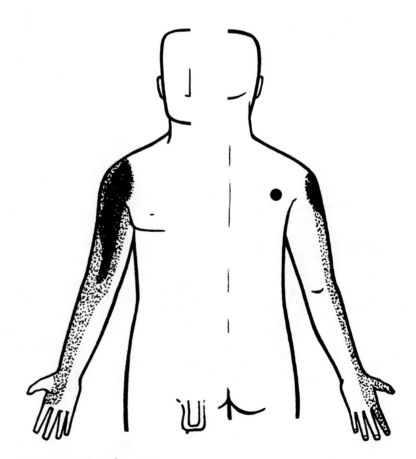

● Trigger points
■::: Referral zones

Figure 11–22   Infraspinatus.

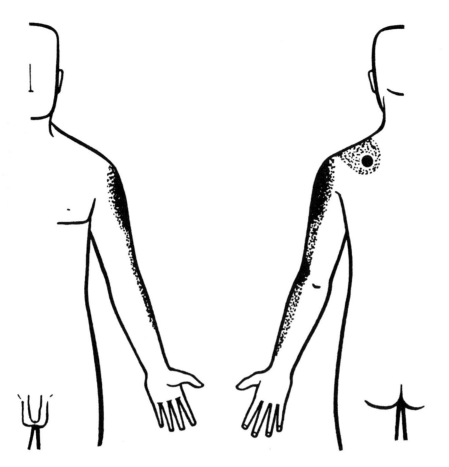

Figure 11–23   Supraspinatus.

●   Trigger points
■⦂⦂⦂ Referral zones

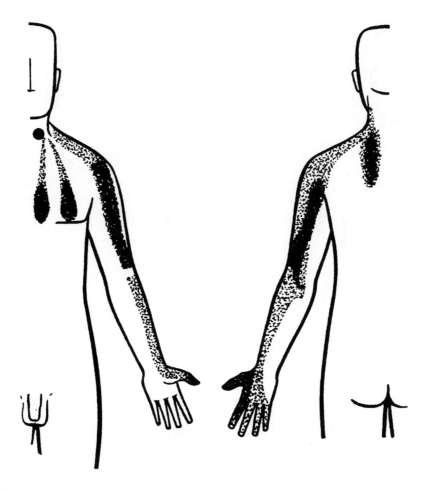

Figure 11–24   Scalenes.

● Trigger points
■∷ Referral zones

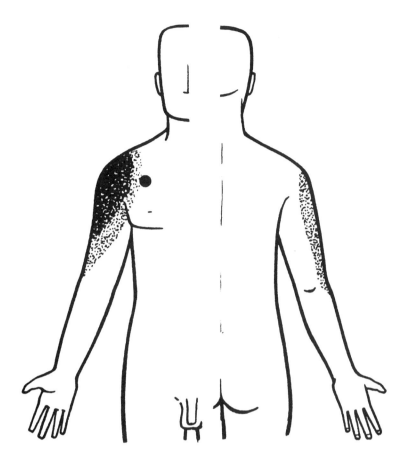

Figure 11–25 Deltoid.

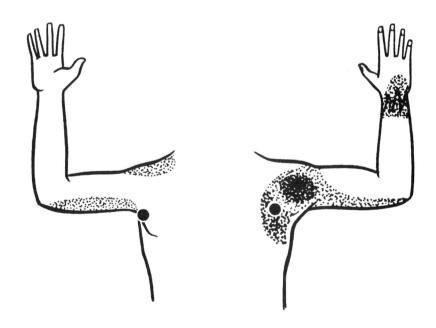

● Trigger points
■░ Referral zones

Figure 11–26 Subscapularis.

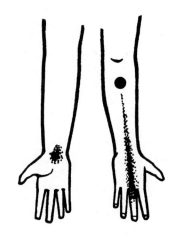

Figure 11–27   Extensor digitorum longus.

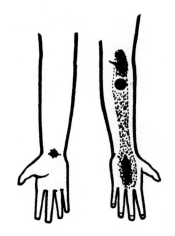

Figure 11–28   Extensor carpi radialis.

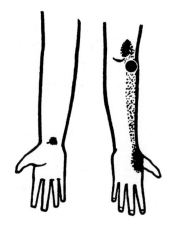

Figure 11–29   Supinator.

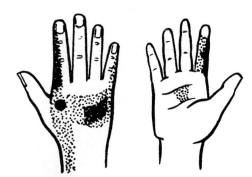

Figure 11–30   Interossei.

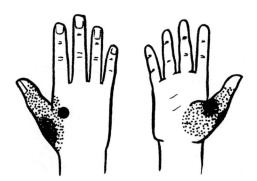

Figure 11–31   Adductor pollicis.

● Trigger points
■ ▦ Referral zones

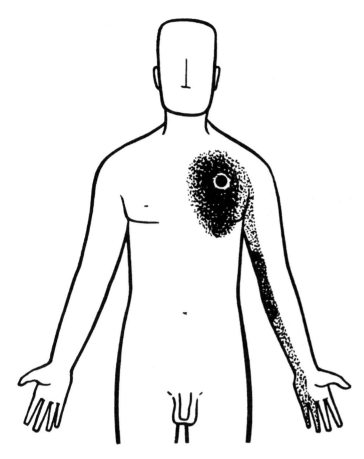

Figure 11–32   Pectorales major and minor.

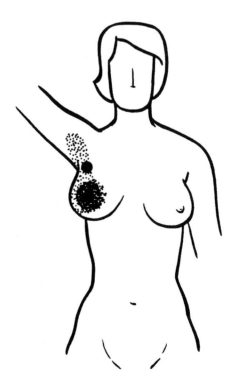

Figure 11–33   Pectorales major.

● Trigger points
■∷ Referral zones

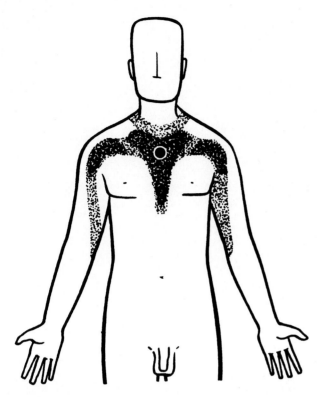

Figure 11–34   Sternalis.

● Trigger points
■∷∷ Referral zones

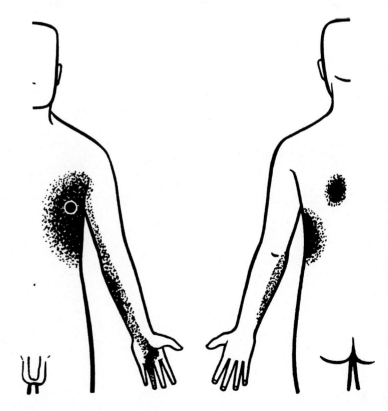

Figure 11–35   Serratus anterior.

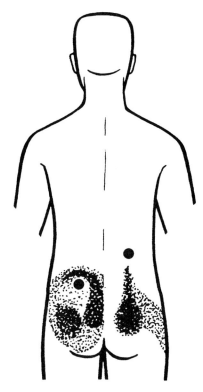

Figure 11–36 Gluteus medius (left side of the body) and iliocostalis (right side of the body).

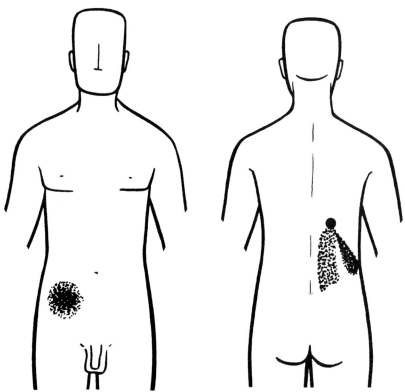

● Trigger points
■∷ Referral zones

Figure 11–37 Iliocostalis.

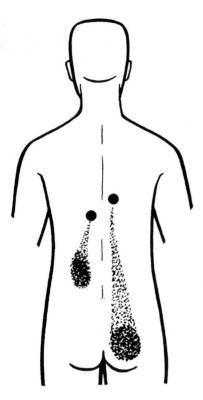

Figure 11–38   Longissimus thoracis.

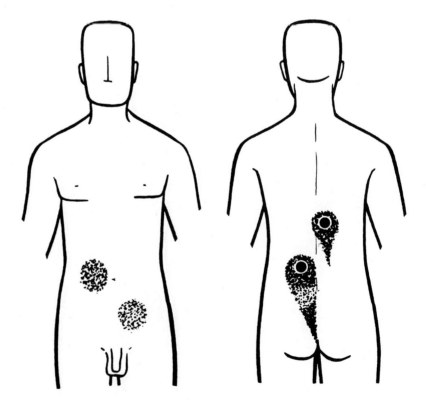

● Trigger points
■▒ Referral zones

Figure 11–39   Multifidi.

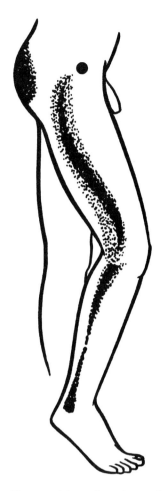

Figure 11–40a   Gluteus minimus (lateral aspect).

Figure 11–40b   Gluteus minimus (dorsal aspect).

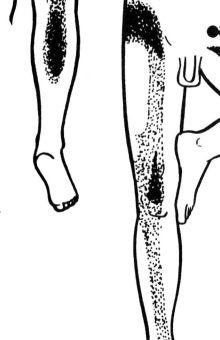

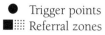
● Trigger points
■⬚ Referral zones

Figure 11–41   Adductor longus.

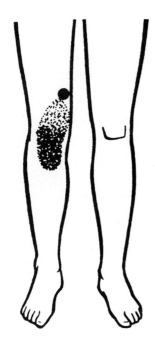

Figure 11–42   Vastus medialis.

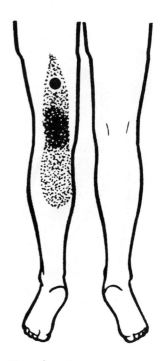

Figure 11–43   Biceps femoris.

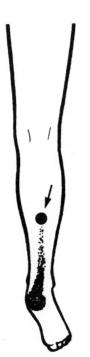

Figure 11–44   Soleus.

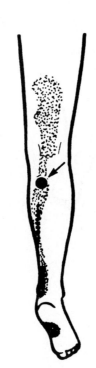

Figure 11–45   Gastrocnemius.

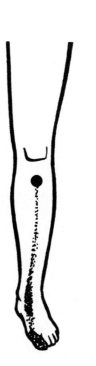

Figure 11–46   Tibialis anterior.

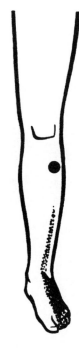

Figure 11–47   Extensor digitorum longus.

● Trigger points
■⠿ Referral zones

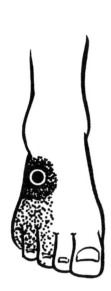

Figure 11–48 Extensor digitorum brevis.

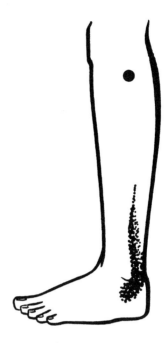

Figure 11–49 Peroneus longus.

● Trigger points
■ Referral zones

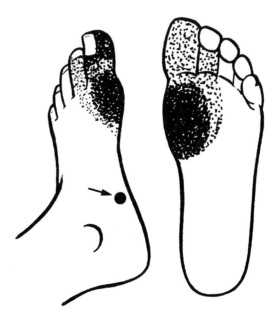

Figure 11–50 Abductor hallucis.

Simons et al. (1999) have expanded on previous clinical operational definitions and proposed essential criteria and confirmatory observations for the diagnosis of myofascial trigger points. Essential criteria include the following:

- Taut band palpable (where muscle is accessible)
- Exquisite spot tenderness of a nodule in a taut band
- Patient recognition of current pain complaint by pressure on the tender nodule (identifies an active trigger point)
- Painful limit to full stretch range of motion

Confirmatory observations are these:

- Visual or tactile identification of a local twitch response
- Imaging of a local twitch response induced by needle penetration of tender nodule
- Pain or altered sensation (in the distribution expected from a trigger point in that muscle) on compression of tender nodule
- Electromyographic demonstration of spontaneous electrical activity characteristic of active loci in the tender nodule of a taut band

Using the preceding diagnostic characteristics, McEvoy and Huijbregts (2008) provide a best evidence synthesis based on their systematic review of the literature with regard to the reliability of manual trigger point palpation and note the following:

- Sufficient intrarater reliability has been established for identification of spot tenderness, taut band, jump sign, and recognized pain, and referred pain for all four rotator cuff muscles and for the local twitch response in the infraspinatus and teres minor.
- Sufficient interrater reliability has been established for identification of local tenderness, taut band, recognized pain, and jump signs for both the gluteus medius and the quadratus lumborum muscles, whereas identification of referred pain has sufficient interrater reliability for the gluteus medius only.
- Sufficient interrater reliability has been established for identification of tenderness in the upper trapezius, infraspinatus, and the axillary portion of the latissimus

dorsi; taut band in the upper trapezius, infraspinatus, the axillary portion of the latissimus dorsi, and extensor digitorum; referred and patient recognized pain, and absence or presence of latent or active trigger points in the sternocleidomastoid, upper trapezius, infraspinatus, the axillary portion of the latissimus dorsi, and extensor digitorum; and local twitch response in the latissimus. Operational definition in this case for an active trigger point includes point tenderness and a taut band with palpation reproducing the patient's recognized pain, whereas a latent trigger point is characterized only by a tender point and taut band.

- If a latent trigger point is defined as needing to have two of the following characteristics present: taut band, nodule, and/or spot tenderness, accuracy of trigger point location in the upper trapezius is highly reliable between raters.
- If the criteria for trigger point presence include 1. a nodule in a taut band, 2. referred pain, 3. local twitch response, and 4. a jump sign, trigger point identification in the posterior deltoid, biceps brachii, and infraspinatus is highly reliable between raters. Identification of referred pain and the jump sign are the most reliable individual diagnostic characteristics in these muscles.

McEvoy and Huijbregts (2008) note as a caveat with these findings that reliability seems dependent on a high level of rater expertise, intensive training and consensus discussion on technique and operational definitions, and possibly higher levels of patient-reported pain.

Tendomyoses

Following are dorsal lumbopelvic region tendomyoses and their proposed segmental relationships (based on Dvorak and Dvorak, 1983; see **Figure 11–51**):

LL: Longissimus, parslumborum
GMA1: Gluteus maximus
GMA2: Gluteus maximus
GMA3: Gluteus maximus
GMA4: Gluteus maximus
GME: Gluteus medius

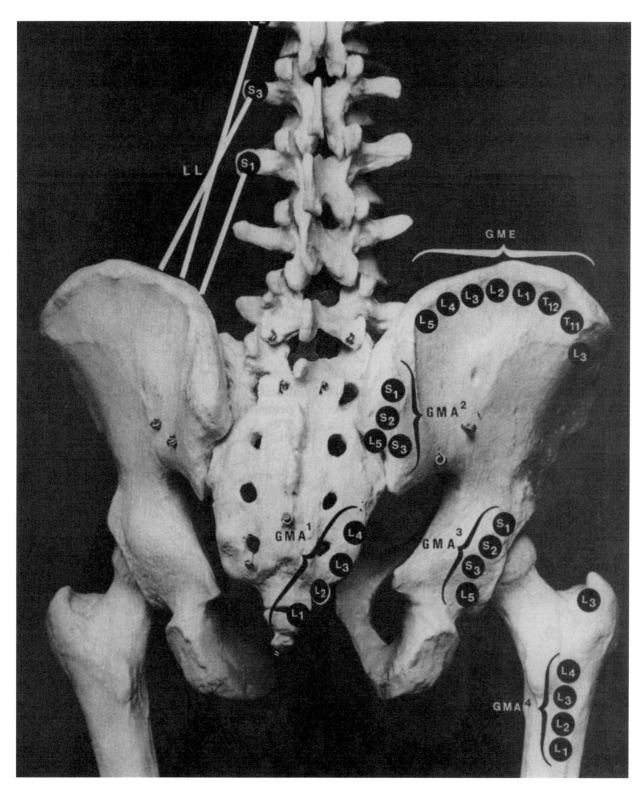

Figure 11–51

Following are ventral lumbopelvic region tendomyoses and their segmental relationships (**Figure 11–52**):

LL: Longissimus, pars lumborum

IL: Iliacus

SA: Sartorius

RE: Rectus femoris

GME: Gluteus medius

GMI: Gluteus minimus

QF: Quadratus femoris

AMA: Adductor magnus

ALO: Adductor longus

PE: Pectineus

PI: Pyramidalis

RA: Rectus abdominis

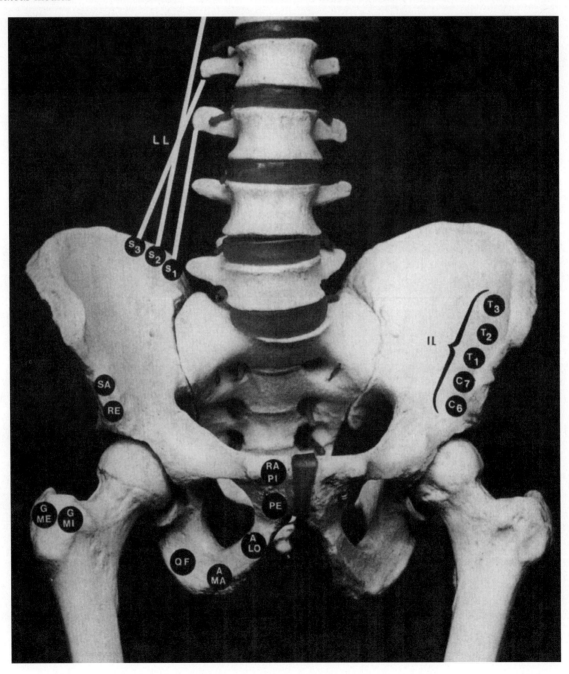

Figure 11–52

Following are the more common ventral thoracic origin and insertion tendinopathies (**Figure 11–53**):

PM: Pectoralis major

PMI: Pectoralis minor

STC: Sternocleidomastoid

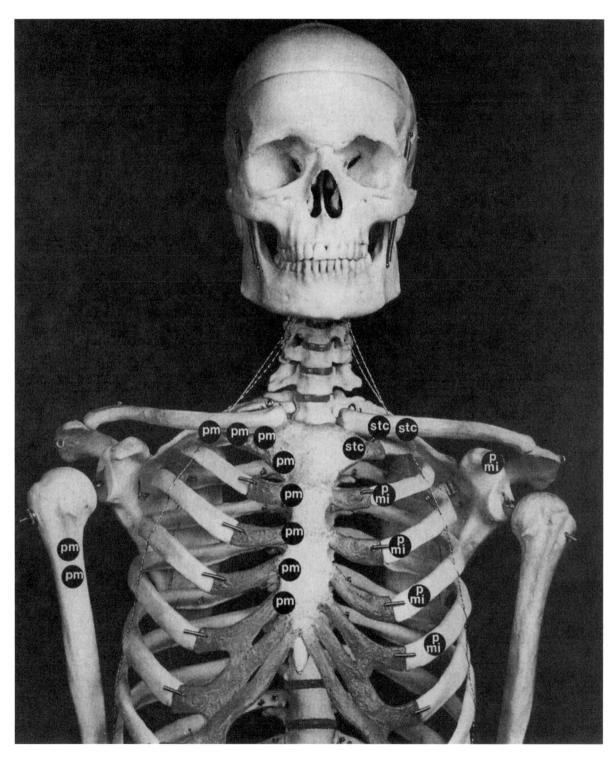

Figure 11–53

Following are the more common lumbar origin and insertion tendinopathies (**Figure 11–54**):

R: Rotatores
M: Multifidi

IS: Interspinales
LD: Latissimus dorsi
LT: Thoracis
QL: Quadratus lumborum

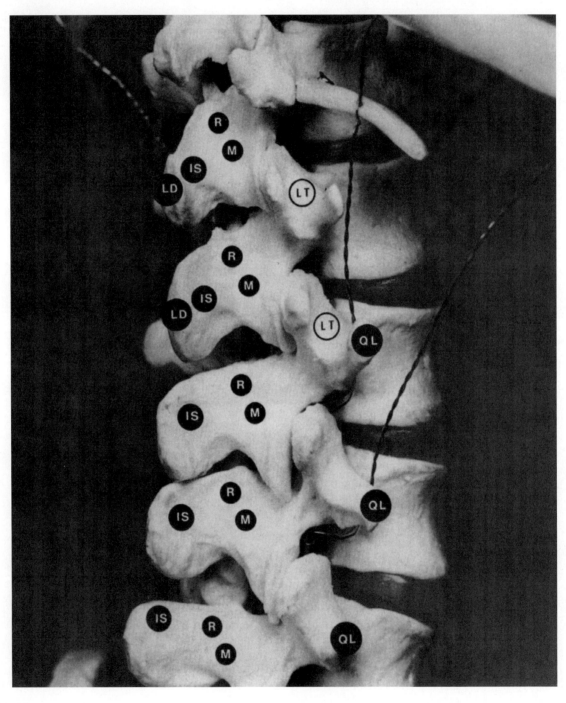

Figure 11–54

Following are common cervical origin and insertion tendinopathies (**Figure 11–55**):

1: Rectus capitis minor

2: Rectus capitis major

3: Obliquus capitis superior

4: Obliquus capitis inferior

R:Rotatores

IS: Interspinales

LC: Longissimi capitis

SC: Semispinalis capitis

I: Intertransversarii

T: Trapezius

RH: Rhomboid

M: Multifidi

LT: Longissimi thoracis

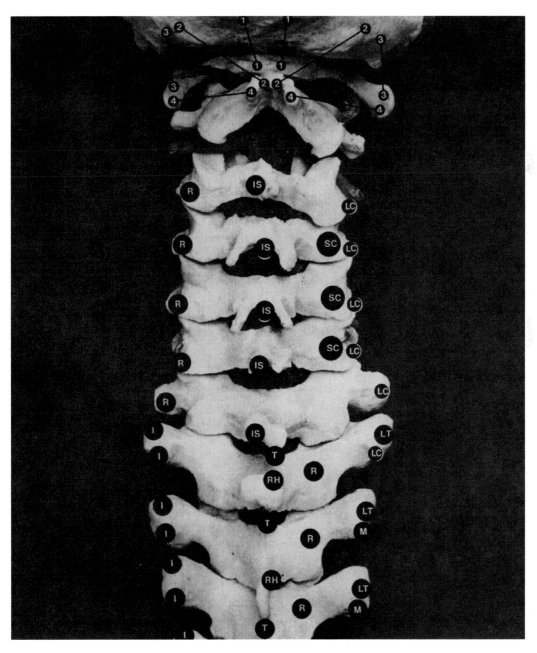

Figure 11–55

Following are additional cervical origin and insertion tendinopathies (**Figure 11–56**):

IS: Interspinales

R: Rotatores

SC: Semispinalis

IT: Intertransversarii

RH: Rhomboid

T: Trapezius

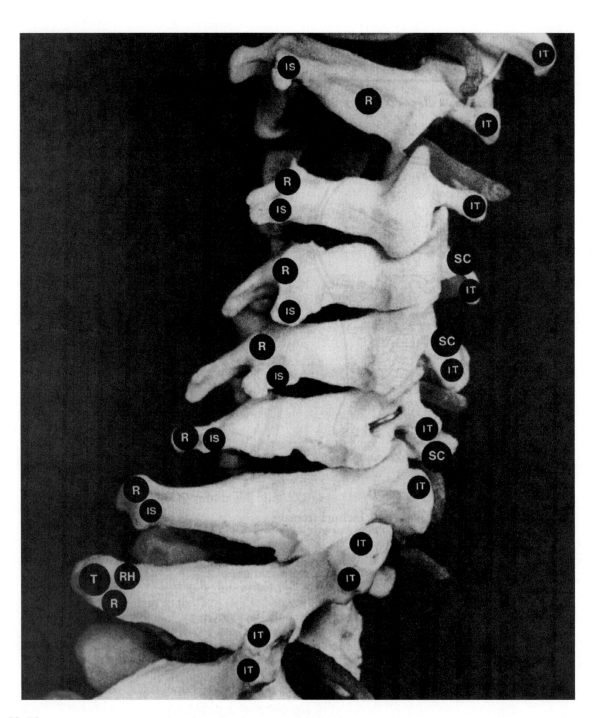

Figure 11–56

Nerve Pressure Points

Nerve pressure points of the head and cervical spine (**Figure 11–57**) are presented in **Table 11–4**.

Table 11–4   Nerve Pressure Points of the Head and Cervical Spine

Region/Nerves	Location of Pressure Point	Examination Position

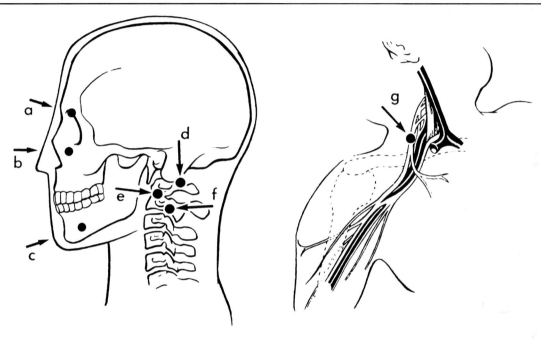

Figure 11–57   Nerve pressure points of head and cervical spine.

Region/Nerves	Location of Pressure Point	Examination Position
Trigeminal nerve: VI Supraorbital nerve	a. Incisura frontalis	Seated or supine
Trigeminal nerve: V2 Infraorbital nerve	b Foramen infraorbitale	Seated or supine
Trigeminal nerve: V3 Mentalis nerve	c. Foramen mentale	Seated or supine
Minor occipital nerve (C2–C3)	d. Between mastoid process and posterior arch C1	Seated or supine
Major occipital nerve (C2)	e Lateral to atlantoaxial joint	Seated or supine
Greater auricular nerve Posterior ramus (C2–C3)	f. Lateral to 2nd and 3rd intervertebral joints	Seated or supine
Brachial plexus (C4 to T1)	g. Between trapezius and m. Sternocleidomastoid muscles above clavicle (Erb's point)	Seated or supine

Nerve pressure points of the arm (**Figure 11–58**) are presented in **Table 11–5**.

Table 11–5   Nerve Pressure Points of the Arm

Region/Nerves	*Location of Pressure Point*	*Examination Position*

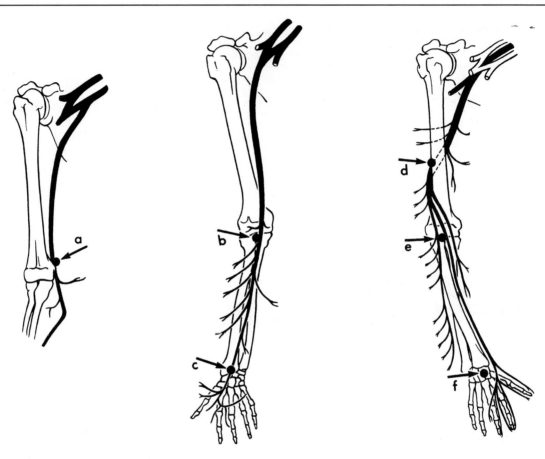

Figure 11–58   Nerve pressure points of the arm.

Region/Nerves	Location of Pressure Point	Examination Position
Ulnar nerve (C8–T1)	a. Between olecranon and medial epicondyle	Seated or supine
Median nerve (C5 to T1)	b. Ventral to elbow joint, lateral to to the tendon of biceps brachii	Seated or supine
	c. Flexor retinaculum	
Radial nerve (C5 to T1)	d. Middle of lateral aspect of upper arm	Seated or supine
	e. Medial to radial head	
	f. Intermetacarpal II and III	

Nerve pressure points of the thoracic spine (**Figure 11–59**) are presented in **Table 11–6**.

Table 11–6 Nerve Pressure Points of the Thoracic Spine

Region/Nerves	*Location of Pressure Point*	*Examination Position*

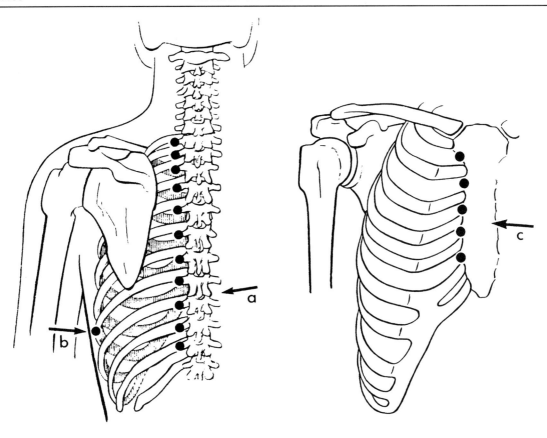

Figure 11–59 Nerve pressure points of the thoracic spine.

| Intercostal nerves (T1 to T11) | a. Directly caudal to costovertebral joint
b. Lateral and central, directly caudal to the rib
c. Lateral to the sternum | Seated or prone

Seated or supine |

Nerve pressure points of the lumbar spine, pelvis, and upper leg (**Figure 11–60**) are presented in **Table 11–7**.

Table 11–7   Nerve Pressure Points of the Lumbar Spine, Pelvis, and Upper Leg

Region/Nerves	Location of Pressure Point	Examination Position

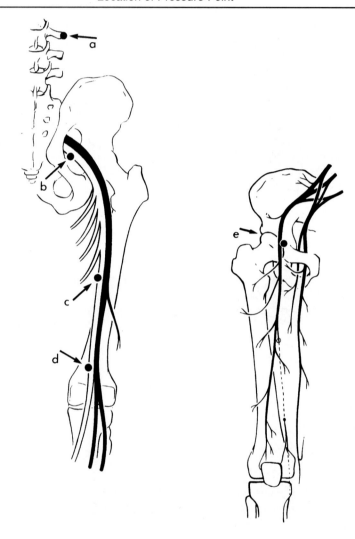

Figure 11–60   Nerve pressure points of the lumbar spine, pelvis, and upper leg.

Region/Nerves	Location of Pressure Point	Examination Position
Sciatic nerve (L4 to S1)	a. Transverse process L3 b. Caudal edge of sciatic foramen c. Middle of dorsal aspect of thigh d. Cranial to middle of popliteal fossa	Prone
Femoral nerve	e. Medial to hip joint	Supine

Nerve pressure points of the lower leg and foot (**Figure 11–61**) are presented in **Table 11–8**.

Table 11–8 Nerve Pressure Points of the Lower Leg and Foot

Region/Nerves	Location of Pressure Point	Examination Position
	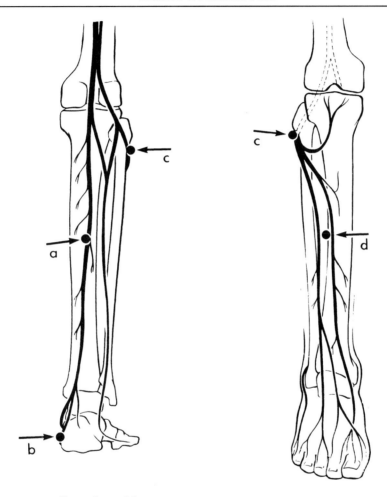	

Figure 11–61 Nerve pressure points of lower leg and foot.

Region/Nerves	Location of Pressure Point	Examination Position
Tibial nerve (L4 to S1)	a. Middle of dorsal aspect of lower leg	Seated or prone
	b. Medial aspect of calcaneus	
Common peroneal nerve (L4 to S2)	c. Dorsal to head of fibula	Seated or supine
Deep peroneal nerve (L4 to S2)	d. Middle of muscle belly tibialis anterior	Seated or supine

Using a 4-point tenderness rating scale from 0 (normal) to 4 (marked mechanical allodynia), Jepsen et al. (2006) report interrater reliability for palpation for nerve mechanosensitivity. Palpation of the brachial plexus at the upper trunk level in the scalene triangle yielded a κ value (95% CI) of 0.48 (0.27–0.70), and at the cord level infraclavicular behind the pectoralis minor muscle this was 0.63 (0.47–0.8). Palpation of the suprascapular nerve in the suprascapular notch yielded κ = 0.29 (0.1–0.48), and of the axillary nerve in the quadrilateral space, 0.52 (0.34–0.7). Palpation of the musculocutaneous in the coracobrachialis muscle, the radial nerve in the triceps or brachioradialis arcades, and the posterior interosseus at the supinator tunnel yielded κ values of 0.56 (0.37–0.75); 0.54 (0.37–0.71); and 0.41 (0.22–0.60). The median nerve palpated at the elbow yielded a κ = 0.54 (0.32–0.77), and at the carpal tunnel κ = 0.47 (0.1–0.83). Palpation of the ulnar nerve at the elbow produced a κ value of 0.69 (0.4–0.98).

CHAPTER 12

Active Examination

GRAPHIC REPRESENTATION OF MOVEMENT IMPULSE OR MOVEMENT DIRECTION

Notations or graphic representations can be used as a shorthand for movement directions or impulse imparted during examination and treatment, thereby cutting down on time required for documentation and communication with other orthopaedic manual therapy colleagues. Used throughout the remainder of this book, this shorthand notation is introduced here in **Figure 12–1**.

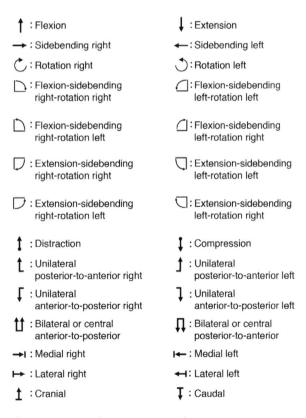

↑ : Flexion
→ : Sidebending right
↻ : Rotation right
⊐ : Flexion-sidebending right-rotation right
⊐ : Flexion-sidebending right-rotation left
⊐ : Extension-sidebending right-rotation right
⊐ : Extension-sidebending right-rotation left
↑ : Distraction
↑ : Unilateral posterior-to-anterior right
↓ : Unilateral anterior-to-posterior right
↑↑ : Bilateral or central anterior-to-posterior
→| : Medial right
↦ : Lateral right
↑ : Cranial

↓ : Extension
← : Sidebending left
↺ : Rotation left
⊏ : Flexion-sidebending left-rotation left
⊏ : Flexion-sidebending left-rotation right
⊏ : Extension-sidebending left-rotation left
⊏ : Extension-sidebending left-rotation right
↓ : Compression
↑ : Unilateral posterior-to-anterior left
↓ : Unilateral anterior-to-posterior left
↓↓ : Bilateral or central posterior-to-anterior
|← : Medial left
↤ : Lateral left
↓ : Caudal

Figure 12–1   Graphic representation of movement impulse or movement direction.

ACTIVE EXAMINATION

For the purpose of the active examination, the spine is divided into two regions, namely, the lumbar–thoracic spine and the upper-thoracic and cervical spine. Initially, the movements are performed freely, i.e., without specific instructions to the patient as to performance of these movements. If specific movement instructions are required to gain or confirm information, this can be done as a second stage.

The criteria used during the active examination are the following:

- Willingness to perform the movement
- Movement path; locations where deviation or torsion occurs
- Rhythm of movement; locations where the rhythm (or smooth movement performance) is disturbed

- Active instability and its location
- Compensatory movements in peripheral joints
- Preferred movements
- Preferred pivotal points
- Pain: location, nature, moment of onset, increase, or decrease
- Referred sensations
- Noises, such as crepitation and clicking

Active Examination: Lumbar/Thoracic

Active examination of the lumbar and thoracic spine is done in both standing (depicted in **Figures 12–2 through 12–13**) and in sitting (as shown in **Figures 12–14 through 12–25**). The only cardinal plane motions examined are flexion and extension; all other motions look at three-dimensional movement combinations.

Standing

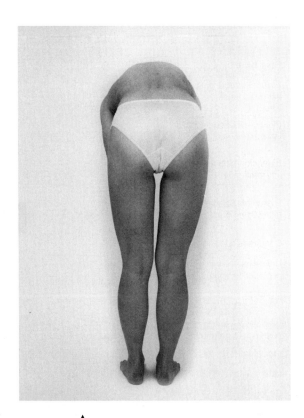

Figure 12–2 ↑

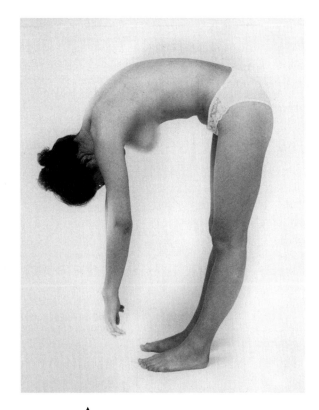

Figure 12–3 ↑

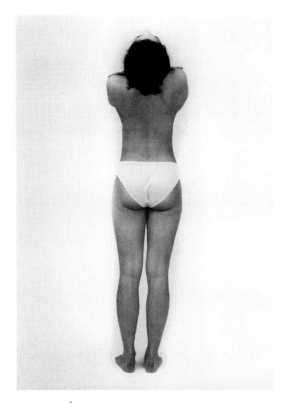

Figure 12–4   ↓

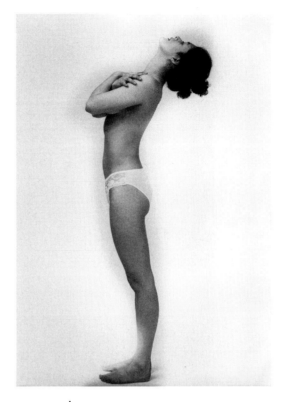

Figure 12–5   ↓

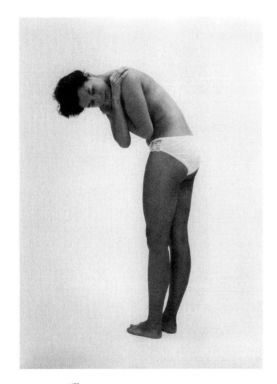

Figure 12–6

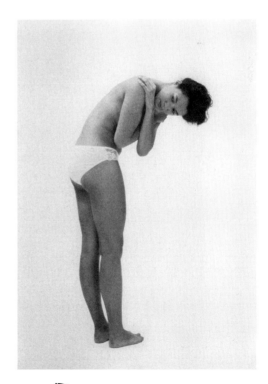

Figure 12–7

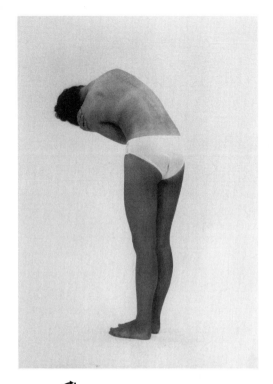

Figure 12–8

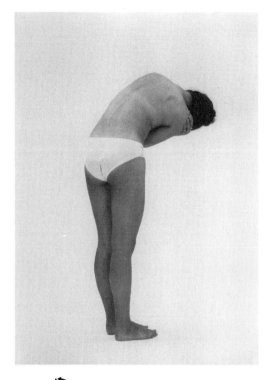

Figure 12–9

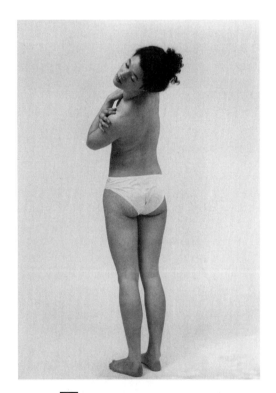

Figure 12–10

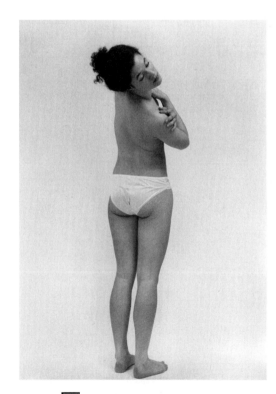

Figure 12–11

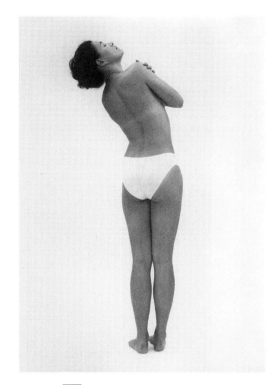

Figure 12–12

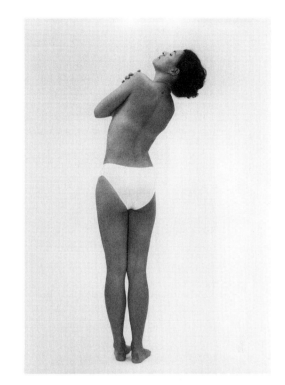

Figure 12–13

Sitting

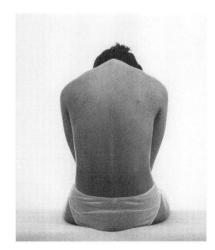

Figure 12–14

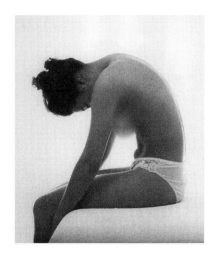

Figure 12–15

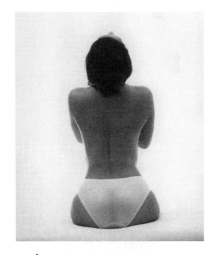

Figure 12–16 ↓

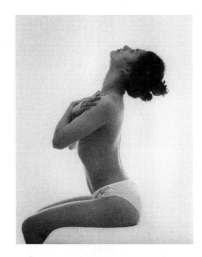

Figure 12–17 ↓

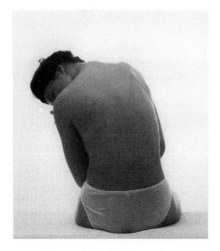

Figure 12–18

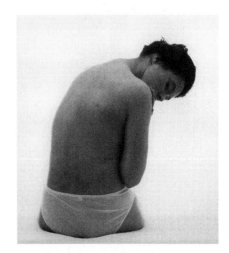

Figure 12–19

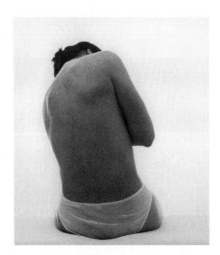

Figure 12–20

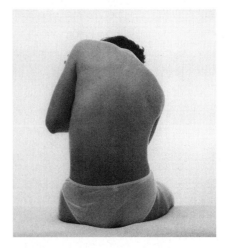

Figure 12–21

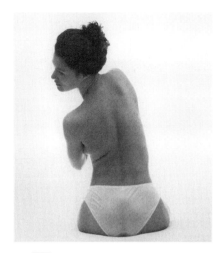

Figure 12–22

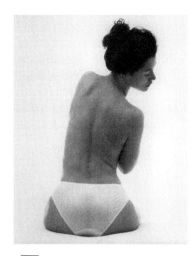

Figure 12–23

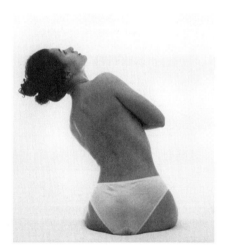

Figure 12–24

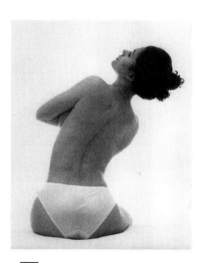

Figure 12–25

Fritz et al. (2005b) established interrater reliability for mobility of lumbar flexion and end extension active range of motion assessment. Flexion yielded an ICC of 0.60 (95% CI: 0.33–0.69); extension yielded an ICC of 0.61 (95% CI: 0.37–0.78). Cleland (2005) provides further interrater reliability data on instrumental range of motion assessment for the thoracolumbar spine. Peret et al. (2001) report ICC = 0.99 for intra- and interrater agreement of the fingertip-to-floor test, where the distance between the floor and the fin-

gertips is measured with a tape measure; correlation with radiographs was high ($r = 0.96$) and responsiveness with a standardized mean response of 0.97 and effect size of 0.87 was noted to be excellent. Haswell et al. (2004) report interrater reliability data for symptom provoking active range of motion assessment of the lumbar spine. Sidebending yielded 81.4% agreement and a κ value of 0.60 (95% CI: 0.40–0.79). Rotation showed 70% agreement with a κ value of 0.17 (95% CI: –0.08–0.42). Sidebending–rotation yielded 64.3% with κ = 0.29 (95% CI: 0.06–0.51), flexion–sidebending–rotation 70% and κ = 0.39 (95% CI: 0.18–0.61), and extension–sidebending–rotation 67.1% and a κ = 0.29 (95% CI: 0.06–0.52). Cleland et al. (2006) established interrater reliability for symptom provocation with seated thoracic rotation testing: 14% agreement for right rotation (κ = −0.03, 95% CI: −0.11–0.04) and 86% agreement for left rotation (κ = 0.7, 95% CI: 0.4–1.0).

Active Examination: Cervicothoracic/Cervical

Active examination of the cervico-thoracic and cervical spine is done in sitting (as shown in **Figures 12–26 through 12–37**). The only cardinal plane motions examined are flexion and extension; all other motions look at three-dimensional movement combinations.

Sitting

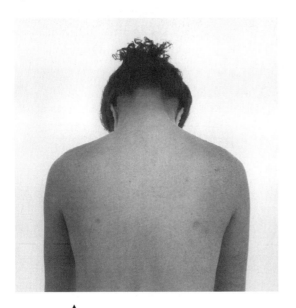

Figure 12–26   ↑

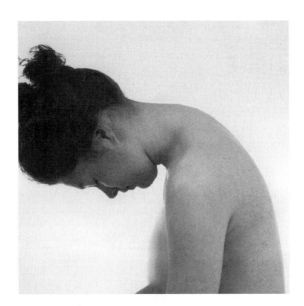

Figure 12–27   ↑

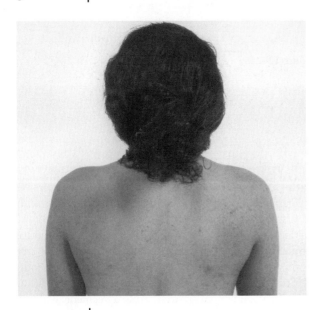

Figure 12–28   ↓

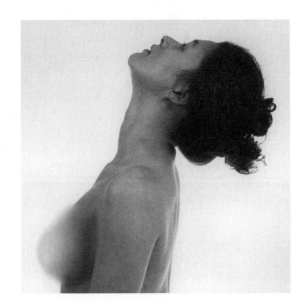

Figure 12–29   ↓

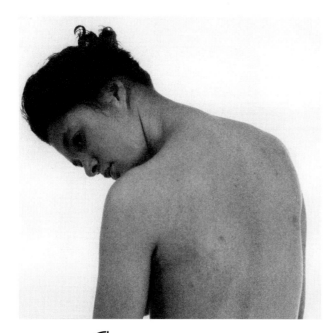

Figure 12–30

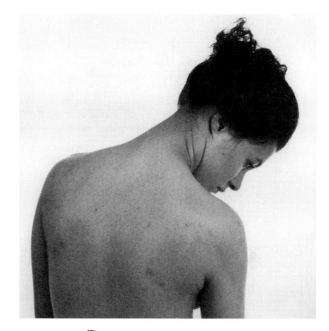

Figure 12–31

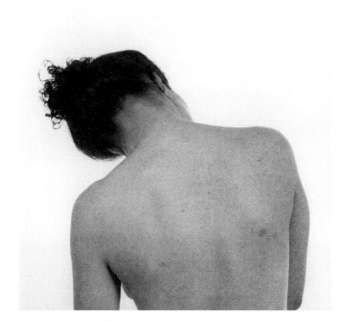

Figure 12–32

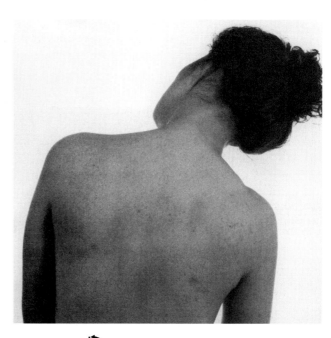

Figure 12–33

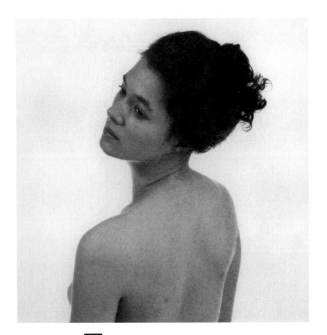

Figure 12–34

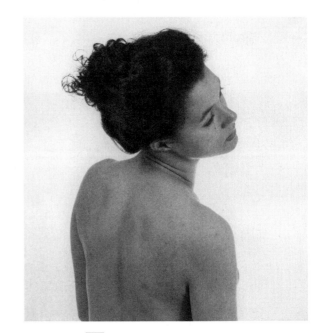

Figure 12–35

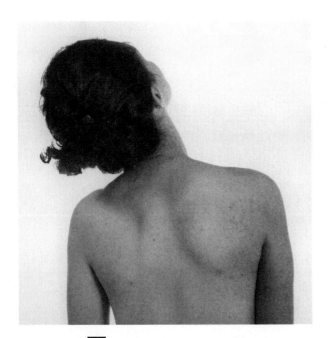

Figure 12–36

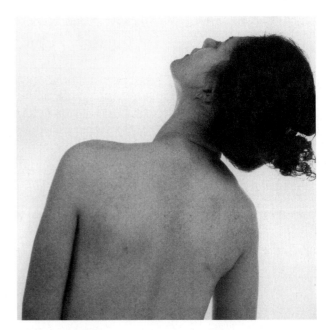

Figure 12–37

Table 12–1 Reliability and responsiveness of visual estimation of cervical active range of motion tests

	ICC	SD	SEM	MDC_{95}
Flexion	0.42	10	7.60	21.1
Left rotation	0.69	13	7.28	20.2
Right rotation	0.82	15	6.30	17.5
Left sidebending	0.63	9	5.49	15.2
Right sidebending	0.70	10	5.50	15.2

ICC = Intraclass correlation coefficient; SD = Standard deviation; SEM = Standard error of measurement; MDC_{95} = Minimal detectable change at 95% confidence

Youdas et al. (1991) provide reliability data on active cervical range of motion assessment using two instrumental methods and visual assessment. Graziano et al. (2007) used the formulas discussed in Chapter 5 and calculated responsiveness data for the commonly used method of visual motion assessment for the cervical spine. Data on reliability and responsiveness are provided in **Table 12–1**.

Pool et al. (2004) provide interrater agreement data on the active cervical examination using visual assessment and a dichotomous rating scale of normal or limited: interrater agreement on cervical flexion was 71% (κ = 0.19), on extension 71% (κ = 0.39), and on extension–sidebending–ipsilateral rotation 55% right (κ = 0.15) and left 81% (κ = 0.61).

Active Examination: Upper Cervical

The upper cervical spine is specifically evaluated separate from the rest of the cervical spine. Again, forward and backward nodding (flexion and extension, respectively) are the only cardinal plane motions assessed (**Figures 12–38 and 12–39**) with all other active motions consisting of three-dimensional movement combinations (**Figures 12–40 through 12–47**).

Sitting

Pool et al. (2004) provide reliability data on the active upper cervical examination using visual assessment and a dichotomous rating scale of normal or limited: interrater agreement for upper cervical flexion was 97% and for upper cervical extension 79%.

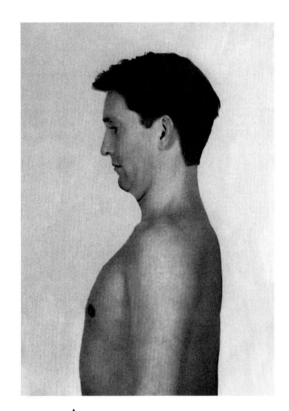

Figure 12–38 ↑

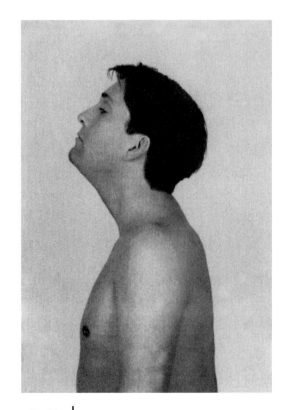

Figure 12–39 ↓

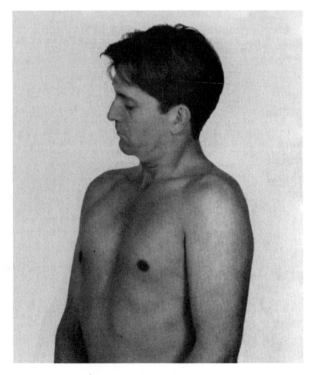

Figure 12–40

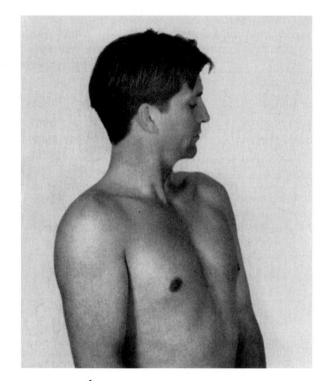

Figure 12–41

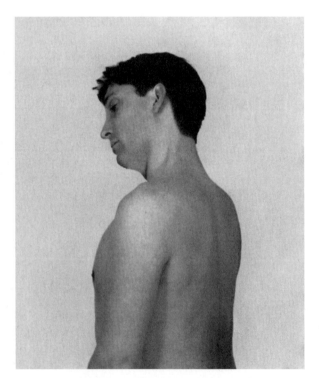

Figure 12–42

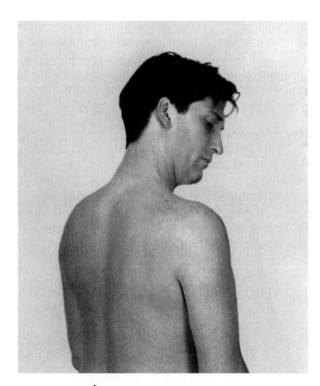

Figure 12–43

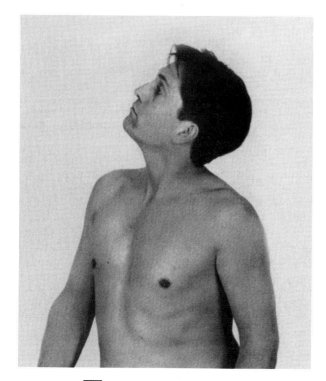

Figure 12–44

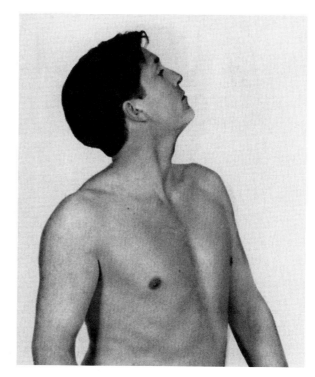

Figure 12–45

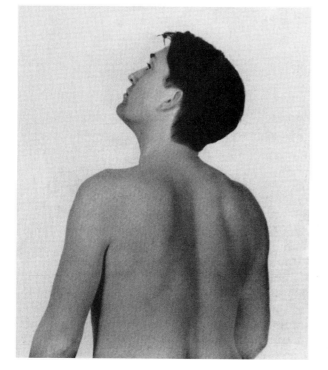

Figure 12–46

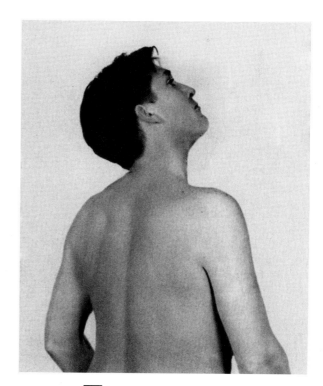

Figure 12–47

CHAPTER 13

Examination of the Pelvic Region

PELVIS

Functional Aspects of the Pelvis

The pelvis forms the connection between the spinal column and the lower extremities. It functions as a springlike base that receives the forces from the spine and transmits them to the lower extremities, and vice versa. The interplay of the forces exerted by the spine and lower limbs activates the self-locking system in the pelvis (**Figure 13–1**).

The force that the spine exerts on the sacrum creates a caudoventral movement impulse. The force exerted by the

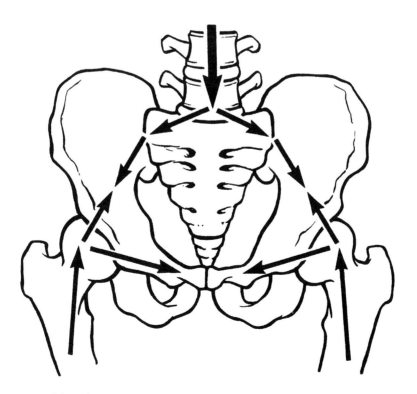

Figure 13–1 Self-locking system of the pelvis.

legs on the two innominate bones causes a craniodorsal movement impulse. The axis of these two opposing movements in the sacroiliac joint is at the level of S2.

The opposing forces exerted on the sacrum and the two innominate bones are curbed in the neighboring joints by the ligamentous structures, which include the iliolumbar ligaments, the superficial and deep dorsal sacral ligaments, the ventral iliosacral ligaments, and the sacrospinous and sacrotuberous ligaments. According to Cramer (1958) and Weisl (1955), the more cranially situated ligaments inhibit the ventrally directed component of sacral movement.

Because the sacroiliac joint surfaces diverge ventrally, the two innominate bones are pushed away from each other dorsally when functional tension of the dorsal ligaments is normal. This causes compression of the ventral pubic symphysis.

If the dorsal ligaments are too lax, the sacrum is displaced in a ventrocaudal direction relative to the two innominate bones, which move closer together dorsally because of the ventral divergence of the joint surfaces. This can change the compression in the symphyseal joint into tension, which in serious cases can cause the ligamentous structures of this joint to tear (**Figure 13–2**).

There are periods when functional laxity is a necessity, for example, during the descending and expelling stages of childbirth, when first the pelvic entrance and then the pelvic exit need to enlarge. Enlargement of the pelvic entrance is achieved through extension of the spine, during which the sacrum flexes ventrally relative to L5 and moves dorsally relative to the two innominate bones. This causes

an increase in the length of the true conjugate and a decrease in the sagittal diameter. The two innominate bones move away from each other at the top and toward each other at the bottom. This causes the pelvic entrance to enlarge and the exit to become smaller.

The pelvic exit becomes larger during flexion of the spine, in which the sacrum bends in a dorsal direction relative to L5 and moves in a ventral direction relative to the two innominate bones. This causes a decrease in the true conjugate and a decrease in the sagittal diameter. The two innominate bones are pushed closer together at the top and away from each other at the bottom. This causes the pelvic entrance to become smaller and the exit to become larger.

These two movements have been described by Zaglas and Duncan (Kapandji, 1974). The movement during which the true conjugate loses about 6 mm in length and the sagittal diameter gains about 15 mm is called nutation ("nodding"). The movement during which the true conjugate increases in length and the sagittal diameter decreases is called counternutation (**Figure 13–3**).

Research by Faraboef (Kapandji, 1974) indicates that nutation and counternutation take place around a turning point at the level of S2. Faraboef discovered a bow-shaped crest on the irregular cartilaginous joint surface of the ilium; the midpoint of the crest was situated at the level of the sacral tuberosity of S2 (**Figure 13–4A**).

On the joint surface of the sacrum he discovered two bow-shaped crests, the midpoints of which lay at the level of the transverse tuberosity of S2. The crest on the joint surface of the ilium was thought to work like a tram rail in the channel formed by the two crests on the sacral joint surfaces. The common turning point was located in the axial ligaments at the level of S2. However, an examination of three sections through the sacroiliac joint did not reveal such a structure in its entirety (Kapandji, 1974).

Bonnaire (Kapandji, 1974) developed a theory according to which a tubercle located on the iliac joint surface between the upper and lower poles or aspects of the joint (Bonnaire's tubercle) is the turning point of the sacroiliac joint (**Figure 13–4B**). Weisl (1954) proposed two theories, the first of which is based on linear displacement in the lower pole, which would allow the sacrum to move in a cranioventral direction (**Figure 13–4C**). The second theory is based on a rotational movement having its center of rotation ventral to the sacrum (**Figure 13–4D**). Van der Bijl Sr. (1969) proposed a theory based on the possibility that both the upper and the lower poles of the sacroiliac joint are capable of linear displacement.

Marsman (1981) maintains that there are two axes of rotation, located in the separate joints; this view is based on the divergence of the joint surfaces. The axes of rotation of the sacroiliac and hip joints, like the median, are all di-

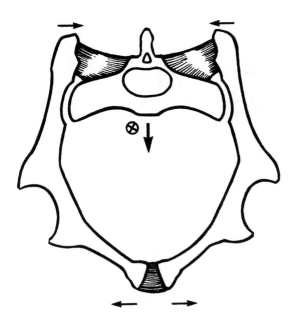

Figure 13–2   Laxity of the dorsal ligaments of the pelvis.

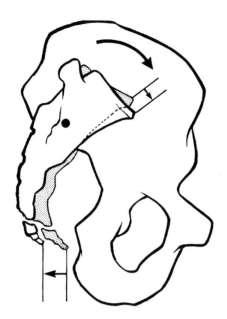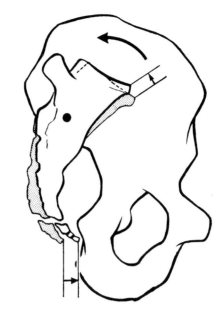

Figure 13–3 Nutation–counternutation.

rected toward the body's center of gravity, which lies about 2 cm in front of S2. The possibility of two axes of rotation implies the existence of a third axis to prevent rotation of the sacrum relative to the two innominate bones in the sagittal plane.

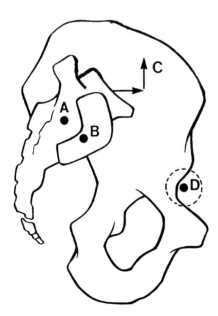

Figure 13–4 Axis of rotation of the sacroiliac joint (Faraboef, Bonnaire, and Weisl) and the linear displacement in the lower pole (Weisl).

Of the many theories about the movement mechanism of the sacroiliac joint, the one based on nutation and contranutation seems the most plausible. It will, therefore, be used here as the basis for describing examination of the pelvis.

Pelvic Types

Erdmann (1965) and Gutmann (1965) describe three types of pelves:

- High assimilation or unstable pelvis
- Normal or fixation pelvis
- Horizontal or strained pelvis

High Assimilation Pelvis

The high assimilation pelvis (**Figure 13–5**) is characterized by the steep position of the sacrum. The sacral promontory stands high between the two innominates. The disk between L4 and L5 often lies above a line connecting the two iliac crests. The dorsal aspect of the sacrum forms an angle (δ) of 50° to 70° with the horizontal, while the angle of inclination of the sacrum (α) is 15° to 30°.

The posterior superior iliac spine projects dorsally only a little in relation to the sacrum. The lever arm of the dorsal musculature is short. The L5–S1 disk is generally high,

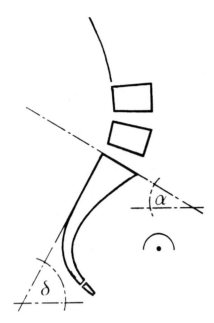

Figure 13–5   High assimilation pelvis.

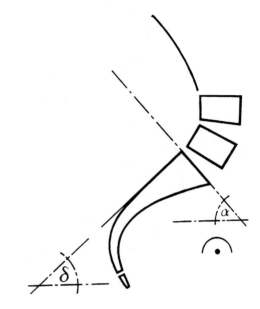

Figure 13–6   Normal pelvis.

while the iliolumbar ligaments are less developed. The divergence of the joint surfaces is less marked. Clinically, it is not unusual to find hypermobility of the lumbosacral junction and the sacroiliac joint. This may lead to osteochondrosis or a prolapse at the level of L5–S1.

This type of pelvis seems to occur most often in hypermobile women. A plumb line both from the head and the promontory run posterior to the hip joint.

Normal Pelvis

The normal pelvis (**Figure 13–6**) occupies an intermediate position between the assimilation pelvis and the strained pelvis. Both the angle of inclination of the sacrum (α) and the angle between the dorsal side of the sacrum and the horizontal (δ) are 35° to 45°. The L4–L5 disk lies at the level of a line connecting the two iliac crests. L5 is somewhat trapezoidal in shape. The L5–S1 disk is somewhat narrower than the L4–L5 disk and somewhat lower dorsally than ventrally. The transverse processes of L5 and the iliolumbar ligaments are strongly developed. If a prolapse develops with this type of pelvis, it is in most cases in the L4–L5 segment.

The plumb line descending from the head lies behind the hip, and that from the promontory lies dorsally within the hip.

Strained or Overloaded Pelvis

The strained or overload pelvis (**Figure 13–7**) is characterized by the more horizontal position of the sacrum. The dorsal surface of the sacrum forms an angle (δ) of 15° to 30° with the horizontal; the same is true of the disk. The

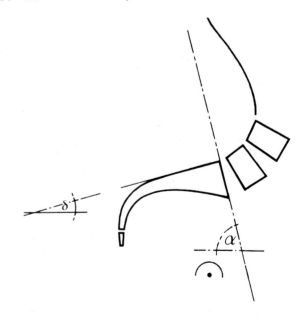

Figure 13–7   Strained pelvis.

angle of inclination of the sacrum (α) is 50° to 70°. The transverse processes of the lower lumbar vertebrae, like the iliolumbar ligaments, are especially strongly developed.

The L4–L5 disk usually lies below the line connecting the iliac crests. The posterior superior iliac spines project markedly posterior relative to the sacrum. The lever arm of the back muscles is relatively long.

The most important clinical consequences of this type of pelvis are overloading of the lumbosacral junction and of the hip and knee joints. Fixations in the lumbosacral and sacroiliac joints are also common. The plumb lines from the head and the promontory lie in front of the hip joint.

Strain Analysis of the Intervertebral Disk, the L5–S1 Intervertebral Joints, and the Hip Joints With the Different Pelvic Types

The information given by Gutmann (1956) is too limited to form a basis for calculating the different levels of strain imposed on L5–S1 and the hip joints by each of the three types of pelvis. To enable us to make some very general calculations, the following assumptions are made:

- The center of gravity of the trunk, arms, and head, which determines the static load on L5–S1, lies along a vertical line indicated in the diagrams by L.
- Vertebra L5 has an axis of rotation relative to S1 that lies in the center of disk L5–S1.
- A system of ligaments at the front of the spine is assumed to be responsible for mechanical balance (anterior longitudinal ligament). From this follow the moments of the forces relative to the central point of rotation. The moment of the force of gravity is aI, aII, and aIII for the three types of pelvis.

The lever arm of the force in the anterior longitudinal ligament is c; it is the same for all three pelvis types.

The lever arm of the force of gravity relative to the midpoint of the hip joint is bI, bII, and bIII, respectively.

The lever arm of the force of gravity relative to the midpoint of the hip joint is d and is the same for all three pelvic types.

- When calculating the load on L5–S2, the influence of muscular forces is not taken into account.
- When calculating the load on the hip joint, the forces in the ligamentous system surrounding it are not taken into account because their moments are small.

Strain on the L5–S1 Intervertebral Disk

The moments of the ligamentary force F_{lig} must balance the force of gravity L, so

$$L \times a = F_{lig} \times c$$

(See **Figure 13–8**.) It follows from this that:

$$F_{lig} = L / c \times a$$

For the forces to balance, the disk force F_{disk} must balance the two forces L and F_{lig} via the center of rotation. This means that:

$$F_{disk} = L + F_{lig} = L + L / c \times a = L / c \times (c + a)$$

According to Gutmann's findings (1965) (**Figure 13–9**), we have the following actual situations:

c = 3.5 mm
I: aI = 0mm $F_{disk} = (L / c) \times 3.5$
II: aII = 3.5mm $F_{disk} = (L / c) \times 7$
III: aIII = 9mm $F_{disk} = (L / c) \times 12.5$

The vertical load on disk L5–S1 in situation II is about twice that in situation I. In situation III, it is about 3.5 times that in situation I.

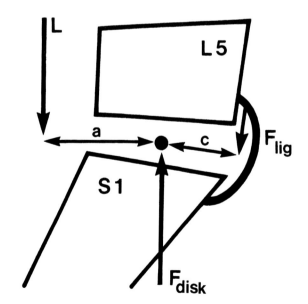

Figure 13–8 Load on the intervertebral disk L5–S1.

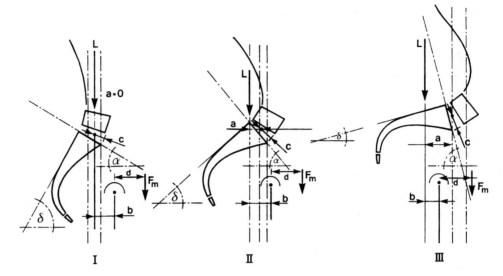

Figure 13–9   Load differences on the intervertebral disk L5–S1 in the three pelvic types.

Strain on the L5–S1 Intervertebral Joints

The direction of the forces is important here. (See **Figure 13–10**.) The normal perpendicular force on the endplate of S1 is

$$F_{norm} = F_{disk} \times \cos \alpha$$

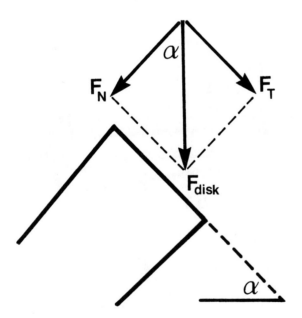

Figure 13–10   Load in the intervertebral joints L5–S1.

The tangential force on the disk is

$$F_{tang} = F_{disk} \times \sin \alpha$$

For the three situations, this yields:

I. $\alpha = 20°$ $\cos \alpha = 0.94$ $\sin \alpha = 0.34$ $F_{disk} = 3.5 \times L / c$
II. $\alpha = 40°$ $\cos \alpha = 0.77$ $\sin \alpha = 0.64$ $F_{disk} = 7 \times L / c$
III. $\alpha = 60°$ $\cos \alpha = 0.5$ $\sin \alpha = 0.87$ $F_{disk} = 12.5 \times L / c$

$F_{norm} = 3.3 \times L / c$ $F_{tang} = 1.2 \times L / c$
$F_{norm} = 5.4 \times L / c$ $F_{tang} = 4.5 \times L / c$
$F_{norm} = 6.3 \times L / c$ $F_{tang} = 10.8 \times L / c$

The normal force varies relatively little and is absorbed by the disk. The tangential force must be absorbed by the L5–S1 intervertebral joints. This force is about nine times greater in situation III than in situation I.

Strain on the Hip Joint

The force of gravity L exerts a moment M_L on the hip joint (See **Figure 13–11**). This moment must be compensated by a contrary moment M_{comp}, which is provided by the postural muscles to preserve balance of moments:

$$F_M \times d = L \times b \qquad F_M = L / d \times b$$

The total of forces in the hip joint F_H is, therefore:

$$F_H = L + F_M = L + L / d \times b = L / d \times (d + b)$$

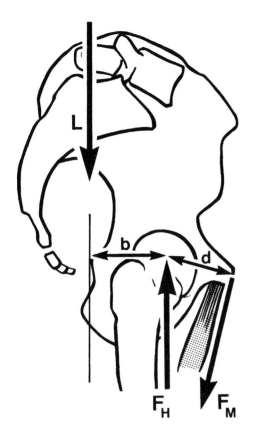

Figure 13–11   Load of the hip joint in the three pelvic types.

If we assume a value for d, for example, 10 mm, we have the following:

I. b = 6.5 mm $F_H = L / d \times 16.5$ $F_M = L / d \times 6.5$

II. b = 7 mm $F_H = L / d \times 17$ $F_M = L / d \times 7$

III. b = 4.5 mm $F_H = L / d \times 14.5$ $F_M = L / d \times 4.5$

The strain on the hip joint is thus approximately the same in all three situations. These rough calculations indicate that the differences between the three types of pelvis described by Gutmann (1956) have little effect on the strain on the hip joint. However, the strain on the connections between the vertebrae, both the disk and the intervertebral joints, varies greatly with the type of pelvis.

Strain on the Pelvis When Standing on Two Legs

Drukker and Jansen (1969) describe the stress on the pelvis when the individual stands on two legs as a "bow mechanism" (see **Figure 13–12**). In this position, compressive forces are exerted on the upper sides of both sacroiliac joints, both acetabuli, and the symphysis, while tractional forces are exerted on the underside of these joints.

Strain on the Pelvis When Standing on One Leg

Drukker and Jansen (1969) describe the stress on the pelvis when the individual stands on one leg as a "beam mechanism" (see **Figure 13–13**). In this position, compressive forces are exerted on the undersides of both sacroiliac joints, the loaded acetabulum, and the pubic symphysis, and traction forces are exerted on the upper sides of these joints. Considerable compressive force is exerted on the underside of the acetabulum of the supporting leg and on the underside of the symphysis.

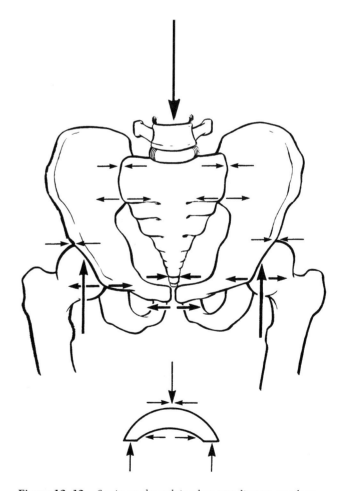

Figure 13–12   Strain on the pelvis when standing on two legs.

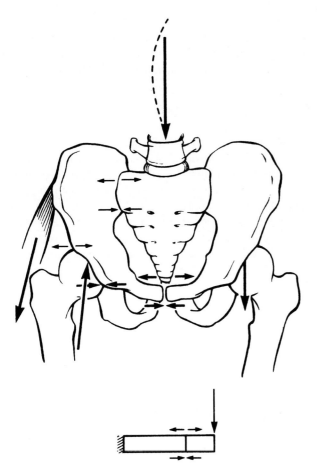

Figure 13–13 Strain on the pelvis when standing on one leg.

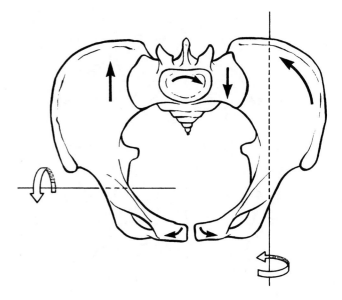

Figure 13–14 Movement mechanism of the sacroiliac joint when standing on one leg.

Movement Mechanism of the Sacroiliac Joint When Standing on One Leg

According to Cramer (1958), when the individual stands on the left leg, the following movements take place (**Figure 13–14**):

- The sacrum on the left side moves ventrally and caudally and rotates in a ventral direction (right rotation).
- The ilium on the left side moves in a dorsocranial direction relative to the sacrum. The posterior superior iliac spine moves in a caudal direction. The anterior superior iliac spine moves in a cranial direction.

There is also external rotation around a vertical axis.

- The sacrum on the right side moves dorsally and cranially and rotates in a dorsal direction (right rotation).

- The ilium on the right side moves ventrocaudally (relative to the sacrum) around a horizontal axis.
- The posterior superior iliac spine moves in a cranial direction.
- The anterior superior iliac spine moves in a caudal direction.

These twisting movements can cause a step to form in the symphysis. This happens if there is laxity in the connective tissues (pre- and postpartum hypermobility). Under normal circumstances, given the relatively low mobility of this synchondrosis, there is no step formation that can be clearly seen on X-ray. The step is leveled as a result of the external rotation of the ilium at the side of the supporting leg. The external rotation can be confirmed on X-ray because the obturator foramen becomes smaller on the side of the supporting leg.

The traction, bending, and compression forces exerted on the pubic symphysis are absorbed, respectively, by the horizontal fibers, the oblique fibers, and the cartilage (**Figure 13–15**).

The distortion of the pelvis also affects the spine, specifically the L5–S1 segment.

Pelvic Torsion

In pelvic torsion, the posterior superior iliac spine on one side is lower dorsally than the other is, and the anterior

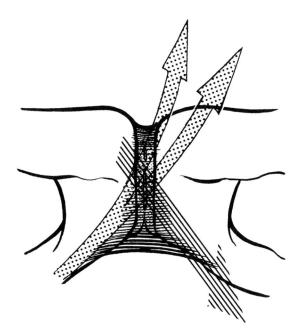

Figure 13–15 Traction, bending, and compression forces on the pubic symphysis.

superior iliac spine on one side is higher ventrally than the other is. The reverse is also possible (**Figure 13–16**).

In the case of fixated left pelvic torsion in a posterior direction, where the ilium on the same side shows a slight external rotation, the leg will follow the external rotation in a supine position. The extent of the external rotation is thus greater on the left side than on the right. If torsion is suspected, it must be verified by means of supplementary information. Investigations will also be needed to establish whether the torsion has a muscular or an arthrogenic basis.

The following points describe the relationship between pelvic torsion and fixation of the sacroiliac joint:

- Torsion with arthrogenic fixation
- Torsion with muscular fixation
- Torsion without fixation
- Fixation without torsion

Following are causes of pelvic torsion:

- Anatomic anomaly; this can only be confirmed by X-ray.
- Arthrogenic limitation of a sacroiliac joint.
- Unilateral shortening of a muscle (unilateral muscular spasm).

Sacroiliac Joint Fixation

The possible arrangements of the sacroiliac joint are the following:

- Ilium is posterior to the sacrum.
- Ilium is anterior to the sacrum.
- Ilium is in a neutral position relative to the sacrum.

Differences in Leg Length

Where there is a difference in leg length, both the anterior and posterior superior iliac spines will be lower on the side of the shorter leg than on the side of the longer leg.

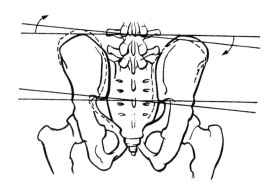

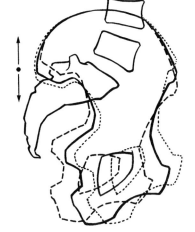

Figure 13–16 Pelvic torsion.

Following are causes of differences in leg length during the growing period (Taillard and Morscher, 1965):

	Growth inhibited	Growth stimulated
Congenital	Atrophy (essential hypoplasia)	Partial gigantism with blood vessel
	Atrophy with skeletal anomaly (fibular atrophy,	anomalies (Klippel–Trenaunay, Parker–Weber)
	femoral atrophy, coxa vara, etc.)	Hemarthrosis associated with hemophilia
	Dyschondroplasia (Ollier's disease)	
	Dysplasia with epiphyseal punctate calcifications	
	Congenital hip dislocation	
	Pes equinovarus adductus	
Infections	Growth plate dysfunction due to osteomyelitis	Osteomyelitis of the diaphysis of femur
	(femur, tibia, knee joint, foot)	Brodie abscess
	Tuberculosis of the hip, knee, and/or foot joints	Tuberculosis of the metaphysis of the tibia and
	Purulent arthritis	femur (tumor albus genus)
		Syphilis of femur and tibia
		Elephantiasis following soft tissue infections
		Thrombosis of femoral and iliac veins
Paralyses	Poliomyelitis	
	Other paralyses (spastic)	
Tumors	Osteochondroma (solitary exostoses)	Hemangioma
	Generalized arthritic cystic fibrosis	Lymphangioma
	Generalized neurofibromatosis	Giant cell tumors
	(Von Recklinghausen disease)	Localized osseous cystic fibrosis
		Von Recklinghausen neurofibromatosis
		Fibrous dysplasia (Jaffé–Lichtenstein)
Trauma	Damage to the growth plates (displacement,	Fractures of the femoral and tibial diaphysis and
	operations)	metaphysis
	Diaphysis fractures with long-axis dislocation	Diaphysis surgery (periosteal loosening,
	Serious burns	osteotomy, etc.)
Mechanical	Prolonged rest	
	Prolonged post-fracture traction	
Other causes	Femoral head epiphysiolysis	
	Leg-Calvé-Perthes disease	
	Radiation exposure of femoral and tibial growth	
	plates	

If the legs are of different lengths, the pelvis will tilt, and the sacrum, which forms the base of the spine, follows this tilt. The result is a lumbar scoliosis, which may or may not be compensated by the part of the spine lying above it. Gait is altered, and the act of walking places higher demands on muscles (Taillard and Morscher, 1965). During normal walking, the center of gravity of the body describes a flat sinusoidal curve. The limp that can result from a difference in leg length of 1 to 2 cm causes sharp peaks in the curve, which indicate a rise in energy consumption. The pelvic tilt can also disturb the function of the hip and knee joints and of the spine.

The load imposed on the hip joint of the shorter leg decreases (Pauwels, 1976). The tilt causes the contact surface of the femur head in the acetabulum on the shorter side to increase. The angle of the load-bearing part of the acetabulum on the side of the shorter leg (γ) increases by twice the angle of pelvic tilt (β) relative to angle (α) on the side of the longer leg. The moment of the body weight about the head of the femur is reduced because the center of gravity of the trunk (L) is shifted in the direction of the shorter leg. The moment lever arm (a) thus becomes shorter.

The opposite is true of the longer leg. The moment lever arm (b) becomes longer. At the side of the longer leg, the abductor muscles of the hip are placed under stronger tension (F_{ab}) (**Figure 13–17**).

The increased distance between the origin and the insertion of the hip abductors places an extra load on the hip joint by increasing pressure of the iliotibial tract on the greater trochanter. According to Bopp (1971), this can cause chronic bursitis. Bopp also discovered tendinopathies at the origin and insertion of the iliopsoas muscle, for example, on the transverse processes of the lumbar vertebrae and at the origin of the adductors on the pubic bone. Although it seems logical that the convexity of the lumbar scoliosis would be at the side of the shorter leg, this is not always the case. Ingelmark and Lindström (1963) found convex scoliosis in 75% of cases where the right leg was shorter and in 87% where the left leg was shorter.

In addition to the static forces, the dynamic forces exerted during walking probably play an important additional part (Morscher, 1972). Pelvic tilt usually causes deviation in the sagittal as well as the frontal plane. The lower ilium usually rotates in a ventral direction (Seidel, 1969). Where there have been morphologic changes to the vertebrae as a result of scoliosis that developed during the growth period, the scoliosis can probably not be fully corrected by conservative means.

The following are important mechanical consequences of the difference in leg length and the resultant scoliosis:

- The position of the line through the center of gravity of the body in the direction of the force of gravity (gravity plumb line)
- The click-clack phenomenon (Snijders, Snijder, Schijvens, and Seroo, 1975)

The tilt of the pelvis and the sacrum shifts the center of gravity of the body toward the shorter leg. The gravity plumb line shifts by the same distance (**Figure 13–18**).

The centers of gravity of the parts of the body are also partly shifted in the same direction. Because of the symmetrical position of the lower limbs, the shift in the center of gravity of the trunk is even greater than that of the center of gravity of the whole body. The weight of the trunk and the upper limbs exerts a bending moment on the L5–S1 disk, which increases the intervertebral space at the side of the longer leg. This increases the tilt. The moment causes a redistribution of compressive and tensile forces in the annulus fibrosus. The tissues are compressed on the side of the shorter leg and stretched on the other side.

The click-clack phenomenon (**Figure 13–19**) can be described in relation to a leaf spring. If a leaf spring is fixed in a vertical position, hinged at the underside and with the upper surface free to move vertically, it has two stable positions when a vertical load is applied, one to the left and one to the right. The two positions can be held without the application of extra external force. To bring the spring from one stable position to the other, a small momentum is needed at the hinge.

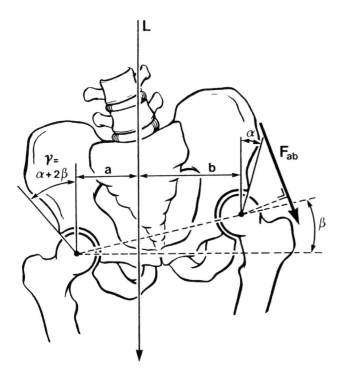

Figure 13–17 Load on hip joints of the shorter and longer leg.

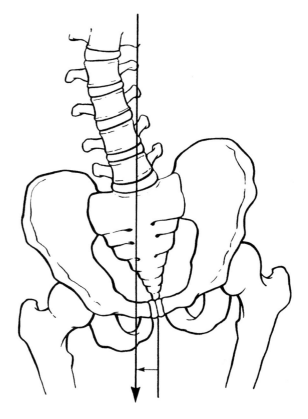

Figure 13–18 Shift of the center of gravity of the body in the direction of the shorter leg.

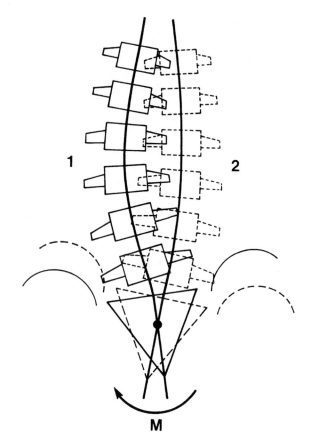

Figure 13–19   Click-clack phenomenon.

The spine behaves in the same way. A left convex scoliosis, for example, can be changed to a mild right convex scoliosis with the aid of a small momentum applied to the sacrum. This momentum can be obtained by a shift in the center of gravity.

In theory, the scoliosis should disappear if the shorter leg is raised to the level of the longer leg. In practice, this does not usually happen because the shift in the center of gravity is not enough to correct the irreversible adaptation of the capsuloligamentous system to the overload discussed.

At the Technical College of Eindhoven, the stabilograph was developed. This is a device for tracking the shift in center of gravity when the heel of the shorter leg is raised, and for identifying the moment when the click-clack phenomenon occurs, which is often not until the heel has been raised by twice the difference in leg length. The overcorrection that is needed initially is reduced in two stages at intervals of 3 months.

Measurement of Leg Length

The following are the usual methods of measuring leg length (Eigler, 1972; Morscher, 1972)

Direct Measurement   The direct measurement method is based on the length of the bones. The distance between points at the ends of one or more bones is measured. The points used for the measurements must be precisely defined.

Indirect Measurement   The indirect measurement method is a static measure. Supports are placed under the shorter leg until the pelvic tilt disappears.

Radiographic Measurement   Several methods exist, of which orthoradiography presents the fewest technical difficulties. It involves taking anteroposterior X-rays of the hip and knee joints. The points from which the measurements are made are the top of the femoral head, the underside of the medial femoral condyle, the intercondylar eminence of the tibia, and the distal underside of the tibia joint surface. This method of measurement is the most accurate.

Leg Length

Figure 13–20 shows different ways leg length can be measured.

Absolute leg length: Top of femoral head to plantar surface of the foot (a)

Anatomic leg length: Upper surface of greater trochanter to most distal aspect of lateral malleolus (b)

Apparent leg length: Navel to most distal aspect of medial malleolus (c)

Clinical leg length: ASIS to most distal aspect of lateral malleolus (d)

Relative leg length: Underside of hip joint space to joint space of talocrural joint (e)

Functional leg length: Shortening or lengthening of leg through joint contractures or leg anomalies

Pelvic Instability

The pelvic girdle plays a key role in transmitting forces between the trunk and the legs (Mens et al., 1996). The sacroiliac joint is a weak link in the chain of transmission. Normally, forces are exchanged between the sacrum and ilium via the interlocking grooves and ridges of the two articular surfaces and by tension in the ligaments and muscles (Vleeming et al., 1990). The articular surfaces of the sacrum and ilium, during weight bearing, are compressed against each other by ligaments, muscles, the force of gravity, and the normal force in reaction to the force of gravity. The ligaments involved are the dorsal sacroiliac and interosseous ligaments, the upper and most ventral sacroiliac capsule,

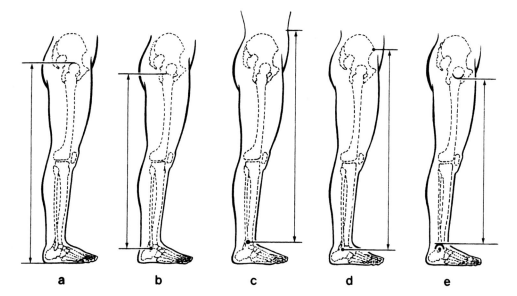

Figure 13–20 Different measurements of leg length.

the sacrotuberous and sacrospinous ligaments, and the iliolumbar and symphyseal ligaments. The polyarticular muscles also play a part in pressing the articular surfaces together.

If mobility increases, the forces of compression can cause a change of position in the sacroiliac joint. A reduction in the force transfer between the articular surfaces leads to instability in the sacroiliac joint. If this happens, a larger proportion of the forces will be conveyed via the ligaments and muscles. In cases of severe instability, it may be impossible for the forces to be transferred.

Causes of Instability

Following are several causes of pelvic instability:

- Hormonal changes during pregnancy (Orvieto et al., 1994). During pregnancy, tissue fluid content increases in the sacroiliac and symphyseal joints, which causes widening of the joint space and weakening of the ligaments. This is a result of the production of the hormone relaxin (Hisaw, 1925).
- Slackening of the oblique and rectus abdominis muscles, which then give too little support to the symphyseal ligaments and to the uppermost and most ventral capsule of the sacroiliac joints.
- Trauma caused during childbirth, work, sport, and intercourse. If the ligaments have been overstretched

or torn, this may result in unilateral or bilateral instability.

Radiography

The most important X-rays are those of the symphysis because they will reveal the extent of the instability. The widening of the joint space is a less important factor here, the more important one being a possible increase in mobility in the vertical direction. X-rays should be taken with the patient standing on the left leg and the right leg separately.

Vertical displacement can be identified by external palpation, and the history and the provocation tests provide sufficient detail, so X-rays add little to the picture in this respect. For details of the history and provocation tests, please see the account of the practical examinations later on in this chapter.

Muscular Influences on the Pelvis

Various muscles in the lumbopelvic-hip region have a movement effect on the pelvis; **Table 13–1** provides more detail on these muscular influences on the pelvis.

Knowledge of the motor and sensory nerves of the lumbopelvic region will allow for a more accurate structure-based diagnosis and identification of possible reasons for further medical-surgical diagnosis and management. **Table 13–2** provides detailed information on the motor and sensory innervation originating in the lumbosacral region.

Table 13–1   Muscular Influences on the Pelvis

Muscle	Bilateral	Unilateral
Ventral		
Rectus abdominis muscle	Extension	
External oblique muscle	Extension	External rotation, medial sidebending
Internal oblique muscle	Extension	Internal rotation, medial sidebending
Rectus femoris muscle	Flexion	Internal rotation, lateral sidebending
Iliacus muscle	Flexion	
Psoas minor muscle	Extension	Internal rotation, medial sidebending
Sartorius muscle	Flexion	Internal rotation, lateral sidebending
Tensor fasciae latae muscle	Flexion	External rotation, lateral sidebending
Psoas major muscle	Flexion/Extension	
Dorsal		
Longissimus muscle	Flexion	Medial sidebending
Iliocostalis muscle	Flexion	Medial sidebending
Intertransversarius muscles	Flexion	Medial sidebending
Interspinal muscle	Flexion	
Rotator muscles	Flexion	Internal rotation
Multifidi muscles	Flexion	Internal rotation
Latissimus dorsi muscle	Flexion	Medial sidebending
Gluteus maximus muscle	Extension	Internal rotation
Semimembranous muscle	Extension	External rotation
Semitendinous muscle	Extension	External rotation
Biceps femoris muscle	Extension	Internal rotation
Medial		
Internal rotators of the hip		External rotation
Pectineus muscle	Flexion	Medial sidebending
Adductor longus muscle	Flexion	Internal/external rotation
Gracilis muscle	Flexion	Medial sidebending
Adductor brevis muscle	Flexion	Medial sidebending
Adductor magnus muscle	Flexion/Extension	Medial sidebending
Lateral		
Gluteus minimus muscle	Flexion	Laterorotation, lateral sidebending
Gluteus medius muscle	Flexion/Extension	External/internal rotation lateral sidebending
External rotators of the hip		External rotation
Quadratus lumborum muscle	Flexion	Medial sidebending

Table 13–2   Motor–Sensory Relationships

Segment Nerve	Motor	Sensory
L4–S2 sacral plexus (ventral rami)	Piriformis muscle Gemellus superior muscle Gemellus inferior muscle Obturator internus muscle Quadratus femoris muscle	
Sciatic nerve (tibial part)	Semitendinous muscle Semimembranous muscle Abductor magnus muscle Biceps femoris muscle Long head	Posterior femoral cutaneous nerve (ventral and dorsal rami): Back of thigh, scrotum, labia majora

Segment Nerve	Motor	Sensory
Dorsal ramus (peroneal part)	Biceps femoris muscle Short head	
L4–S3 tibial nerve	Plantaris muscle Gastrocnemius muscle Popliteus muscle Soleus muscle Tibialis posterior muscle Flexor digitorum longus muscle Extensor hallucis longus muscle	The medial cutaneous nerve of the leg, together with the lateral cutaneous leg nerve of the common peroneal nerve, forms the sural nerve: Dorsolateral part of lower leg, back of lateral malleolus, lateral part of foot
Lateral plantar nerve	Quadratus plantaris muscle Flexor digiti minimi brevis muscle Adductor hallucis Lumbrical muscles III, IV Abductor digiti minimi Opponens digiti minimi Interosseous muscles	Lateral side of sole and back of foot, fifth distal phalanx, and lateral side of fourth phalanx
Medial plantar nerve	Abductor hallucis muscle Flexor digitorum brevis muscle Flexor halluscis brevis muscle Lumbrical muscles I, II	Medial plantar side of sole, distal phalanxes I, II, III, and medial side of IV
Sacral plexus (dorsal ramus)		
Superior gluteal nerve	Gluteus medius muscle Gluteus minimus muscle Tensor fasciae Latae muscle	
Inferior gluteal nerve	Gluteus maximus muscle	
Pudendal nerve	Levator ani muscle Coccygeal muscle Bulbospongiosus muscle External anal sphincter muscle Superficial and deep transverse perineal muscles Ischiocavernosus muscle	Perineum, scrotum, labia, penis, clitoris
Coccygeal nerve	Coccygeal muscle Levator ani muscle	Skin of coccygeal area
L4–S2 common peroneal nerve	Tibialis anterior muscle Extensor hallucis longus muscle Extensor hallucis brevis muscle	Dorsomedial side of second toe and dorso lateral side of first toe
Deep peroneal nerve	Extensor digitorum longus muscle Extensor hallucis brevis muscle Accessory peroneal muscle	Lower ventrolateral part of lower leg, dorsolateral side of foot The lateral cutaneous nerve of the leg, together with the medial cutaneous nerve of the tibia, forms the sural nerve: dorsolateral side of lower leg, back of external, and lateral side of foot
Superficial peroneal nerve	Long peroneal muscle Short peroneal muscle	

PELVIS: INSPECTION

Provided that the two halves of the pelvis are the same size, inspection will reveal whether there is any pelvic tilting or torsion. This is revealed by the position of the superior iliac spines relative to each other.

Pelvic Tilt

If the pelvis is tilted, both the anterior and posterior superior iliac spines will be lower on one side than on the other. (See **Figures 13–21** and **13–22**.) The asymmetry of the pelvis can be a result of a difference in leg length. A difference in height between the two halves of the pelvis can also be a consequence of the ilium on one side being less developed than that on the other. Preece et al. (2008) underlined this possibility: in 30 cadaveric pelves, they noted side-to-side differences in innominate height of up to 16 mm. To make an accurate assessment, the therapist must observe the position of the lumbar spine during the inspection.

Pelvic Torsion

To make a clinical decision on whether pelvic torsion is present, the position of the iliac spines relative to each other must be compared both dorsally and ventrally in the horizontal plane. (See **Figures 13–23** and **13–24**.) If this comparison indicates that pelvic torsion is likely, further examination is needed to establish whether the disturbance is in the left or the right sacroiliac joint. The following picture is found in pelvic torsion:

PSIS lower on the left than on the right
ASIS higher on the left than on the right

    or

PSIS lower on the right than on the left
ASIS higher on the right than on the left

With regard to reliability of landmark palpation of the PSIS and ASIS as discussed previously, Richter and Lawall

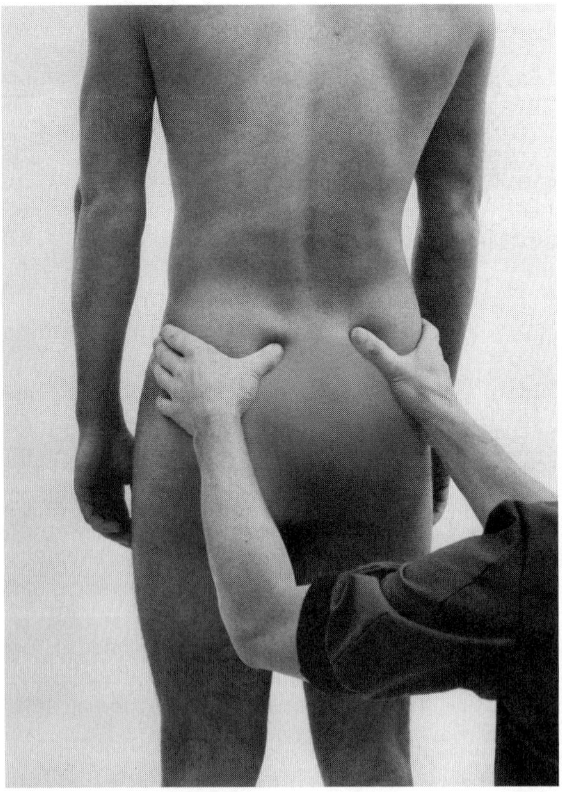

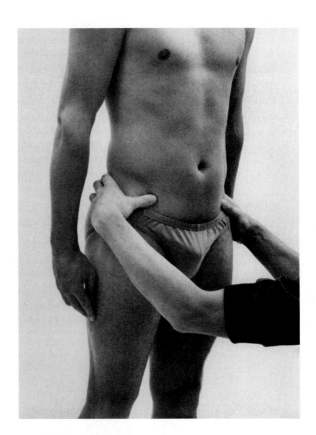

Figure 13–21   PSIS left lower.

Figure 13–22   ASIS left lower.

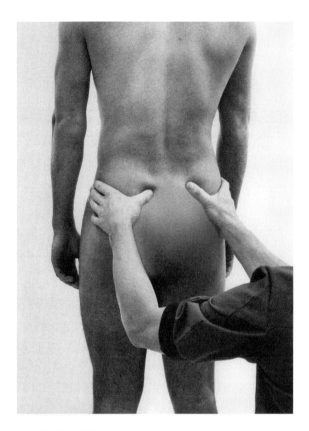

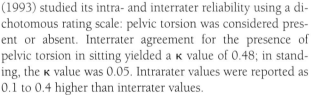

Figure 13–23 PSIS left lower.

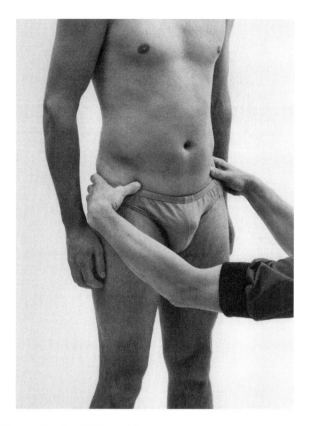

Figure 13–24 ASIS left higher.

(1993) studied its intra- and interrater reliability using a dichotomous rating scale: pelvic torsion was considered present or absent. Interrater agreement for the presence of pelvic torsion in sitting yielded a κ value of 0.48; in standing, the κ value was 0.05. Intrarater values were reported as 0.1 to 0.4 higher than interrater values.

Tullberg et al. (1998) studied concurrent criterion-related validity of palpation of the iliac crest, PSIS, and ASIS height with the patient standing, prone, or supine using a dichotomous rating scale indicating presence or absence of asymmetry on 10 patients with unilateral sacroiliac joint dysfunction. The gold standard test was an assessment of three-dimensional sacroiliac joint position using Roentgen-stereophotogrammetric analysis (RSA) before and after a manipulation to the sacroiliac joint (SIJ). All three raters judged all positional tests indicative of asymmetry prior to manipulation and, with a few exceptions, normalized after manipulation. However, RSA showed no change in positional relationship pre- and postmanipulation, indicating positional palpation tests may not be a valid way to determine sacroiliac joint position.

EXAMINATION OF THE SACROILIAC JOINT

During examination of the pelvis, assessments are made of the load-transfer capacity of the sacroiliac joints, the ligamentous and capsular tissues; the extent and quality of movement; and any pain or referred sensations that may be associated with the latter.

Active Examination of the Sacroiliac Joint

The Vorlauf Phenomenon or Standing Flexion Test

Figures 13–25 and **13–26** show the standing flexion test:

Examination position, patient: Symmetrical standing position.

Starting position, therapist: Sitting or standing behind the patient.

Hand position, therapist: The thumbs are placed against the distal aspects of the left and right posterior superior iliac spines.

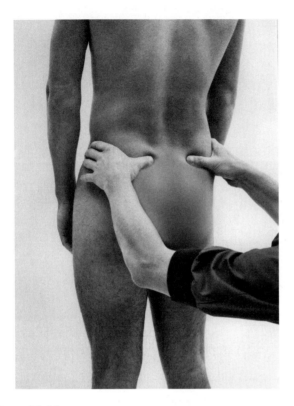

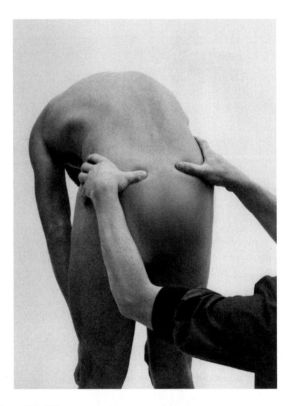

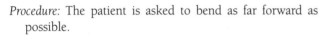

Figure 13–25

Figure 13–26

Procedure: The patient is asked to bend as far forward as possible.

Assessment: The difference in height is measured both before and after the maneuver. When the patient is bending as far forward as possible, if one spine has clearly moved farther than the other in a cranioventral direction compared with the initial position, the test result is positive provided that this difference is the same when the test is repeated.

Remarks: At the fixated side, the ilium follows directly in the path of the sacrum when the patient bends forward. At the nonfixated side, the ilium follows more slowly because of the action of the capsule; this is expressed in the difference between the positions of the two spines. If the difference decreases or disappears when the test is performed repeatedly, the fixation is probably muscular

Various authors have studied the reliability of Vorlauf phenomenon or standing flexion test using a 3-point rating scale. Potter and Rothstein (1985) reported an interrater agreement for the standing flexion test of 43.75%. Bowman and Gribble (1995) reported 52% interrater agreement (κ = 0.2333). Vincent-Smith and Gibbons (1999) found a

mean interrater percentage agreement of 42% with a mean κ of 0.052. Intrarater agreement ranged from 44–88% with a mean of 68%; κ ranged from 0.16–0.72 with a mean κ of 0.46. Riddle et al. (2002) reported an interrater agreement of 55.4% with κ = 0.32.

The Rücklauf Phenomenon: Standing Hip Flexion or Stork Test

Figures 13–27, 13–28, and **13–29** show the standing hip flexion test:

Examination position, patient: Symmetrical standing position.

Starting position, therapist: Sitting or standing behind the patient.

Hand position, therapist: The thumbs are placed against the distal aspects of the left and right posterior superior iliac spines.

Procedure: The patient is asked to bring the knee at the side of the sacroiliac joint being examined to his or her chest. During this maneuver, the patient may support himself or herself with one hand on the treatment bench.

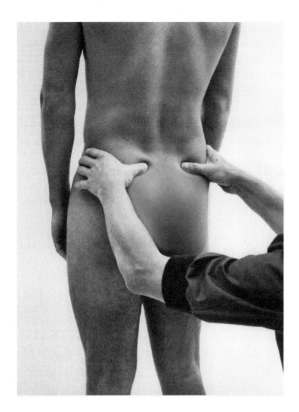

Figure 13–27

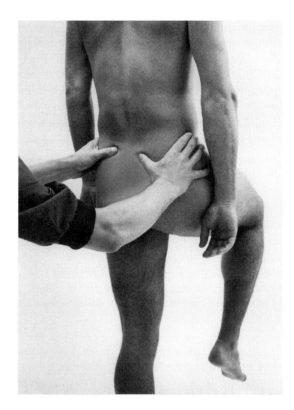

Figure 13–28

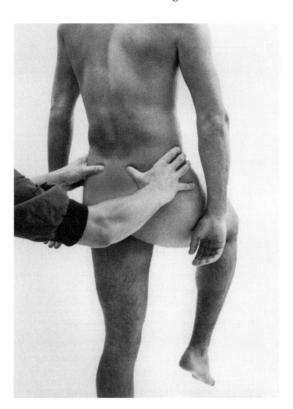

Figure 13–29

Assessment: While the patient performs this movement, the therapist observes whether the PSIS on the side of the moving leg shifts in a caudodorsal direction earlier than the PSIS at the side of the supporting leg, or at the same time. If the PSIS at the side of the moving leg shifts in a caudodorsal direction at the same time as the PSIS at the side of the supporting leg, the test result is positive.

Remarks: The sacroiliac joint at the side of the supporting leg is fixed by the weight of the body. If the joint at the side of the lifted leg is fixated, the ilium will take the sacrum with it, so the two spines will move at the same time in a caudodorsal direction. If the sacroiliac joint is not fixated, the ilium or the spine will move in a caudodorsal direction before the sacrum because of the play in the capsule. If the sacroiliac joint is normal, the spine of the moving leg will have moved farther in a caudodorsal direction at the end of the maneuver than the spine of the supporting leg. Any difference in leg length should be taken into account.

Various authors have also studied the Rücklauf phenomenon or standing hip flexion test. Using a 3-point rating scale, Potter and Rothstein (1985) reported 46.67% interrater agreement. Richter and Lawall (1993) used a dichotomous scale and reported intrarater agreement of $\kappa = 0.86$ (95% CI: 0.56–1.00) for the right and $\kappa = 0.93$ (95% CI: 0.66–1.00) for the left standing hip flexion test. Interrater agreement yielded $\kappa = 0.69$ (95% CI: 0.40–0.97) for the right and $\kappa = 0.65$ (95% CI: 0.42–0.88) for the left test. Dreyfuss et al. (1996) reported 54% interrater agreement

($\kappa = 0.22$). Using a gold standard test of 90–100% reduction in pain after a fluoroscopically guided sacroiliac joint block, these authors also reported a sensitivity of 0.43 and a specificity of 0.68. Perhaps best reflecting current thought on the load transfer function of the sacroiliac joint, Hungerford et al. (2007) reported 91.9% and 89.9% ($\kappa = 0.67, 0.77$) interrater agreement for the left and right test, respectively, when using a 2-point rating scale of cranial versus no or caudal movement of the PSIS in relation to the sacrum on the stance leg side. Using a 3-point rating scale of caudal, cranial, or no movement of the PSIS relative to the sacrum, these values were 82.8 and 79.8% ($\kappa = 0.59, 0.59$), respectively.

Lordosis/Kyphosis Test I

Figures 13–30, 13–31, and **13–32** show the first lordosis/kyphosis test:

Examination position, patient: Sitting on the long side of the treatment table.

Starting position, therapist: Sitting or standing behind the patient.

Hand position, therapist: The thumbs are placed against the distal aspects of the left and right PSIS.

Procedure: The patient is asked to bend forward as far as possible then immediately backward as far as possible.

Assessment: The difference in height is noted both before and after the movement. The test is positive if one spine moves farther in a cranioventral direction following lor-

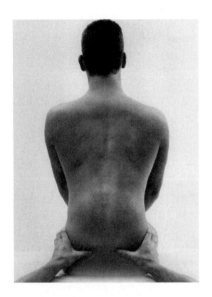

Figure 13–30

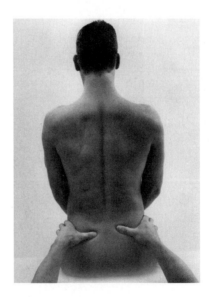

Figure 13–31

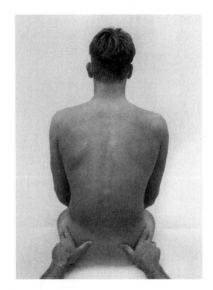

Figure 13–32

dosis, and farther in a caudodorsal direction following kyphosis.

Remarks: During lordosis, the PSIS on the fixated side will follow directly in the path of the sacrum and will move farther in a cranioventral direction. During kyphosis, the PSIS on the fixated side will directly follow the sacrum and will move farther in a caudodorsal direction.

Van Kessel-Cobelens et al. (2008) studied interrater agreement on this test in women aged 20 to 40 years using a dichotomous rating system whereby the test was considered positive if one of the PSIS moved slower from cranial to caudal. In women pregnant for greater than 20 weeks but without pelvic girdle pain interrater agreement was 45% ($\kappa = -0.22$). In women pregnant for greater than 20 weeks with pelvic girdle pain agreement was 55% ($\kappa = 0.0$). In a control group of women that were neither pregnant nor had low back or pelvic pain agreement was 60% ($\kappa = 0.21$). Over all groups combined interrater agreement was 53% ($\kappa = 0.03$).

Lordosis/Kyphosis Test II

Figures 13–33, **13–34**, and **13–35** show the second lordosis/kyphosis test:

Examination position, patient: Sitting on the long side of the treatment table.

Starting position, therapist: Sitting or standing behind the patient.

Hand position, therapist: The thumb of one hand is placed against the distal aspect of the PSIS on the side being examined. The thumb of the other hand is placed at the same height against median sacral crest.

Procedure: The patient is asked to bend forward as far as possible, then backward as far as possible.

Assessment: Any difference in height is noted after each of the two movements. If the sacroiliac joint is functioning normally, the sacrum will move farther relative to the PSIS in a cranioventral direction during lordosis, and farther in a caudodorsal direction during kyphosis. The test is positive if this does not happen.

Supine to Long Sitting Test

Figures 13–36 and **13–37** show the supine to long sitting test:

Examination position, patient: Supine.

Starting position, therapist: Standing at patient's feet.

Hand position, therapist: Both thumbs are placed distally against the two medial malleoli; any asymmetry in a proximal-distal direction is noted.

Procedure: The patient is asked to rise from the supine position to a sitting position, with the legs extended.

Assessment: When the patient has reached a long sitting position, the therapist judges whether one leg has elongated more than the other. If pelvic torsion is present, whether or not in combination with a fixation, the leg at

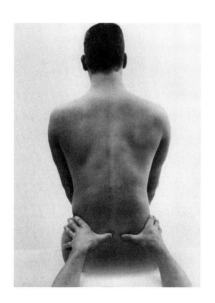

Figure 13–33

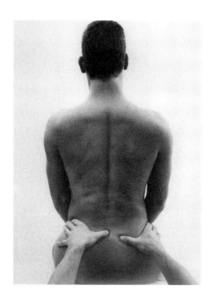

Figure 13–34

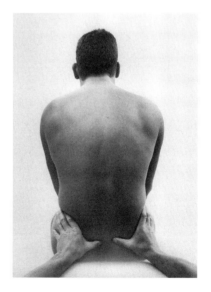

Figure 13–35

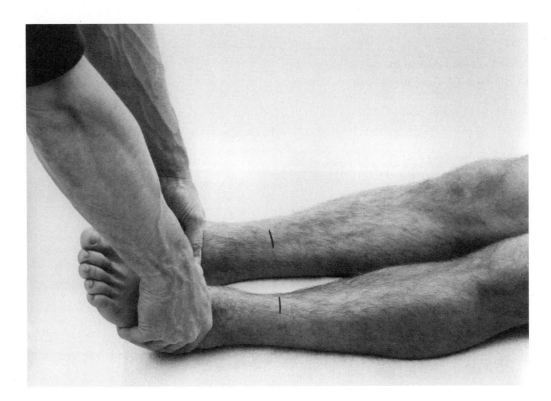

Figure 13–36

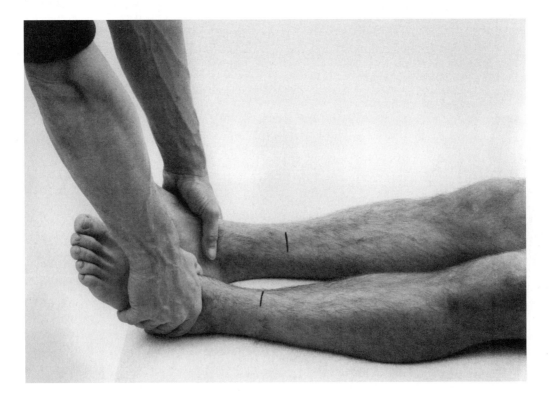

Figure 13–37

the side where the ilium is posteriorly rotated will be relatively longer in a sitting position. The medial malleolus on the side where the ilium rotates backward will move farther distally than the other while the patient is rising to a sitting position.

Remarks: Where there is posterior rotation of the ilium, the acetabulum moves in a cranioventral direction. As a result, the leg at the side of the posterior rotation will be relatively shorter in a supine position and relatively longer in a sitting position.

Using a 3-point rating scale Potter and Rothstein (1985) established an interrater agreement of 40.00% for the supine-to-sit test. Riddle et al. (2002) reported 44.6% interrater agreement with a κ value of 0.19.

Provocation Tests for the Sacroiliac Joint

The symptoms of a dysfunction can be provoked by bringing about physiologic torsion in one or both sacroiliac joints, as in the following examples.

Iliopsoas Muscle Test

Stretching the iliopsoas muscle causes anterior movement of the ilium at the side being examined (**Figure 13–38**).

Straight Leg Raise Test

A straight leg raise causes posterior movement of the ilium at the side being examined (**Figure 13–39**). When us-

ing this test to detect sacroiliac joint dysfunction, it is essential to observe the location and nature of the symptoms.

Piriformis Muscle Test

Where there is sacroiliac dysfunction, the piriformis muscle is often hypertonic. Stretching this muscle passively to its full length often produces traction pain at the affected side. (See **Figure 13–40**.)

Patrick's Test (FABER or Hyperabduction Test)

Applying passive hyperabduction to the hip joint can yield information about dysfunction in the hip and sacroiliac joints (**Figure 13–41**). Pain and limitation of movement may be caused by reflexive spasm of the adductors on the side where there is hip or sacroiliac joint dysfunction.

Patrick's test can cause mechanical stimulation in the sacroiliac joint being examined (Hoppenfeld, 1976).

Various authors have studied the Patrick test, which is most commonly referred to as the flexion-abduction-external rotation, or FABER, test using a dichotomous rating scale of pain present or absent on testing. Dreyfuss et al. (1996) reported 82% interrater agreement (κ = 0.62). Using a gold standard test of 90–100% reduction in pain after a fluoroscopically guided sacroiliac joint block, these authors also reported a sensitivity of 0.69 and a specificity of 0.16. Strender et al. (1997) found 88–96% interrater agreement. Broadhurst and Bond (1998) used a gold standard test of 70% or 90% reduction of pain after a fluoroscopically guided double-blind sacroiliac block. At the 70% criterion, sensitivity and specificity for the FABER test were

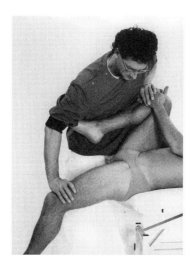

Figure 13–38

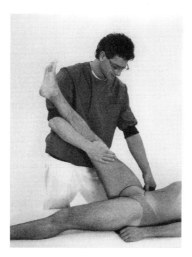

Figure 13–39

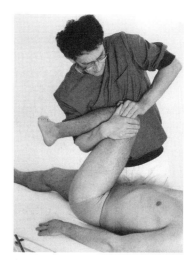

Figure 13–40

77% and 100%; at 90%, they were 50% and 100%, respectively. Albèrt et al. (2000) reported 88% interrater agreement ($\kappa = 0.54$). Kokmeyer et al. (2002) reported 91.32% interrater agreement ($\kappa = 0.62$, 95% CI: 0.33–0.91).

Reverse Lasègue

Depending on fixation, this test can yield information about dysfunctions in the hip and sacroiliac joint and in the lumbar spine. It also stretches the psoas muscle and the L3 nerve root. (See **Figure 13–42**.) To provoke the sacroiliac joint, the apex of the sacrum is fixed in a ventral direction. The hip joint on the side to be examined is brought into the close-packed position. Raising the leg in the direction of extension exerts a ventral rotational impulse on the ilium. This provokes the sacroiliac joint.

Ligament Tests

Figures 13–43, 13–44, and **13–45** illustrate the ligament tests:

Examination position, patient: Supine. The leg on the ipsilateral side is flexed through 90° at the hip and brought into partial adduction.

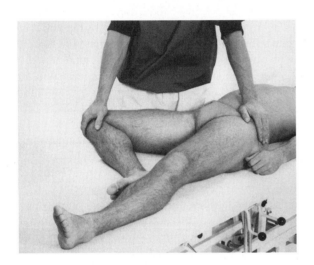

Figure 13–41

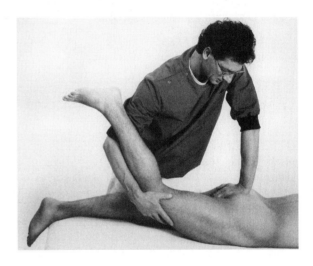

Figure 13–42

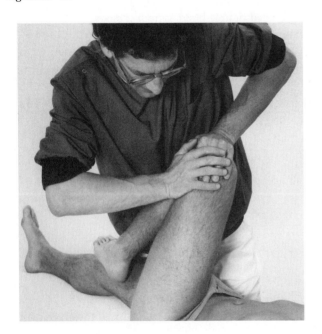

Figure 13–43

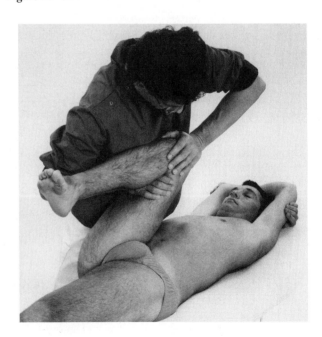

Figure 13–44

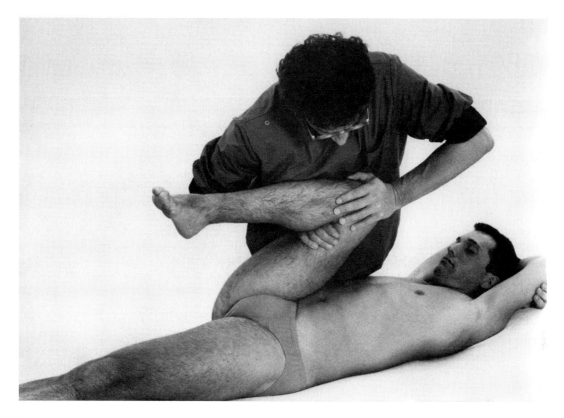

Figure 13–45

Starting position, therapist: Standing beside the patient at the side to be examined.

Hand position, therapist: The therapist's two hands encircle the patient's knee at the side of the flexed hip.

Procedure: While the axial pressure on the hip joint is maintained, the therapist carries out an adduction movement in the direction of the contralateral hip, a flexing movement toward the ipsilateral shoulder, and an adduction and flexing movement toward the contralateral shoulder.

Assessment: If these movements are continued for some time, the therapist will be able to judge the load-bearing capacity of ligaments in terms of endfeel and pain.

Remarks: The adduction movement loads the iliolumbar ligament; the ipsilateral bending loads the vertically extended ligamentary structures; and the contralateral bending loads the diagonal ligamentous structures.

Compression/Gapping Test I

Figure 13–46 shows the gapping test:

Examination position patient: Supine.

Starting position, therapist: Standing beside the patient.

Hand position, therapist: The arms are crossed and the hands are placed medially against the iliac bones.

Procedure: Lateral pressure is applied with both hands.

Assessment: The ventrally stretched ligamentous structures are tested by way of tension.

Remarks: During this test, the dorsal compartments of the sacroiliac joints are compressed, which can cause direct pressure pain. The ventral compartments are opened, which places the ventral capsuloligamentous structures under tension.

Potter and Rothstein (1985) reported 94.12% interrater agreement for the distraction test. Laslett and Williams (1994) reported 88.2% interrater agreement ($\kappa = 0.69$). Albert et al. (2000) noted 97% interrater agreement ($\kappa = 0.84$). Kokmeyer et al. (2002) reported 88.46% ($\kappa = 0.46$, 95% CI: 0.13–0.79). Using verification of sacroiliitis on radiograph or MRI as a gold standard test, Levin and Stenström (2003) reported a sensitivity and negative predictive value of the test performed from the right of 0.55 and 0.69; from the left, these values were 0.55 and 0.67, respectively. The specificity and positive predictive values were 1.0.

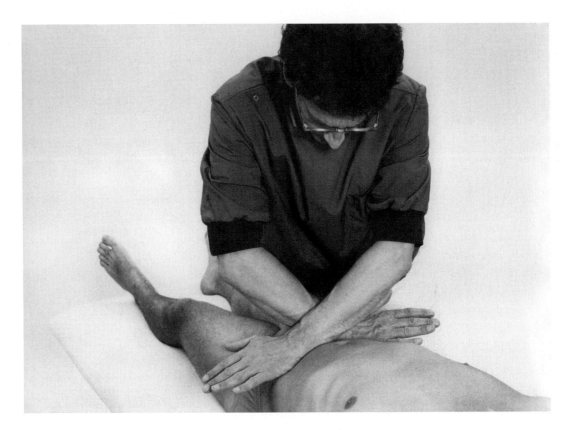

Figure 13–46   ←┤ ├→

Compression/Gapping Test II

Figure 13–47 illustrates the compression test:

Examination position, patient: Supine.

Starting position, therapist: Standing beside the patient.

Hand position, therapist: Both hands are placed laterally against the iliac bones.

Procedure: Pressure is applied with both hands in a medial direction.

Assessment: The dorsally stretched ligamentous structures are tested by way of tension.

Remarks: During this test, the ventral compartments of the sacroiliac joints are compressed, causing direct pressure pain. The dorsal compartments are opened, which puts the dorsal capsuloligamentous structures under tension. Ligament stretch pain will only appear after some time; it will then gradually increase.

Potter and Rothstein (1985) reported 76.47% interrater agreement for the compression test. Laslett and Williams (1994) reported 88.2% interrater agreement ($\kappa = 0.73$). Strender et al. (1997) found 74–79% interrater agreement ($\kappa = 0.26$). Albert et al. (2000) noted 97% interrater agreement ($\kappa = 0.79$). Kokmeyer et al. (2002) reported 93.59% ($\kappa = 0.58$, 95% CI: 0.23–0.94).

Sell's Test I

Figures 13–48 and **13–49** show the first Sell's test:

Examination position, patient: Prone.

Starting position, therapist: Standing beside the patient at the side not to be examined.

Hand position, therapist: The hypothenar of the manipulating hand is placed at the contralateral side of the apex of the sacrum. The index finger of the examining hand is placed on the gluteal muscles in the upper and inner quadrant, directly under the edge of the iliac crest.

Procedure: The manipulating hand applies ventromedial pressure to the apex of the sacrum, and the examining hand palpates changes in tone of the gluteal muscles.

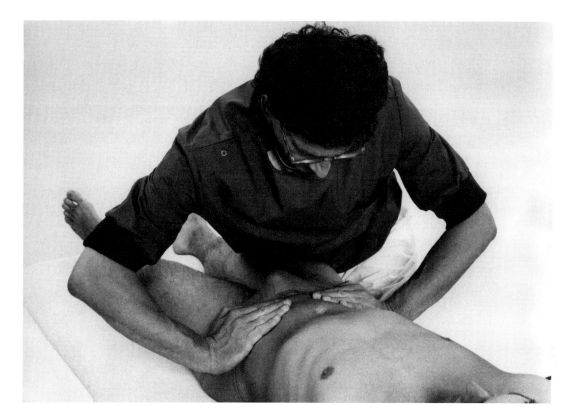

Figure 13–47   →| |←

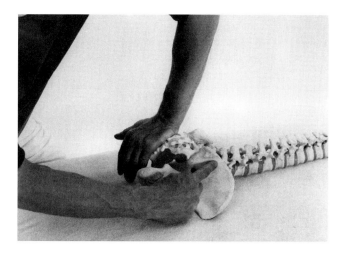

Figure 13–48   ↑

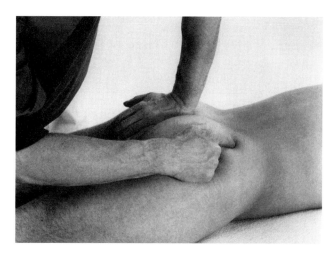

Figure 13–49   ↑

Assessment: During this test, the therapist determines by palpation the increases and decreases in tone in the gluteal muscles, and the relationship of the joint partners of the sacroiliac joint in a posteroanterior direction.

Sell (1969) states that a pathologic dorsoventral change in the position of the ilium relative to the sacrum causes a reflexogenic increase in tone in the upper and inner quadrant of the gluteal muscles. If the position of the sacrum is changed, the pain and hypertonicity in these muscles will either disappear or increase, depending on whether the sacrum is moved in the correcting direction or in the patho-

logic direction. From this, Sell deduces the direction in which correction is necessary.

Modified Sell's Test II

Figures 13–50 and **13–51** show the modified Sell's test:

Examination position, patient: Prone, with the lower legs over the edge of the examination bench.

Starting position, therapist: Standing at the foot end with the patient's leg on the side to be examined between the therapist's thighs.

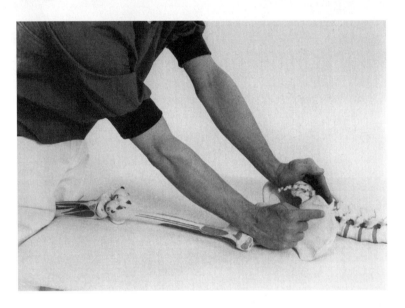

Figure 13–50

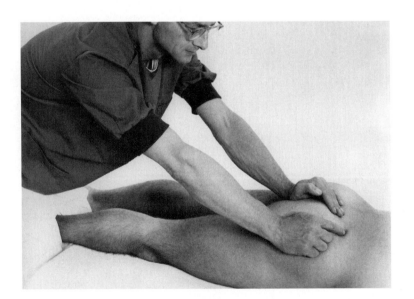

Figure 13–51

Hand position, therapist: The hypothenar of the stabilizing hand is placed at the contralateral side at the apex of the sacrum; the index finger of the examining hand is placed on the gluteal muscles in the upper and inner quadrant, directly below the edge of the crest.

Procedure: The two thighs exert force in a caudal direction on the ipsilateral ilium; the stabilizing hand maintains the position of the sacrum by applying pressure in a ventromedial direction; the examining hand palpates changes in tone in the gluteal muscles.

Assessment: During this test, the therapist determines by palpation the increases and decreases in tone in the gluteal muscles, and the relation of the joint partners of the sacroiliac joint in nutation and counternutation. If the pain and hypertonicity decrease during these maneuvers, the dysfunction is probably caused by a posterior rotation of the ilium relative to the sacrum.

Remarks: Contrary to the theory that the ilium rotates in relation to the sacrum, Sell assumed for the purposes of the original test that the sacrum can move caudally in relation to the ilium. Sell, therefore, places the restraining hand on the ipsilateral side, distally against the apex of the sacrum.

Passive Examination of the Sacroiliac Joint

External/Internal Rotation Test of Hip Joints

Figures 13–52, **13–53**, and **13–54** illustrate the external/internal rotation test of hip joints:

Examination position, patient: Supine.

Starting position, therapist: Standing at the foot end or by the patient's side.

Hand position, therapist: The two hands encircle the patient's lower legs distally.

Procedure: Both the patient's legs are brought into either internal rotation or external rotation.

Assessment: Observation is carried out in the resting state before the test starts. During the test, the endfeel is assessed and the movement trajectories of the two legs are compared. If there is pelvic torsion, whether or not this is accompanied by a fixation, the leg at the side where the ilium has a greater posterior rotation will lie in a more externally rotated position than the other leg. During passive movement, resistance to external rotation

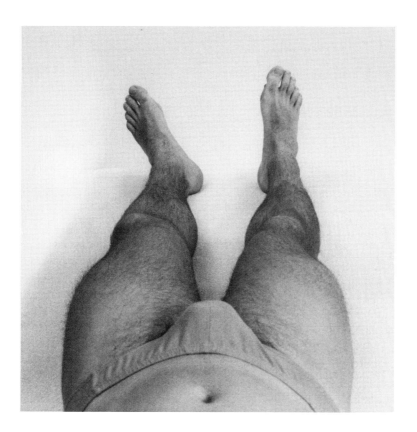

Figure 13–52

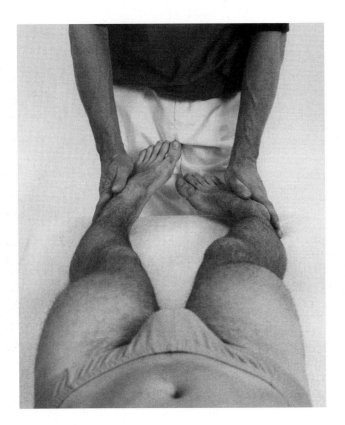

Figure 13–53

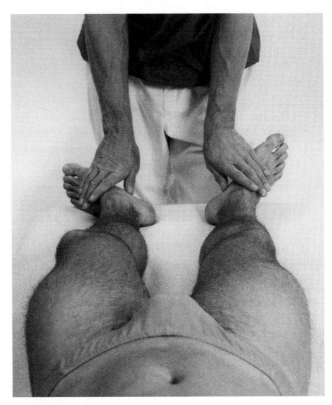

Figure 13–54

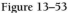

will occur later and resistance to internal rotation earlier than in the other hip joint.

Remarks: A difference in rotation position can indicate posterior rotation in the one joint or anterior rotation in the other. The passive endfeel and the results of additional tests will establish on which side the dysfunction is located.

The results of this test can be judged accurately only if dysfunctions of the hip joint and spine have previously been excluded.

Anterior Innominate Rotation Range of Motion Test

Figures 13–55 and **13–56** illustrate the anterior innominate rotation range of motion test:

Examination position patient: Prone.

Starting position, therapist: Standing at the side of the patient that is not to be examined.

Hand position, therapist: The base of the manipulating hand is placed on the contralateral side on the apex of the

sacrum; the thumb or index finger of the examining hand is placed on the ipsilateral side on the os sacrum against the PIIS.

Procedure: The manipulating hand presses the apex of the sacrum in a ventromedial direction; the examining hand tests the movement between the os sacrum and the PIIS.

Assessment: During this test, the therapist judges the counternutation of the sacroiliac joint.

Remarks: During physiologic movement, the ipsilateral cranial part of the sacrum will move dorsally relative to the PIIS.

Posterior Innominate Rotation Range of Motion Test

Figures 13–57 and **13–58** illustrate the posterior innominate rotation range of motion test:

Examination position, patient: Prone.

Starting position, therapist: Standing beside the patient at the side not being examined.

Hand position, therapist: The manipulating hand encircles the ilium ventrocranially; the thumb or index finger of

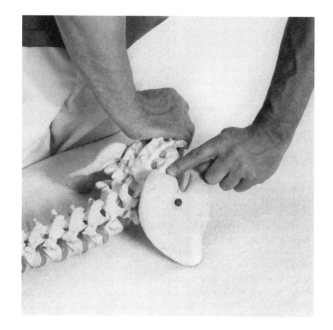

Figure 13–55 $\llcorner$

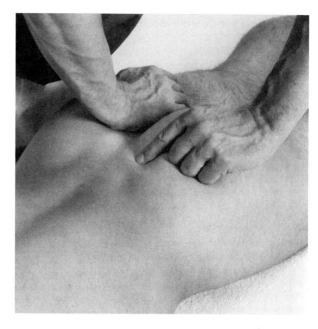

Figure 13–56 $\llcorner$

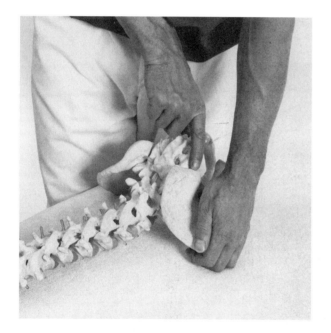

Figure 13–57 $\urcorner$

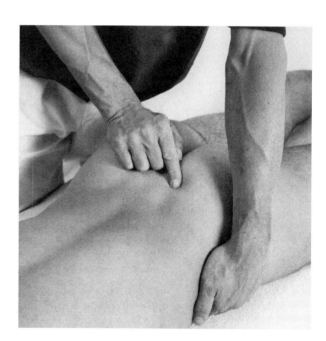

Figure 13–58 $\urcorner$

the examining hand is placed on the ipsilateral side on the sacrum, against the PIIS.

Procedure: The manipulating hand pushes the ilium in a dorsomediocaudal direction; the examining hand tests the movement between the sacrum and the PIIS.

Assessment: This test is used to assess the nutation of the sacroiliac joint.

Remarks: During physiologic movement, the ilium will move in a dorsal direction relative to the cranial ipsilateral part of the sacrum.

Anterior Innominate Rotation Endfeel Test

Figure 13–59 shows the anterior innominate rotation endfeel test:

Examination position, patient: Prone.

Starting position, therapist: Standing beside the patient at the side not being examined.

Hand position, therapist: The restraining hand is placed on the ipsilateral ilium; the base of the hand or the hypothenar of the manipulating hand is placed on the contralateral side, on the apex of the sacrum.

Procedure: The stabilizing hand maintains the position of the ilium; the manipulating hand exerts a ventromedial pressure.

Assessment: The counternutation endfeel is tested in the relevant sacroiliac joint.

Posterior Innominate Rotation Endfeel Test

Figure 13–60 illustrates the posterior innominate rotation endfeel test:

Examination position, patient: Prone.

Starting position, therapist: Standing beside the patient at the side not being examined.

Hand position, therapist: The hypothenar of the stabilizing hand is placed on the ipsilateral side, on the base of the sacrum; the manipulating hand surrounds the ipsilateral ilium ventrocranially.

Procedure: The stabilizing hand maintains the position of the sacrum; the manipulating hand makes a dorsomediocaudal movement.

Assessment: The nutation endfeel is tested in the sacroiliac joint being examined.

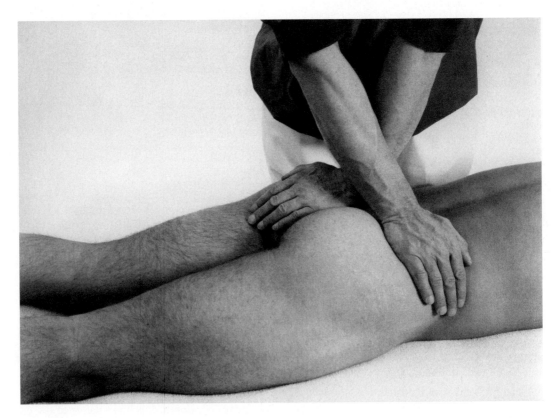

Figure 13–59

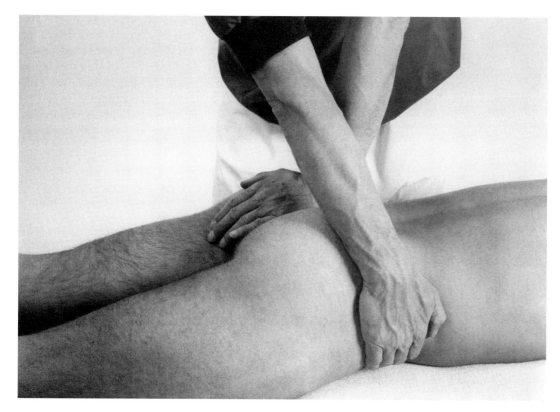

Figure 13–60 ↕

EXAMINATION OF THE PUBIC SYMPHYSIS

The symphysis is a synchondrosis; as such, it has little mobility under normal circumstances. Nevertheless, tensile stresses can arise as a result of pelvic torsion and may lead to irritation in this area. The symphysis sometimes becomes asymmetric following childbirth. A possible consequence of this is inability to stand on one leg.

Asymmetry of the symphyseal synchondrosis can be detected by palpation: the patient stands on both legs and the underside of the symphysis is palpated for unequal height.

Provocation Test

Local Spring Test

Figures 13–61 and **13–62** illustrate the local spring test:

Examination position, patient: Supine.
Starting position, therapist: Standing beside the patient.

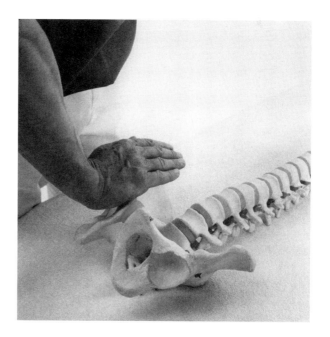

Figure 13–61 ↓

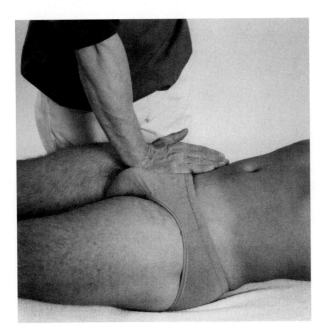

Figure 13–62   ⌐
↓

Hand position, therapist: The hypothenar of the manipulating hand is placed on the ipsilateral side just adjacent to the joint line.

Procedure: The manipulating hand exerts pressure in a dorsal direction.

Assessment: This test is used to test the symphysis for possible dysfunction.

No data are available on the diagnostic accuracy of this test for the diagnosis of symphyseal dysfunction or pathology. However, Maigne et al. (1996) used a gold standard test of 75% or greater reduction of pain with a fluoroscopically guided double sacroiliac joint block. Pain on pressure over the pubic symphysis as a possible indicator of sacroiliac joint dysfunction had no statistically significant association with the gold standard test, and the authors concluded this test was not a useful predictor of sacroiliac joint–related pain.

EXAMINATION OF THE COCCYX

The coccyx forms the distal end of the spine. When patients are being examined because of complaints in the pelvic and lumbar regions, these segments are often neglected. Nevertheless, it is recognized that positional faults in the coccygeal segments, and dysfunctions such as hypo and hypermobility, can lead to problems both local and diffuse in the lumbosacral transitional area.

The function and position of the os coccyx should be examined if there is anything in the history to suggest a possible disorder. A rectal examination is the only way to obtain an accurate result.

Segmental Examination of the Coccyx

Flexion/Extension Test

Figure 13–63 shows the flexion/extension test:

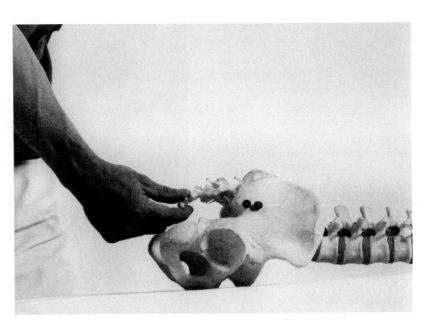

Figure 13–63   ↑ ↓

Examination position, patient: On all fours.

Starting position, therapist: Standing behind the patient.

Hand position, therapist: The gloved index finger of the manipulating hand is introduced into the rectum and placed against the ventral side of the coccygeal bone. The thumb of the same hand is placed on the dorsal side of the bone.

Procedure: The therapist moves the coccygeal bone between his or her thumb and index finger in a ventrodorsal direction.

Assessment: This test is used to assess the position and function of the coccygeal bone.

INSTABILITY EXAMINATION OF THE SACROILIAC JOINT

Significant History Items

- Clinical observations have provided the following history findings as potential indicators of sacroiliac joint instability:
- Posture-dependent pain around the symphysis
- Pain on jolting movements
- Pain when walking, cycling, or sitting
- Increase in pain after an active day
- Pain when standing on one leg
- Inability to stand on one leg
- Increase in pain when running or negotiating stairs
- Increased pain during menses
- Pain during sexual intercourse

Clinical Signs

In addition to the preceding history findings, clinical instability of the sacroiliac joint can also be suspected based on positive findings on the following tests.

Active Straight Leg Raise (ASLR) Test to 5°

The result of the ASLR test is positive if the movement is impossible or painful. (See **Figure 13–64**.) The test can be repeated with a sacroiliac stabilizing belt; this should make it less provocative.

Mens et al. (1999) studied the construct validity of the active straight leg raise test (ASLR) as a test for pelvic joint instability. Using a 4-point rating scale going from no restriction to inability to raise the leg, 21 nonpregnant women with mainly asymmetric peripartum pelvic pain and impaired ASLR were tested with the ASLR test, the same

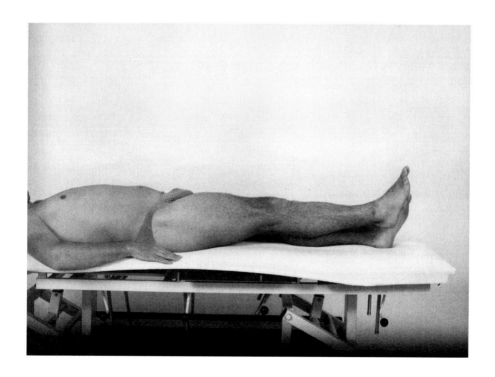

Figure 13–64

test after application of a pelvic belt fastened around the pelvic girdle, and a radiograph as described by Chamberlain. Application of a pelvic belt reduced impairment in 20 patients (significant at $P = 0.0000$). Of 21 patients, 17 had a greater step on standing on the reference side than on the symptomatic side on radiograph and 4 had an equal step (significant at $P = .01$). The authors suggested that the step visible on a radiograph was the result of an anterior innominate rotation on the symptomatic side and proposed a correlation between impaired ASLR and mobility of the pelvic joints in patients with peripartum pelvic girdle pain. Damen et al. (2002) studied the predictive validity of the ASLR test for postpartum pregnancy-related pelvic pain (PRPP). The ASLR test yielded a sensitivity of 76.9%, a specificity of 55.2%, a positive predictive value of 60.6%, a negative predictive value of 66.7%, and a relative risk of 2.4.

Adductor Test

In patients with pelvic problems, the adductor muscles are weakened and the adductor test (**Figure 13–65a–d**) of-

ten causes pain. In healthy persons, the strength of the adductors is roughly equal to that of the abductors. The result of the test is positive if there is a clear difference in strength between the two.

Mens et al. (2002) reported an intra- and interrater ICC of 0.79 for measuring adduction strength in patients with posterior pelvic pain since pregnancy using a handheld dynamometer. Hip adduction strength also correlated strongly with other measures of disease severity and its responsiveness with a standardized response mean of 0.93 was high, making it a sensitive indicator for improvement in this patient group. Somewhat questioning the assertion that in healthy subjects abduction and adduction strength are similar is the fact that pain on hip abduction has been shown to occur in patients with sacroiliac joint dysfunction: Broadhurst and Bond (1998) used a gold standard test of 70% or 90% reduction of pain after a fluoroscopically guided double-blind sacroiliac joint block. Sensitivity and specificity of the resisted abduction test were 87% and 100% at the 70% criterion and 65% and 100% at the 90% criterion.

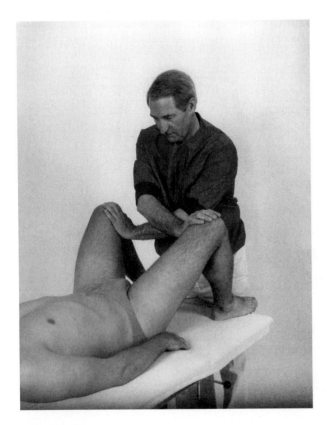

Figure 13–65a

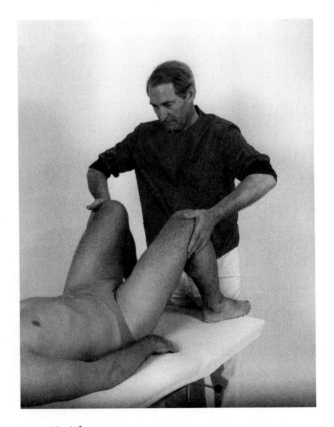

Figure 13–65b

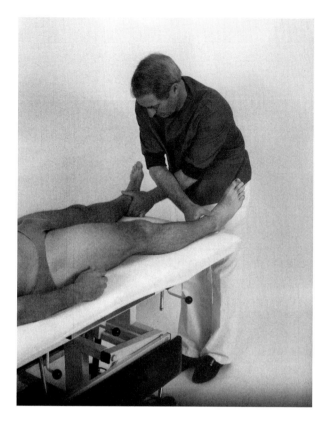

Figure 13–65c

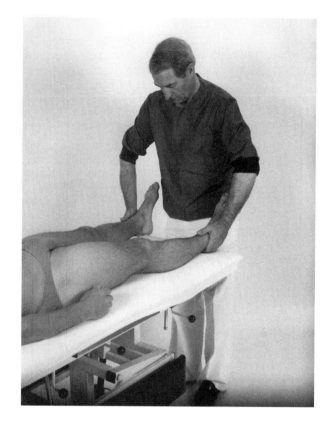

Figure 13–65d

Internal/External Rotation Test

For the internal/external rotation test (**Figure 13–66a and b**), the patient is asked to perform internal and external rotation against the resistance exerted by the therapist. If this is painful or impossible, the test is regarded as positive.

Maigne et al. (1996) used a gold standard test of 75% or greater reduction of pain with a fluoroscopically guided initial and subsequent confirmatory sacroiliac joint block. Pain on resisted external rotation of the hip had no statistically significant association with the gold standard test, and the authors concluded this test was not a useful indicator of SIJ-related pain.

Axial Compression or Thigh Thrust Test

For the axial compression test (**Figure 13–67**), the patient lies supine with the hip joint flexed through 90°. The therapist exerts axial pressure on the pelvis via the thigh. If this pressure causes pain, the test result is positive.

Also known as the thigh thrust test, this test has been studied by various authors. Laslett and Williams (1994) reported 94.1% interrater agreement (κ = 0.88). Dreyfuss et al. (1996) reported 82% interrater agreement (κ = 0.64). Using a gold standard test of 90–100% reduction in pain after a fluoroscopically guided sacroiliac joint block, these authors also reported a sensitivity of 0.36 and a specificity of 0.50. Broadhurst and Bond (1998) used a gold standard test of 70% or 90% reduction of pain after a fluoroscopically guided double-blind sacroiliac joint block. The sensitivity and specificity of the thigh thrust test were 80% and 100% at the 70% criterion; at 90%, they were 69% and 100%, respectively. Albert et al. (2000) found 91% (κ = 0.70) interrater agreement. Kokmeyer et al. (2002) reported 88.46% interrater agreement (κ = 0.69, 95% CI: 0.51–0.88). Damen et al. (2002) studied the predictive validity of the thigh thrust test for postpartum pregnancy-related pelvic pain. The thigh thrust test yielded a sensitivity of 61.5%; a specificity of 72.4%; a positive predictive value of 66.7%; a negative predictive value of 67.7%; and a relative risk ratio of 2.1.

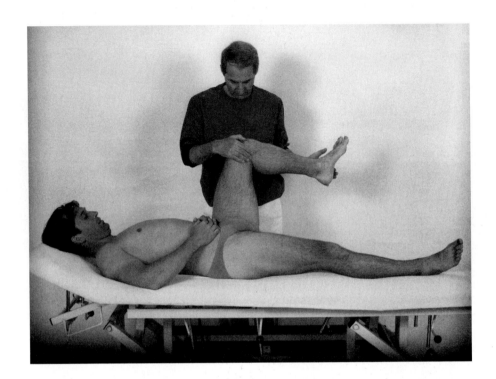

Figure 13–66a

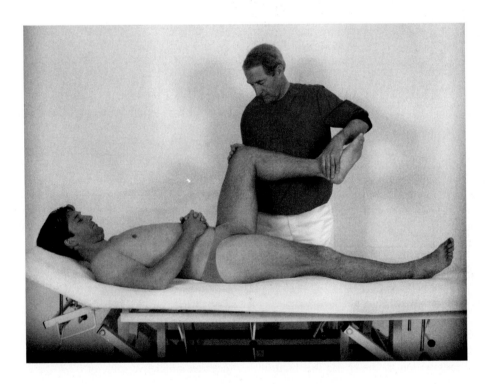

Figure 13–66b

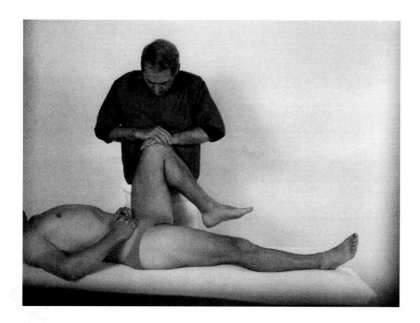

Figure 13–67

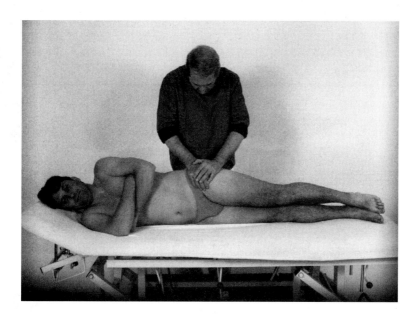

Figure 13–68

Gapping Test

For the gapping test (**Figure 13–68**), the patient lies on his or her side and the therapist exerts pressure on the ventral side of the iliac crest. If this causes pain, the test result is positive.

Bend-Stretch or Pelvic Torsion Test

For the bend-stretch test (**Figure 13–69**), the patient is asked to bend one leg as far as possible while extending the other leg. If this movement cannot be performed correctly or if it is painful, the test result is positive.

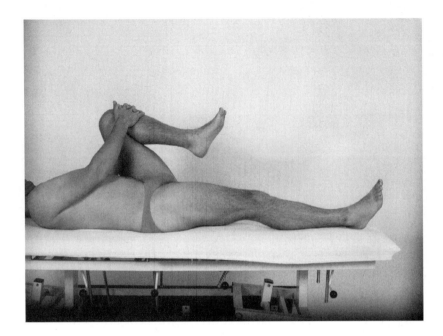

Figure 13–69

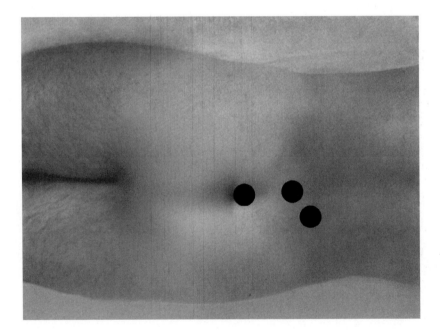

Figure 13–70

This test is also known as the pelvic torsion or Gaenslen test. Laslett and Williams (1994) reported 88.2% interrater agreement (κ = 0.72–0.75). Dreyfuss et al. (1996) reported 85% interrater agreement (κ = 0.61). Using a gold standard test of 90–100% reduction in pain after a fluoroscopically guided sacroiliac joint block, these authors also reported a sensitivity of 0.71 and a specificity of 0.26. Kokmeyer et al. (2002) reported 89.74% interrater agreement (κ = 0.58, 95% CI: 0.32–0.88).

Sacral Ligament Test

For the sacral ligament test (**Figure 13–70**), the patient lies prone and the therapist exerts pressure on the base of the sacrum, the apex of the sacrum, and the iliolumbar ligaments. If this causes pain, the test result is positive.

Knee Flexion Test

For the knee flexion test (**Figure 13–71**), the patient is asked to let one knee go slack, and to alternate the knees. If this is impossible or causes pain, the test result is positive.

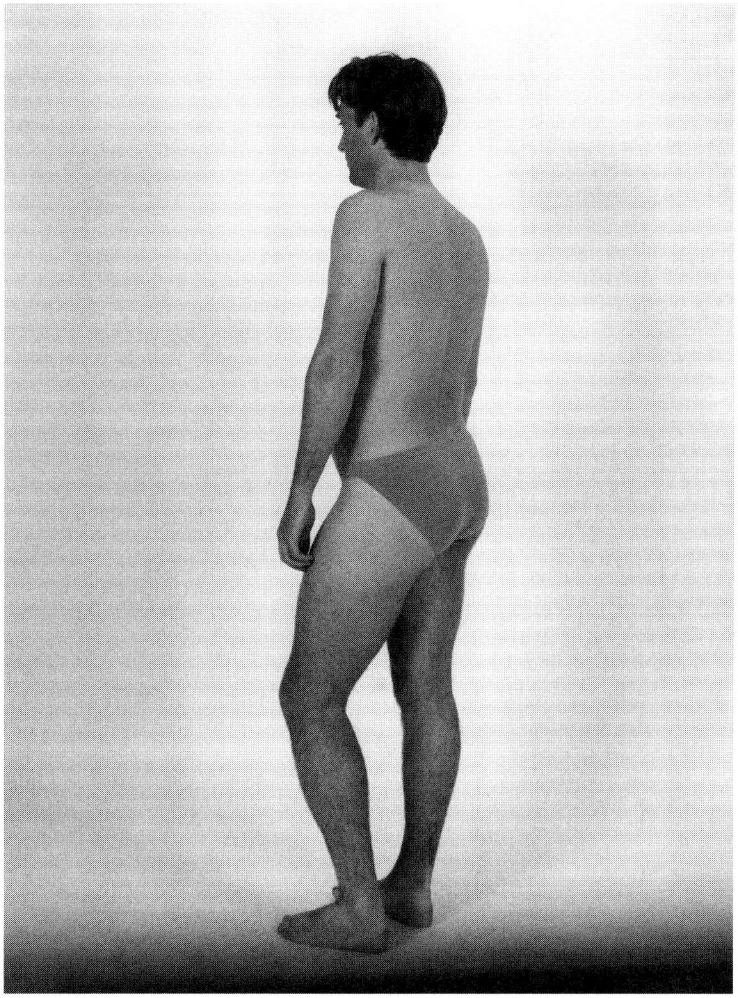

Figure 13–71

CHAPTER 14

Examination of the Lumbar Spine

THE LUMBAR SPINE: T(11)12–S1

Prior to discussing the actual techniques used for examination of the lumbar spine we need to review anatomical, biomechanical, functional, and neurological information pertinent to the lumbar spine.

Functional Features of the Lumbar Spine

The height of the disks in the lumbar spine is on average a third that of the vertebral body. The height increases from L1 to L4, whereas the L5–S1 disk is somewhat lower and wedge-shaped. The height of the disk is related to the extent of possible movement. The position of the vertebral body and the intervertebral articular processes are also functionally important to the movement mechanism.

Putz (1981) made measurements of all the vertebrae in different regions; these are useful for an understanding of function. The average measures for the lumbar spine are (**Figure 14–1**):

Angle of inclination (α): L1 = 82.5°, L2 = 82.5°, L3 = 85°, L4 = 85°, S1 = 87.5°

Opening angle (β): L1 = 25°, L2 = 10°, L3 = 25°, L4 = 35°, L5 = 50°, S1 = 90°

Transverse plane distance: The distance between the articular surfaces of the superior articular processes (a): L1 = 26 mm, L2 = 27 mm, L3 = 29 mm, L4 = 31 mm, L5 = 34.5 mm, S1 = 44 mm

Sagittal plane distance: The distance of the articular surfaces of the superior articular processes to the center of the as-

sociated vertebra (b): L1 = 46 mm, L2 = 47 mm, L3 = 46.5 mm, L4 = 46 mm, L5 = 42 mm

The standard deviation reported by Putz (1981) is not provided in this book.

A common characteristic of the vertebrae belonging to the lumbar region is the special shape of the intervertebral joint surfaces. These consist of a more frontal and a more sagittal area. The intervertebral joint surfaces in the sagittal direction somewhat converge ventrally, but the sagittal parts converge less than the frontal parts do. The sagittal parts also converge in a caudal direction. The frontal part shows a slight ventral inclination in a caudocranial direction. During movement, the articular surfaces do not remain parallel to each other because the joint surfaces of the superior articular processes are larger than those of the inferior articular processes. The intervertebral surfaces are congruent only in certain circumstances, for instance, when the body is in the normal upright standing position. The sacrum forms the base of the lumbar region from which the center of the upper surface of the S1 body, together with the centers of its superior articular processes, form a supporting surface that is almost an equilateral triangle. Its ability to absorb forces is great because of its large opening angle.

Flexion

A significant degree of flexion is possible in the thoracolumbar and the lumbosacral transitional areas (**Figure 14–2**). In the area between these two, the capacity for movement is lower (Putz, 1981). Other authors give different values. From a normal starting position, flexion is

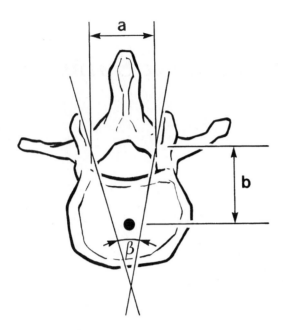
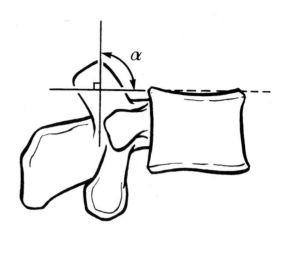

Figure 14–1   Characteristic parameters of the lumbar vertebra.

greater than extension. During flexion, a minimal ventral translation occurs between adjacent vertebrae. The inferior articular processes move in a cranioventral direction relative to the superior articular processes.

The average flexion–extension axis of rotation in this spinal region is located inferiorly within the disk, somewhat dorsal to the center (Reichmann, 1972; Seroo and Penning,

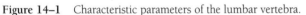
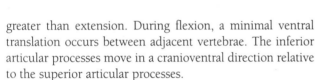
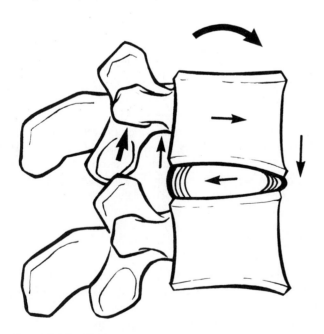

Figure 14–2   Flexion.

1981). During the movement, "gapping" of the intervertebral joint space occurs (Reichmann, Berglund, and Lindgren, 1972). Even during the initial phase of flexion, contact no longer occurs in the dorsal part of the intervertebral joint space. This increases the pressure in the more frontal part. The displacement of the nucleus pulposus is slight; it increases in height dorsally and decreases ventrally.

The oblique outer fibers of the annulus fibrosus that run in the direction of movement, especially the dorsolateral ones, come under tension, while those that run in the opposite direction, especially the ventrolateral ones, relax. The joint capsule is also under tension, especially the reinforcing fibers and the dorsal ligamentous structure, whereas the anterior longitudinal ligament, which lies ventral to the axis of rotation, relaxes. The posterior longitudinal ligament, despite having fibers that branch obliquely toward the base of the vertebral arches, offers insufficient support to the dorsal fibers of the annulus fibrosus.

In the end phase of flexion, the tops of the joint surfaces of the inferior articular processes slide over the cranial edge of the joint surfaces of the superior articular processes of the vertebra below in such a way that a narrow contact area remains. This is the fulcrum of the prevailing moments.

Because of their more frontal position and their large angles of inclination, the front parts of the intervertebral joints absorb the greater part of the flexion forces. Transmission of forces by the intervertebral joint bodies, which involves significant widening of the intervertebral joint space in a caudodorsal direction, is limited primarily by the interspinous

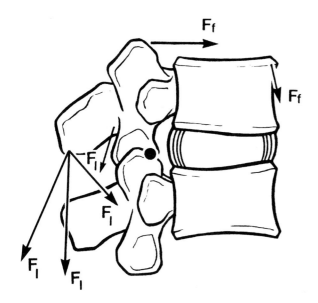

Figure 14–3   Balance of forces.

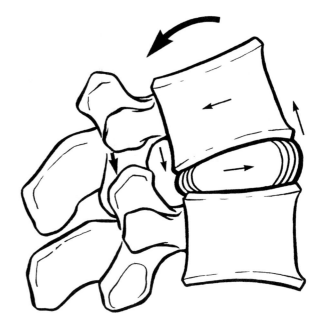

Figure 14–4   Extension.

ligament. The ligamentous forces (F_l) must balance the flexion forces (F_f) (**Figure 14–3**).

The fibers of the interspinous ligament run in an S shape from the base of the spinous process of a lower vertebra to the top of the spinous process of the vertebra above. This means that these fibers will only be stretched when the spinous processes have moved a certain distance apart. Because they are attached caudally to the base of the lower spinous process, the dorsal moment arm is shortened during the end phase and the pressure on the contact area of the intervertebral joint surfaces is increased. The average movement trajectory is 40° (Kapandji, 1974). According to G. S. Tanz (Kapandji, 1974), the segmental distribution of movement in the 35–49 year age group is L1–L2: 6°; L2–L3: 8°; L3–L4: 9°; L4–L5: 12°; L5–S1: 8°.

Extension

During extension (**Figure 14–4**), translation occurs in a dorsal direction between the adjacent vertebral bodies. In the end phase, they show a slight step alignment dorsally. The inferior articular processes move in a dorsocaudal direction relative to the superior articular processes. The axis of the movement is located in the same place as for flexion. During extension, the nucleus pulposus shows little displacement, though it increases in height ventrally and decreases dorsally. The oblique outer fibers of the annulus that run in the direction of movement, especially the ventrolateral ones, are tensed, while those that run in the opposite direction, especially the dorsolateral ones, relax. The liga-

mentous structure that lies dorsal to the axis of movement also relaxes.

In the end phase of extension, the tops of the inferior articular processes slide somewhat over the caudodorsal edge of the superior articular processes. At the same time, the intervertebral joint spaces widen in the cranioventral direction. When strong forces are applied, or when the opening angle of the superior/inferior articular processes approaches zero, the reinforcing fibers often offer insufficient resistance. The tops of the inferior articular processes are then pressed into the grooves that border the joint surfaces of the superior articular processes. These grooves often occur in the lordotic spinal regions. They are covered by the synovial membrane and filled with nonrigid material that, however, is not suited to absorbing pressure.

When the opening angle is zero, the contact between the intervertebral articular surfaces that are approximating each other can come to a standstill with a sudden jolt. If the opening angle is more than zero—that is, if the intervertebral articular surfaces are not in a purely sagittal position—then part of the pressure can be transferred in the end phase to the dorsal parts of the intervertebral articular surfaces.

According to Reichmann (1971a, 1972), the end position in which the tops of the intervertebral joint surfaces end in the grooves is normal in extension. At the same time, all the fibers that are capable of limiting extension must be fully tensed. Among these are the annular fibers, the reinforcing fibers of the capsule, the anterior longitudinal ligament, and the interspinous ligament (F_l). Because of its

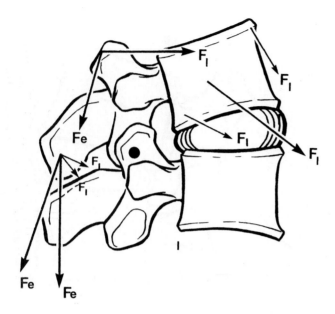

Figure 14–5 Balance of forces.

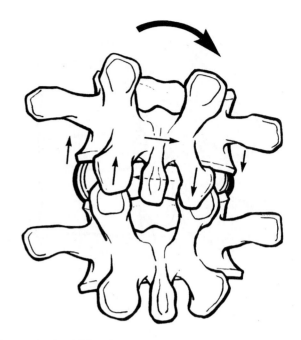

Figure 14–6 Sidebending.

S-shaped upward course in a dorsal and cranial direction, the interspinous ligament is stretched during dorsal translation. The forces that limit extension must balance those that cause it (**Figure 14–5**).

A jerk-like limitation of extension by the tops of the inferior articular processes in the bony grooves exerts a bending stress on the caudal vertebral arch, primarily in the area of the isthmus. This has given rise to new theories about the development of spondylolysis. Runge and Zippel (1976) maintain that structural changes in the vertebral arch are responsible for the development of spondylolysis in adults. A number of investigations have suggested that these changes are caused and maintained by microtrauma. The total extent of extension is about 30° (Kapandji, 1974). The greatest movement has been measured at the level of L4–L5. The extent of movement decreases toward the cranial end.

Sidebending

A greater degree of sidebending (**Figure 14–6**) is possible in the thoracolumbar transition and the upper lumbar vertebrae than in the lower lumbar vertebrae. The segment that is most limited with regard to movement is the lumbosacral transitional segment. The reason for this is the relative width of the load-bearing triangle and the rigid fixation by the iliolumbar ligaments (Lumsden and Morris, 1968).

Sidebending is possible because the dorsal parts of the intervertebral articular surfaces are generally not in a fully sagittal position, and they often have groove-shaped con-

cavities. Even a small caudal convergence of the intervertebral joint space creates the play needed for sidebending. This increases during simultaneous flexion. Movement in the sagittal plane also causes a wedge-shaped widening of the intervertebral joint space (Reinhardt, 1963). During the course of the movement, there is a forced rotation in the motion segments that, according to Putz (1981), is in the direction of the sidebending (in the neutral and flexion positions). The axis of sagittal plane sidebending, which is situated in the middle of the disk, during the end phase equals the line joining the concave-side edge of the disk and the associated intervertebral joint.

During the movement, the nucleus pulposus shows little displacement. It increases in height on the convex side and decreases on the concave side. The outer oblique fibers that run in the direction of movement, especially those on the ventral and dorsal convex sides, are tensed, while those that run contrary to the direction of movement, especially at the ventral and dorsal concave sides, relax. On the concave side, the vertebral bodies approach each other, while on the convex side they move away from each other. The articular surfaces approximate each other on the concave side and move away from each other on the convex side. The capsular reinforcing fibers come under increasing tension because of the opposing displacement of the intervertebral joint surfaces.

The ligamentous structures (F_1) that lie to the convex side of the axis, such as the intertransverse ligaments, the anterior and posterior longitudinal ligaments, and the flaval ligaments, are also stretched. These ligamentous forces must balance the forces (F_s) that cause sidebending (**Figure 14–7**).

In the end phase, the axis that lies along a line joining the concave-side edge of the disk and the associated vertebral joint determines the length of the moment arm. In this phase, locking occurs through combined boney and ligamentous restriction.

During sidebending and in the starting position for extension, if the opening angle is zero, pure boney restriction can occur in the intervertebral joint. This is supported by the bony edges of these joints.

Groove-shaped concavities in the lateral parts of the joint surfaces of the superior articular processes often permit sidebending, during which the capsular fibers that run in a transverse direction and the outer oblique fibers of the annulus fibrosus are placed under tensile stress.

The forced rotation that occurs during sidebending in a flexion position can be explained in terms of the intervertebral articular surfaces and the position of the more anterior sloping position of the frontal parts. The rotation takes place in the concave direction. The forced rotation that occurs before the end phase of sidebending while in an extension position is explained by the transverse pressure on the most dorsal parts of the intervertebral joint surfaces. This pressure opposes sidebending. Since the intervertebral joint surfaces diverge in a dorsal direction, the rotation will be in the convex direction.

Rotation

Opinions differ about whether the lumbar spine is capable of rotation. According to Sieglbauer (1958), it is not. Braus and Elze (1954) and Heine (1957) detected minimal movement. Later researchers, for example, Gregersen and Lucas (1967), Lumsden and Morris (1968), and Putz (1981), found that in a standing position, rotation of 3° to 7° per segment is possible. Rotation is possible only if the intervertebral joint surfaces can move away from each other (**Figure 14–8**).

The lateral parts of the joints of the superior and inferior articular processes have an acute opening angle that faces backward and converge caudally to some extent. When translating sagittally (during flexion), the caudal intervertebral joint surfaces of the upper vertebra move in a ventrocranial direction, and the intervertebral joint space widens, which increases the capability for the segment to rotate.

In the lumbosacral motion segment, which has an opening angle of about 90°, there is a significant increase in rotational capability during flexion. According to Kapandji (1974), the axis of upper lumbar rotation is located centrally at the level of the dorsal side of the intervertebral joints, whereas the axis of low lumbar rotation is at the level of the base of the spinous process. The translation component of the lower lumbar spine is, therefore, greater than that of the upper lumbar spine. During rotation, the contralateral joint surface of the inferior articular process will

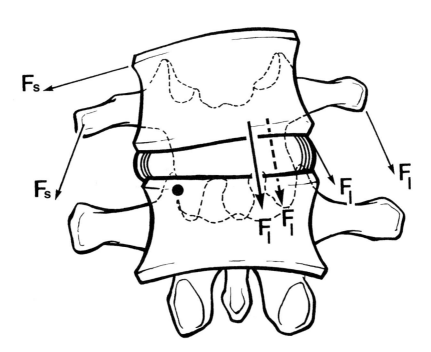

Figure 14–7 Balance of forces.

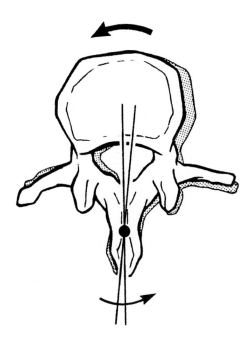

Figure 14–8   Rotation.

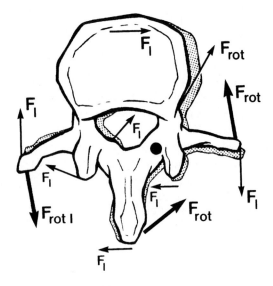

Figure 14–9   Balance of forces.

move in a ventral direction, and the ipsilateral one in a dorsal direction. The disk is exposed to a degree of central compressive force, although there is a small amount of translation (screw effect).

The oblique outer fibers of the annulus fibrosus that run in the direction of the movement show an increase in tension, while those that run in the opposite direction relax. The compressive force in the intervertebral joint that is contralateral to the direction of movement will increase, as will the tension in the joint capsule and the intertransverse ligaments in the ipsilateral joint.

Tension will also increase in the interspinous and supraspinous ligaments, the anterior/ posterior longitudinal ligaments, and the flaval ligaments. The ligamentous inhibiting forces must balance those that cause rotation (F_{rot}) (**Figure 14–9**).

In the end phase of rotation, considerable force is exerted on the more frontally situated part of the intervertebral joint surface that lies contralateral to the direction of movement. The moments of force use this contact area as a fulcrum. Because the opening angle in the lumbosacral movement segment is about 90°, the dorsoventral pressures can be distributed there over a wider surface area.

Rotation places a bending stress on the parts of the superior articular processes that diverge dorsally, which is expressed in the trabecular morphology resembling a pointed arch. Bending stress in both lateral directions can be absorbed because the reinforcing ligamentous fibers as well as

the muscles are attached to the tops of the intervertebral joint protuberances and the mamillary processes. The particularly strong transverse reinforcing ligamentous fibers in the lumbar region counteract the unilateral dorsal shift that occurs during rotation. As a result there is bending stress in the end position of rotation on both the superior articular processes. Moments are in balance in the end position of rotation because of the compressive forces generated on the one side and the tensile forces exerted on the other.

The total extent of rotation in the lumbar spine varies between 15° and 35°.

Transitional Vertebrae in the Lumbar Region

Thoracolumbar Junction

The thoracic and lumbar parts of the spine have their transition at T(11)12. The superior articular processes are oriented in the same way as in the other thoracic vertebrae, while the inferior ones are oriented in the same manner as in the lumbar vertebrae. The vertebral body is strongly developed in relation to the vertebral arch, which is consistent with its function. There are fewer muscular attachments, and this transitional vertebra functions like a ball bearing between the thoracic and lumbar areas (Delmas as referenced in Kapandji, 1974). Where there is pelvic tilt with resultant scoliosis, this transitional segment often seems to be the point where curve reversal occurs (**Figure 14–10**).

Maigne (1980) directs attention to the important role that dysfunction in the thoracolumbar transitional area can play in lower back complaints. Most low lumbar complaints

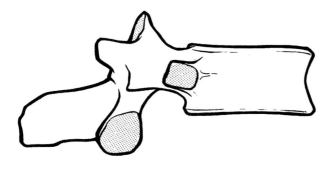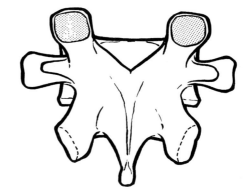

Figure 14–10 Lateral and dorsal view of T12.

can be explained in terms of dysfunctions of local structures; however, Maigne believes that there are low lumbar symptoms for which no cause can be identified in the lumbar region.

Maigne's (1980) clinical experience is that pain in the lumbosacral or gluteal area can be caused by irritation of the dorsal rami of the low thoracic (iliohypogastric) nerve or the first lumbar spinal nerve (ilioinguinal and genitofemoral nerves). The irritation could be caused by dysfunction of the intervertebral joints in the thoracolumbar or first lumbar movement segments (**Figure 14–11**). The dorsal ramus of the spinal nerve splits into a medial and a lateral branch. The medial branch, which is almost completely motor in function, innervates the multifidus, rotator, and interspinal muscles. The lateral branch passes through the lumbar fascia and reaches the skin via the subcutaneous tissues; it ends in the skin of the lower lumbar area and has many anastomoses. The classic view is that the lateral branches of L1–L2 and L3 innervate the skin of the lower lumbar and gluteal areas. The branches from T11–L1 with their anastomoses are also involved.

The following are essential features of lower back complaints caused by dysfunctions in the thoracolumbar junction (Maigne, 1980):

- The point at the iliac crest is a pressure pain point that corresponds to the skin area innervated by the most dorsal branch of the irritated spinal nerve (12th thoracic nerve). Pressure causes a sharp pain. The point, once identified, must be examined symmetrically.

- Positive Kibler or skin rolling test. This test is carried out in the region of the iliac crest and the gluteal muscle. If the area seems thickened and hypersensitive, the test is positive. Here, too, symmetrical comparisons must be made.

- Clear clinical evidence of dysfunction of the segment in question. The segments T11–L5 are provoked vertically and tangentially on both sides via the spinous processes. This test must be positive in the thoracolumbar transitional area.

- Provocation by palpatory pressure on the intervertebral joints. These joints are provoked about 1 cm lateral to the spinous process by exerting pressure. The test must also yield a positive result in the thoracolumbar area.

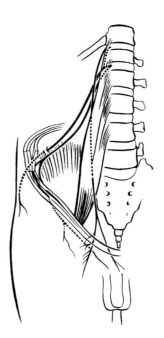

Figure 14–11 Dorsal branches of the spinal nerves in the thoracolumbar region.

- Diagnostic block induced by procaine around the painful intervertebral joint. The block must cause the symptoms to disappear within a few minutes.

Recent studies have indicated that dysfunction of the sympathetic nervous system caused by dysfunction in the thoracolumbar junction produces the same symptoms as those described by Maigne (1980). Furthermore, there are neuroanatomic connections between the segments L1–L5 and T8–T12. If the selectivity of the central nervous system is inadequate, dysfunction in the lower lumbar spine can lead to problems at the level of the thoracolumbar junction. This kind of dysfunction can also lead to the symptoms described by Maigne (1980).

Upper Lumbar–Lower Lumbar Junction

L3 is the junction between the upper and lower lumbar regions. This vertebra is also regarded as a transitional one by Delmas (Kapandji, 1974; Bourdiol, 1980). It is seen as a "relay station" between the cranial and the caudal parts of the spine, and as the first mobile lumbar vertebra in relation to L4 and L5, which are anchored by the iliolumbar ligaments to the two iliac crests. The vertebral arch of L3 is strongly developed because of the muscle attachments that it supports (**Figure 14–12**). Observed from the caudal end, the latissimus dorsi muscle, which stretches from the lumbar fascia and the iliac crest, is attached by a number of fibers to the transverse process of L3. Observed from the cranial end, L3 is the lowest level to which the spinalis muscle inserts. In the standing position, L3 is horizontal and forms the apex of lumbar curvature. In sidebending, it is the deepest point in the concave curve.

Lumbosacral Junction

Finally, L5 forms the important junction between the mobile lumbar spine and the immobile sacrum (**Figures 14–13, 14–14,** and **14–15**). Its shape is congruent with the sloping cranial surface of the sacrum. In a lateral projection, the vertebral body is trapezoid, and the transverse processes are strongly developed. The intervertebral foramen is often smaller than that of the other vertebral segments. The opening angle is generally larger (90°) than that of the other lumbar vertebrae. This is functionally related to the ventrally directed load-bearing component. The strongly developed iliolumbar ligaments, which course between the transverse processes and the crests, are also important in this context, because they act as a buffer between the innominates and the lumbar vertebrae. There is a certain similarity between the lumbosacral junction and the

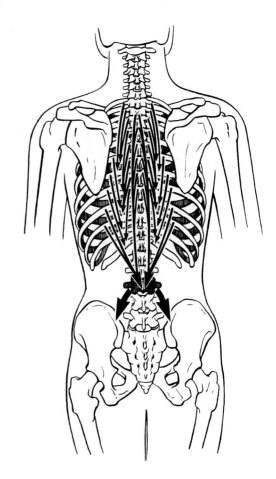

Figure 14–12   Transitional vertebra L3.

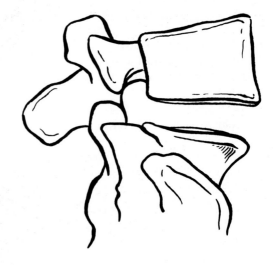

Figure 14–13   Lateral view L5.

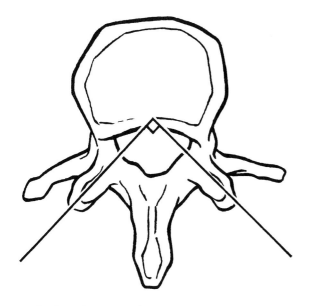

Figure 14–14   Opening angle L5.

cervico-occipital juncton. L5 and the two innominate bones move opposite to the sacrum because they are joined by the iliolumbar ligaments. The same is seen in the upper cervical area: C0 and C2 can move in the opposite direction to C1 because they are joined by the alar ligaments.

The lumbosacral junction, like the cervico-occipital junction, is the area where the most anomalies occur, for example:

- Lumbarization
- Hemisacralization
- Sacralization
- Spondylolysis
- Spondylolisthesis (**Figure 14–16**)
- Abnormalities in the position of the joint facets

Lumbar Segmental Instability

It is estimated that 20–30% of patients with lower back complaints have segmental instability (White and Panjabi, 1990). However, definitions of *segmental instability* and *clinical segmental instability* vary a good deal in the literature (White and Panjabi, 1990; Frymoyer, 1996, Manabu et al., 1993). Before discussing the views of some leading researchers on segmental instability and relating them to manual diagnosis, it will be useful to provide a short overview of the stabilizing factors in the lumbosacral region.

The functional spinal unit (FSU) is the smallest functional unit of the spine that has the same biomechanical functions as the whole spinal column (Keessen, 1988). The

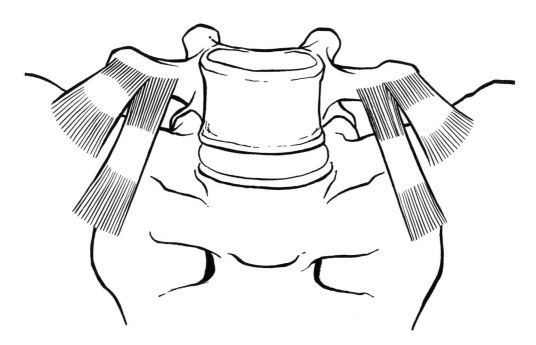

Figure 14–15   Iliolumbar ligaments.

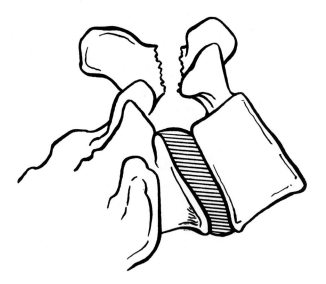

Figure 14–16   Spondylolisthesis L5.

FSU of the lumbosacral region is formed by the body of S1, the superior articular processes of S1, the body of L5, the inferior articular processes of L5, the intervertebral disk L5–S1, and all the ligamentous structures that run between L5 and S1. The stability of the L5–S1 FSU depends heavily on the position of the sacrum and the body of L5. A high assimilation pelvis is less stable than a strained pelvis. Under normal circumstances, stability is ensured by the mainly frontally positioned facet joints and by the strong lumbosacral ligamentous system, in which the iliolumbar ligaments are the most important stabilizing component. In the first 10 years of life, the iliolumbar ligament is part of the lumbar quadratus muscle and consists mainly of contractile elements. Around the 10th year, the dorsocaudal part of this muscle changes into very strong collagenous connective tissue, which is then called the iliolumbar ligament. Research findings indicate that this ligament is thicker and has a higher stiffness modulus in people who have a more horizontally oriented sacrum.

The intervertebral disk L5–S1 is wedge-shaped in the sagittal plane. It provides little contribution to lumbosacral stability. The intervertebral disk of L4–L5, which is significantly thicker than that of L5–S1, has a more important stabilizing role. The endplates of the L4–L5 disk lie more or less in the transverse plane. The annular fibers that stretch between them must withstand significant traction during all physiologic movements; this affects one part more than the other. In people with a high assimilation pelvis, the L4–L5 disk lies outside the pelvic girdle. In these people, the stability of L4–L5 FSU is at greater risk than in people with a more horizontally oriented sacrum. Active stability is provided by the muscles of the back and abdomen, and the muscles that extend from the pelvis to the lower limbs. In this context the most important muscles are the multifidus and the oblique and transverse abdominal muscles attached to the thoracolumbar fascia.

Lumbar Segmental Instability/Clinical Lumbar Segmental Instability

In 1944, Knutsson described a relationship between degeneration of the lumbar disk and an increase in translation during extension and flexion. The increase in translation during these movements was noted on X-rays. Knutsson's publication of his findings was the start of a long series of studies and publications on the topic of lumbar instability.

There is no consensus on the diagnosis of lumbar instability or on appropriate therapies. Pope and Panjabi (1985) describe the concept of instability using the terminology of physics: they speak of "stable balance" or "unstable balance" (**Figure 14–17**). The absence of adequate stabilizing factors in the spine results, according to Pope and Panjabi, in a labile or unstable balance.

Pope and Panjabi's description is not consistent with present-day biomechanical insights and current knowledge of the pathokinesiology of the spine. The whole of the spine, or a functional part of it (FSU), can be in stable balance in some instantaneous positions and in labile balance in others.

White and Panjabi (1990) defined clinical instability as follows: "Clinical instability is the loss of the ability of the spine under physiologic loads to maintain its pattern of displacement so that there is no initial or additional neurological deficit, no major deformity, and no incapacitating pain." Following further research, they produced a definition of clinical segmental instability: "Clinical instability is defined as a significant decrease in the capacity of the stabilizing system of the spine to maintain the intervertebral neutral zones within the physiologic limits so that there is no neurological dysfunction, no major deformity, and no incapacitating pain."

Although White and Panjabi's (1990) definitions are frequently quoted and seem to be generally accepted in orthopaedic medicine, they are not useful in a clinical setting. They do not address the fact that instability can exist in an FSU without the associated clinical symptoms. Furthermore, "major deformity" and "incapacitating pain" are difficult to quantify. The authors offer no basis for defining objective parameters that would make their definition clinically useful.

Gertzbein et al. (1984) and Weiler et al. (1990) introduced the concept of instantaneous centers of rotation. These are determined from a series of lateral X-rays taken in a variety of positions involving flexion and extension. They calculated the so-called centrode by mathematical addition of the instantaneous centers of rotation. An abnormal cen-

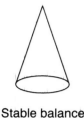
Stable balance

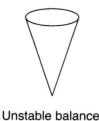
Unstable balance

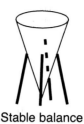
Stable balance

Figure 14–17   Stable balance; unstable balance; stable balance.

trode pattern was thought to indicate instability. The method was tried on cadavers and then adapted for use in vivo. Because of major measurement errors, the centrode patterns proved difficult to determine and interpret in the in vivo situation (Weiler et al.). Because the measuring of centrodes was not clinically useful, other measurement methods were introduced. Weiler et al. introduced the instability factor (IF). This is defined as the total translation between maximum extension and maximum flexion, divided by the total angulation between maximal extension and maximal flexion, expressed in mm/rad (millimeters per radian):

$$IF = \text{total translation/total angulation (mm/rad)}$$

The authors examined 36 patients with chronic low back problems and 12 healthy controls. The diagnoses in the patient group were idiopathic low back pain, lumbar disk prolapse, and degenerative disk disease. The findings were that the IF in patients with degenerative conditions of the lumbar disk was significantly greater than in the healthy controls. No significant differences were found between the group of patients with idiopathic low back pain and the group with a lumbar disk prolapse.

The definition of the instability factor offered by Weiler et al. (1990) appears to be clinically useful. It does not involve the *clinical symptomatology,* which means that it can be used in the context of both *clinical* and *nonclinical* instability. However, Weiler bases his method on objectively calculable parameters, which means that it is not suitable for use in the manual therapy clinical situation: it is not desirable to X-ray every patient who might be suffering from lumbar instability. The diagnosis of pathophysiology by radiographic means is not acceptable because of the relatively high radiation dose involved.

The Association for Education in Manual Therapy in Amersfoort has sought definitions of lumbar segmental instability and clinical lumbar segmental instability that could be used in manual diagnosis and manual therapy. In addition to the material found in the literature, the following considerations were taken into account:

- Instability of the FSU should be central to the definition because the FSU is the smallest functional unit that has the same biomechanical properties as the whole spinal column. It is also the specific starting point for manual therapy. The term chosen was *lumbar segmental instability,* whereby *segmental* is used as a synonym for FSU, borrowed from Junghanns's concept of spinal motion segment.

- A distinction is made between lumbar segmental instability and clinical lumbar segmental instability. The latter is used where there is a lower back complaint in which the instability plays an important part. The two terms are defined as follows:

  Lumbar segmental instability is the occurrence during physiologic postures and/or movements of a pathologic increase in transverse, and/or sagittal, and/or frontal translation motility of the upper vertebra relative to the one beneath it in a lumbar motion segment as a result of a nonphysiologic position of the IAR (instantaneous axis of rotation).

  Clinical lumbar segmental instability is the complex of disturbances and limitations of which a patient complains as a result of a nonphysiologic position of the IAR of a lumbar motion segment in the presence of reduced local, general, and/or spinal segment load-bearing capacity.

Classification of Lumbar Segmental Instability According to Cause

Frymoyer (1996) gives the following classification of types of lumbar segmental instability:

- Fractures.
- Infections affecting the ventral vertebral column. This refers to progressive decrease in the height of the vertebral body as a result of infection.
- Primary tumors and metastases.
- Spondylolisthesis. A distinction is made here between the isthmic spondylolisthesis and L4–L5 deformities.

- Degenerative instability.
- Scoliosis.

Of Frymoyer's (1996) types of lumbar segmental instability, degenerative instability, and, to some extent, isthmic spondylolisthesis belong to the range of dysfunctions for which manual therapy is indicated. Because degenerative instability occurs more frequently, it is described in more detail.

Degenerative Lumbar Segmental Instability

A distinction is made between primary forms of degenerative lumbar instability and secondary forms. Primary forms arise as a result of normal and pathologic aging. Secondary forms are caused by invasive procedures such as diskectomy, laminectomy, spondylodesis, and chemonucleolysis. The risk of the secondary form will probably become lower as the use of lumbar microsurgery increases. Frymoyer (1996) distinguishes the following forms of primary lumbar segmental instability:

- Axial rotatory instability
- Translatory rotatory instability
- Retrolisthesis
- Progressive degenerative scoliosis
- Disk disruption

Frymoyer (1996) appears to be using both pathophysiologic criteria (first two) and pathomorphologic criteria (last three).

The literature contains descriptions of many causal factors involved in lumbar segmental instability and clinical lumbar segmental instability. Degeneration of the lumbar motion segment, trauma, and pathophysiologic factors are all given as causes. Degenerative processes and pathophysiologic changes in the lumbar spine are discussed as etiological factors. Trauma as a cause is not discussed here because the consequences of trauma to the lumbar area are not part of the primary focus of manual therapy.

Degeneration of Lumbar Motion Segments

Kirkaldy-Willis (1982) described three phases in the degenerative process:

- The dysfunction phase
- The unstable phase
- The stabilization phase

Dysfunction Phase   Kirkaldy-Willis states that degeneration takes place simultaneously in the disk and in the facet joints. These two kinds of degeneration form the starting point for his description of pathomorphologic and pathophysiologic processes.

Nonspecific low back complaints are typical of the dysfunction phase. These complaints are dependent on posture and movement, but cannot be evoked by specific postures, movements, or loads. At the beginning of the dysfunction phase, the multifidus muscle is clearly hypertonic. This painful hypertonicity imposes a nonphysiologic load on the intervertebral disk and the facet joints. Kirkaldy-Willis describes changes in the disk and facet joints as the degeneration proceeds. The annular fibers of the disk show decreased resistance to tensile forces; later, the annular material may tear. At the same time, the cartilage in the facet joints becomes weaker, resulting ultimately in a reduction of the thickness of the joint cartilage and a slackening of the joint capsule.

Unstable Phase   The clinical picture is more specific during the unstable phase. By now, the disk has lost its stabilizing capacity and the joint capsule offers insufficient resistance to external forces. The result is an abnormal position and/or abnormal movements of the upper vertebra of the FSU relative to the one below it. This is known as degenerative spondylolisthesis. There may also be a progressive increase in translation of the upper vertebra, both in adorsal and ventral direction. Degenerative spondylolisthesis is three to six times more common in women than in men (Brown, 1983). According to Brown, the L4–L5 FSU is affected in 80% of cases; Frymoyer (1991), however, says that L5–S1 is the motion segment most commonly affected. Degenerative spondylolisthesis is seldom found in people under the age of 50.

Stabilization Phase   The stabilization phase is the body's reaction to instability. It is marked by sclerotic formations in the endplates, increased flattening of the disk, and the appearance of osteophytes growing from the facet joints and the vertebral body. The whole process of degeneration of the lumbar region can be symptom-free. However, during the instability phase, the load-bearing capacity of the region is so low that clinical signs are extremely probable. It may result, for instance, in a protrusion or prolapse of the disk.

Pathophysiologic Factors Involved in the Development of Lumbar Segmental Instability

Displacement of the Instantaneous Axis of Rotation   A number of authors believe that displacement of the instantaneous axis of rotation (IAR) in both the sagittal and the transverse planes is an etiological factor (Weiler et al., 1990; Gertzbein et al., 1984; Manabu et al., 1993). The changed position of the IAR is thought to lead to changes in the loading of the connective tissue structures that control the FSU, such as the annular fibers of the intervertebral disk and the longitudinal ligaments. During movements involving flexion or extension, for example, the inadequate physiologic processing of forces and moments is thought to change the movement of the upper vertebra relative to the lower one. The shift in the IAR also leads to changes in arthrokinetic reflex activity (Stokes et al., 1988). These reflexes can be described as spinal and supraspinal reflex activities initiated by stimulation of mechanoreceptors in and around the joint capsules of the facet joints. The arthrokinetic reflexes are responsible for the fine control of tension in the paravertebral muscles during active movements of the spine. A change in the movement path of the upper vertebra relative to the one below leads to nonphysiologic stimulation of the mechanoreceptors in and around the fibrous capsules of the spinal joints. The result is a change in muscle contraction patterns.

Local Muscle Fatigue and Emotional Factors   Local muscle fatigue and emotional factors reduce the stability of the lumbar spine (Kirkaldy-Willis, 1982; Holstege, 1991). If local muscles are fatigued, they provide an inadequate response to the sudden movements that can occur during daily living activities. This increases the load on the FSU.

Emotional factors appear to influence sensorimotor processes. In times of psychological stress, fine motor skills are partly inhibited, and gross motor skills predominate. This hinders fine positioning of the vertebrae relative to each other.

Reduction in Trophic Levels in the Spinal Segment
Lowering of trophic levels in the spinal segment can be a factor in the development of lumbar segmental instability. Trophic disturbances may be caused by systemic illnesses, local inflammatory processes, or disturbances in segmental homeostasis. Regulatory disturbances within the segment are significant in the framework of manual therapy.

The term *segment* may be defined as follows: a segment is the complex of tissues and organs innervated by one spinal nerve in conjunction with the postganglionic sympathetic innervation.

The initial processing of the nociceptive activity that arises during actual or threatened damage to the tissues takes place at the spinal level. The activity of the spinal interneurons in the dorsal horn determines whether there will be excitation of secondary neurons and further transmission of the input.

If nociceptive activity continues and there is an alarm situation in the central nervous system (nonspecific arousal), electrical activity increases in the lateral horn of the spinal canal and in the origin segments of the sympathetic innervation of structures affected by the (threatened) damage.

This increased postganglionic sympathetic activity leads to a reduction in effective tissue circulation in the tissues and organs with a segmental relationship, and to an increase in sensitivity in the peripheral receptors, including the nociceptors. Activity also increases in the ventral horn of the segment; this results in hypertonicity in the muscles innervated by the segment. Segmental dysregulation occurs when circulation in the tissues is deficient as a result of prolonged sympathetic activity within the affected segment. When this happens, the nutritional level of the tissues and organs falls off sharply. We may assume that a reduction in effective circulation in the tissues belonging to the lumbar FSUs leads to a reduction in the mechanical load-bearing capacity. Furthermore, the condition and endurance of the intrinsic back musculature is reduced by the trophic disturbances. This hinders the lumbar spine musculature in adapting adequately to different postures and movements.

General Lowering of Load-Bearing Capacity   Deterioration in general bodily condition leads to a reduction in fine motor capability. The consequences of this have already been discussed.

Manual Diagnosis and Lumbar Segmental Instability

A mismatch between load and adaptation mechanisms occupies a special place in manual therapy. When describing disorders of the postural and locomotor apparatus, manual therapy makes use of the concepts found in the ICF, where the consequences of these disorders are classified as *impairments, limitations in activities,* or *restrictions in participation*.

It is important in manual diagnosis to identify the clinical manifestations of *impairments*. A number of impairments are specific to certain diagnoses, that is, they are characteristic of the diagnosis. However, a large number of impairments are not specific to a particular diagnosis. Lumbar segmental instability does not come with diagnosis-specific impairments; there are no clinical manifestations that only occur in cases of lumbar segmental instability. An attempt is made here to chart the disturbances that frequently occur in association with lumbar segmental instability; however, it must be stressed that these dysfunctions also occur with other diagnoses. The dysfunctions are listed in the section titled "Instability Examination" at the end of this chapter.

The point has already been made that manual diagnosis is directed at identifying the consequences of disease or dysfunction. Although some tests of instability have been described, it is difficult, if not impossible, to diagnose segmental instability with certainty by way of manual methods. It is also impossible to determine the position of the instantaneous axis of rotation (IAR) by manual diagnostic methods. It is only the consequences of lumbar instability that can be mapped.

A *reduction in arthrokinetic reflex activity* is more or less characteristic of lumbar segmental instability. Manual diagnosis can be specifically directed toward identifying this. Disturbances in arthrokinetic reflex activity are identified by active guided three-dimensional examination of the lumbar motion segments. The quality of eccentric contractions of the lumbar muscles is assessed. A discontinuous movement course and en masse undifferentiated contraction in parts of the spinal erector muscle are typical of disturbances in arthrokinetic reflex activity.

Manual diagnosis is also directed toward identifying movement dysfunctions in the lumbar FSUs, namely, the endfeel of physiologic segmental movements. A distinction is made between fixation of the intervertebral joints and protective joint fixation. In protective joint fixation, the protective tension reduces during non-weight-bearing three-dimensional physiologic movements. It is thought that subtle physiologic movements starting from a non-weight-bearing position cause a shift in the IAR such that the tissues belonging to the damaged FSU are not loaded. The tone and strength of the intrinsic segmental musculature and the endurance of the oblique and transverse abdominal muscles are also examined.

Please see the section titled "Instability Examination" at the end of this chapter for details on history taking and clinical examination. For the therapeutic approach to segmental instability, please see *Mobilization, Stabilization, and Coordination in Non-Specific Back and Neck Complaints'* (van der El, 2002).

Muscular Influences on the Lumbar Spine

The following muscles exert an influence in the ventral area:

Rectus abdominis muscle
Transverse abdominis muscle
Internal oblique muscle
External oblique muscle

During simultaneous contraction, the abdominal muscles reduce the distance between the sternum and the symphysis. Because of the considerable distances between the promontory and symphysis, and between the thoracic spine and sternum, the moment arm during flexion is long. During unilateral activity, the abdominal muscles cause sidebending. Contraction of the internal oblique muscle causes ipsiexternal rotation, which is supported synergistically by the external oblique on the contralateral side. Increased bilateral tone in the internal and external oblique abdominal muscles reduces the size of the triangle formed by the shoulders as the base and the sacrum as the apex.

In the dorsal area:

Deep layer:
- Rotatores muscles
- Multifidus muscles
- Intertransversal muscles
- Interspinal muscles

Middle layer:
- Posterior inferior serratus muscle

Superficial layer:
- Spinalis muscle
- Longissimus muscle
- Iliocostalis muscle
- Latissimus dorsi muscle

When these muscles contract bilaterally, they bring about extension of the lumbar spine relative to the lumbosacral segment. They pull the lumbar spine in a dorsal direction and increase the curvature.

With unilateral contraction, depending on the origin and insertion of the muscles, sidebending or rotation takes place. They are also active during expiration. The rotatores and multifidus muscles have a symmetric stabilizing function. When they work unilaterally, they cause contraexternal rotation.

In the lateral area:

- Quadratus lumborum muscle

When it contracts symmetrically, the quadratus lumborum muscle causes extension. When it contracts unilaterally, it causes ipsilateral sidebending.

Muscles That Connect With the Lower Limbs

When the psoas muscle contracts bilaterally, depending on the position of the lumbar spine, this muscle causes flexion or extension ("psoas paradox"). When it contracts unilaterally, it brings about ipsilateral sidebending and contralatderal rotation. In addition to the muscles named previously, which are directly connected to the lumbar spine, the rest of the body musculature works at a distance to support the static and dynamic function of the lumbar spine.

Motor–Sensory Relationships

When examining patients with lumbosacral and lower extremity complaints it is pertinent to be intimately familiar with the motor and sensory relationships of the lumbar spine with the leg.

Segment	Nerve	Motor	Sensory
	Lumbar plexus		
	Ventral part:		
T12–L1	*Iliohypogastric nerve (ventral ramus)*	Internal oblique muscle Transverse abdominis muscle	Skin, symphysis area
L1	*Ilioinguinal nerve*	Internal oblique muscle Transverse abdominis muscle	Penis, upper medial area of scrotum and inguinal area
L1–L2	*Genitofemoral nerve*	Scrotal cremaster muscle	Middle of upper thigh
L2–L3–L4	*Obturator nerve*	Abductor brevis muscle Adductor longus muscle Gracilis muscle Adductor magnus muscle Pectineus muscle Adductor minimus muscle Obturator externus muscle	Lower medial part of thigh
	Dorsal part:		
T12–L1	*Iliohypogastric nerve*		Lateral part of gluteus and thigh
L2–L3– L4–L5	*Femoral nerve*	Sartorius muscle Pectineus muscle Quadratus femoris muscle Psoas major muscle Psoas minor muscle Iliacus muscle	*Femoral nerve* *Saphenous nerve* *Infrapatellar branch* Anteromedial part of thigh, infrapatellar Medial side of lower leg, medial side of ankle, medial side of foot to proximal Phalanx of big toe *Lateral femoral cutaneous nerve* Lateral aspect thigh

REGIONAL EXAMINATION

Active-Assisted Regional Examination: Lumbar

The assessment criteria used during the active assisted regional examination are the following:

- Endfeel
- Symptom provocation
- Confirmation of findings of the active examination
- Increased intensity or distribution of symptoms present during the active examination

Flexion, Weight-Bearing

Examination position, patient: Sitting on the short side of the examination table with lower legs hanging down; the hands are placed on the neck or the arms are crossed in front of the chest; the spine down to and including the lumbar region is flexed ventrally.

Starting position, therapist: Standing beside the patient.

Stabilization: The stabilizing hand, the base of which is placed on the patient's back against the sacrum, maintains the position of the latter.

Procedure: The manipulating hand/arm, which encircles the arms of the patient, brings about the flexion (**Figure 14–18**).

Flexion, Sidebending, Ipsilateral Rotation, Weight-Bearing

Examination position, patient: Sitting on the short side of the examination table with the lower legs hanging down; the arms are crossed in front of the chest; the spine down to

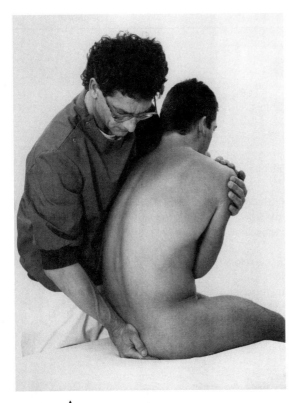

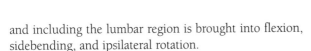

Figure 14–18 ↑

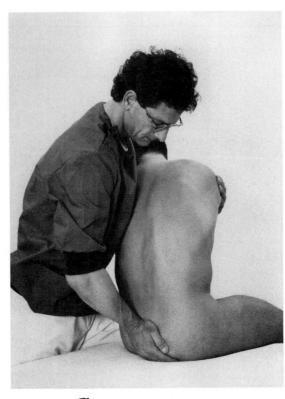

Figure 14–19 ⌐

and including the lumbar region is brought into flexion, sidebending, and ipsilateral rotation.

Starting position, therapist: Standing beside the patient at the side to be examined.

Stabilization: The stabilizing hand, the base of which is placed on the patient's back against the sacrum, maintains the position of the latter.

Procedure: The manipulating hand/arm, which passes between the patient's crossed arms from the cranial end and encircles the dorsal edge of the armpit on the contralateral side, brings about flexion, sidebending, and ipsilateral rotation (**Figure 14–19**).

Flexion, Sidebending, Contralateral Rotation, Weight-Bearing

Examination position, patient: Sitting on the short side of the examination table with the legs hanging down; the arms are crossed in front of the chest; the spine down to and including the lumbar region is brought into flexion, sidebending and contralateral rotation.

Starting position, therapist: Standing beside the patient at the side to be examined.

Stabilization: The base of the stabilizing hand is placed on the patient's back against the sacrum to maintain the position of the latter.

Procedure: The manipulating hand/arm, which passes through the patient's crossed arms from the caudal end to hold the shoulder at the contralateral side, carries out flexion, sidebending, and contralateral rotation (**Figure 14–20**).

Extension, Weight-Bearing

Examination position, patient: Sitting on the short side of the examination table with lower legs hanging down; the hands are placed on the neck or the arms are crossed in front of the chest; the spine is extended down to and including the lumbar region.

Starting position, therapist: Standing beside the patient.

Stabilization: The base of the stabilizing hand is placed on the patient's back against the sacrum to maintain its position.

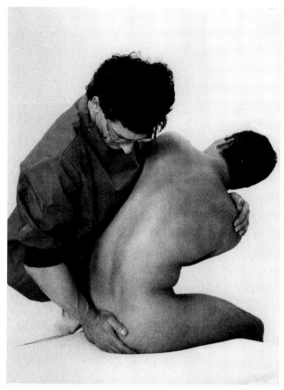

Figure 14–20

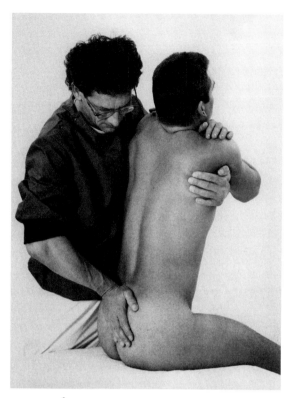

Figure 14–21

Procedure: The manipulating hand/arm, which passes under the patient's arms and round the thorax at the opposite side, extends the patient's spine (**Figure 14–21**).

Remarks: To carry out this test efficiently, the therapist asks the patient to lean forward a little. To avoid the hips flexing to more than 90° when the patient bends forward, and thus bringing the lumbar spine into kyphosis, the movable head end of the examination table can be set in a downward-sloping position.

Extension, Sidebending, Ipsilateral Rotation, Weight-Bearing

Examination position, patient: Sitting on the short side of the examination table with lower legs hanging down; the hands are placed on the neck and the arms crossed in front of the chest; the spine down to and including the lumbar region is brought into extension, sidebending, and ipsilateral rotation.

Starting position, therapist: Standing beside the patient at the side to be examined.

Stabilization: The base of the stabilizing hand is placed on the back against the sacrum to maintain its position.

Procedure: The manipulating hand/arm, which passes through the patient's crossed arms from the cranial end and round the thorax on the contralateral side, moves the spine into extension, sidebending, and ipsilateral rotation (**Figure 14–22**).

Extension, Sidebending, Contralateral Rotation, Weight-Bearing

Examination position, patient: Sitting on the short side of the examination table with lower legs hanging down; the hands are placed on the neck and the arms crossed in front of the chest; the spine down to and including the lumbar region is brought into extension, sidebending, and contralateral rotation.

Starting position, therapist: Standing beside the patient at the side to be examined.

Stabilization: The base of the stabilizing hand is placed on the patient's back against the sacrum to maintain its position.

Procedure: The manipulating hand/arm, which passes through the patient's crossed arms from the caudal end and around the shoulder at the contralateral side, brings

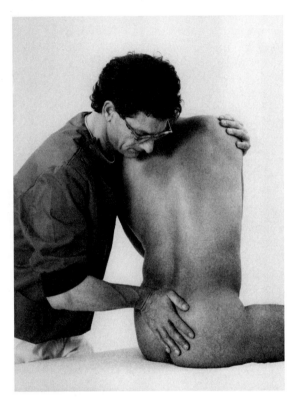

Figure 14–22

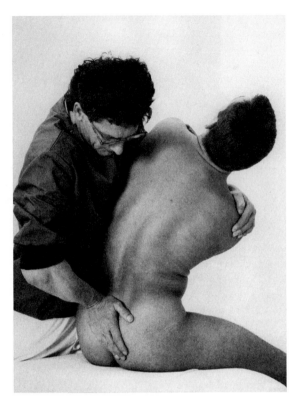

Figure 14–23

the spine into extension, sidebending, and contraexternal rotation (**Figure 14–23**).

Flexion, Non-Weight-Bearing

Examination position, patient: Lying on the side with hips and knees flexed through 90°.

Starting position, therapist: Standing in front of patient.

Stabilization: The thumb and index finger of the stabilizing hand grasp the spinous process of T12 and stabilize the thoracic spine. The therapist's forearm rests on the patient's thoracic spine for support.

Procedure: The therapist places the base of the manipulating hand against the sacrum and uses that hand/arm and his or her thighs, which support the patient's lower legs, to flex the patient's spine (**Figure 14–24**).

Flexion, Sidebending, Ipsilateral Rotation, Non-Weight-Bearing

Examination position, patient: Lying on the side with hips and knees flexed through 90°.

Starting position, therapist: Standing in front of the patient.

Stabilization: The stabilizing hand and arm rest on the patient's thoracic spine. The thumb and index finger of the therapist's hand hold the spinous process of T12 to maintain the position of the thoracic spine.

Procedure: The manipulating hand/arm passes behind the pelvis to hold the contralateral ilium. The therapist uses that arm and his or her thighs, which support the patient's lower legs, to bring the patient's spine into flexion, sidebending, and ipsilateral rotation (**Figure 14–25**).

Remarks: The legs accentuate the flexion component and the hand/arm accentuate the sidebending and rotation components.

Flexion, Sidebending, Contralateral Rotation, Non-Weight-Bearing

Examination position, patient: Lying on the side with hips and knees flexed through 90°.

Starting position, therapist: Standing in front of the patient.

Stabilization: The stabilizing hand/arm rest on the patient's thoracic spine. The thumb and index finger of that hand

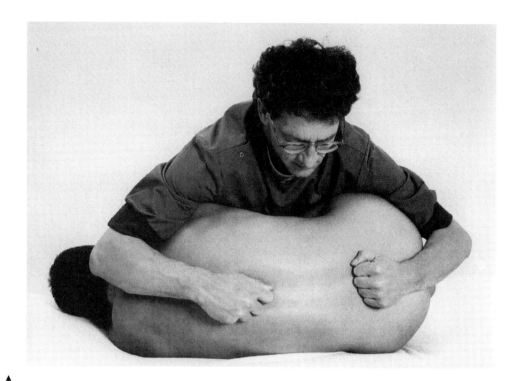

Figure 14–24

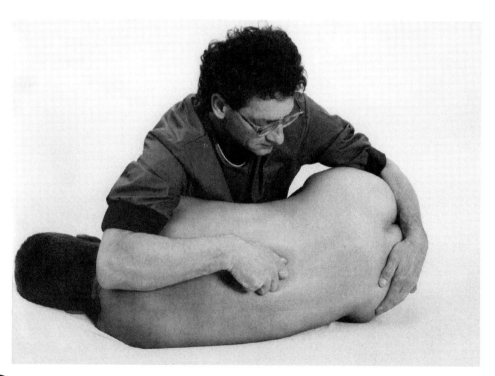

Figure 14–25

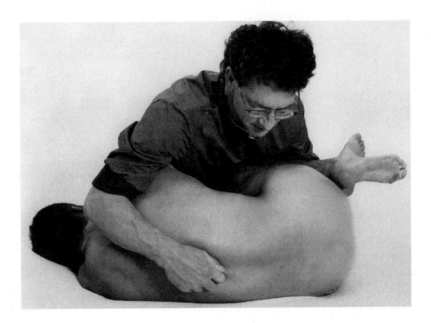

Figure 14–26 ⌐

hold the spinous process of T12 and maintain the position of the thoracic spine.

Procedure: The manipulating hand/arm passes under the pelvis to hold the contralateral ilium. The therapist uses that arm and his or her thighs, which support the patient's lower legs, to bring the patient's spine into flexion, sidebending, and contralateral rotation (**Figure 14–26**).

Extension, Non-Weight-Bearing

Examination position, patient: Prone.

Starting position, therapist: Standing beside the patient.

Stabilization: The restraining hand, the base of which is placed on the spinous process of T12, maintains the position of the thoracic spine.

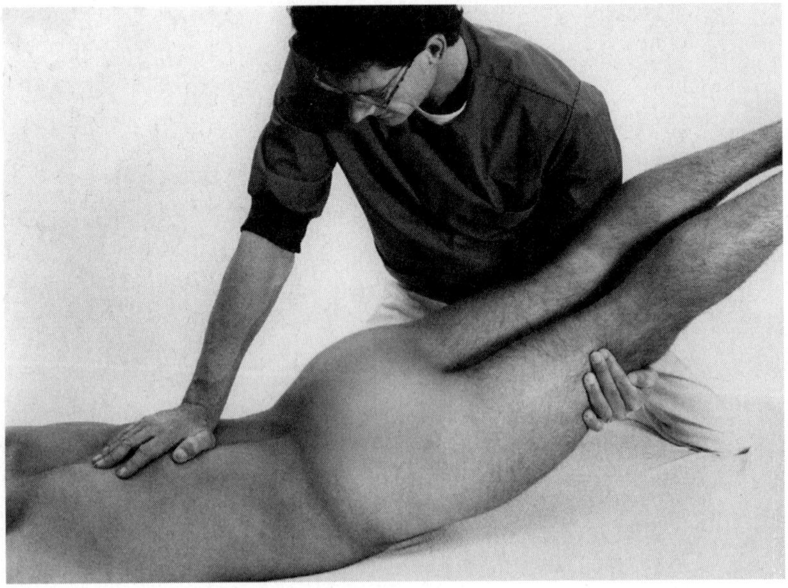

Figure 14–27 ↓

Procedure: The manipulating hand/arm passes under the patient's thighs and extends the spine (**Figure 14–27**).

Extension, Sidebending, Ipsilateral, Non-Weight-Bearing

Examination position, patient: Prone.

Starting position, therapist: Standing beside the patient at the side to be examined.

Stabilization: The stabilizing hand, the base of which is placed on the spinous process of T12, maintains the position of the thoracic spine.

Procedure: The manipulating hand/arm holds the contralateral thigh at its lateral aspect and brings about extension, sidebending, and ipsilateral rotation (**Figure 14–28**).

Extension, Sidebending, Contralateral Rotation, Non-Weight-Bearing

Examination position, patient: Prone.

Starting position, therapist: Standing beside the patient at the side not to be examined.

Stabilization: The stabilizing hand, the base of which is placed on the spiny process of T12, maintains the position of the thoracic spine.

Procedure: The manipulating hand/arm passes under both thighs and brings about extension, sidebending, and contralateral rotation (**Figure 14–29**).

Regional Provocation Tests: Lumbar

The assessment criteria used in regional provocation tests are the following:

- Regional mobility
- Symptom provocation or reduction
- Increased intensity or distribution of symptoms

Regional Springing Test

Examination position, patient: Prone.

Starting position, therapist: Standing beside the patient.

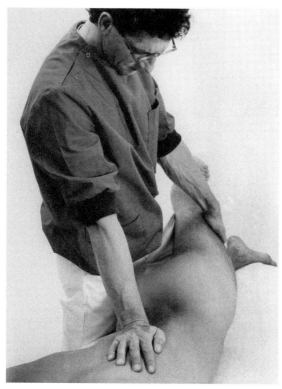

Figure 14–28

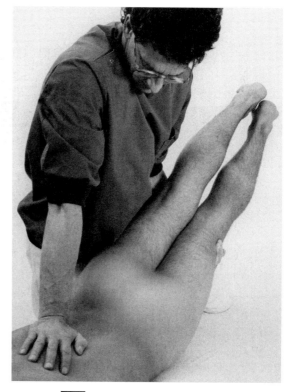

Figure 14–29

Procedure: The manipulating hand is placed on the lumbar spine and, supported by the other hand, exerts a rhythmic posteroanterior springing movement (**Figure 14–30**).

Regional Traction Test

Examination position, patient: Sitting or standing with arms folded below the ribs; the thoracic spine flexed down to and including the lumbar region.

Starting position, therapist: The therapist stands behind the patient with one foot in front of the other and places the front foot behind the patient's heels.

Procedure: The therapist's arms pass under the patient's arms and hold his or her lower arms. The therapist applies traction by moving the upper body straight backward (**Figures 14–31** and **14–32**).

Regional Compression Test

Examination position, patient: Sitting on a stool or the examination bench.

Starting position, therapist: Standing behind the patient.

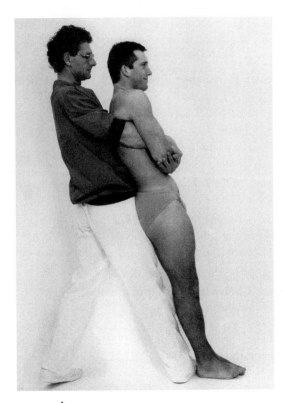

Figure 14–31 ↕

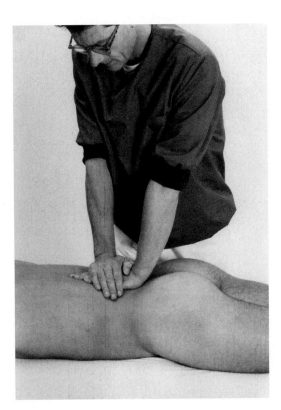

Figure 14–30 ↕↕

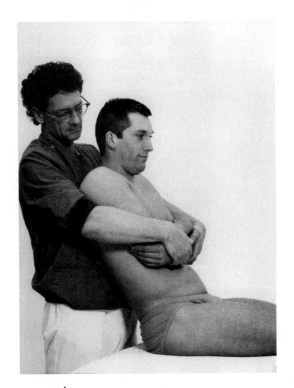

Figure 14–32 ↕

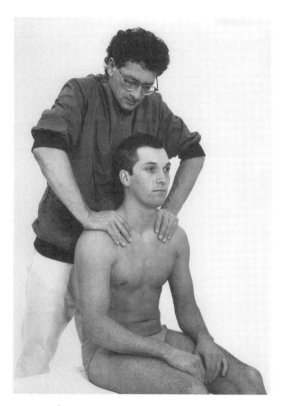

Figure 14–33 ⬍

Procedure: With both hands on the patient's shoulders, the therapist exerts force in a caudal direction (**Figure 14–33**).

Remarks: Alternatively, intense compression can be exerted if the patient stands on tiptoes and then falls to his or her heels.

SEGMENTAL EXAMINATION

Segmental Tissue–Specific Examination: Lumbar

The assessment criteria used during the segmental tissue–specific examination are the following:

- Sensory abnormality
- Elasticity of the subcutaneous tissue
- Muscle tone
- Coordination
- Referred sensations

Pinwheel Sensory Examination

Examination position, patient: Prone.

Starting position, therapist: Standing beside the patient.

Procedure: Holding the pinwheel between his or her thumb and index finger, the therapist examines the skin segment at the level being assessed for surface sensitivity to pain, directly lateral to the spinous process (**Figure 14–34**).

Remarks: This test is used to examine the medial branch of the dorsal ramus.

Kibler Test

Examination position, patient: Prone.

Starting position, therapist: Standing beside the patient.

Procedure: The therapist takes the skin at the level being examined between the thumb and the index fingers of both hands, unilaterally or bilaterally, and tests by way of a rolling movement (**Figure 14–35**).

Muscle Tone Palpation

Examination position, patient: Prone.

Starting position, therapist: Standing beside the patient.

Procedure: The therapist places his or her index fingers at the level being examined bilaterally lateral to the spinous process, on the muscles that span the segment. Muscle tone is assessed by palpation and compared with the tone at adjacent levels (**Figure 14–36**).

Using a dichotomous rating scale of normal versus abnormal, Boline et al. (1988) reported percentage agreement and κ values for interrater agreement for muscle tone palpation. Their study yielded agreements of 70% (κ = 0.31) at T12–L1, 68% (κ = 0.16) at L1–L2, 70% (κ = 0.18) at L2–L3, 65% (κ = 0.27) at L3–L4, 68% (κ = 0.17) at L4–L5, and 70% (κ = 0.10) at L5–S1.

Segmental Coordination Test and Variation

Examination position, patient: Prone (alternatively done in supine or crouching).

Starting position, therapist: Standing beside the patient.

Procedure: The therapist places his or her thumbs on the spinous process or the transverse processes of the vertebra above the level being examined. The patient is asked to resist light pressure exerted by the therapist (**Figure 14–37**).

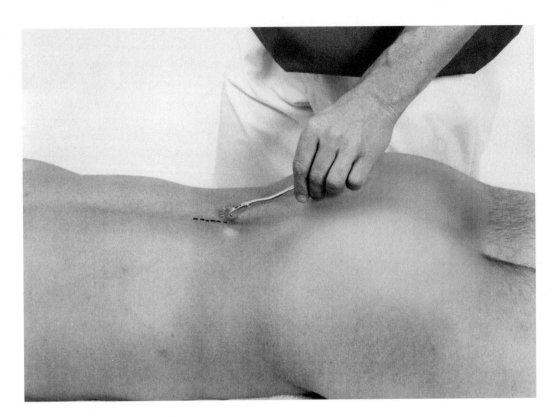

Figure 14–34

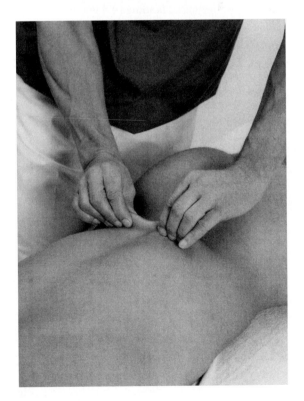

Figure 14–35

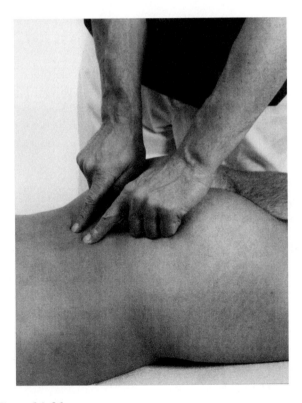

Figure 14–36

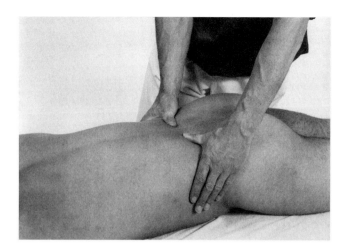

Figure 14–37

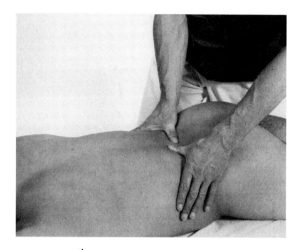

Figure 14–39

Variations

Examination position, patient: Prone.

Starting position, therapist: Standing beside the patient.

Procedure: The therapist places his or her thumbs against both lateral aspects of the spinous process of the vertebra above the level being examined. The patient is asked to resist light pressure exerted alternately on the left and right by the therapist (**Figure 14–38**).

Remarks: Alternatively, the thumbs can be placed on both sides of the spinous process of the vertebra below the level and above the level being examined. During a rhythmic stabilization the pressure exerted and subsequent release by the therapist should be alternated evenly (**Figure 14–39**).

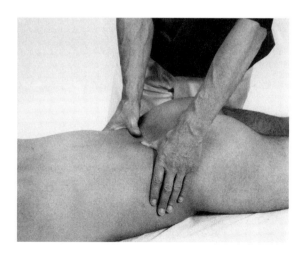

Figure 14–38

Specific Pain Point Palpation

Examination position, patient: Prone.

Starting position, therapist: Standing beside the patient.

Procedure: The therapist places his or her index finger on the pain point associated with the level being examined and exerts light pressure (**Figures 14–40** and **14–41**).

Remarks: Depending on the type of pain point, the patient will experience localized or referred pain.

Using a dichotomous rating scale of present or absent, Boline et al. (1988) reported percentage agreement and κ values for interrater agreement for segmental palpation for pain. Their study yielded agreements of 94% ($\kappa = 0.37$) at T12–L1, 94% ($\kappa = -0.03$) at L1–L2, 96% ($\kappa = 0.49$) at L2–L3, 94% ($\kappa = 0.37$) at L3–L4, 92% ($\kappa = -0.03$) at L4–L5, and 90% ($\kappa = -0.03$) at L5–S1.

Segmental Provocation Tests: Lumbar

The assessment criteria used in segmental provocation tests are the following:

- Segmental mobility
- Symptom provocation or reduction
- Increased intensity or distribution of symptoms

Segmental Springing Test

Examination position, patient: Prone.

Starting position, therapist: Standing beside the patient.

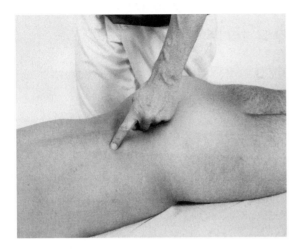

Figure 14–40

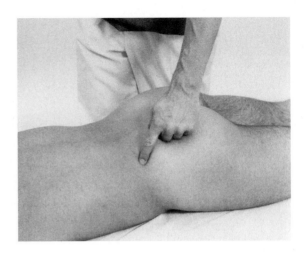

Figure 14–41

Procedure: The manipulating hand, which is placed with its hypothenar on the spinous process, performs a posteroanterior springing movement. The therapist uses the other hand to support the manipulating hand (**Figures 14–42** and **14–43**).

Remarks: Pressure on the spinous process can also be exerted using a pinch grip or with the two thumbs supporting each other.

Variation

Examination position, patient: Prone.

Starting position, therapist: Standing beside the patient.

Procedure: The manipulating hand, which is placed with the index and middle fingers on the two transverse

processes, produces a posteroanterior springing movement. The therapist uses the other hand to support the manipulating hand (**Figures 14–44** and **14–45**).

Phillips and Twomey (1996) showed similar interrater percentage agreement for the prone springing test when judging presence or absence of pain (60–99%, κ = −0.15–0.28) and assessing for mobility (74–99%, κ = 0.14–0.24). However, the findings by Maher and Adams (1994) of greater interrater agreement when assessing for pain (31–43%; ICC = 0.67–0.72) than for mobility (21–29%; ICC = 0.03–0.37) seem more representative of the findings in the research literature on this technique (Huijbregts, 2002). Landel et al. (2008) seem to have definitively invalidated the prone springing test as a test of seg-

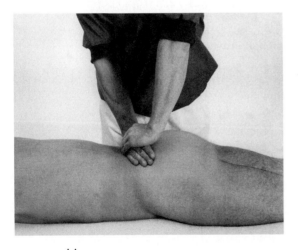

Figure 14–42 ⬆⬇

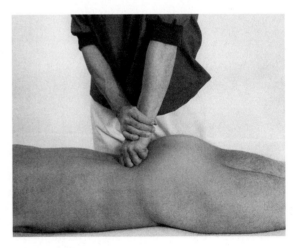

Figure 14–43 ⬆⬇

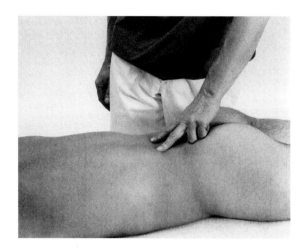

Figure 14–44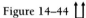

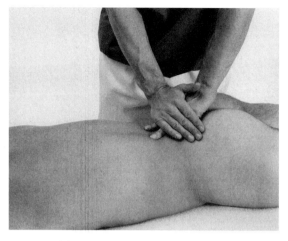

Figure 14–45 ⬆⬇

mental mobility: they reported a poor level of agreement between MRI assessment and manual assessment of segmental motion with κ = 0.04 (95% CI: −0.16–0.24) for the least mobile segment and κ = 0.00 (95% CI: −0.09–0.08) for the most mobile segment.

Recent research has used the segmental test but collapsed findings by not assessing for segmental but rather for regional findings. Using flexion-extension radiographic measurements as a gold standard and a three-point rating scale of hypomobile, normal, or hypermobile, Abbott and Mercer (2003) reported a sensitivity of 0.75 (90% CI: 0.36–0.94), a specificity of 0.35 (90% CI: 0.20–0.55), a positive likelihood ratio of 1.16 (90% CI: 0.44–2.03), and a negative likelihood ratio of 0.71 (0.12–2.75) for using the prone springing test in the diagnosis of a subgroup of patients with lumbar hypomobility, albeit not specified to segmental level. Using a similar three-point rating, Abbott et al. (2005) also compared the prone springing test to flexion-extension radiographs and reported a sensitivity of 0.29 (95% CI: 0.14–0.50) but a specificity of 0.89 (95% CI: 0.83–0.93), giving a positive test a positive likelihood ratio of 2.52 (95% CI: 1.15–5.53) for the diagnosis of lumbar segmental instability. Fritz, Piva, and Childs (2005b) reported interrater reliability of the prone segmental springing test scored as hypermobile, normal, and hypomobile. Interrater agreement on the presence of hypomobility was 77% (κ = 0.38, 95% CI: 0.22–0.54); agreement for the presence of hypermobility was 77% (κ = 0.48, 95% CI: 0.35–0.61). Using a gold standard of instability assessed by way of radiographic flexion-extension images yielded a sensitivity of 0.43 (95% CI: 0.27–0.61), a specificity of 0.95 (95% CI: 0.77–0.99), a positive likelihood ratio of 9.0 (95% CI:

1.3–63.9), and a negative likelihood ratio of 0.60 (95% CI: 0.43–0.84) for the absence of hypomobility of the segmental springing test; values for the presence of segmental hypermobility on this test were, 0.46 (95% CI: 0.30–0.64); 0.81 (95% CI: 0.60–0.92); 2.4 (95% CI: 0.93–6.4), and 0.66 (95% CI: 0.44–0.99), respectively. Fritz, Whitman, and Childs (2005c) further supported validity of the lumbar springing test in treatment planning by showing that patients judged to be hypermobile using this test benefited more from stabilization, whereas patients judged to be hypomobile benefited more from a manipulation with stabilization combination.

Segmental Rotation Test

Examination position, patient: Prone.

Starting position, therapist: Standing beside the patient.

Procedure: The therapist places his or her thumbs against the lateral aspect of the upper spinous process of the level being examined, and on the opposite lateral aspect of the spinous process of the inferior vertebra. The therapist exerts pressure by pushing his or her thumbs toward the midline. By changing thumb position, the therapist can test rotation in the opposite direction. (**Figures 14–46** and **14–47**).

Phillips and Twomey (1996) showed greater interrater agreement for the prone segmental rotation or transverse pressure test when judging presence or absence of pain (51–100%, κ = 0.16–0.22) as compared to assessing for mobility (76–100%, κ = −0.15–0.23).

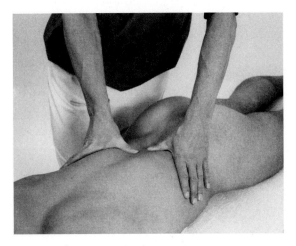

Figure 14–46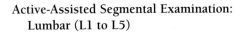

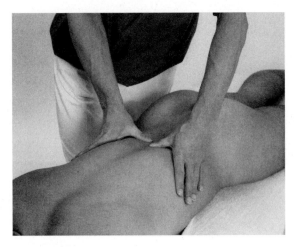

Figure 14–47

Active-Assisted Segmental Examination: Lumbar (L1 to L5)

When making a qualitative assessment of active assisted segmental function, the therapist will pay particular attention to the following factors:

- The patient's willingness to perform/allow the movements
- Endfeel
- Pain provocation or reduction
- Pseudoradicular symptomatology
- Radicular symptomatology
- Passive instability
- Muscular spasm, hypertonicity
- Tender points
- Referred sensations

Flexion, Weight-Bearing

Examination position, patient: Sitting on the short side of the examination table with lower legs hanging down; the hands are placed on the neck and the arms crossed in front of the chest; the spine is flexed down to the level to be examined.

Starting position, therapist: Standing beside the patient.

Stabilization: The therapist holds the spinous process of the lower vertebra of the level being examined between the thumb and index finger of the stabilizing hand and maintains its position.

Procedure: The manipulating hand/arm encircles the patient's thorax above his or her arms and introduces segmental flexion (**Figure 14–48**).

Richter and Lawall (1993) reported $\kappa = 0.18$–0.33 for interrater agreement on active-assisted segmental examination of seated L1–S1 flexion.

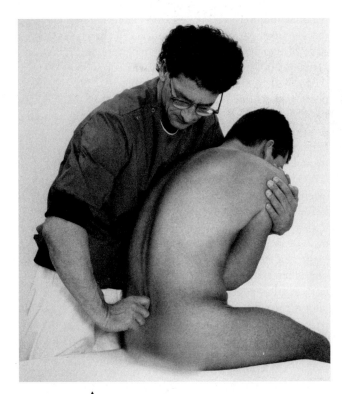

Figure 14–48

Flexion, Sidebending, Ipsilateral Rotation, Weight-Bearing

Examination position, patient: Sitting on the short side of the examination table with lower legs hanging down; the arms are crossed in front of the chest; the spine is brought into flexion, sidebending, and ipsilateral rotation down to the level to be examined.

Starting position, therapist: Standing beside the patient at the side to be examined.

Stabilization: The therapist holds the spinous process of the lower vertebra of the level being examined between the thumb and index finger of the stabilizing hand and maintains its position.

Procedure: The manipulating hand and arm, which pass between the patient's crossed arms from the cranial end and round the outer edge of the contralateral armpit, introduces segmental flexion, sidebending, and ipsilateral rotation (**Figure 14–49**).

Flexion, Sidebending, Contralateral Rotation, Weight-Bearing

Examination position, patient: Sitting on the short side of the examination table with lower legs hanging down; the arms are crossed in front of the chest; the spine is brought into flexion, sidebending, and contralateral rotation down to the level to be examined.

Starting position, therapist: Standing beside the patient at the side to be examined.

Stabilization: The therapist holds the spinous process of the lower vertebra of the level being examined between the thumb and index finger of the stabilizing hand and maintains its position.

Procedure: The manipulating hand and arm, which pass between the patient's arms from the caudal end and around the contralateral shoulder, introduces segmental flexion, sidebending, and contralateral rotation (**Figure 14–50**).

Extension, Weight-Bearing

Examination position, patient: Sitting on the short side of the examination table with lower legs hanging; the arms are crossed in front of the chest and the hands placed on the neck; the spine is brought into extension down to the level to be examined.

Starting position, therapist: Standing beside the patient.

Stabilization: The therapist holds the spinous process of the lower vertebra of the level being examined between the

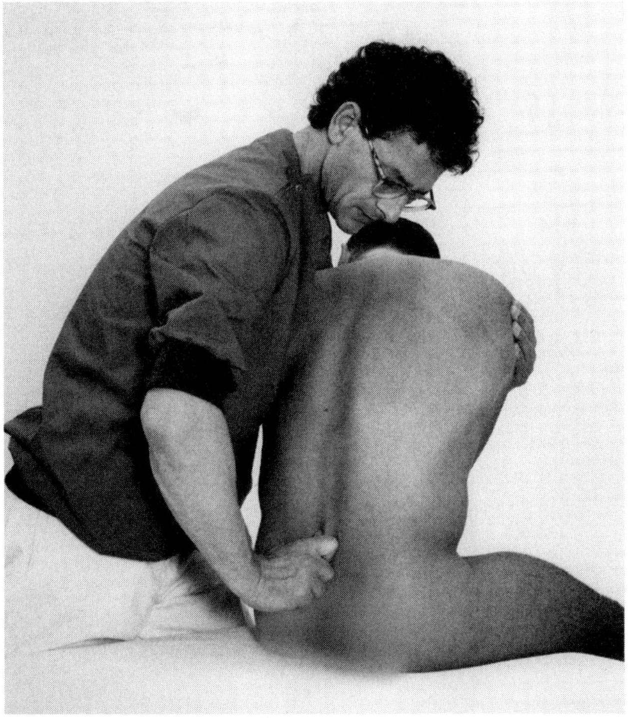

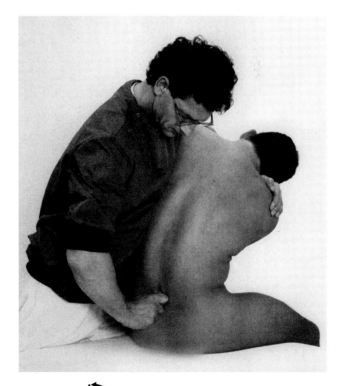

Figure 14–49

Figure 14–50

thumb and index finger of the stabilizing hand and maintains its position.

Procedure: The manipulating hand and arm, which pass under the patient's arms and around the thorax on the contralateral side, introduce segmental extension (**Figure 14–51**).

Richter and Lawall (1993) reported κ = 0.14–0.36 for interrater agreement on active-assisted segmental examination of seated L1–S1 extension.

Extension, Sidebending, Ipsilateral Rotation, Weight-Bearing

Examination position, patient: Sitting on the short side of the examination table with lower legs hanging down; the arms are crossed in front of the chest; the spine is brought into extension, sidebending, and ipsilateral rotation down to the level being examined.

Starting position, therapist: Standing beside the patient at the side to be examined.

Stabilization: The therapist holds the spinous process of the lower vertebra of the level being examined between the thumb and index finger of the stabilizing hand and maintains its position.

Procedure: The manipulating hand and arm, which pass between the patient's arms, from the cranial end, and around the thorax on the contralateral side, introduce segmental extension, sidebending and ipsilateral rotation (**Figure 14–52**).

Extension, Sidebending, Contralateral Rotation, Weight-Bearing

Examination position, patient: Sitting on the short side of the examination table with lower legs hanging down; the arms are crossed in front of the chest; the spine is brought into extension, sidebending, and contralateral rotation down to the level being examined.

Starting position, therapist: Standing beside the patient at the side to be examined.

Stabilization: The therapist holds the spinous process of the lower vertebra of the level being examined between the thumb and index finger of the stabilizing hand and maintains its position.

Procedure: The manipulating hand and arm, which pass between the patient's crossed arms, from the caudal end, and around the contralateral shoulder, introduces seg-

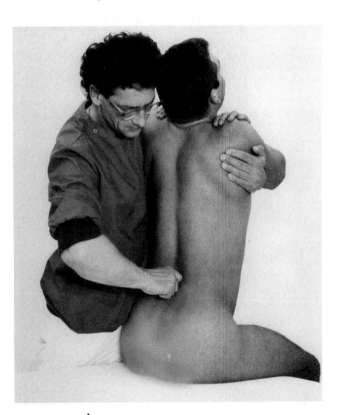

Figure 14–51

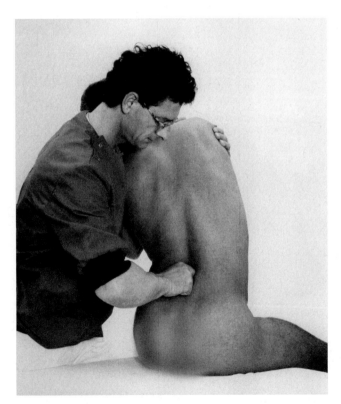

Figure 14–52

mental extension, sidebending, and contralateral rotation (**Figure 14–53**).

Flexion, Non-Weight-Bearing

Examination position, patient: Lying on one side with the hips and knees flexed to 90°.

Starting position, therapist: Standing in front of the patient.

Stabilization: The lower part of the stabilizing arm rests along the upper part of the patient's spine. With the thumb and index finger of the same hand, the therapist holds the spinous process of upper vertebra of the level being examined and maintains its position.

Procedure: The base of the manipulating hand is placed against the sacrum; the therapist holds the spinous process of the lower vertebra of the level being examined between his or her thumb and index finger. The therapist uses the manipulating arm—together with his or her thighs, which support the patient's lower legs—to bring the spine into a flexed position (**Figure 14–54**).

Qvistgaard et al. (2007) reported an intrarater κ value of 0.31 for this technique judging the absence or presence of segmental dysfunction indicative of the need for manipula-

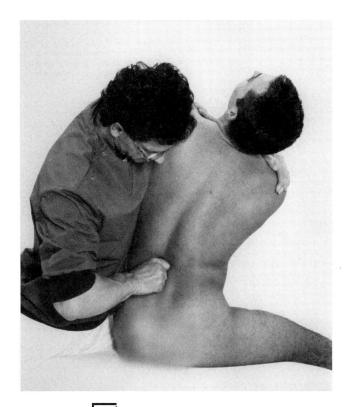

Figure 14–53

tion; interrater agreement yielded a κ value of 0.22. Phillips and Twomey (1996) reported 55–98% interrater agreement for this technique (κ = −0.11–0.32). Using flexion-extension radiographic measurements as a gold standard and a five-point rating scale giving two options for hypo- and hypermobility and anchored in the middle for normal mobility, Abbott and Mercer (2003) reported a sensitivity of 0.42 (90% CI: 0.19–0.71), a specificity of 0.89 (90% CI: 0.71–0.96), a positive likelihood ratio of 3.86 (90% CI: 0.89–16.31), and a negative likelihood ratio of 0.64 (0.28–1.04) for using mobility findings on sidelying active-assisted flexion segmental examination in the diagnosis of a subgroup of patients with lumbar hypomobility, albeit not specified to segmental level. Using a similar rating scale and gold standard test, Abbott et al. (2005) established sensitivity of 0.05 (95% CI: 0.01–0.22) and specificity of 0.995 (95% CI: 0.97–1.00) yielding a positive likelihood ratio of 8.73 (95% CI: 0.57–134.7) for the diagnosis of segmental translational lumbar instability, albeit it not specified to segmental level.

Flexion, Sidebending, Ipsilateral Rotation, Non-Weight-Bearing

Examination position, patient: Lying on one side with hips and knees flexed to 90°.

Starting position, therapist: Standing in front of the patient.

Stabilization: The lower part of the stabilizing arm rests along the upper part of the patient's spine. With the thumb and index finger of the same hand, the therapist holds the spinous process of upper vertebra of the level being examined and maintains its position.

Procedure: The manipulating hand lies along the back of the contralateral ilium. The therapist uses this hand and arm—together with his or her thighs, which support the patient's lower legs—to bring the spine into flexion, sidebending and ipsilateral rotation (**Figure 14–55**).

Flexion, Sidebending, Contralateral Rotation, Non-Weight-Bearing

Examination position, patient: Lying on one side with the hips and knees flexed to 90°.

Starting position, therapist: Standing in front of the patient.

Stabilization: The lower part of the stabilizing arm lies along the upper part of the patient's spine. With the thumb and index finger of the same hand, the therapist holds the spinous process of upper vertebra of the level being examined and maintains its position.

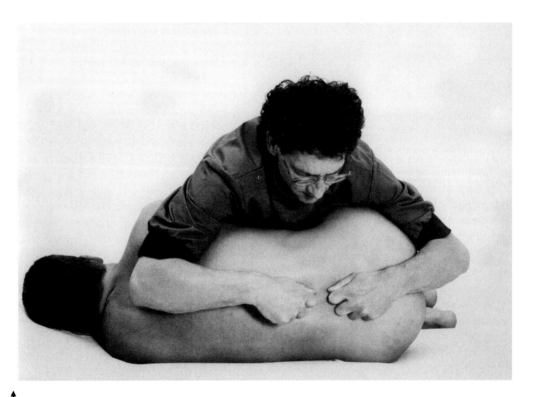

Figure 14–54

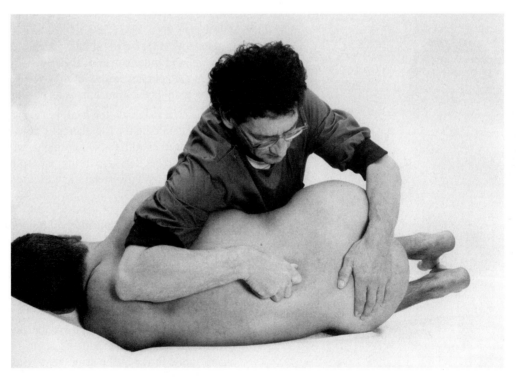

Figure 14–55

Procedure: The manipulating hand and arm lie along the lower edge of the ipsilateral ilium. The therapist uses this hand and arm—together with his or her thighs, which support the patient's lower legs—to bring the spine into flexion, sidebending, and contralateral rotation (**Figure 14–56**).

Although not specific to the two preceding techniques, Brismée et al. (2005) reported on the interrater reliability of a similar L4–L5 flexion-sidebending-rotation segmental motion test to see if raters could agree whether ipsilateral or contralateral sidebending produced the greatest excursion into rotation. Questioning the reliability of the preceding two tests, these authors noted only poor to slight agreement with pair-wise interrater percentage agreement from 46.3–62.9% and κ values ranging only from –0.16–0.04.

Extension, Non-Weight-Bearing

Examination position, patient: Lying on one side with the hips and knees flexed to 90°.

Starting position, therapist: Standing in front of the patient.

Stabilization: The lower part of the stabilizing arm rests along the upper part of the patient's spine. With the

thumb and index finger of the same hand, the therapist holds the spinous process of upper vertebra of the level being examined and maintains its position.

Procedure: The base of the manipulating hand is placed against the sacrum and the therapist holds the spinous process of the lower vertebra of the level being examined between his or her thumb and index finger. The therapist uses this hand and arm—together with his or her thighs, which support the patient's lower legs—to bring the spine into extension (**Figure 14–57**).

Variation

Examination position, patient: Prone.

Starting position, therapist: Standing beside the patient.

Stabilization: The stabilizing hand maintains the position of the upper vertebra.

Procedure: The manipulating hand and arm pass under the patient's thighs and move the spine into extension (**Figure 14–58**).

Qvistgaard et al. (2007) reported an intrarater κ value of 0.54 for the sidelying technique judging the absence or

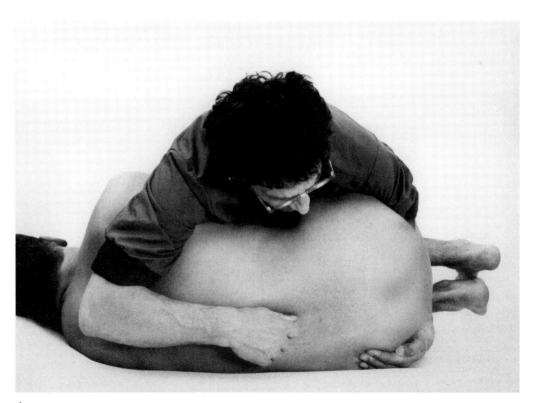

Figure 14–56

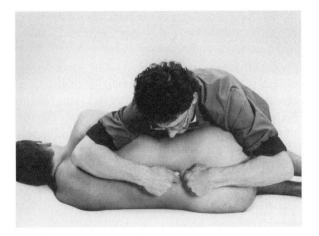

Figure 14–57 ↓

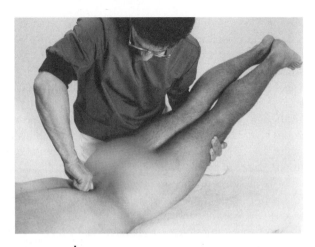

Figure 14–58 ↓

presence of segmental dysfunction indicative of the need for manipulation; interrater agreement yielded a κ value of 0.23. Phillips and Twomey (1996) reported 61–99% interrater agreement for this technique (κ = −0.02–0.23). Using flexion-extension radiographic measurements as a gold standard and a five-point rating scale giving two options for hypo- and hypermobility and anchored in the middle for normal mobility, Abbott et al. (2005) established sensitivity of 0.16 (95% CI: 0.06–0.38) and specificity of 0.98 (95% CI: 0.94–0.99) yielding a positive likelihood ratio of 7.07 (95% CI: 1.71–29.2) for the diagnosis of translational segmental lumbar instability, albeit it not specified to segmental level.

Extension, Sidebending, Ipsilateral Rotation, Non-Weight-Bearing

Examination position, patient: Prone.

Starting position, therapist: Standing beside the patient at the side to be examined.

Stabilization: The thumb and index finger of the restraining hand grasp the spinous process of the upper vertebra of the level being examined and maintain its position.

Procedure: The manipulating hand and arm pass around the contralateral thigh or ilium. The therapist uses this hand and arm to bring the patient's spine into extension, sidebending, and ipsilateral rotation (**Figure 14–59**).

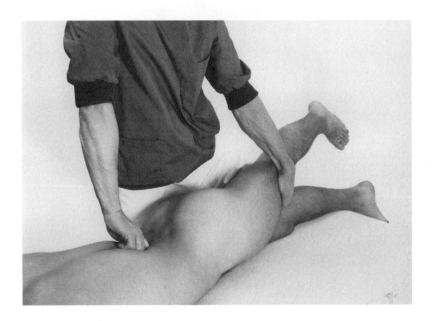

Figure 14–59 ⤵

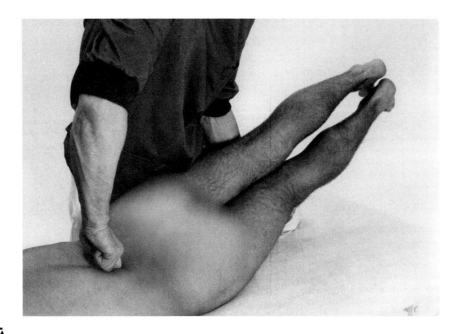

Figure 14–60

Extension, Sidebending, Contralateral Rotation, Non-Weight-Bearing

Examination position, patient: Prone.

Starting position, therapist: Standing beside the patient at the side not being examined.

Stabilization: The thumb and index finger of the stabilizing hand grasp the spinous process of the upper vertebra of the level being examined and maintain its position.

Procedure: Coming from a medial position, the manipulating hand and arm pass under both the patient's thighs and move the spine into extension, sidebending, and contralateral rotation (**Figure 14–60**).

INSTABILITY EXAMINATION

Earlier we discussed the lack of specificity of symptoms and signs proposed for the identification of patients with lumbar instability.

Features in Patient History

The following symptoms can be found in the examination of patients with lumbar instability:

- Pain after prolonged standing
- Pain after prolonged sitting
- Pain when walking or strolling for prolonged periods
- Pain when maintaining spinal flexion for prolonged periods
- Pain after prolonged sleeping
- Pain when standing up from a low sitting position

Clinical Signs

Similarly, clinical observation has us include the following symptoms as possibly indicative of lumbar instability:

- Increased tone in the intrinsic musculature
- Hyperesthesia of the dorsal ramus of the affected segment
- Reduced mobility in L4–L5, L5–S1
- Reduced mobility in the thoracolumbar junction
- Deviation and/or disturbance of the course of the movement during active spinal flexion and/or deflexion. Any instability will be seen more clearly if the patient is carrying weights in the hands (**Figure 14–61**).
- Placing the hands on the knees during active spinal flexion and deflexion, also known as Gower's sign (**Figure 14–62**)
- Disturbed course of movement when actively tilting the pelvis while sitting with legs hanging (**Figure 14–63a,b**)

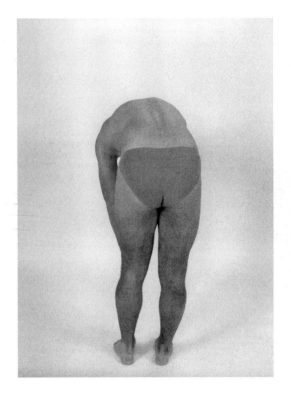

Figure 14–61

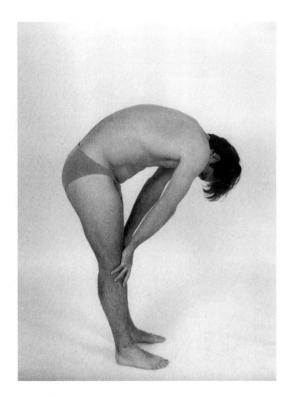

Figure 14–62

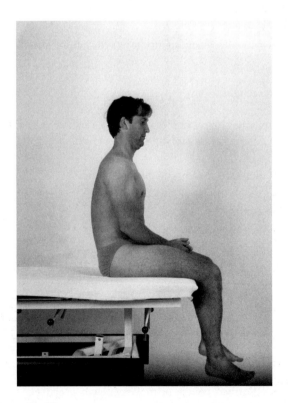

Figure 14–63a

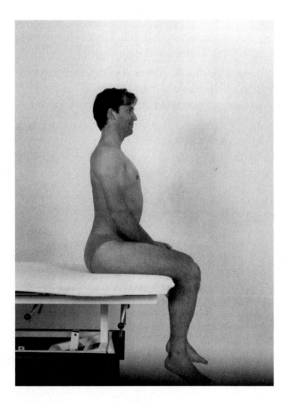

Figure 14–63b

- Tendency to bend the knees during active spinal extension (**Figure 14–64**)
- Inability to take long steps backward (**Figure 14–65**)
- Disturbed course of movement when raising both extended legs while lying on the side (**Figure 14–66**)
- Inability to maintain lumbar stability when lifting, carrying

- Reduced or absent segmental isometric three-dimensional rotation (**Figure 14–67**)
- Reduced power in the gluteal muscle when resisting pressure on an extended/ abducted/internally rotated leg while lying on the side (**Figure 14–68**)
- Reduced local muscular coordination
- Reduced left–right coordination
- Reduced general conditioning

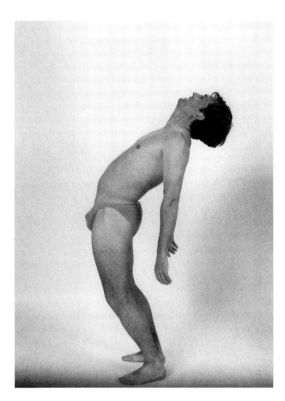

Figure 14–64

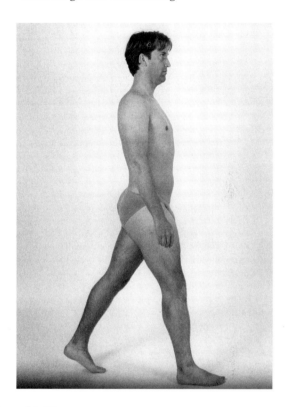

Figure 14–65

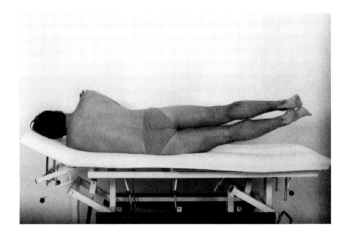

Figure 14–66

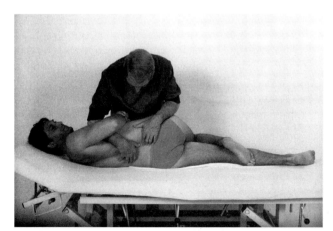

Figure 14–67

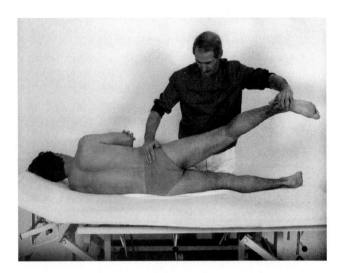

Figure 14–68

Possible Weak Links

Lumbar instability may be the result of various combinations of impairments or so-called weak links:

- Sensorimotor function
- Stability
- Dynamic strength
- Muscular reactivity
- Muscular endurance

Changes in the neural control system caused by pain lead to changes in timing, contractions when balance is challenged, changes in reflexes, and dysfunctions in the neuromuscular system.

Where there is a *painful flexion/rotation* instability, the lower lumbar spine shows accentuated flexion and the thoracolumbar spine accentuated lordosis. The lower lumbar spine shows reduced extension during movements of which it is a component.

Where there is a *painful extension/rotation* instability, the lower lumbar spine shows an increased lordosis and hypertonicity in the multifidus muscles. The gluteal muscle and the deep abdominal musculature exhibit a degree of inactivity.

Muscles That May Be Involved

In the global muscle system, the following muscles might be involved:

- Rectus abdominis muscle
- External oblique muscle
- Iliocostalis muscle (pars thoracis)

In the local muscle system, the following muscles might be involved:

- Pelvic floor muscles
- Iliopsoas muscle
- Quadratus lumborum muscle
- Iliocostalis muscle (pars lumborum)
- Longissimus muscle
- Diaphragm muscle
- Latissimus dorsi muscle
- Piriformis muscle
- Gluteal muscle
- Transverse abdominis muscle
- Internal oblique muscle

In the segmental muscle system, the following muscle might be involved: multifidus muscle.

10-Point Test

During the whole test procedure, diaphragmatic breathing should be maintained and the navel drawn in. This test may serve as a quick albeit non-validated assessment of the active subsystem involved in lumbar stability.

1. The patient is on all fours and the navel is drawn in (contraction of transverse abdominis muscle), then relaxed. This is repeated several times.
2. The patient lies prone with a stabilizer inflated to 70 mmHg under the abdomen. The navel is drawn in for 10 seconds. During this time, the pressure should fall by about 10 mmHg. Ten repetitions.
3. The patient lies supine with the knees drawn up and holds the navel in for 1 minute.
4. The patient lies supine with the knees drawn up and the navel drawn in. The right and left hip joints alternately are abducted/rotated through 45° for 1 minute.
5. The patient lies supine with the knees drawn up and the navel drawn in. The left and the right hip joints are flexed alternately through 90°. This continues for 1 minute.
6. The patient lies supine with the knees drawn up and the navel drawn in. The two hip joints are flexed alternately through 90° for 1 minute.

7. The patient lies supine with the knees drawn up and the navel drawn in. The left and right legs are alternately flexed and extended, the heel sliding over the surface of the bench, for 1 minute.
8. The patient lies supine with the knees drawn up and the navel drawn in. Both legs together are alternately flexed and extended, sliding over the surface of the bench, for 1 minute.
9. The patient lies supine with the knees drawn up and the navel drawn in. The right and left legs are flexed and extended alternately while held free of the bench surface. This is repeated 10 times.
10. The patient lies supine with the knees drawn up and the navel drawn in. The two legs together are held free of the bench and are alternately flexed and extended 10 times.

Assessment Criteria

During the exercises, care is taken to ensure that the navel remains pulled in, that there is no undesired activity in the global musculature, and that diaphragmatic breathing is maintained. The assessment occurs by observation and palpation.

Therapy

The treatment of instability is described in *Mobilization, Stabilization and Coordination in Non-Specific Back and Neck Complaints* (van der El, 2002).

Clinical Research into Lumbar Segmental Instability
Peter A. Huijbregts

The preceding information with regard to the diagnosis of lumbar segmental instability is based mainly on authority-based and experiential knowledge and on a pathophysiologic rationale. Although these sources of knowledge continue to be of value within evidence-informed OMT clinical practice, this same paradigm also requires that they be supplemented by and integrated with data based on research.

Hicks et al. (2003) established the interrater reliability of clinical examination measures commonly used in the examination of patients suspected of lumbar segmental instability. They described the posterior shear test, whereby the subject stands with arms crossed over the lower abdomen. The examiner stands at the side of the subject and places one arm around the abdomen of the subject, over the subject's crossed hands. The heel of the examiner's other hand is placed on the subject's pelvis for stabilization and the in-

dex or middle finger palpates L5–S1. The examiner then produces a posterior shear force through the subject's abdomen and a simultaneous anterior stabilizing force with the opposite hand repeating this test at each lumbar level. A positive test was defined as provocation of symptoms but was not based on the amount of intersegmental motion detected. With the prone instability test the subject was prone with the torso on the examination table and legs over the edge with the feet resting on the floor. While the subject rests in this position, the examiner performs a prone lumbar springing test and the patient is asked to report pain provocation. In case of pain provocation, the subject lifts the legs off the floor with hand-holding to the table permitted to maintain position, The springing test is reapplied to any segments that were identified as painful. A positive test was defined as pain provoked during the first part of the test that disappeared when the test was repeated with the legs off the floor. These researchers also studied the interrater reliability of pain using a dichotomous rating scale (pain present or absent) and mobility using a three-point rating scale (hypermobile, normal, hypomobile) on the lumbar prone springing test, and looked at the interrater agreement for painful arc in flexion painful arc upon return, Gower sign or thigh climbing, instability catch, and reversal of lumbopelvic rhythm; presence of one or more of these movement patterns was used to score for the presence of aberrant motions on active trunk flexion. Assessment of pain provocation with the springing test had greater interrater agreement ($\kappa = 0.25$–0.55) than assessment of mobility with this test ($\kappa = -0.02$–0.26). Interrater agreement values for the other tests are provided in **Table 14–1**.

Hicks et al. (2003) also studied interrater reliability for the Beighton Ligamentous Laxity Scale (Beighton and Horan, 1969). This nine-point scale attributes one point on each side for passive elbow extension $> 10°$, passive knee extension $> 10°$, passive little finger extension $> 90°$, and abduction of the thumb to where it touches the forearm, and one point for being able to bend forward at the waist and touch the hands flat on the ground without bending the knees. Interrater agreement yielded an ICC of 0.79 (95% CI: 0.68–0.87).

Based on the interrater reliability findings, Hicks et al. (2005) developed a preliminary clinical prediction rule for lumbar stabilization discussed in Chapter 4 in the context of treatment-based diagnostic classification systems relevant to OMT clinical practice. These researchers identified four variables relevant to predicting success with stabilization exercises:

- Age < 40
- Average range of motion on the straight-leg raise test $> 91°$

Table 14–1   Interrater Agreement Physical Examination Signs With Regard to Lumbar Segmental Instability

Physical Examination Sign	Percent Agreement	κ Value (95% CI)
Painful arc in flexion	92	0.69 (0.54–0.84)
Painful arc upon return from flexion	90	0.61 (0.44–0.78)
Instability catch	92	0.25 (−0.10–0.60)
Gower sign	98	0.00 (−1.09–1.00)
Reversal of lumbopelvic rhythm	87	0.16 (−0.15–0.46)
Aberrant movement pattern	84	0.60 (0.47–0.73)
Posterior shear test	74	0.35 (0.20–0.51)
Prone instability test	91	0.87 (0.80–0.94)

- Presence of aberrant motions
- Positive prone instability test

The presence of three or more variables indicated the greatest likelihood of success with a positive likelihood ratio of 4.0 (95% CI: 1.6–10.0).

Variables associated with failure of a stabilization approach were the following (Hicks et al., 2005):

- Negative prone instability test
- Absence of aberrant motions
- Absence of hypermobility on lumbar spring testing
- Fear Avoidance Beliefs Questionnaire Physical Activity (FABQ-PA) subscale score of < 9

Two or more of these variables present carried a negative LR of 0.18 (95% CI: 0.08–0.38).

Fritz, Piva, and Childs (2005b) reported interrater agreement for the prone instability test (85%, κ = 0.69, 95% CI: 0.59–0.79), the posterior shear test (64%, κ = 0.27, 95% CI: 0.14–0.41), and the presence of aberrant motions during lumbar range of motion tests (87%, κ = −0.07, 95% CI: −0.45–0.31). We discussed interrater reliability findings for the prone springing test in the section titled "Segmental Springing Test" earlier in this chapter. These authors also used flexion-extension radiographic findings as a gold standard test to establish the diagnostic accuracy of clinical examination findings in the diagnosis of patients with lumbar instability. Based on significant between-group differences six variables were further analyzed for diagnostic accuracy. Data on diagnostic accuracy are presented in **Table 14–2**. Of these variables, logistic regression analysis yielded two variables as most relevant: lack of hypomobility during the lumbar springing test and lumbar flexion range > 53°. If one of these two variables was present, sensitivity was 0.82 (95% CI: 0.64–0.92), specificity 0.81 (95% CI: 0.60–0.92), positive likelihood ratio 4.3 (5% CI: 1.8–10.6), and negative likelihood ratio 0.22 (95% CI: 0.10–0.50). With both variables present sensitivity for detecting radiographic instability by way of the physical examination was 0.29 (95% CI: 0.13–0.46), specificity was 0.98 (95% CI: 0.91–1.0), positive likelihood ratio 12.8 (95% CI: 0.79–211.6), and negative likelihood ratio 0.72 (95% CI: 0.55–0.94).

As discussed in the preceding chapters on segmental provocation tests and active-assisted segmental examination, Abbott et al. (2005) used flexion-extension radiographic measurements as a gold standard to establish diagnostic accuracy statistics for segmental springing tests and sidelying active-assisted flexion and extension segmental mobility tests in the diagnosis of lumbar segmental instability. Using kinematic parameters from flexion-extension radiographs of a sample of 30 asymptomatic volunteers, they defined translational and rotational lumbar segmental instability as values exceeding two standard deviations above the mean of the parameters derived from this asymptomatic sample. **Table 14–3** provides diagnostic accuracy data from this study. Rel-

Table 14–2   Diagnostic Accuracy Statistic of Clinical Examination to Detect Radiographic Instability

Clinical Examination Findings	Sensitivity (95% CI)	Specificity (95% CI)	+ LR (95% CI)	− LR (95% CI)
Age < 37	0.57 (0.39–0.74)	0.81 (0.60–0.92)	3.0 (1.2–7.7)	0.53 (0.33–0.85)
Lumbar flexion range > 53°	0.68 (0.49–0.82)	0.86 (0.65–0.94)	4.8 (1.6–14.0)	0.38 (0.21–0.66)
Lumbar extension range > 26°	0.50 (0.33–0.67)	0.76 (0.55–0.89)	2.1 (0.9–4.9)	0.66 (0.42–1.0)
Beighton scale > 2	0.36 (0.21–0.54)	0.86 (0.65–0.94)	2.5 (0.78–8.0)	0.75 (0.54–1.0)
No hypomobility on springing test	0.43 (0.27–0.61)	0.95 (0.77–0.99)	9.0 (1.3–63.9)	0.60 (0.43–0.84)
Hypermobility on springing test	0.46 (0.30–0.64)	0.81 (0.60–0.92)	2.4 (0.93–6.4)	0.66 (0.44–0.99)

Table 14–3   Diagnostic Accuracy Statistics for Segmental Tests in the Diagnosis of Radiographic Lumbar Instability

Technique	Type of Instability	Sensitivity (95% CI)	Specificity (95% CI)	+ LR (95% CI)	– LR (95% CI)
Prone springing test	Rotational	0.33 (0.12–0.65)	0.88 (0.83–0.92)	2.74 (1.01–7.42)	0.76 (0.48–1.21)
	Translational	0.29 (0.14–0.50)	0.89 (0.83–0.93)	2.52 (1.15–5.53)	0.81 (0.61–1.06)
Sidelying segmental flexion test	Rotational	0.05 (0.01–0.36)	0.99 (0.96–1.00)	4.12 (0.21–80.3)	0.96 (0.83–1.11)
	Translational	0.05 (0.01–0.22)	0.995 (0.97–1.00)	8.73 (0.57–134.7)	0.96 (0.88–1.05)
Sidelying segmental extension test	Rotational	0.22 (0.06–0.55)	0.97 (0.94–0.99)	8.4 (1.88–37.55)	0.80 (0.56–1.13)
	Translational	0.16 (0.06–0.38)	0.98 (0.94–0.99)	7.07 (1.71–29.2)	0.86 (0.71–1.05)

evant in the clinical context is that this study supports the value of a positive springing or segmental flexion and extension test in the diagnosis of both translational and rotational segmental instability of the lumbar spine but that a negative finding does not exclude this pathology.

CHAPTER 15

Examination of the Thoracic Spine

THORACIC SPINE T1(2)–T(11)12

Before discussing the clinical examination of the thoracic spine it is important to review pertinent aspects of thoracic spine anatomy, biomechanics, muscular influences on the thoracic spine, and rib cage, and clinical neurology of this spinal region to allow for the clinical reasoning required when evaluating the examination findings.

Functional Aspects of the Thoracic Spine

The thoracic spine is regarded as a single movement region because it exhibits certain internal consistencies. Despite the fact that vertebrae 1 to 12 are attached to the ribs, there are individual variations among them in the transitional areas. The first thoracic vertebra, for example, is sometimes regarded as belonging functionally to the cervical spine because of its shape; similarly, the 12th thoracic vertebra can be seen as part of the lumbar spine. According to Putz (1981), a distinction can be made between two parts of the thoracic region, namely, T1(2) to T8 and T8 to T(11)12. In the first of these areas, the ribs have a direct connection with the sternum; the extent of spinal flexion and extension is, therefore, significantly less than in the lower thoracic area. The two areas join at approximately the turning point of rotation during walking.

Alternatively, the thoracic spine can be divided into three areas, namely, high, middle, and low, based on the direction of the axes of movement of the ribs. A third possibility is to make a tripartite subdivision as follows: cervicothoracic as far as T4, because cervical movements are manifest to that level; midthoracic to T8, because the ribs are directly connected

with the sternum to that level; and low thoracic, because in this part, the connection with the sternum is indirect or absent, which means that increased movement is possible.

Putz (1981) gives some average values for the thoracic vertebrae (**Figure 15–1**):

Angle of inclination (α): T1 = 64°, T2 = 69°, T3 = 71°, T4 = 74°, T5 = 75°, T6 = 76°, T7 = 77.5°, T8 = 80°, T9 = 81°, T10 = 82°, T11 = 82°, T12 = 82.5°

Opening angle (β): T1 = 195°, T2 = 215°, T3 = 220°, T4 = 217.5°, T5 = 215°, T6 = 217.5°, T7 = 215°, T8 = 215°, T9 = 213°, T10 = 213°, T11 = 213°, T12 = 179°

Transverse distance: Distance between the joint surfaces of the superior articular processes (a):

T1 = 36 mm, T2 = 31 mm, T3 = 26 mm, T4 = 24 mm, T5 = 23 mm, T6 = 23 mm, T7 = 23 mm, T8 = 24 mm, T9 = 25 mm, T10 = 26 mm, T11 = 27 mm, T 12 = 28 mm

Sagittal distance: Distance between the joint surfaces of the superior articular surfaces and the center of the associated vertebral body (b): T1 = 20 mm, T2 = 22 mm, T3 = 25 mm, T4 = 30 mm, T5 = 33 mm, T6 = 36 mm, T7 = 38 mm, T8 = 39 mm, T9 = 40 mm, T10 = 39 mm, T11 = 39 mm, T12 = 43 mm

The standard deviation of values given by Putz is not provided in this book.

Other characteristics that distinguish the thoracic spine from the remaining regions are the insertion, size, and direction of the spinous and transverse processes, and the presence of the ribs, which are attached to the thoracic vertebrae.

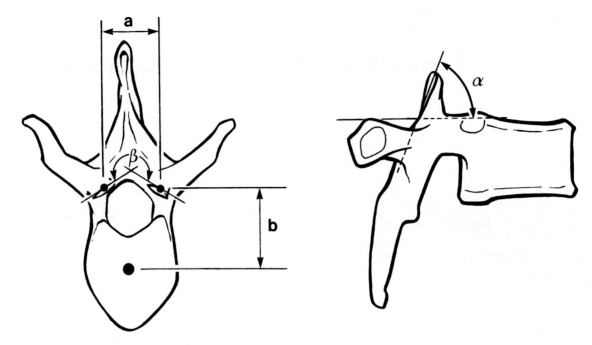

Figure 15–1   Characteristic parameters of the thoracic vertebra.

Ribs 1 to 10 also have direct or indirect contact with the sternum. These characteristics influence the functioning of the thoracic region. The relationship between the costotransverse joints and the sympathetic chain is also a distinguishing characteristic of this region. The movement of the ribs in the costovertebral and costotransverse joints depends on the

direction of the axes of movement that run through the centers of those joints (**Figure 15–2**).

The axis of movement of the upper ribs approaches the frontal plane (A). Elevation of these ribs increases the anteroposterior thoracic diameter. The axis of movement of the middle ribs forms an angle of about 45° with sagittal

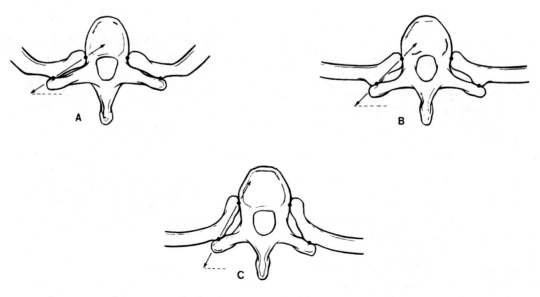

Figure 15–2   Axes of movement of the costovertebral and costotransverse joints.

plane (B). Elevation of these ribs increases both the transverse diameter and the anteroposterior diameter. The axis of movement of the lower ribs is almost in the sagittal plane (C), which means that elevation of these ribs increases the transverse diameter.

Movement also takes place in the sternocostal joint and in the costochondral attachments. The chondrosternal attachment is wedge-shaped, which permits vertical movement but not rotation. The costochondral attachment is cone-shaped, so some lateral and vertical movement is possible, but not rotation (Kapandji, 1974).

During inhalation, there is movement in vertical, transverse, and sagittal directions because the ribs rotate around the axis that runs through the centers of the costovertebral and costotransverse joints. As a result, the sternum moves in a cranial and ventral direction, while torsion occurs in the cartilaginous part of the costosternal attachment. This torsional force helps to ensure that the rib will return to its original position during exhalation. When the cartilage loses elasticity as a result of aging, this function is reduced.

During inhalation, the ventral movement of the sternum is greater at the cranial than at the caudal end. The angle between the first rib and the sternum becomes smaller, whereas the angle between the manubrium and the body of the sternum becomes larger. The angle between the 10th rib and its cartilaginous attachment enlarges, as does the angle between this attachment and the sternum (**Figure 15–3**).

The changes in the sizes of the angles are caused by axial rotation of the cartilage located between the bony part of the rib and the sternum. Exhalation produces the reverse pattern.

Flexion

The axis of flexion/extension appears to lie ventral to the vertebral body. The greatest amount of flexion/extension range of motion is found in the lowest part of the thoracic spine. Here, contact is maintained between the joint surfaces even in the extreme positions, so the upper edges of the superior articular processes of the vertebra below are not exposed to peak forces.

The amount of flexion in the middle and upper parts is somewhat lower. During flexion, there is a minimal translation between adjacent vertebrae in a ventral direction, and the ventral aspects of the vertebral bodies approximate, while the dorsal aspects move farther apart. The nucleus pulposus shows little displacement, but it increases in height dorsally and decreases ventrally (**Figure 15–4**).

The oblique annular fibers that run in the direction of movement, especially those on the dorsolateral side, are tensed, while those that run in the opposite direction, especially those on the ventrolateral side, relax. The intervertebral joints slide apart; the lower intervertebral joint surfaces of the upper vertebra move in a cranioventral direction relative to the upper intervertebral joint surfaces of the lower vertebra.

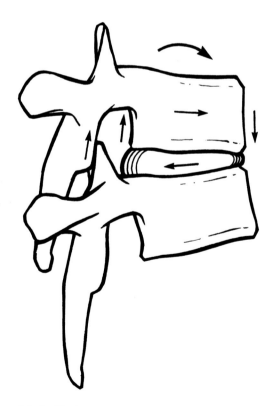

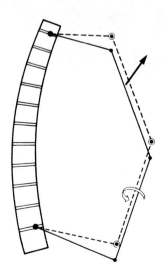

Figure 15–3 Changes in the size of the angles during inhalation.

Figure 15–4 Flexion.

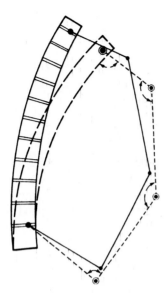

Figure 15–5   Changes in the size of the angles during flexion.

During flexion, the costovertebral angle, the superior and inferior sternocostal angles, and the chondrocostal angle all increase (**Figure 15–5**). If the movement coincides with exhalation, these changes in angle size will be reduced to some extent, with the exception of the angle between the first rib and the sternum, which increases. The ribs move in a more caudodorsal or more caudomedial direction depending on the direction of their axes. The intercostal space decreases.

The structures that inhibit flexion are the annular fibers, the joint capsule, the intra and supraspinous ligaments, the flaval ligaments, the intertransverse ligaments, the posterior longitudinal ligaments, the ligaments that span the joints between the vertebrae and ribs, and any compressive forces exerted by the ribs.

The outer oblique annular fibers that run opposite to the direction of movement relax, as does the anterior longitudinal ligament. In the end phase of flexion, it is probable that wedge-shaped openings appear caudally in the joint spaces in the middle and high thoracic parts of the spine. This is associated with the slope of the intervertebral joint surfaces. It does not, however, show on X-rays. The average range of movement is 45° (Kapandji, 1974).

Extension

During extension, there is minimal translation between the vertebrae in a dorsal direction. The intervertebral space increases ventrally and decreases dorsally. The nucleus pulposus moves little, but it increases in height ventrally and decreases dorsally. The outer oblique annular fibers that run

in the direction of movement, especially the ventrolateral ones, are tensed. Those that run in the opposite direction, especially the dorsolateral ones, relax. The joint partners of the intervertebral joints slide into each other. The lower intervertebral joint surfaces of the upper vertebra move in a caudal, and to some extent dorsal, direction (**Figure 15–6**).

During extension, the costovertebral angle, the superior and inferior sternocostal angles, and the chondrocostal angles all become smaller (**Figure 15–7**). As noted earlier, if extension coincides with inhalation, the angle changes are reduced, except for the angle between the first rib and the sternum, which decreases even further.

The ribs move in a more cranioventral or more craniolateral direction depending on the direction of their axes. The intercostal space increases. The structures that limit extension are the annular fibers, the capsule, the anterior longitudinal ligament, the interspinous ligaments, the tone of the abdominal muscles, the bony impact of the lower articular processes of the upper vertebra, and the spinous processes of the adjacent vertebrae, which may approach each other. When extension coincides with inhalation, the torsional forces in the cartilage that stretches between the ribs and the sternum may have a certain limiting effect. The posterior longitudinal ligament, the flaval ligaments, and the supraspinous ligaments all relax.

In the end phase of extension, it is probable that a wedge-shaped opening appears caudally in the joint spaces of the middle and higher thoracic areas. This would be as-

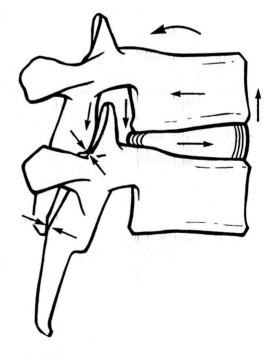

Figure 15–6   Extension.

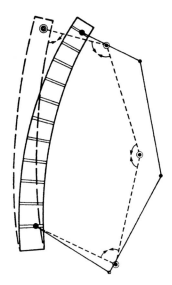

Figure 15–7 Changes in the size of the angles during extension.

sociated with the slope of the intervertebral joint surfaces. The average range of movement is 25° (Kapandji, 1974).

Sidebending

Opinions vary on whether sidebending is possible in the thoracic region. Heine (1957) distinguished three types of thoracic sidebending, based on high mobility, no mobility, and mixed forms. According to Heine, the relative rigidity of the upper thoracic vertebrae is due to the suspension of the muscles. Putz (1981) argues that limited sidebending is possible because of the shape of the intervertebral joint surfaces.

The compressive forces that arise unilaterally during sidebending cause a forced rotation. This rotation is least in the lowest part of the thoracic spine because of the angle of inclination, which increases toward the caudal end. The vertebral bodies move in the concave direction relative to each other. The intervertebral spaces become lower on the concave side during sidebending and higher on the convex side. The nucleus pulposus shows little displacement, but it increases in height on the convex side and decreases in height on the concave side (**Figure 15–8**).

The outer oblique annular fibers that run in the direction of movement are tensed, primarily on the ventral and dorsal convex sides, while those which run in the opposite direction, especially on the ventral and dorsal concave sides, relax. The intervertebral joint surfaces slide into each other on the concave side and away from each other on the convex side. The lower intervertebral joint surface of the upper vertebra moves in a caudodorsal direction on the concave side and in a cranioventral direction on the convex side.

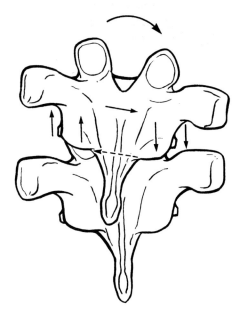

Figure 15–8 Sidebending.

Displacement will be the least in dorsal and ventral directions in the lower thoracic area because of the greater angle of inclination.

On the concave side, the rib cage will move downward and become narrower, the intercostal spaces will become smaller, and the chondrocostal angle of the 10th rib will decrease. The convex side will show the opposite pattern (**Figure 15–9**).

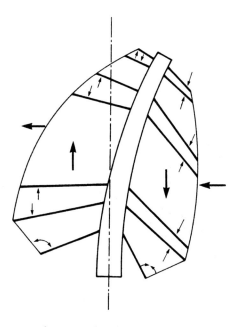

Figure 15–9 Changes in the rib cage during sidebending.

The structures that inhibit sidebending are the annular fibers, the joint capsule, the intra and supraspinous ligaments, the flaval and intertransverse ligaments, the anterior and posterior longitudinal ligaments, the ligaments that stretch between the vertebrae and the ribs, and the muscles that are involved on the convex side. Other factors are the impact of the lower facet joint surfaces of the upper vertebrae and compression of the ribs on the concave side.

The flaval and intertransverse ligaments on the concave side and the annular fibers described previously will relax. In the end phase, sidebending is limited in an elastic fashion in the absence of strong local compressive forces by the ligamentous structures, some of which, including the costovertebral connections, have long moment arms. The movement range is 20° (Kapandji, 1974).

Rotation

In most segments the axis of rotation runs in a longitudinal direction, approximately through the centers of the vertebral bodies and the disks. Taking into account the slight curvature in the sagittal plane, the facet joint surfaces of a motion segment may be regarded as part of the upper surface of a rotational ellipsoid. The facet joint surfaces in this region thus create very favorable conditions for rotational movement (**Figure 15–10**).

In the cervical and lumbar spine, the extent of movement is limited mainly by the shape of the facet articular

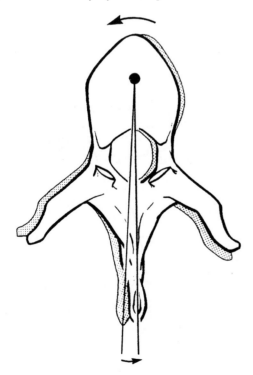

Figure 15–10   Rotation.

surfaces. In the thoracic spine, these have no such role. In the thoracic region, the transverse processes and the attached ribs, with their ligaments, offer a favorable transmission system for limiting the sagittal forces that arise primarily in the end phase. One, therefore, finds hardly any reinforcing fibers in the joint capsule. From T3 on, there is no associated sidebending in the neutral position because of the circular curvature of the facet joint surfaces in the transverse plane (Putz, 1981).

Because the center of curvature coincides with the axis of rotation, no compressive forces are exerted along the body's longitudinal axis in the end phase of rotation that could cause sidebending. Above T3, there is a slight forced sidebending because the center of curvature of the intervertebral joint surfaces does not coincide with the axis of rotation. Rotation above T3 is important for the final degrees of elevation of the arm (Stenvers and Overbeek, 1981).

During the course of the movement, there are no shearing forces in the thoracic region. The nucleus will be somewhat compressed centrally by the increase in tension of the outer annular fibers that run in the direction of movement; these exert a screw effect.

The outer annular fibers that run in the opposite direction relax. The upper facet joint surfaces within the segment move relative to the facet joint surfaces below them in a mediodorsal direction on the side of the direction of rotation, and medioventrally on the other side.

The transverse processes of the upper vertebra move in the same way relative to the vertebra below as do the upper facet joint surfaces within the segment. The spinous process of the upper vertebra moves relative to that of the lower vertebra in the direction opposite to that of movement. The presence in the thoracic area of the ribs and their attachments to the sternum has a marked effect on the course of the movement. During rotation, every pair of ribs is exposed, through the connection with the sternum, to distorting forces that have an effect on the rib cartilage. These forces cause the following changes in the rib cage during rotation (**Figure 15–11**):

- Dorsolateral increase in concavity at the side of the direction of rotation
- Decrease in the concavity of the chondrocostal angle at the same side
- Increase in concavity of the chondrocostal angle at the side opposite to the direction of rotation
- Dorsolateral decrease in concavity on the other side

The distorting forces cause a position of slight ventrodorsal obliquity of the sternum in the direction of rotation. The displacement is difficult to see on X-rays. The movement-limiting influence of the ribs and their attach-

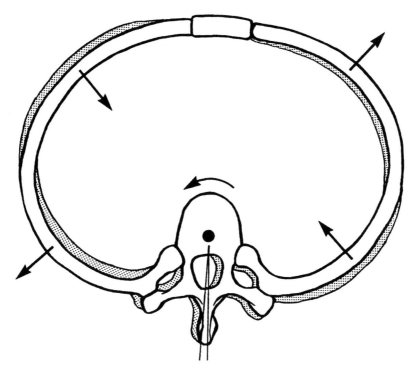

Figure 15–11   Changes in the rib cage during rotation.

ments increases as the cartilage becomes less elastic. The other structures that limit rotation are the outer oblique annular fibers that run in the direction of movement, the joint capsule, the intertransverse and flaval ligaments, the intra and supraspinous ligaments, the posterior and anterior longitudinal ligaments, the ligaments that span the vertebra and rib, the intercostal membrane, and the muscles that are involved.

In the end phase, the balance of forces is determined entirely by the forces exerted on the processes and ribs, and the opposing tensile forces that arises in the ligamentous structures. In every phase of the movement, the axis of rotation is located within the associated vertebral disk.

The average extent of movement is 35° (Kapandji, 1974).

Muscular Influences on the Thoracic Spine

The following muscles in the ventral area are relevant in this context:

- Abdominal muscles
- Pectoralis major and minor muscles
- Sternocleidomastoid muscle
- Anterior, middle, and posterior scalene muscles

When the abdominal muscles contract bilaterally, they have a flexion effect on both the thoracic and the lumbar spine. When they contract unilaterally, they cause sidebending or rotation, depending on their orientation. To bring about rotation, the internal oblique muscle on one side must work in coordination with the external oblique abdominal muscle on the other side. When their insertions are fixated, the chest and neck muscles listed previously have an extension effect when they contract bilaterally and a sidebending effect when they contract unilaterally.

In the deep layer of the dorsal area:

- Rotatores muscles
- Multifidus muscles
- Semispinalis muscles
- Intertransverse muscles
- Interspinales muscles

When these muscles contract bilaterally, they have a flexion effect. Just as important is their finely tuned stabilizing function. When they contract unilaterally, the first three in the list cause contraexternal rotation. When the intertransverse muscles contract unilaterally, they bring about ipsilateral sidebending.

In the intermediate layer:

- Posterior inferior serratus muscle
- Posterior superior serratus muscle
- Rhomboid minor and major muscles

When the first of these muscles contracts, it moves the lowest four ribs in a caudodorsal direction, so when it contacts bilaterally, it has a flexion effect on the lower part of the thoracic spine. When the second muscle contracts, it moves ribs 2 to 5 in a cranioventral direction. When the second and third muscles contract bilaterally, they cause a degree of flexion in the upper thoracic region. When they contract unilaterally, all these muscles bring about ipsilateral sidebending.

In the superficial layer:

- Spinalis muscle
- Longissimus muscle
- Iliocostalis muscle
- Latissimus dorsi muscle
- Middle and lower trapezius muscles

Bilateral contraction of these muscles causes extension; unilateral contraction causes ipsilateral sidebending.

In the lateral area:

- Quadratus lumborum muscle
- Serratus anterior muscle

Bilateral contraction of these muscles causes extension. Unilateral contraction causes ipsilateral sidebending.

Muscles Involved in Respiration

Inhalation

During inhalation, there is an increase in tone in the scalene muscles, which raise the first and second ribs. This movement is followed as far down as the sixth rib, bringing about an expansion consistent with the axes of movement of the vertebral joints. The diaphragm is also active. The highest level of activity occurs before the end of inspiration, causing expansion in three directions. The thoracic spinal erector muscle, which often seems to become insufficient, has an important role in inhalation, as do the intercostal muscles, which, according to MacConnail and Basmajian (1969) always maintain a constant basic level of activity that neither increases nor decreases. During vigorous inhalation, however, the activity of the intercostal muscles does in-

crease to some extent. These muscles maintain a constant spatial separation of the ribs.

The quadratus lumborum muscle becomes active at the same moment as the diaphragm; one of its functions is to stabilize the lower ribs. Both inhalation and exhalation are important as aspects of normal functioning of the thoracic spine.

Muscles that assist inhalation, especially when it is vigorous, are the following:

- Sternocleidomastoid muscle
- Pectoralis muscles

Exhalation

During exhalation, the basic tone of the intercostal muscles remains constant. Murphy (1959) (in MacConnail and Basmajian, 1969) states that during relaxed exhalation, the diaphragm shows a lower level of activity over a longer period than during inhalation. One reason for this could be that during passive exhalation, the activity of the diaphragm has an inhibiting effect on the elastic contraction of the lung tissues. During vigorous exhalation, there appears to be no activity in the diaphragm. Exhalation is normally brought about by the force of gravity, the elasticity of the rib cartilage, the quadratus lumborum muscles, and the abdominal muscles.

Muscles that assist in exhalation, especially when vigorous, are the following:

- Rectus abdominis muscle
- Internal oblique muscle

Motor and Sensory Relationships

The 12 pairs of thoracic nerves all branch to form the following structures:

- Ventral ramus
- Dorsal ramus
- A small recurrent meningeal branch

The ventral rami form the intercostal nerves, which innervate the intercostal muscles, while the dorsal rami innervate the sacrospinal muscles. These nerves have many sensory branches. The thoracic muscles, which are innervated from the brachial plexus, are described in the section on "Motor-Sensory Relationships" in Chapter 17. The meningeal nerve plays an important part in the nerve supply to the intervertebral joint.

REGIONAL EXAMINATION

The regional examination consists of an active-assisted regional examination and regional provocation tests.

Active-Assisted Regional Examination: Thoracic

For assessment criteria, see the section titled "Active-Assisted Regional Examination: Lumbar" in Chapter 14. The active-assisted regional examination of the thoracic spine is in many respects the same as that of the lumbar spine, so only illustrations, and not further descriptions of the techniques, are provided here (**Figures 15–12** through **15–21**).

The thoracic examination differs from the lumbar one in the following ways:

- The non-weight-bearing active-assisted regional examination is not included.
- The stabilizing hand is placed on the spinous process of L1.

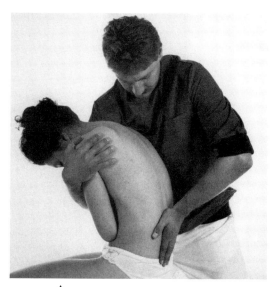

Figure 15–12

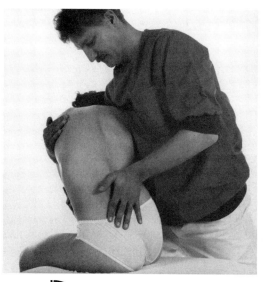

Figure 15–13

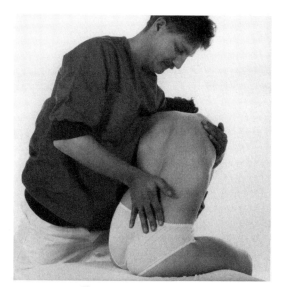

Figure 15–14

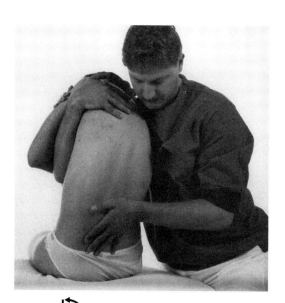

Figure 15–15

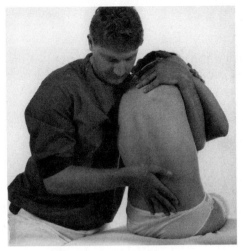

Figure 15–16

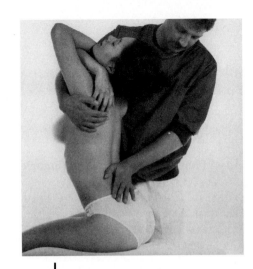

Figure 15–17

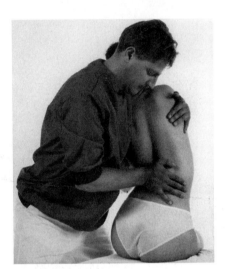

Figure 15–18

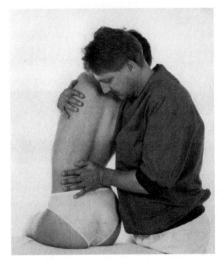

Figure 15–19

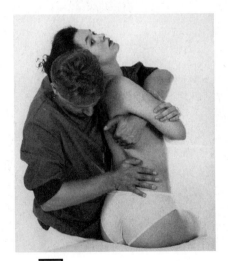

Figure 15–20

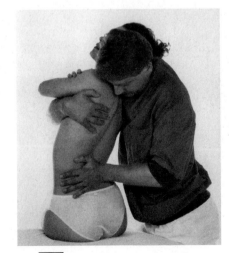

Figure 15–21

Regional Provocation Tests

For the assessment criteria and a description of the thoracic regional provocation tests, please see the section titled "Regional Provocation Tests: Lumbar" in Chapter 14. For the regional traction test, the patient crosses his or her arms in front of the chest, with the hands on shoulders. The therapist crosses his or her hands so that each holds the opposite elbow of the patient. For the regional compression test, the patient's spine should be in the extended position. (See **Figures 15–22, 15–23, 15–24**).

SEGMENTAL EXAMINATION

The thoracic segmental examination consists of a segmental tissue-specific examination, segmental provocation tests, and an active-assisted segmental examination.

Segmental Tissue–Specific Examination

For the assessment criteria and a description of the thoracic segmental tissue–specific tests, please see the section

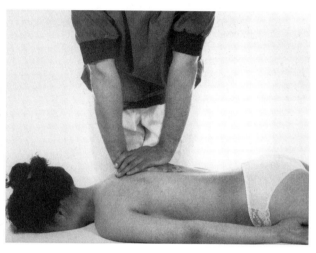

Figure 15–22 ⇅

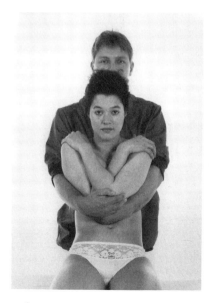

Figure 15–23 ↕

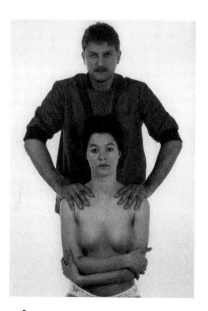

Figure 15–24 ↕

titled "Segmental Tissue–Specific Examination: Lumbar" in Chapter 14. See **Figures 15–25** through **15–30**. Figure 15–26 shows the examination of the lateral branch of the dorsal ramus.

Christensen et al. (2002) reported a κ value of 0.57 (95% CI: 0.13–1.00) for intrarater agreement on palpation for pain at the left T1–T8 zygapophyseal joints when all subjects were reexamined within 1.5–2 hours; palpation on the right yielded κ = 0.50 (95% CI: 0.21–0.92). If subjects were reexamined on two consecutive days, the intrarater κ value left was 0.34 (95% CI: −0.16–0.84) and right was 0.45 (95% CI: 0.02–0.88). The interrater study yielded κ =

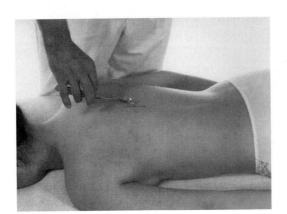

Figure 15–25

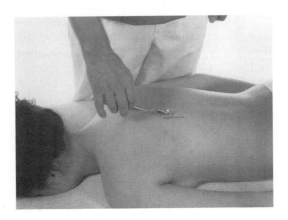

Figure 15–26

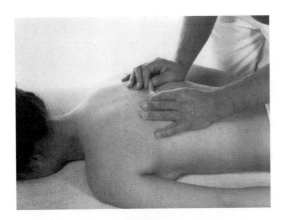

Figure 15–27

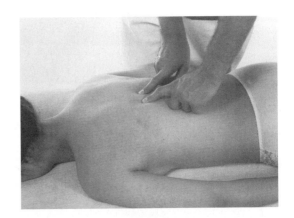

Figure 15–28

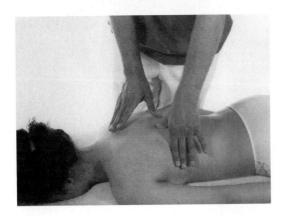

Figure 15–29

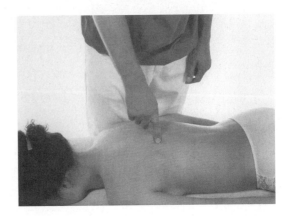

Figure 15–30

0.38 (95% CI: 0.07–0.69) on the left and κ = 0.38 (95% CI: 0.08–0.68) for palpation of a painful zygapophyseal joint on the right. Keating et al. (2001) reported on differences in tenderness to palpation at the C4, T4, T6, and L4 levels in asymptomatic subjects and noted significant ($P <$ .001) differences in tenderness at the various levels with pressure pain thresholds increasing in a caudal direction. The authors indicated that clinically greater thoracic as compared to cervical tenderness should be interpreted as an abnormal finding. Bertilson et al. (2003) studied interrater reliability of palpation for tenderness at the T1–T3 and T4–T7 spinal processes and reported 78% (κ = 0.55) and

72% (κ = 0.43) agreement, respectively. Palpation for tenderness at the T1–T3 and T4–T7 joints yielded 70 (κ = 0.41) and 76% (κ = 0.5) agreement, respectively.

Segmental Provocation Tests

For the assessment criteria and a description of the thoracic segmental provocation tests, please see the section titled "Segmental Provocation Tests: Lumbar" in Chapter 14. See also **Figures 15–31, 15–32, 15–33**.

Christensen et al. (2002) reported a κ value of 0.33 (95% CI: −0.21–0.87) for intrarater agreement on prone

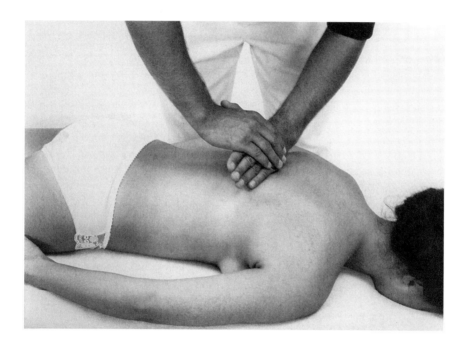

Figure 15–31

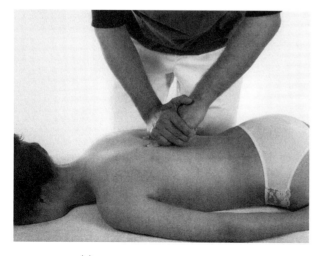

Figure 15–32

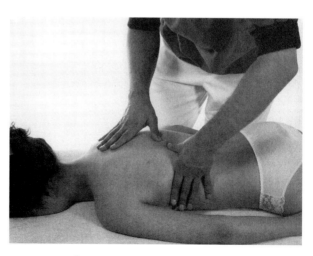

Figure 15–33

Table 15–1   Data on Interrater Agreement Prone T1–T9 Springing Test

Level	K_w, 95% CI (mobility)	PA (mobility)	K_w, 95% CI (pain)	PA (pain)
T1	0.67 (0.33–1.0)	86%	0.72 (0.43–1.0)	86%
T2	0.68 (0.36–0.99)	86%	0.54 (0.23–0.85)	76%
T3	0.49 (0.05–0.98)	86%	−0.11 (−0.50–0.29)	50%
T4	0.72 (0.43–1.0)	86%	0.90 (0.73–1.0)	95%
T5	0.49 (0.19–0.79)	72%	0.22 (0.00–0.45)	54%
T6	0.89 (0.59–1.0)	90%	0.30 (0.05–0.55)	59%
T7	0.13 (−0.26–0.53)	72%	0.36 (0.02–0.71)	64%
T8	0.39 (−0.07–0.87)	81%	0.24 (−0.14–0.62)	64%
T9	0.52 (0.16–0.89)	77%	0.0 (−0.51–0.31)	45%

T1–T8 springing test when all subjects were reexamined within 1.5–2 hours. If subjects were reexamined on two consecutive days, the intrarater κ value was 0.45 (95% CI: −0.01–0.91). The interrater study yielded κ = −0.03 (−0.42–0.36). Using a three-point rating scale of hypermobile, normal, hypomobile, Cleland et al. (2006) reported on interrater agreement for the prone T1–T9 springing test; these authors also provided interrater agreement data with regard to absence or presence of pain for this test. **Table 15–1** provides data on interrater percentage agreement (PA) and weighted κ values for the prone springing test.

Active-Assisted Segmental Examination: Thoracic (T4 to T12)

The clinician must determine the position of the transverse process relative to the spinous process (**Figures 15–34** and **15–35**).

The end of the spinous process of a thoracic vertebra lies lower than the corresponding transverse process. The difference in vertical position increases from the cranial to the caudal end of the spine, though it decreases again to some extent in the lowest region. Overall, it can be said that the end of the spinous process of a given vertebra lies at the same height as the transverse process of the vertebra below. The following test is used to determine the exact position of the transverse process of a thoracic vertebra:

The spinous process of the thoracic vertebra is palpated with the index finger of one hand. With the thumb of the other hand, pressure is applied in a ventral direction near the vertebra on the expected location of its transverse process. When the thumb is placed on the exact position of the transverse process, the ventral pressure will cause the vertebra to rotate. This movement will displace the associated spinous process in an ipsilateral direction relative to the thumb exerting the pressure, and it will then be felt by the palpating finger.

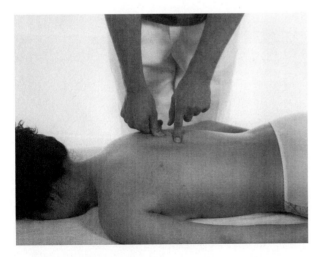

Figure 15–34 ⌐

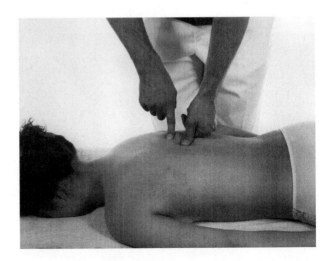

Figure 15–35 ⊢—

It is also possible to move the spinous process in a rotatory direction and to determine by observation the position of the corresponding contralateral transverse process.

Remarks

Because of the ligamentous connections between the vertebrae, the ventral pressure on the transverse process will cause other vertebrae to move with it. However, when the thumb has located the exact position of the transverse process, the associated spinous process will show a greater range of movement than the other spinous processes.

For assessment criteria of active-assisted segmental examination of the thoracic spine, please see the section titled "Active-Assisted Segmental Examination: Lumbar (L1 to L5)" in Chapter 14.

Flexion, Weight-Bearing

Examination position, patient: Sitting on the short side of the examination table with the lower legs hanging down; the arms are crossed in front of the chest; the spine is brought into flexion down to and including the level to be examined.

Starting position, therapist: Standing beside the patient.

Stabilization: The therapist holds the spinous process of the lower vertebra at the level to be examined between the thumb and the index finger of the stabilizing hand and keeps the vertebra in position.

Procedure: The manipulating hand and arm surround the patient's arms and introduce flexion. (See **Figure 15–36**.)

Flexion, Lateral Flexion, Ipsilateral Rotation, Weight-Bearing

Examination position, patient: Sitting on the short side of the examination table with the lower legs hanging down; the arms are crossed in front of the chest; the spine is brought into flexion, lateral flexion, and ipsilateral rotation down to and including the level to be examined.

Starting position, therapist: Standing beside the patient at the side to be examined

Stabilization: The therapist holds the spinous process of the lower vertebra of the level to be examined between the

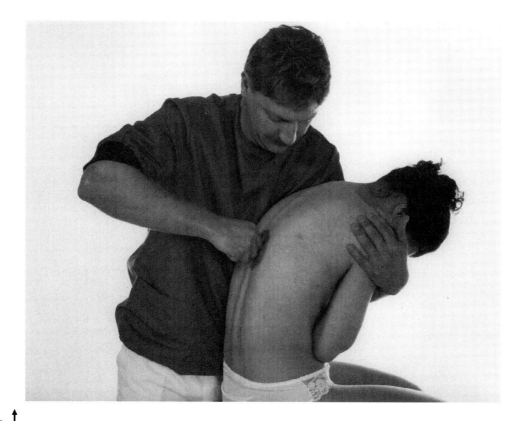

Figure 15–36

thumb and the index finger of the stabilizing hand and keeps the vertebra in position.

Procedure: The manipulating hand and arm pass between the patient's crossed arms from the cranial end and surround the contralateral side of the thorax. The therapist introduces ventral flexion, lateral flexion, and ipsilateral rotation. (See **Figure 15–37**.)

Flexion, Lateral Flexion, Contralateral Rotation, Weight-Bearing

Examination position, patient: Sitting on the short side of the examination table with the lower legs hanging down; the arms are crossed in front of the chest; the spine is brought into flexion, lateral flexion, and contralateral rotation down to and including the level to be examined.

Starting position, therapist: Standing beside the patient at the side not being examined, or at the other side as preferred.

Stabilization: The therapist holds the spinous process of the lower vertebra at the level to be examined between the

thumb and the index finger of the stabilizing hand and keeps the vertebra in position.

Procedure: The manipulating hand and arm pass between the patient's crossed arms from the cranial end and surround the contralateral side of the thorax. The therapist introduces ventral flexion, lateral flexion, and contralateral rotation. (See **Figure 15–38**.)

In Figure 15–38, the examiner is standing at the side not being examined. If the examiner stands at the side to be examined, that is, turning back toward him- or herself, the manipulating hand and arm pass between the patient's crossed arms from the caudal end and hold on to the contralateral shoulder.

Extension, Weight-Bearing

Examination position, patient: Sitting on the short side of the examination table with the lower legs hanging down; the hands are placed on the neck or the arms are crossed in

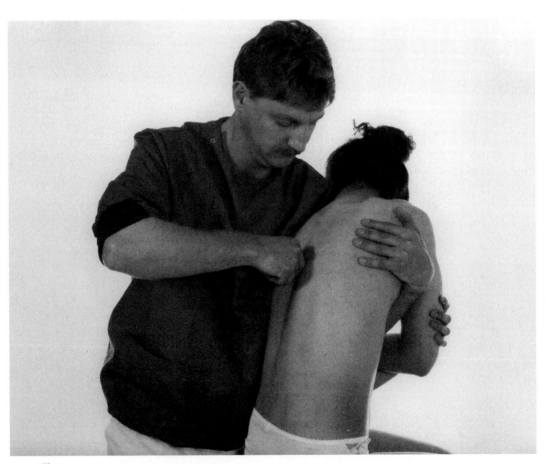

Figure 15–37

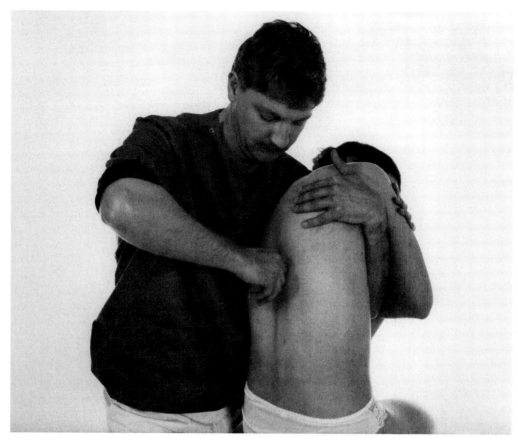

Figure 15–38

front of the chest; the spine is brought into extension down to and including the level to be examined.

Starting position, therapist: Standing beside the patient.

Stabilization: The therapist holds the spinous process of the lower vertebra at the level to be examined between the thumb and the index finger of the stabilizing hand and keeps the vertebra in position.

Procedure: The manipulating hand and arm pass under the patient's arms, surround the contralateral side of the thorax, and introduce extension. (See **Figure 15–39**.)

Extension, Lateral Flexion, Ipsilateral Rotation, Weight-Bearing

Examination position, patient: Sitting on the short side of the examination table with the lower legs hanging down; the arms are crossed in front of the chest; the spine is brought into extension, lateral flexion, and ipsilateral rotation down to and including the level to be examined.

Starting position, therapist: Standing beside the patient at the side to be examined.

Stabilization: The therapist holds the spinous process of the lower vertebra of the level to be examined between the thumb and the index finger of the stabilizing hand and keeps the vertebra in position.

Procedure: The manipulating hand and arm pass between the patient's crossed arms from the cranial end and surround the contralateral side of the thorax. The therapist introduces extension, lateral flexion, and ipsilateral rotation. (See **Figure 15–40**.)

Extension, Lateral Flexion, Contralateral Rotation, Weight-Bearing

Examination position, patient: Sitting with the lower legs hanging down on the short side of the examination table; the arms are crossed in front of the chest; the spine is brought into extension, lateral flexion and contralateral rotation down to and including the level to be examined.

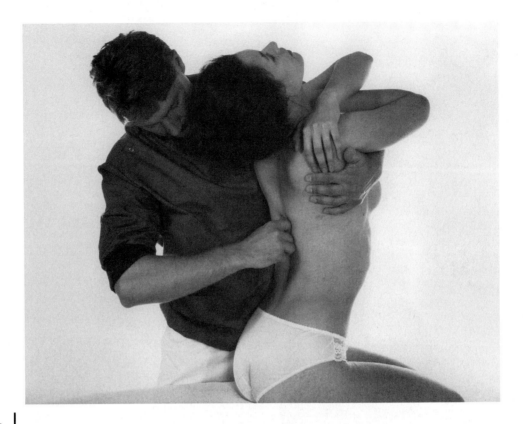

Figure 15–39

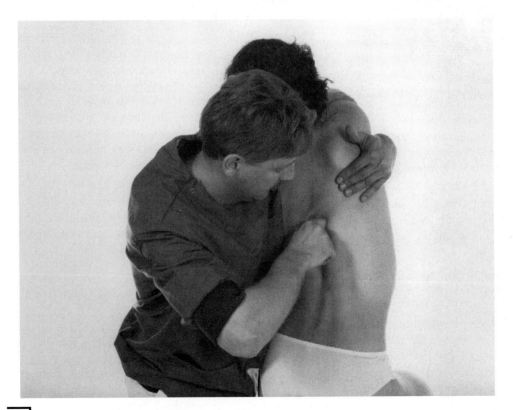

Figure 15–40

Starting position, therapist: Standing beside the patient at the side not to be examined or at the other side.

Stabilization: The therapist holds the spinous process of the lower vertebra at the level to be examined between the thumb and the index finger of the stabilizing hand and keeps the vertebra in position.

Procedure: The manipulating hand and arm pass between the patient's crossed arms from the cranial end and surround the contralateral side of the thorax. The therapist introduces extension, lateral flexion, and contralateral rotation. (See **Figure 15–41**.)

If the examiner stands at the side being examined, turning back toward him- or herself, the manipulating hand and arm pass between the patient's arms from the caudal end and the hand is placed on the contralateral shoulder.

Although not specific to the two preceding techniques, Brismée et al. (2006) reported on the interrater reliability of a similar T6–T7 extension-rotation segmental motion test to see if raters could agree whether ipsilateral or contralateral

sidebending produced the greatest excursion. Somewhat supporting the reliability of the two preceding tests, these authors noted fair to substantial agreement with pair-wise interrater percentage agreement from 63.4–82.5% and κ values from 0.27–0.65.

Ribs

In the complex thoracic region, with its many rib attachments, dysfunctions can arise in the following structures (see **Figures 15–42** and **15–43**):

- Costovertebral joints (a)
- Costotransverse joints (b)
- Costocartilaginous attachments (c)
- Chondrosternal attachments (d)
- Interchondral attachments (e)
- Intercostal musculature (f)

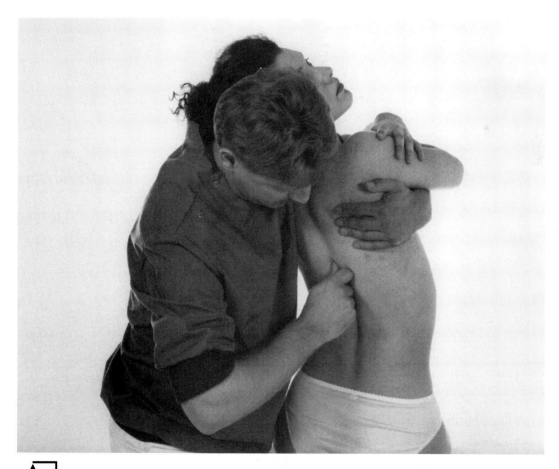

Figure 15–41

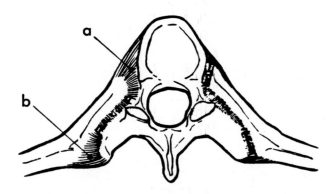

Figure 15–42   Costovertebral and costotransverse joints.

The examination of the ribs is subdivided as follows:

General examination: Observation of thorax excursion during respiration, both when resting and during maximum inhalation and exhalation, and in different starting positions. Examination by inspection can be supported by palpation of the intercostal spaces.

Examination 1st rib: with or without palpation of the sternocostal joint.

Examination 2nd to 5th ribs: intercostal spaces (ventral), costovertebral joints, chondrosternal attachments.

Examination 6th to 10th ribs: intercostal spaces (lateral), costovertebral joints, chondrosternal attachments, interchondral attachments.

Examination 11th and 12th ribs: costovertebral joints.

Assessment of general function:

The patient sits on the examination table with arms hanging. The therapist observes individual breaths in a resting condition from ventral, lateral, and dorsal positions (**Figures 15–44, 15–45, 15–46**).

In a second phase of the examination, the patient can be asked to breathe in and out as far as possible on request. The extent of thorax excursion is then observed in supine and prone positions. Next, the therapist may palpate the intercostal spaces symmetrically on both sides during maxi-

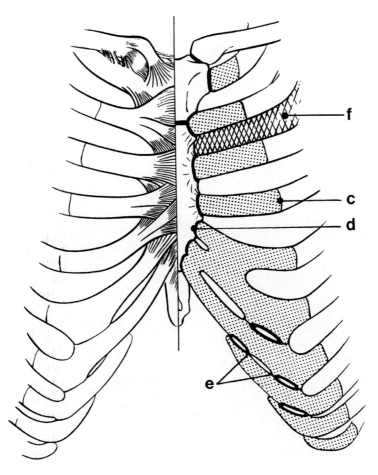

Figure 15–43   Costosternal connections and structures.

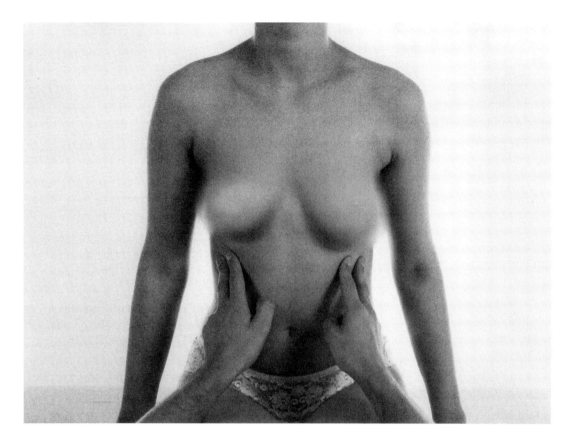

Figure 15–44

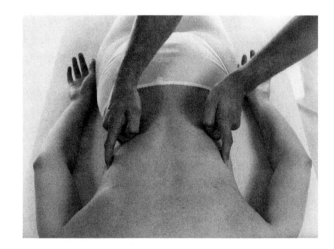

Figure 15–45

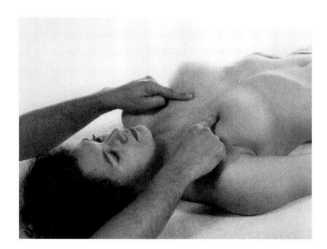

Figure 15–46

mal respiration. The intercostal spaces from the 2nd to the 5th rib are assessed in a more ventral position, and those from the 6th to 10th rib more laterally. During palpation, the therapist examines the spreading of the ribs (symmetrical or asymmetrical); this indicates whether a particular rib tends toward the inhalation or exhalation position. Adjacent intercostal spaces are also compared. For the assessment criteria used in local examination of the costovertebral attachments, please see the section titled "Active-Assisted Segmental Examination: Lumbar (L1 to L5)" in Chapter 14.

Examination of the rib attachments involves *primarily:*

- The intercostal spaces
- The costotransverse joints
- The costosternal attachments

and *secondarily:*

- The interchondral attachments

Because of the close connections between the ribs and the spine, disturbances in the costovertebral joints can lead to problems in thoracic or adjacent lumbar and cervical spinal segments.

The assessment criteria are as follows:

- Position
- Endfeel
- Sensitivity to pressure and pain
- Compression of nerves and blood vessels
- Autonomic reactions
- Swelling
- Increased muscle tone
- Specific pain points

First Rib, Weight-Bearing

Examination position, patient: Sitting on the long side of the examination table; the cervical spine is brought into flexion and ipsiexternal rotation down to T2.

Starting position, therapist: Standing behind the patient.

Stabilization: The upper part of the stabilizing arm rests on the patient's contralateral shoulder. The hand encircles the patient's head and maintains the position of the cervical spine.

Procedure: The ventral side of the index finger of the manipulation hand is placed on the dorsocranial aspect of the first rib and performs the movement in a ventro-medio-caudal direction. (See **Figure 15–47**.)

Remarks: To obtain good contact with the first rib, the overlying part of the trapezius muscle must be moved in a dorsal direction.

First Rib, Non-Weight-Bearing

Examination position, patient: Supine; the head and the cervical spine are brought into ipsiexternal rotation and sidebending.

Starting position, therapist: Standing by the patient's head.

Stabilization: The stabilizing arm is placed on the patient's head and maintains the position of the cervical spine; the index finger is used to assess sternocostal mobility by means of palpation.

Procedure: The ventral side of the index finger of the manipulating hand is placed on the dorsocranial side of the first rib and moves it a ventro-medio-caudal direction. The therapist may use his or her thigh as support if needed. (See **Figures 15–48** and **15–49**.)

Remarks: The overlying part of the trapezius muscle is manually moved ventrally during this examination. Cervical extension must be avoided.

Ribs, Non-Weight-Bearing (Second to Fifth)

Examination position, patient: Supine; the arm on the side to be examined is elevated as far as possible.

Starting position, therapist: Standing by the patient's head.

Stabilization: The index finger of the stabilizing hand is placed ventrally in the intercostal space on the lower rib of the level to be examined; the hand maintains the position of the rib.

Procedure: The patient's lower arm is held between the therapist's upper arm and thorax. The manipulating hand and arm enclose the patient's elevated upper arm and perform extension under traction. (See **Figure 15–50**.)

Remarks: The patient can be asked to breathe in or out as far as possible, in which case the therapist must adapt his or her actions to the patient's breathing.

Ribs, Non-Weight-Bearing (6th to 10th)

Examination position, patient: Lying on the side; the arm at the side to be examined is elevated as far as possible.

Starting position, therapist: Standing by the patient's head.

Stabilization: The index finger of the stabilizing hand is placed ventrally in the intercostal space on the lower rib

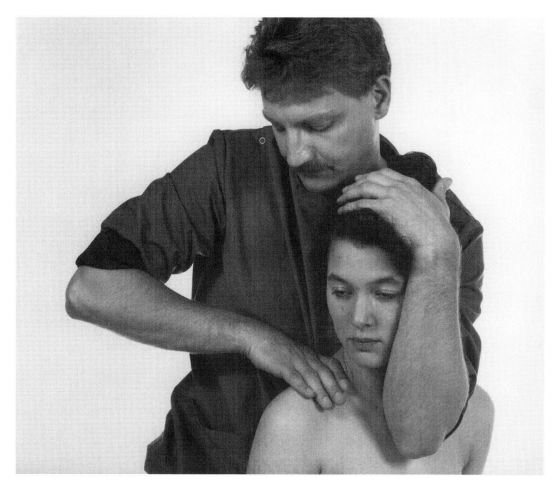

Figure 15–47 ⌊ ↤ ⌶

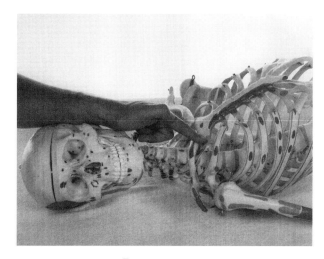

Figure 15–48 ⌊ ↤ ⌶

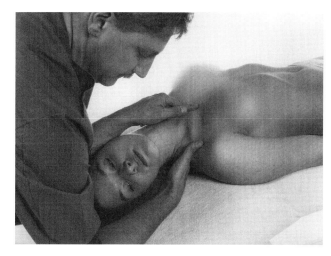

Figure 15–49 ⌊ ↤ ⌶

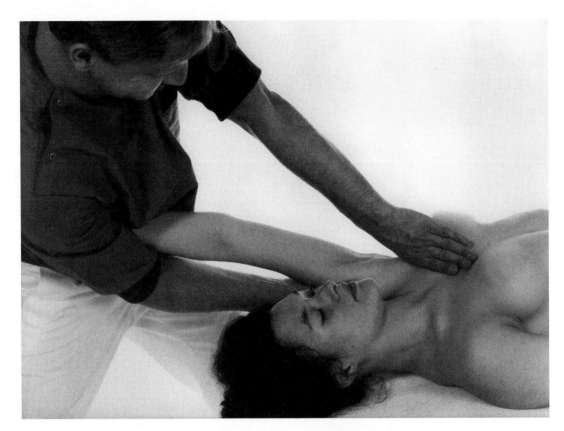

Figure 15–50 ↕ ↓

of the level to be examined. The hand maintains the position of the lower rib.

Procedure: The patient's lower arm is held between the therapist's upper arm and thorax. The manipulating hand and arm enclose the patient's elevated upper arm and perform contralateral sidebending. (See **Figure 15–51**.)

Remarks: The shoulder on which the patient is lying, and which functions as an anchoring point, must be directly below the upper shoulder and in line with it.

Ribs, Weight-Bearing (6th to 10th)

Examination position, patient: Sitting on the short side of the examination table with the legs hanging down; the hand at the side to be examined is placed on the neck, while the elbow is moved in a dorsal direction.

Starting position, therapist: Stands behind the patient with one leg on top of the examination table.

Stabilization: the index finger of the stabilizing hand is placed ventrally in the intercostal space on the lower rib of the level to be examined. The hand maintains the position of the lower rib.

Procedure: The manipulating hand passes through the crook of the patient's arm, encircles the elbow, and brings about contralateral sidebending. (See **Figure 15–52**.)

Costovertebral Joints (2nd to 10th)

Examination position, patient: Prone, with arms hanging down beside the bench.

Starting position, therapist: Depending on the level to be examined, the therapist stands either by the patient's head or beside the patient at the side not being examined.

Stabilization: The hypothenar of the stabilizing hand is placed contralaterally on the transverse process of the level to be examined. The hand maintains the position of this transverse process.

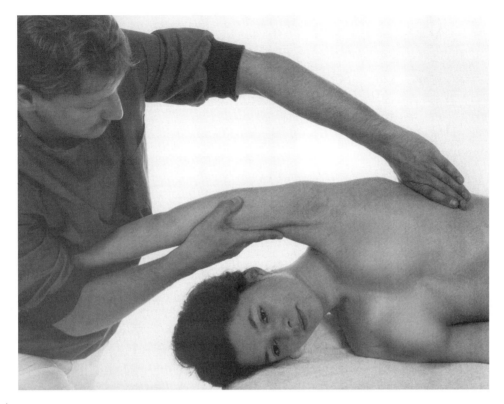

Figure 15–51 $\updownarrow$ $\longrightarrow$

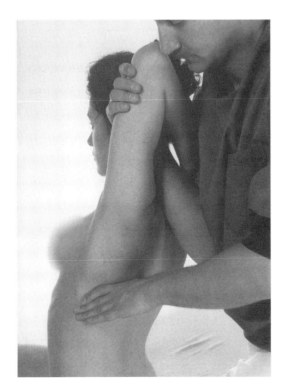

Figure 15–52 $\updownarrow$ $\longrightarrow$

Procedure: The thumb or the hypothenar of the manipulating hand is placed on the rib of the costotransverse joint to be examined, just to the side of the transverse process. The hand exerts light pressure in a ventral direction. (See **Figures 15–53** and **15–54**.)

Costovertebral Joints (11th and 12th Ribs)

Examination position, patient: Prone.

Starting position, therapist: Standing beside the patient at the side not to be examined.

Stabilization: The hypothenar of the stabilizing hand is placed contralaterally on the transverse process of the level to be examined. The hand maintains the position of this transverse process.

Procedure: The thumb or the hypothenar of the manipulating hand is placed on the rib just to the side of the transverse process. The hand exerts light pressure in a ventral direction. (See **Figure 15–55**.)

Remarks: The 11th and 12th ribs have no costotransverse or costosternal joints. They can, therefore, normally move much more than the other ribs.

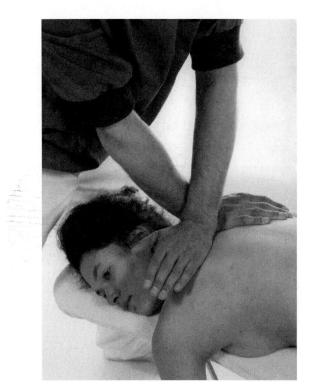

Figure 15–53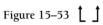

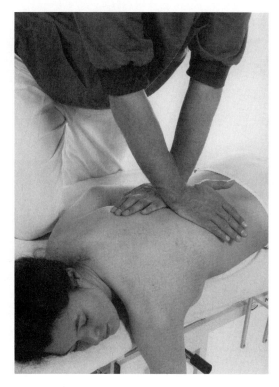

Figure 15–54

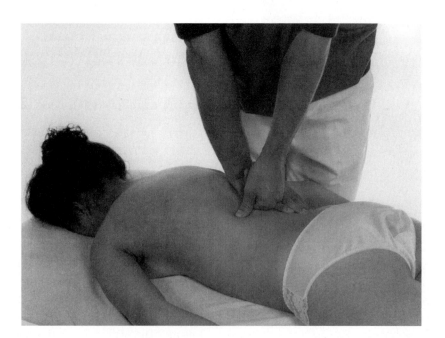

Figure 15–55

Chondrosternal Attachments (Second to Sixth Ribs)

Examination position, patient: Supine.

Starting position, therapist: Standing beside the patient on the side not being examined.

Stabilization: The stabilizing hand, the little finger of which is placed on the sternum at the contralateral side, maintains the position of the sternum.

Procedure: The thumb of the manipulating hand is placed on the rib directly lateral to the chondrosternal attach-

ment. This hand exerts light pressure in a dorsal direction. (See **Figures 15–56** and **15–57**.)

Interchondral Attachments

The interchondral attachments are palpated only for sensitivity to pressure pain (**Figures 15–58** and **15–59**). They seldom are victim to independent dysfunctions. In most cases, dysfunctions of the interchondral attachments indicate problems in the associated ribs and their costovertebral connections.

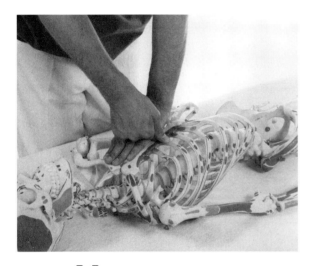

Figure 15–56 ⌐⌐

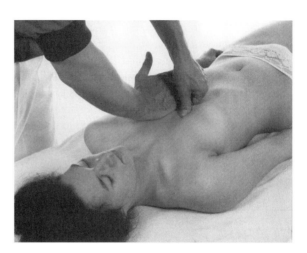

Figure 15–57 ⌐⌐

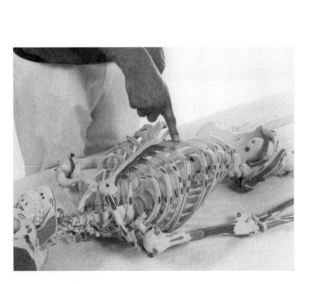

Figure 15–58 ⌐

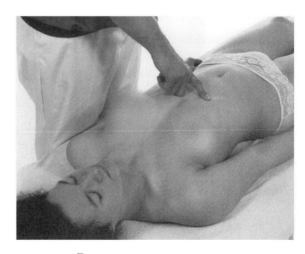

Figure 15–59 ⌐

CERVICOTHORACIC SPINE (C7 TO T4)

From a biomechanical point of view, the cervicothoracic spine is the transitional area between the thoracic and cervical parts. Normal functioning of this region is extremely important for the proper function of the cervical spine and of the upper limbs. Normal function in the upper thoracic vertebral segments is essential for full elevation of the arms.

The cervicothoracic area also has important autonomic connections with the cervical spine because the preganglionic sympathetic neurons of the upper cervical supply area are located in this region.

The active-assisted regional examination of the cervicothoracic transition is performed at the same time as the regional examination of the cervical spine. That examination is described in the section titled "Active-Assisted Regional Examination: Cervicothoracic/Cervical," which follows. During the active-assisted segmental examination of the cervicothoracic transition, the manipulating hand/arm, which is placed on the patient's head, uses the cervical spine as a lever. If there are dysfunctions in the cervical spine, the manipulating hand will need to be placed as close as possible to the upper thoracic spine.

REGIONAL EXAMINATION

Active-Assisted Regional Examination: Cervicothoracic/Cervical

For assessment criteria, please see the section titled "Active-Assisted Regional Examination: Lumbar" in Chapter 14.

Flexion, Weight-Bearing

Examination position, patient: Sitting on the short side of the examination table with the lower legs hanging.

Starting position, therapist: Standing beside the patient.

Stabilization: The thumb and index finger of the stabilizing hand hold the spinous process of T4. This hand maintains the position of this vertebra.

Procedure: The patient leans his or her head against the upper part of the therapist's manipulating arm. The therapist holds the spinous process of C2 with the little finger of the same hand and moves the patient's spine into a flexed position while the upper cervical spine is held in extension. (See **Figure 15–60**.)

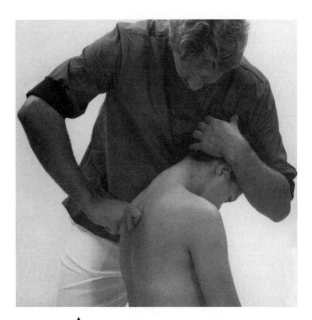

Figure 15–60 ↑

Flexion, Sidebending, Ipsilateral Rotation, Weight-Bearing

Examination position, patient: Sitting on the short side of the examination table with the lower legs hanging down.

Starting position, therapist: Standing beside the patient at the side to be examined.

Stabilization: The thumb and index finger of the stabilizing hand hold the spinous process of T4. This hand maintains the position of this vertebra.

Procedure: The patient leans his or her head against the upper part of the therapist's manipulating arm. The therapist holds the contralateral lamina of C2 with the little finger of the same hand and moves the patient's spine into flexion, sidebending, and ipsilateral rotation, while the upper cervical spine is held in extension and contralateral sidebending. (See **Figure 15–61**.)

Flexion, Sidebending, Contralateral Rotation, Weight-Bearing

Examination position, patient: Sitting on the short side of the examination table with the lower legs hanging down.

Starting position, therapist: Standing beside the patient either on the side to be examined, or on the other side if appropriate.

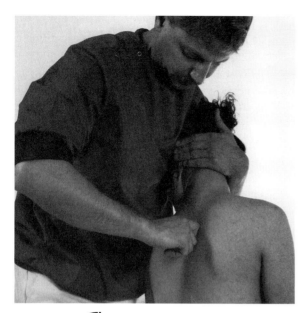

Figure 15–61

Stabilization: The thumb and index finger of the stabilizing hand hold the spinous process of T4. This hand maintains the position of this vertebra.

Procedure: The patient leans his or her head against the upper part of the therapist's manipulating arm. The therapist holds the contralateral lamina of C2 with the little finger

of this hand, and moves the patient's spine into flexion, sidebending and contralateral rotation, while the upper cervical spine is held in extension. (See **Figure 15–62**.)

Remarks: The sidebending and rotation components can also be performed the other way around, in which case the examiner stands at the side to be examined.

Extension, Weight-Bearing

Examination position, patient: Sitting on the short side of the examination table with the lower legs hanging down.

Starting position, therapist: Standing beside the patient.

Stabilization: The thumb and index finger of the stabilizing hand hold the spiny process of T4. This hand maintains the position of this vertebra.

Procedure: The patient leans his or her head against the upper part of the therapist's manipulating arm. The therapist holds the spinous process of C2 with the little finger of this hand and brings the patient's spine into extension, while the upper cervical spine is held in the neutral position. (See **Figure 15–63**.)

Extension, Sidebending, Ipsilateral Rotation, Weight-Bearing

Examination position, patient: Sitting on the short side of the examination table with the lower legs hanging down.

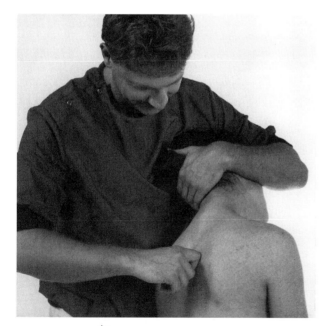

Figure 15–62

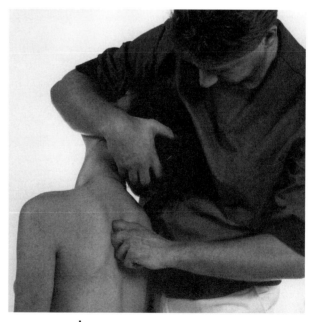

Figure 15–63

Starting position, therapist: Standing beside the patient at the side to be examined.

Stabilization: The thumb and index finger of the stabilizing hand hold the spinous process of T4. This hand maintains the position of this vertebra.

Procedure: The patient leans his or her head against the upper part of the therapist's manipulating arm. The therapist holds the contralateral lamina of C2 with the little finger of the same hand and moves the patient's spine into extension, sidebending, and ipsilateral rotation, while the upper cervical spine is held in the neutral position and contralateral sidebending. (See **Figure 15–64**.)

Extension, Sidebending, Contralateral Rotation, Weight-Bearing

Examination position, patient: Sitting on the short side of the examination table with lower legs hanging down.

Starting position, therapist: Standing beside the patient at the side not to be examined, or at the other side if appropriate (see *Remarks*).

Stabilization: The therapist holds the spinous process of T4 between the thumb and index finger of the stabilizing hand and keeps the vertebra in position.

Procedure: The patient's head leans against the therapist's upper arm. The therapist surrounds the contralateral

lamina of C2 with the little finger of the manipulating hand and brings about extension, sidebending, and contralateral rotation, while the upper cervical spine is held in the neutral position. (See **Figure 15–65**.)

Remarks: The sidebending and rotation components can also be carried out the other way around, in which case the therapist stands at the side being examined.

Ventral-Dorsal Slide, Weight-Bearing

Examination position, patient: Sitting on the short side of the examination table with lower legs hanging down.

Starting position, therapist: Standing in front of the patient.

Stabilization: The therapist holds the spinous process of T4 between the thumb and index finger of the stabilizing hand and keeps the vertebra in position.

Procedure: The patient's head leans against the therapist's upper arm. The therapist encircles the superior nuchal line with the little finger of the manipulating hand and induces a posterior-to-anterior and anterior-to-posterior sliding movement. The position of the head should be maintained. (See **Figures 15–66** and **15–67**.)

Remarks: The posterior-to-anterior slide causes extension of the upper cervical part of the spine and flexion of the lower cervical/high thoracic part. The anterior-to-posterior slide produces the opposite pattern.

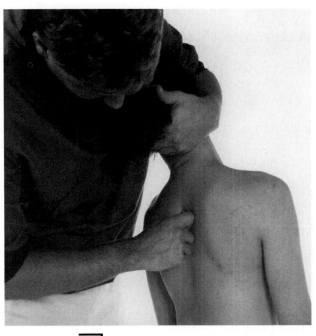

Figure 15–64

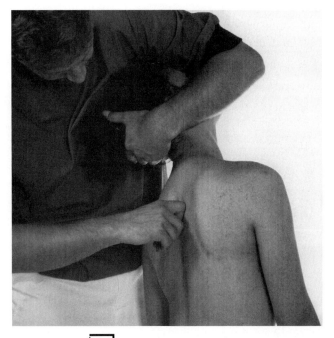

Figure 15–65

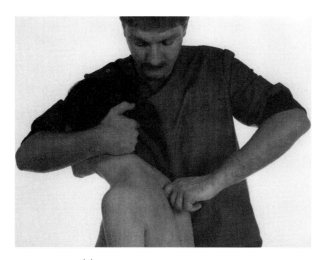

Figure 15–66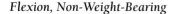

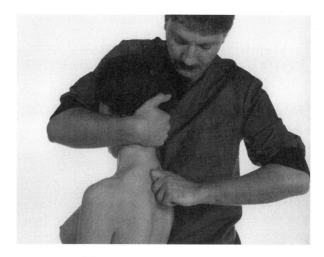

Figure 15–67

Flexion, Non-Weight-Bearing

Examination position, patient: Lying on one side with the hips and knees flexed through 90°.

Starting position, therapist: Standing in front of the patient.

Stabilization: The therapist holds the spinous process of T4 between the thumb and index finger of the stabilizing hand and keeps the vertebra in position.

Procedure: The patient's head leans against the therapist's upper arm. The therapist encircles the spinous process of C2 with the little finger of the manipulating hand and brings about flexion, while the upper cervical spine is held in extension. (See **Figure 15–68**.)

Flexion, Sidebending, Ipsilateral Rotation, Non-Weight-Bearing

Examination position, patient: Lying on one side with the hips and knees flexed through 90°.

Starting position, therapist: Standing in front of the patient.

Stabilization: The therapist holds the spinous process of T4 between the thumb and index finger of the stabilizing hand and keeps the vertebra in position.

Procedure: The patient's head leans against the therapist's upper arm. The therapist encircles the contralateral lamina of C2 with the little finger of the manipulating hand and carries out flexion, sidebending, and ipsilateral rotation, while the upper cervical spine is held in extension and contralateral sidebending. (See **Figure 15–69**.)

Flexion, Sidebending, Contralateral Rotation, Non-Weight-Bearing

Examination position, patient: Lying on one side with the hips and knees flexed through 90°.

Starting position, therapist: Standing in front of the patient.

Stabilization: The therapist holds the spinous process of T4 between the thumb and index finger of the stabilizing hand and keeps the vertebra in position.

Procedure: The patient's head leans against the therapist's upper arm. The therapist encircles the contralateral lamina of C2 with the little finger of the manipulating hand and carries out flexion, sidebending, and contralateral rotation, while the upper cervical spine is held in extension. (See **Figure 15–70**.)

Extension, Non-Weight-Bearing

Examination position, patient: Lying on one side with the hips and knees flexed through 90°.

Starting position, therapist: Standing in front of the patient.

Stabilization: The therapist holds the spinous process of T4 between the thumb and index finger of the stabilizing hand and keeps the vertebra in position.

Procedure: The patient's head leans against the therapist's upper arm. The therapist encircles the spinous process of C2 with the little finger of the manipulating hand and uses his or her upper arm to bring about extension, while the upper cervical spine is held in the neutral position. (See **Figure 15–71**.)

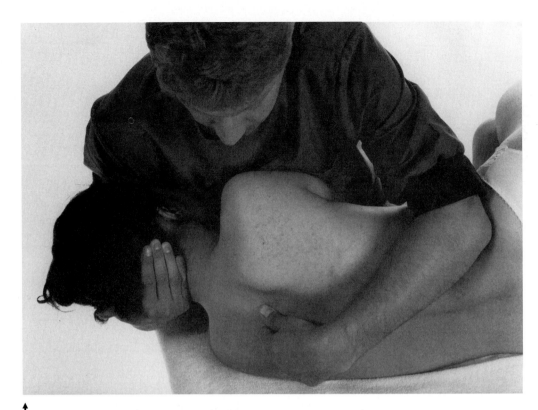

Figure 15–68

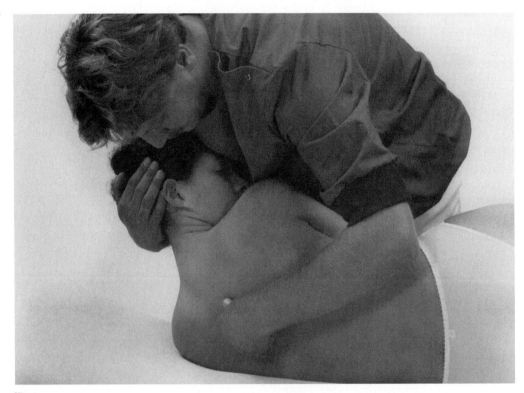

Figure 15–69

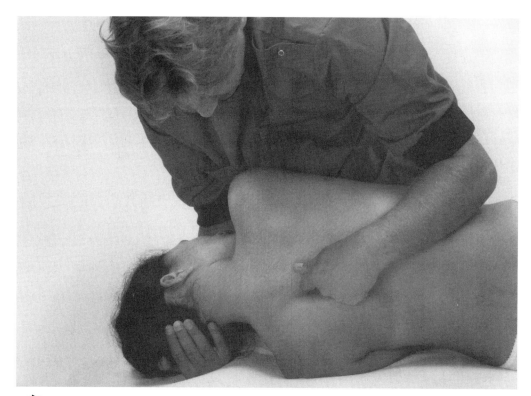

Figure 15–70

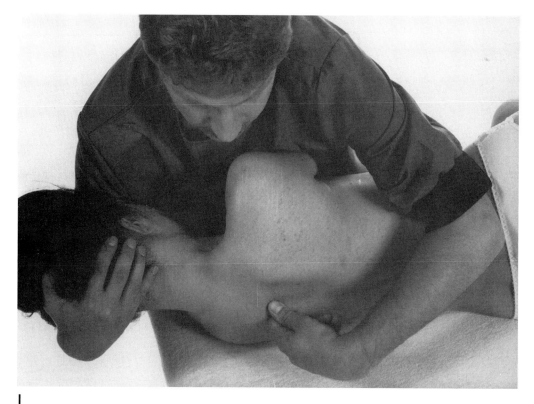

Figure 15–71

Extension, Sidebending, Ipsilateral Rotation, Non-Weight-Bearing

Examination position, patient: Lying on one side with the hips and knees flexed through 90°.

Starting position, therapist: Standing in front of the patient.

Stabilization: The therapist holds the spinous process of T4 between the thumb and index finger of the stabilizing hand and keeps the vertebra in position.

Procedure: The patient's head leans against the therapist's upper arm. The therapist encircles the contralateral lamina of C2 with the little finger of the manipulating hand and carries out extension, sidebending, and ipsilateral rotation, while the spine is held in the neutral position and contralateral sidebending. (See **Figure 15–72**.)

Extension, Sidebending, Contralateral Rotation, Non-Weight-Bearing

Examination position, patient: Lying on one side with the hips and knees flexed through 90°.

Starting position, therapist: Standing in front of the patient.

Stabilization: The therapist holds the spinous process of T4 between the thumb and index finger of the stabilizing hand and keeps the vertebra in position.

Procedure: The patient's head leans against the therapist's upper arm. The therapist encircles the contralateral lamina of C2 with the little finger of the manipulating hand and brings about extension, sidebending, and contralateral rotation, while the upper cervical spine is held in the neutral position. (See **Figure 15–73**.)

Ventral-Dorsal Slide, Non-Weight-Bearing

Examination position, patient: Supine, with the head and the spine as far as T4 extending beyond the edge of the examination table.

Starting position, therapist: Standing by the patient's head.

Procedure: One hand is placed under the back of the patient's head and the other on the forehead, the mandible, or the maxilla. The therapist uses both hands to induce a posterior-to-anterior and anterior-to-posterior sliding movement. (See **Figures 15–74** and **15–75**.)

Remarks: The sliding movement can also be carried out with the patient lying on one side.

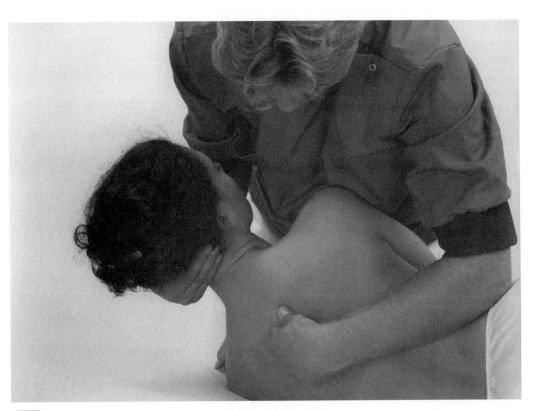

Figure 15–72

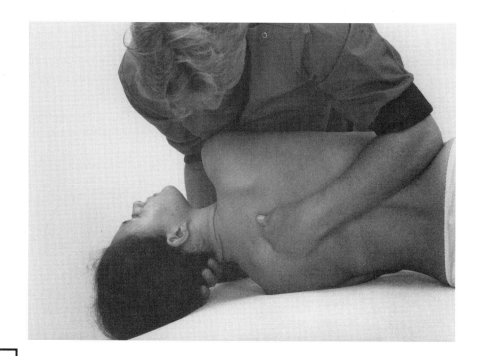

Figure 15–73

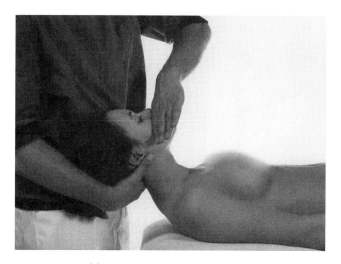

Figure 15–74

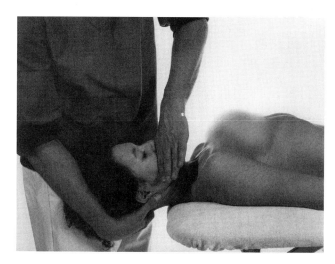

Figure 15–75

Lateral Slide, Non-Weight-Bearing

Examination position, patient: Supine.

Starting position, therapist: Standing by the patient's head.

Procedure: The therapist places his or her hands on each side of the patient's head and moves it in a right to left lateral glide while the head is held in the neutral position. (See **Figures 15–76** and **15–77**.)

Remarks: This movement brings about contralateral sidebending of the upper cervical spine and ipsilateral sidebending of the middle and lower cervical spine.

Regional Provocation Tests: Cervicothoracic/Cervical

For assessment criteria, see the section titled "Regional Provocation Tests: Lumbar" in Chapter 14.

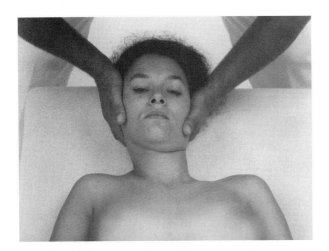

Figure 15–76 ⟼

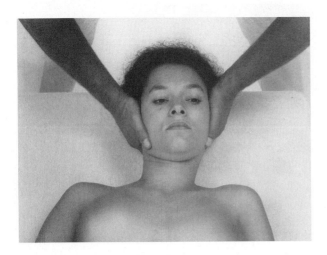

Figure 15–77 ⟻

Regional Traction Test

Examination position, patient: Sitting on the long side of the examination table with the lower legs hanging down.

Starting position, therapist: Standing behind the patient.

Procedure: The therapist supports his or her arms against the patient's shoulders and places his or her hands on each side of the patient's head. The therapist performs the traction test by adducting his or her forearms. (See **Figure 15–78**.)

Bertilson et al. (2003) reported κ values of 78–90% for the interrater agreement on the seated traction test being painful (κ = 0.41–0.56); for pain relief with traction, these values were 82–90% (κ = 0.63–0.8). Wainner et al. (2003) reported on the interrater reliability of a variant of the traction test in supine. When applying some 14 kilograms of distractive force, a positive test was defined as reduction or elimination of symptoms. The κ value reported for this test variant was 0.88 (95% CI: 0.64–1.0). Using electrodiagnostic testing as a gold standard test, these authors also reported a sensitivity of 0.44 (95% CI: 0.21–0.67), specificity of 0.90 (95% CI: 0.82–0.98), positive likelihood ratio of 4.4 (95% CI: 1.8–11.1), and negative likelihood ratio of 0.62 (95% CI: 0.40–0.90).

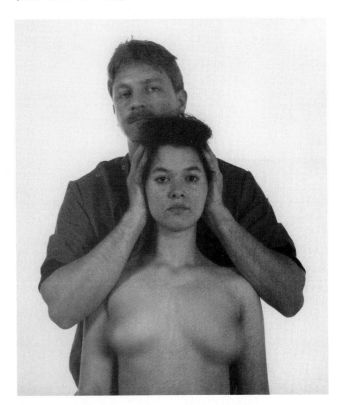

Figure 15–78 ↕

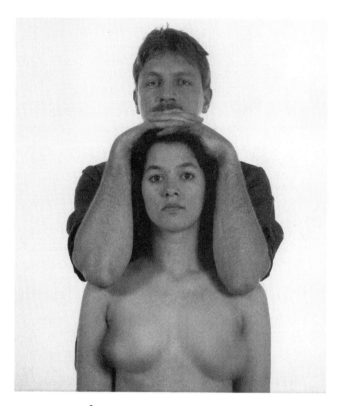

Figure 15–79 ⬍

Regional Compression Test

Examination position, patient: Sitting on the long side of the examination table with the lower legs hanging.

Starting position, therapist: Standing behind the patient.

Procedure: The therapist places both hands, either folded or one on top of the other, on the patient's head, with the forearms adducted. The therapist exerts a compressive force in a caudal direction. (See **Figure 15–79.**)

Bertilson et al. (2003) reported κ values of 70–73% for the interrater agreement on the compression test (κ = 0.34–0.44) using a dichotomous scale on absence or presence of pain on compression.

SEGMENTAL EXAMINATION

The segmental examination of this spinal region consists of segmental tissue-specific and segmental provocation tests and the active-assisted segmental examination.

Segmental Tissue–Specific Examination

For more information on segmental tissue-specific tests, see the section titled "Segmental Tissue–Specific Examination: Cervical" in Chapter 16.

Segmental Provocation Tests

For more information on segmental provocation tests, see the section titled "Segmental Provocation Tests: Cervical" in Chapter 16.

Active-Assisted Segmental Examination: Cervicothoracic (C7–T4)

For assessment criteria, see the section titled "Active-Assisted Segmental Examination: Lumbar (L1 to L5)" in Chapter 14.

Flexion, Weight-Bearing

Examination position, patient: Sitting on the short side of the examination table with the lower legs hanging down; the upper cervical spine is extended; the middle and lower parts of the cervical spine are brought into flexion as far as the level to be examined.

Starting position, therapist: Standing beside the patient.

Stabilization: The therapist holds the spinous process of the lower vertebra of the level to be examined with the thumb and index finger of the stabilizing hand and keeps the vertebra in position.

Procedure: The patient's head rests against the therapist's upper arm. The therapist places the little finger of the manipulating hand just above the level to be examined and uses that hand and arm to bring about flexion. (See **Figure 15–80.**)

Smith et al. (1992) reported on the intra- and interrater reliability of seated C6–T4 active-assisted segmental examination. Intrarater agreement ranged from 51.9–100.0% (κ = 0.291–1.00); interrater agreement ranged from 33.3–92.6% (κ = −0.057–0.602).

Flexion, Sidebending, Ipsilateral Rotation, Weight-Bearing

Examination position, patient: Sitting on the short side of the examination table with the lower legs hanging down; the upper cervical spine is brought into extension and the

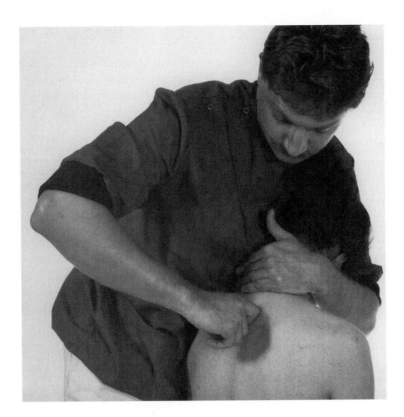

Figure 15–80 ↑

middle and lower cervical spine into flexion, sidebending, and ipsilateral rotation as far as the level to be examined.

Starting position, therapist: Standing beside the patient at the side to be examined.

Stabilization: The therapist holds the spinous process of the lower vertebra of the level to be examined with the thumb and index finger of the stabilizing hand and keeps the vertebra in position.

Procedure: The patient's head rests against the therapist's upper arm. The therapist encircles the cervical spine with the manipulating hand and arm, placing the little finger just above the level to be examined, and carries out flexion, sidebending, and ipsilateral rotation. (See **Figure 15–81**.)

Flexion, Sidebending, Contralateral Rotation, Weight-Bearing

Examination position, patient: Sitting on the short side of the examination table with the lower legs hanging down; the upper cervical spine is brought into extension, the middle and lower cervical spine into flexion, and the whole of the cervical spine as far as the level to be examined into sidebending and contralateral rotation.

Starting position, therapist: Standing beside the patient at the side not being examined, or at the other side, as appropriate (see *Remarks*).

Stabilization: The therapist holds the spinous process of the lower vertebra of the level to be examined between the thumb and index finger of the stabilizing hand and keeps the vertebra in position.

Procedure: The patient's head rests against the therapist's upper arm. The therapist encircles the cervical spine with the manipulating hand and arm, placing the little finger just above the level to be examined, and carries out flexion, sidebending, and contralateral rotation. (See **Figure 15–82**.)

Remarks: The sidebending and rotation components can also be carried out the other way around, in which case the therapist stands at the side being examined.

Extension, Weight-Bearing

Examination position, patient: Sitting on the short side of the examination table with the lower legs hanging down; the upper cervical spine is brought into flexion and the middle and lower cervical spine into extension as far as the level to be examined.

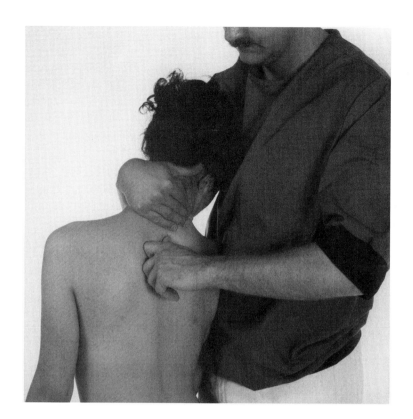

Figure 15–81

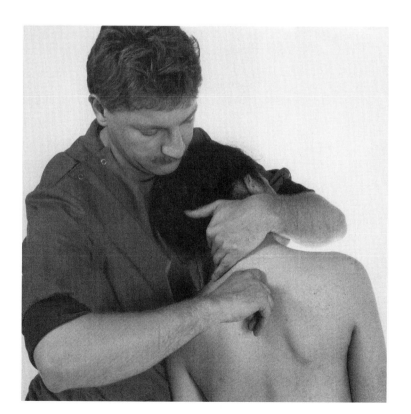

Figure 15–82

Starting position, therapist: Standing beside the patient.

Stabilization: The therapist holds the spinous process of the lower vertebra of the level to be examined between the thumb and index finger of the stabilizing hand and keeps the vertebra in position.

Procedure: The patient's head rests against the therapist's upper arm. The therapist encircles the cervical spine with the manipulating hand and arm, placing the little finger just above the level to be examined, and carries out extension. (See **Figure 15–83**.)

Extension, Sidebending, Ipsilateral Rotation, Weight-Bearing

Examination position, patient: Sitting on the short side of the examination table with the lower legs hanging; the upper cervical spine is brought into flexion and the middle and lower cervical spine into extension, sidebending, and ipsilateral rotation, as far as the level to be examined.

Starting position, therapist: Standing beside the patient at the side to be examined.

Stabilization: The therapist holds the spinous process of the lower vertebra of the level to be examined between the

thumb and index finger of the stabilizing hand and keeps the vertebra in position.

Procedure: The patient's head rests against the therapist's upper arm. The therapist encircles the cervical spine with the manipulating hand and arm, placing the little finger just above the level to be examined, and carries out extension, sidebending, and ipsilateral rotation. (See **Figure 15–84**.)

Extension, Sidebending, Contralateral Rotation, Weight-Bearing

Examination position, patient: Sitting on the short side of the examination table with the lower legs hanging down. The upper cervical spine is brought into flexion and the middle and lower cervical spine into extension. The whole of the cervical spine as far as the level to be examined is brought into sidebending and contralateral rotation.

Starting position, therapist: Standing beside the patient at the side not being examined, or at the other side, as appropriate (See *Remarks*).

Stabilization: The therapist holds the spinous process of the lower vertebra of the level to be examined with the

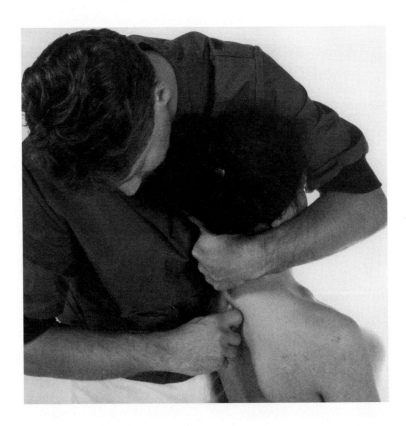

Figure 15–83

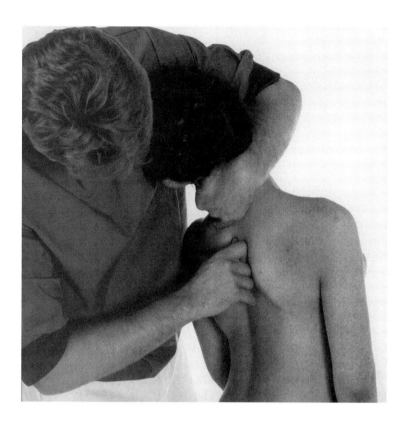

Figure 15–84

thumb and index finger of the stabilizing hand and holds the vertebra in position.

Procedure: The patient's head rests against the therapist's upper arm. The therapist encircles the cervical spine with the manipulating hand and arm, placing the little finger just above the level to be examined, and carries out extension, sidebending, and contralateral rotation. (See **Figure 15–85**.)

Remarks: The sidebending and rotation components can also be carried out the other way around, in which case the therapist stands at the side being examined.

Flexion, Non-Weight-Bearing

Examination position, patient: Lying on one side with the hips and knees flexed. The upper cervical spine is extended and the middle and lower cervical spine flexed as far as the level to be examined.

Starting position, therapist: Standing in front of the patient.

Stabilization: The therapist holds the spinous process of the lower vertebra of the level to be examined between the thumb and index finger of the stabilizing hand and holds the vertebra in position.

Procedure: The patient's head rests against the therapist's upper arm. The therapist encircles the cervical spine with the manipulating hand and arm, placing the little finger just above the level to be examined, and carries out flexion. (See **Figure 15–86**.)

Smedmark et al. (2000) reported on a sidelying C7–T1 combined flexion and extension segmental mobility test judged as hypomobile versus normal or hypermobile when compared to adjacent segments. Interrater agreement was 79 % ($\kappa = 0.36$).

Flexion, Sidebending, Ipsilateral Rotation, Non-Weight-Bearing

Examination position, patient: Lying on one side with the hips and knees flexed; the upper cervical spine is extended and the middle and lower cervical spine, as far as the level to be examined, is brought into flexion, sidebending, and ipsilateral rotation.

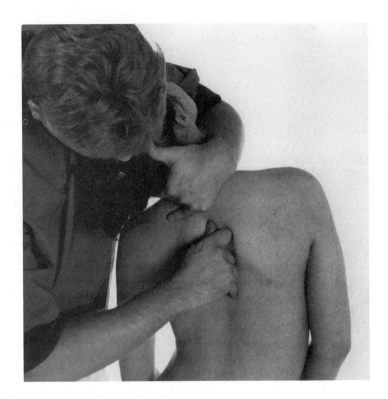

Figure 15–85

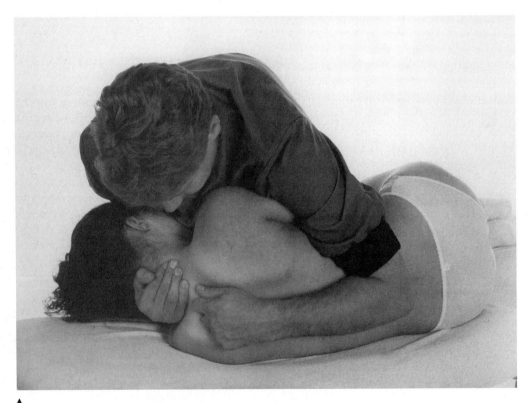

Figure 15–86

Starting position, therapist: Standing in front of the patient.

Stabilization: The therapist holds the spinous process of the lower vertebra of the level to be examined between the thumb and index finger of the stabilizing hand and holds the vertebra in position.

Procedure: The patient's head rests against the therapist's upper arm. The therapist encircles the cervical spine with the manipulating hand and arm, placing the little finger just above the level to be examined, and carries out flexion, sidebending, and ipsilateral rotation. (See **Figure 15–87**.)

Flexion, Sidebending, Contralateral Rotation, Non-Weight-Bearing

Examination position, patient: Lying on one side with the hips and knees flexed; the upper cervical spine is extended and the middle and lower cervical spine flexed. The whole of the cervical spine as far as the level to be examined is brought into sidebending and contralateral rotation.

Starting position, therapist: Standing in front of the patient.

Stabilization: The therapist holds the spinous process of the lower vertebra of the level to be examined between the

thumb and index finger of the stabilizing hand and holds the vertebra in position.

Procedure: The patient's head rests against the therapist's upper arm. The therapist encircles the cervical spine with the manipulating hand and arm, placing the little finger just above the level to be examined, and carries out flexion, sidebending, and contralateral rotation. (See **Figure 15–88**.)

Remarks: The sidebending and rotation components can also be carried out in reverse order.

Extension, Non-Weight-Bearing

Examination position, patient: Lying on one side with the hips and knees flexed. The upper cervical spine is flexed and the middle and lower parts of the cervical spine, as far as the level to be examined, are extended.

Starting position, therapist: Standing beside the patient.

Stabilization: The therapist holds the spinous process of the lower vertebra of the level to be examined between the thumb and index finger of the stabilizing hand and holds the vertebra in position.

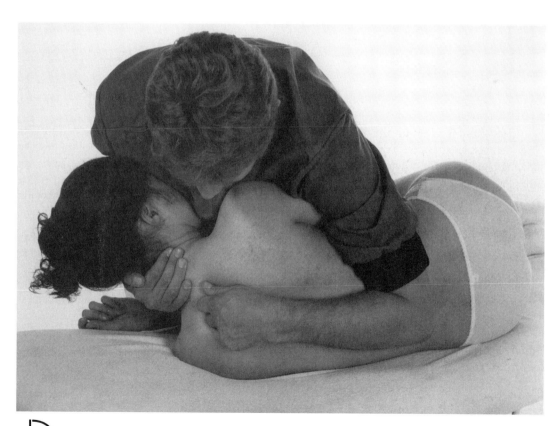

Figure 15–87

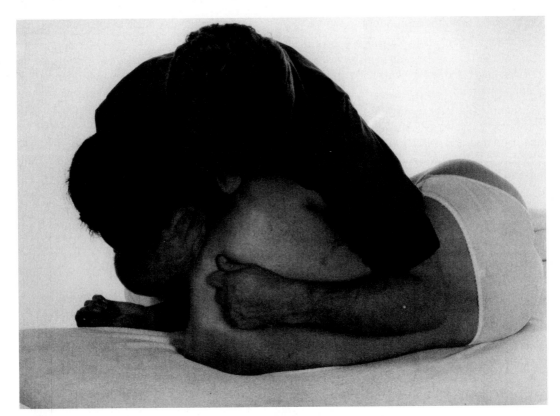

Figure 15–88

Procedure: The patient's head rests against the therapist's upper arm. The therapist encircles the cervical spine with the manipulating hand and arm, placing the little finger just above the level to be examined, and carries out extension. (See **Figure 15–89**.)

Extension, Sidebending, Ipsilateral Rotation, Non-Weight-Bearing

Examination position, patient: Lying on one side with the hips and knees flexed. The upper cervical spine is flexed and the middle and lower cervical spine, as far as the level to be examined, is brought into flexion, sidebending, and ipsilateral rotation.

Starting position, therapist: Standing in front of the patient.

Stabilization: The therapist holds the spinous process of the lower vertebra of the level to be examined between the thumb and index finger of the stabilizing hand and holds the vertebra in position.

Procedure: The patient's head rests against the therapist's upper arm. The therapist encircles the cervical spine with the manipulating hand and arm, placing the little finger just above the level to be examined, and carries out extension, sidebending, and ipsilateral rotation. (See **Figure 15–90**.)

Extension, Sidebending, Contralateral Rotation, Non-Weight-Bearing

Examination position, patient: Lying on one side with the hips and knees flexed. The upper cervical spine is flexed and the middle and lower cervical spine extended. The whole of the cervical spine as far as the level to be examined is brought into sidebending and contralateral rotation.

Starting position, therapist: Standing in front of the patient.

Stabilization: The therapist holds the spinous process of the lower vertebra of the level to be examined between the

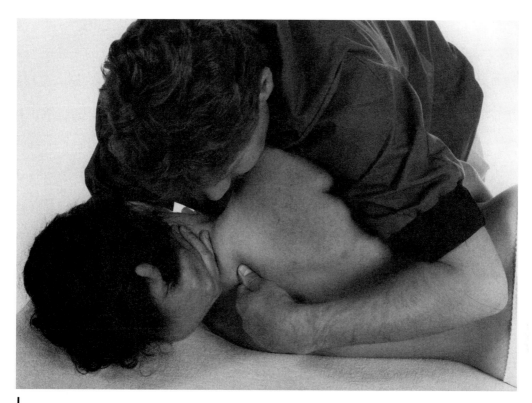

Figure 15–89

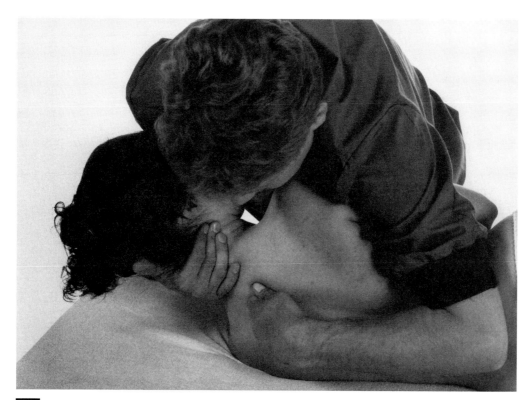

Figure 15–90

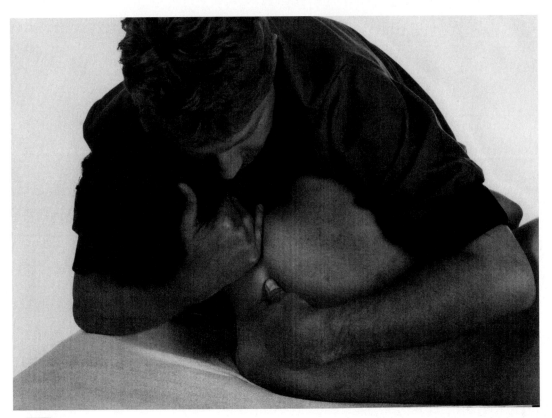

Figure 15–91

thumb and index finger of the stabilizing hand and holds the vertebra in position.

Procedure: The patient's head rests against the therapist's upper arm. The therapist encircles the cervical spine with the manipulating hand and arm, placing the little finger just above the level to be examined, and carries out extension, sidebending, and contralateral rotation. (See **Figure 15–91**.)

Remarks: The sidebending and rotation components can also be carried out in the reverse order.

CHAPTER 16

Examination of the Lower and Mid-Cervical Spine

MIDDLE AND LOWER CERVICAL SPINE (C2–T1)

Before discussing the clinical examination of the lower and mid-cervical spine we need to review relevant anatomy, biomechanics, cervical instability, and neurology.

Functional Aspects of the Middle and Lower Cervical Spine

The middle and lower cervical spine is normally considered to consist of segments C2–T1. T1 forms a stable basis for this movement region, as does C3 for the upper cervical area.

Morphologically, T1 bears a closer resemblance to the seventh cervical vertebra than to the thoracic vertebrae. According to Markuske (1971) and Putz (1981), the mobility of the segment C7–T1 is relatively limited in the sagittal and frontal planes. They relate this to the size and position of the intervertebral joint spaces.

The scalene muscles, which stretch between the first two ribs and the cervical spine, play an important part in the functioning of the cervicothoracic transitional area: they are the means by which the thorax is suspended from the cervical spine (Wolff, 1963). The intrinsic muscles of the middle and lower cervical spine span several segments, which makes independent movement impossible in this region (Penning, 1978). An exception is the forward–backward movement of the cervical spine, though this does not include flexion and extension of the head.

During forward movement, the upper part of the cervical spine goes into extension and the lower part into flexion. The opposite pattern appears during backward movement.

The specific characteristics of the middle and lower cervical spine are as follows (Putz, 1981; **Figure 16–1**):

Angle of inclination (α): C3 = 66°, C4 = 58°, C5 = 54°, C6 = 54°, C7 = 63°

Angle of opening (β): C3 = 143°, C4 = 184°, C5 = 186°, C6 = 200°, C7 = 187°

Transverse distance: The distance between the joint surfaces of the superior articular processes (a): C3 = 38 mm, C4 = 40 mm, C5 = 41.5 mm, C6 = 42.5 mm, C7 = 42 mm

Sagittal distance: The distance between the joint surfaces of the superior articular processes and the center of the associated vertebral body (b): C3 = 15.5 mm, C4 = 12.5 mm, C5 = 12 mm, C6 = 12 mm, C7 = 14 mm

The standard deviation of values given by Putz is not reproduced in this book.

Other characteristics that distinguish the middle and lower cervical spine from the other regions are as follows:

- The relatively high intervertebral disks, which permit a considerable degree of movement in all directions.
- The tearing of the intervertebral disk, which begins in about the ninth year and is often complete in later life. The cervical disk then functions like two brushes with the bristles opposing each other (Hoogland, 1988).
- The presence of uncovertebral joints, which have a stabilizing function, but which also limit movement.
- The spinous processes of C2–C6, which are bifurcate.
- The transverse processes, which have transverse foramina and sulci.

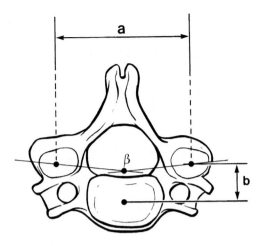

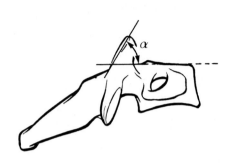

Figure 16–1   Characteristic parameters of the cervical vertebra.

Flexion and Extension

According to Penning (1964, 1968, 1978) the frontal axis of movement for flexion and extension is located in the lower vertebral body (**Figure 16–2**). The axis of the segment C2–C3 turns out to be located low in the vertebral body of C3. Moving toward the caudal end of the spine, the axis moves progressively toward the cranial end of the lower vertebra, such that the axis of the segment C6–C7 is located high in the body of C7. One consequence of this is that the translatory component decreases progressively from C2 to C7, the upper vertebra of the segment becoming in-

creasingly unable to translate in the ventral direction in relation to the lower vertebra (**Figure 16–3**).

These points are important for the interpretation of X-rays. According to Penning (1978), lateral projections show the joint surfaces of the articular processes as cylinders with the axis of movement as their center. The endplate of the upper vertebra is also seen as a cylinder with the axis of movement at its center (**Figure 16–4**). Studies of the spines of giraffes have shown that these animals have a diarthrodial joint between two vertebral bodies.

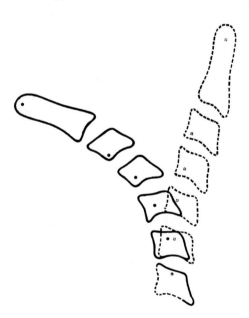

Figure 16–2   Axes of flexion–extension.

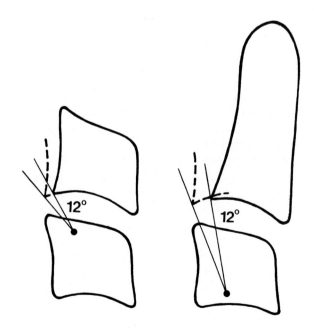

Figure 16–3   Connection between axis of movement and translation component.

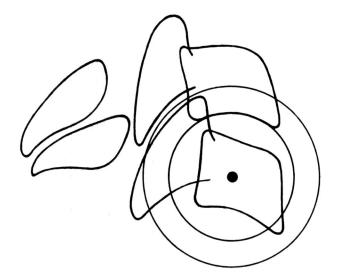

Figure 16–4   The endplate and the joint surfaces of the articular processes are part of a cylinder with the axis of movement in its center.

This means that the disk becomes the articular convexity of the lower vertebral body; it articulates with the concavity formed by the caudal surface of the upper vertebral body. The fact that the intervertebral joint surfaces and the endplate of the upper vertebral body are parts of cylinders with the axis of movement at their center suggests that the intervertebral joint surfaces remain in contact with each other during flexion.

Radiographs of movement have not, however, confirmed this theory under all circumstances. In extreme flexion, a wedge-shaped opening appears dorsocaudally in the intervertebral joint. During the course of flexion, the ventral sides of the vertebrae move closer together, and, depending on where the axis of movement lies, they are displaced in a more or less ventral direction relative to each other. The dorsal sides move apart. The nucleus pulposus does not move to any great extent. The outer oblique annular fibers that lie in the direction of movement, especially the dorsolateral ones, come under tension. Those that run in the opposite direction, especially the ventrolateral ones, relax. The intervertebral joints slide apart, with the upper intervertebral joint surfaces within the segment moving in a cranioventral direction relative to lower surfaces. The spinous and transverse processes separate. The uncovertebral joints have a stabilizing effect during the movement. The structures that inhibit flexion are the annular fibers, the joint capsule, the posterior longitudinal ligament, the flaval and intertransverse ligaments, and the nuchal ligament, which has elastic fibers in humans but not in quadrupeds. The anterior longitudinal ligament and the outer ventrolateral annular fibers that run obliquely in the direction opposite to that of movement relax.

In the end phase of flexion, the upper intervertebral joint surfaces within the segment extend in a ventrocranial direction above the lower joint surfaces. When dorsocaudal gapping appears in the intervertebral joints, there is a small contact surface between a narrow part of the upper intervertebral joint surfaces and the cranial edges of the lower ones within the segment. These function as points of rotation. Because forces are transmitted across them, the tension in the tendons and the joint capsule fibers that lie dorsal to the pivot point is raised significantly. In the end position, they must absorb the torque produced. The magnitude of the pressure on the narrow contact surfaces depends on the angle of inclination: as this angle increases, the tendons and joint capsule need to exert less tensile force to oppose the ventral displacements.

During extension, the dorsal sides of the vertebrae approximate and, depending on where the axis of movement lies, move in a more or less dorsal direction relative to each other. The ventral sides of the vertebrae separate from each other. The nucleus pulposus does not move to any great extent, though its height increases ventrally and decreases dorsally. The outer annular fibers that run obliquely in the direction of movement, especially the ventrolateral ones, come under tension, while those that run in the opposite direction, especially the dorsolateral ones, relax. The two halves of the intervertebral joints slide into each other, with the lower intervertebral joint surfaces of the upper vertebra moving in a caudodorsal direction relative to the upper intervertebral joint surfaces of the lower vertebra. The spinous and transverse processes approximate. The uncovertebral joints also have a stabilizing function in this situation.

The structures that inhibit extension are the joint capsule, the anterior longitudinal ligament, and the outer ventrolateral fibers that run obliquely in the direction of movement. In the extreme extension position, some bony obstruction occurs because the transverse processes of the upper vertebra come into contact with the upper edges of the lower intervertebral joint surfaces within the segment. The outer dorsolateral annular fibers that run opposite to the direction of movement relax, as do the ligaments that lie dorsal to the axis. In the end phase of extension, the upper intervertebral joint surfaces within the segment extend in a dorsocaudal direction over the lower intervertebral joint surfaces. When ventrocranial gapping occurs in the intervertebral joints, there is a small contact surface between the narrow part of the upper intervertebral joint surfaces and the caudal edges of the lower intervertebral joint surfaces within the segment.

The transmission system, with the caudal edges of the lower intervertebral joint surfaces as centers of rotation, brings about a considerable increase in the tension of the capsular structures that lie ventral to these points.

The average range of flexion–extension, as measured by Penning (1978), is C2–C3 = 12°, C3–C4 = 18°, C4–C5 and C5–C6 = 20°, and C6–C7 = 15°. According to Penning (1978), these values show considerable variation and differ markedly from those found in children. The following values have been measured in children: C2–C3 = 23°, C3–C4 and C4–C5 = 38°, C5–C6 = 34°, and C6–C7 = 29°.

Sidebending

Penning (1964, 1968, 1978) states that sidebending does not differ from rotation in the C2 to T1 region. He bases this argument on the fact that the slope of the intervertebral joint surfaces in this area is 45°. During sidebending, the upper intervertebral joint surfaces within the segment move in a cranioventral direction at the convex side and in a caudodorsal direction on the concave side (**Figure 16–5**). During sidebending in a purely frontal plane, there would be a caudal focal loading and cranial gapping.

In sidebending of the whole spine, with the head held in the anterior/posterior position, C1 must make a counterrotation of about 35° relative to C2 to compensate for the rotation that takes place in C2–T1. This is shown in **Figure 16–6**.

It is true that sidebending and rotation in the C2–T1 region are similar in range. However, it may safely be assumed that there are some differences because of the variation in slope of the intervertebral joint surfaces, the

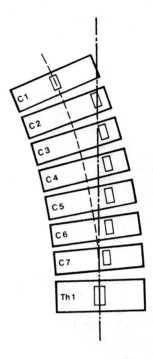

Figure 16–6   Schematic projection of sidebending.

presence of the uncovertebral joints, and differences in movement impulse.

According to Kapandji (1974), the axis of movement for combined sidebending and rotation runs from the middle of a line joining the two lower intervertebral joint surfaces, passing perpendicular to the slope of these surfaces and through the lower vertebral body. Kapandji also draws distinctions between the flat intervertebral joint surfaces of C4–C5, the convex surfaces of C6–C7, and the concave surfaces of C3–C4. Depending on whether the lower intervertebral joint surfaces within the segment are convex or concave, the center of movement of sidebending within the segment lies below (A) or above (B) the motion segment (**Figure 16–7**). According to Kapandji, the slope of the intervertebral joint surfaces decreases from the cranial to the caudal end.

Putz (1981) places the axis of movement within the segment. He argues that sidebending is accompanied by a forced rotation, depending on the angle of inclination of the segment. He also states that the upper vertebra cannot translate in the concave direction over the lower vertebra because of the presence of the uncovertebral joints, which have a limiting effect on cervical sidebending.

During sidebending, the intervertebral spaces become smaller on the concave side and larger on the convex side. The nucleus pulposus does not move to any extent. Its

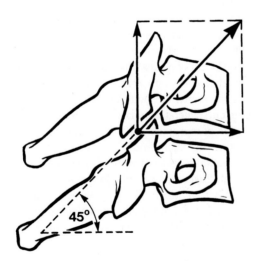

Figure 16–5   Vectorial dissolution of joint movement.

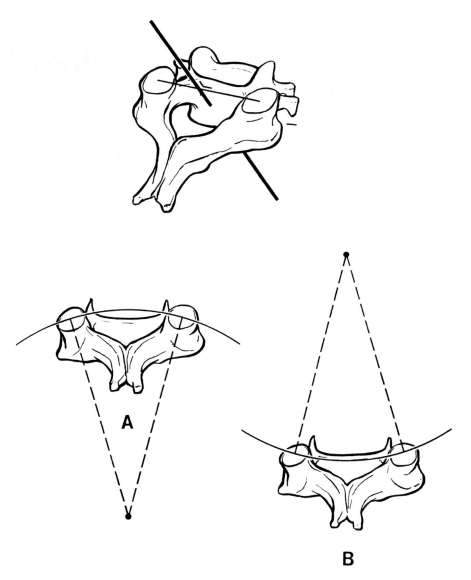

Figure 16–7 Position of axis of sidebending.

height increases on the convex side and decreases on the concave side. The outer oblique annular fibers that lie in the direction of movement, especially those on the ventral and dorsal convex side, come under tension. Those that run in the opposite direction, especially on the ventral and dorsal concave side, relax.

The intervertebral joint surfaces on the concave side slide in a caudodorsal direction into each other; on the convex side, they slide apart in a cranioventral direction. The transverse processes move in the same way as the intervertebral joint surfaces. The spinous processes move relative to each other in a convex direction. The uncovertebral joint

surfaces on the concave side show mediocaudal gapping. The uncovertebral joint surfaces on the convex side separate at an angle (**Figure 16–8**).

The structures that inhibit sidebending are the outer oblique annular fibers that run in the direction of movement, particularly those on the ventral and dorsal convex side; the joint capsules of the intervertebral and uncovertebral joints; and the flaval, longitudinal, and intertransverse ligaments. The supraspinous and nuchal ligaments play a less important part.

In the end phase of sidebending, the axis moves abruptly in the concave direction to a position in the uncovertebral

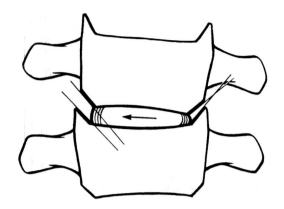

Figure 16–8   Course of movement in the uncovertebral joints during sidebending.

joint. The uncinate process of the lower vertebra then functions as the center of rotation. According to Penning (1964, 1968, 1978), the average extent of sidebending from left to right in young adults is 70°.

Rotation

The difference between sidebending and rotation is the associated rotation in C1–C2 (Penning, 1978; **Figure 16–9**). Putz (1981) states that from a normal starting position, the longitudinal axis of rotation runs through the nu-

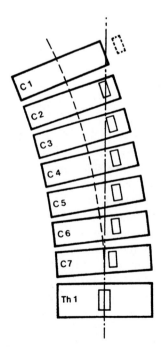

Figure 16–9   Rotation.

cleus pulposus, just dorsal to the midpoint of the vertebral body. During rotation, the slope of the intervertebral joint surfaces causes a forced sidebending in the same direction. As a consequence, the extent of rotation is greater in maximal flexion than in extension. A ventrally directed force operates in the intervertebral joints that lie in the direction opposite to that of rotation. This force can be resolved into a compressive vertical force on the intervertebral joint surfaces and a force in the direction of the intervertebral joint space. The former component increases with the angle of inclination (**Figure 16–10**).

Because of the forced sidebending that accompanies rotation and occurs in the same direction, the intervertebral space becomes smaller on the concave side and larger on the convex side. The nucleus, which is compressed to some extent, decreases in height on the side of rotation and increases on the other side. The outer annular fibers that run obliquely in the direction of rotation come under increased tension, especially on the convex side. Those that run in the opposite direction relax, especially those on the concave side. The intervertebral joint surfaces slide together in a caudodorsomedial direction on the concave side and apart in a cranioventromedial direction on the convex side. The transverse processes move in the same way as the intervertebral joint surfaces. The spinous processes move relative to each other in the direction opposite to that of rotation.

The structures that inhibit rotation are the outer annular fibers that run obliquely in the direction of movement, especially those on the convex side; the joint capsules; the flaval, longitudinal, and intertransverse ligaments; and to a lesser extent, the supraspinous ligaments and the nuchal ligament.

In the end phase of rotation, the point of rotation moves to the lateral part of the intervertebral joint opposite to the direction of movement. This greatly increases the tension in the ligaments that run between the vertebrae. It particularly affects the longitudinal and intertransverse ligaments.

The average range of left–right rotation is about 80°.

Morphology of the Cervical Intervertebral Disk

Research carried out by Töndury (1974), Hoogland (1988), and Bogduk (1990) has shown that the cervical intervertebral disk undergoes extensive changes during life. At birth and during the early years, the cervical intervertebral disks do not differ from those in other regions. In about the ninth year, however, a pseudodegenerative process begins in the fibers of the annulus. The fibers tear in the middle, between the two vertebral bodies; this breaks the firm connection between adjacent vertebrae (**Figure 16–11**). The tearing is progressive; in many cases, it seems

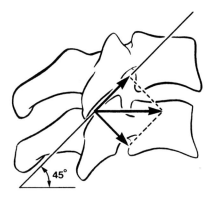 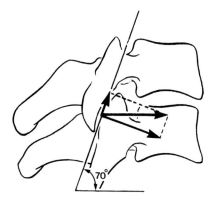

Figure 16–10   Dissolution of forces in ventral direction in the contralateral intervertebral joint with different angles of inclination.

to be complete by middle age. When this happens, the cranial and caudal fibers behave like two brushes with the bristles oriented toward each other. Bogduk (1990) states that the more ventral fibers remain intact, and that the connection, therefore, persists at the ventral side. One consequence of the tearing of the annular fibers is that the nucleus pulposus is no longer enclosed; this has implications for the location and nutrition of the nuclear material. In later life, the nucleus pulposus of the cervical disks seems to have disappeared partially or completely.

The morphologic changes to the cervical disks greatly increase mobility, but they also reduce passive stability. Extra mechanisms are present that protect the cervical spine

from excessive mobility and support passive and active stability; these include the uncinate processes and the extensive musculature of the region. Hypertonicity, which causes shortening of the cervical muscles, pushes the annular fibers against each other; this increases stability and decreases mobility.

A particular consequence of the unusual morphology of the disk is that it allows the cervical spine to lengthen or shorten in a relatively short time. The changes in length, which can amount to several centimeters, affect the tissue structures that are closely associated with the cervical spine, such as the spinal cord, the nerves that enter and leave the spine, and the vertebral artery. A sudden lengthening of the cervical spine (whiplash injury) can cause overstretching of the spinal cord and the attached nerves. Shortening of the cervical spine can also affect the attached tissue structures. It also means that the intervertebral joints carry a greater load in the end position, the joint capsule comes under greater tension, and the intervertebral foramina are narrowed.

The changes in spinal length that occur under various circumstances are in the most part because of the cervical spine (Hoogland, 1988). According to a report in a national newspaper, space travelers showed an increase in height of 1 to 1½ centimeters during the weightless period. Hoogland (1988) believes that most of this is a result of an increase in the height of the cervical disks. When the travelers returned to earth, gravity initially caused the spine to decrease in length to below normal levels. A few months later, the normal body length was restored.

Hoogland's explanation (1988) is that the increase in disk height during the weightless period lengthens the ligamentous structures by placing them under constant tension. Subsequently, gravity and the reduced resistance of neighboring ligaments cause the disks to become flatter than normal. With the passage of time, the surrounding ligaments return to their previous length and the disks are no

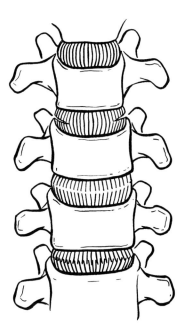

Figure 16–11   Cervical intervertebral disk.

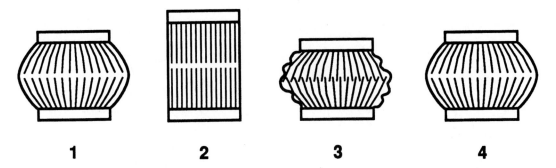

1   **2**   **3**   **4**

Figure 16–12   Changes in height of the cervical intervertebral disk of space travelers.

longer flattened. The body will then return to its normal length (**Figure 16–12**).

The advantage of the unusual structure of the cervical spine is that it permits a greater range of movement. However, it is also responsible for the particular kinds of pathology that occur in this region.

For the cervical spine to perform its autonomic and biomechanical functions efficiently, the thoracic spine must have normal static and dynamic capability. The factors that place a load on the intervertebral cervical disks include the relative positions of the cervical and thoracic spine (forward head position); reduced mobility in the thoracic spine; loading of the thoracic spine; and a psychologically induced increase in tone in the muscles that span the cervical and thoracic regions.

Under normal circumstances, these muscles exert a compressive force on the cervical spine. Where pathology is present, for example, a marked and rigid kyphosis of the thoracic spine, or when there is excessive physiologic stress, for instance, when heavy loads are carried, this compressive force on the cervical spine—and, therefore, on the disks—increases. In cases of cervical dysfunction, therefore, the state of the thoracic spine must be carefully considered as well as that of the cervical spine.

Sequence of Movements in C0–C7 During Movement in the Sagittal Plane

Van Mameren (1988) used videofluoroscopy to examine the pattern of movement of the cervical spine in 10 healthy subjects. He identified the sequence of movements in cervical segments in the sagittal plane. Using an intricate and accurate method of measurement, he also determined the average centers of movement in segments C0–C7 throughout motion. His findings in relation to the upper cervical segments differ somewhat from those of Penning (1978). However, the findings on the centers of movement in the

middle and lower cervical segments show reasonable agreement (**Figure 16–13**).

Measurements were taken at three points: initially, after 2 weeks, and after 10 weeks. The study showed extensive intra- and interindividual variation in range of movement, both for the whole of the cervical spine and for individual segments. It was also found that the largest measurements (in degrees) of active segmental movement could not always be deduced from the extreme positions of the cervical spine. Measuring the range of segmental movement in X-rays that show the static final position does not, there-

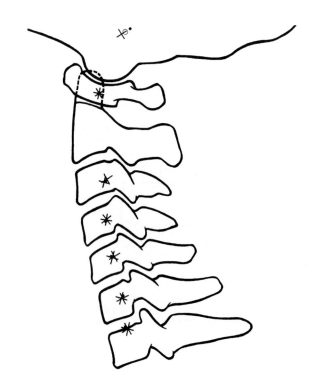

Figure 16–13   Flexion–extension axes.

fore, always yield an accurate result. van Mameren's studies (1988) lead to the following conclusions:

- The size of the variations between individuals suggests that norms for the range of cervical movement would not be meaningful.
- The variation among measurements taken from the same individual at different times indicates that range of movement does not constitute a reliable criterion for evaluating therapies.
- The sequence of movements in the cervical spine during motion in the sagittal plane is consistent.

Sequence of Movements

Flexion Starting From the Extended Position   Flexion always appears to begin in the C4–C7 block, proceeding from the caudal to the cranial end. At the instant when the center of gravity of the head is located dorsal to the sella turcica at the transition to the clivus, vertically above the body of C7, and above or somewhat ventral to the axis of C0–C1, the C0–C1 segment becomes involved in the movement. The C1–C2 segment follows a fraction later.

Although the sequence of movements in the C2–C4 block is difficult to identify, it seems to occur between the two phases of movement in the C4–C7 block. At a certain point in the course of the movement, inversion (countermovement) occurs in segment C0–C1 and/or C1–C2. The moment when this occurs is determined by the onset of tension in the funicular part of the nuchal ligament, which stretches between C5 and the external occipital protuberances (van Mameren, 1988; **Figure 16–14**).

The final locking movement takes place in the C4–C7 block and proceeds from the cranial to the caudal end. Flexion that starts from the extended position always begins and ends in the caudal part of the cervical spine, never in the middle. The sequence of movements can be summarized as follows:

- C6–C7, C5–C6, C4–C5
- C0–C1, C1–C2
- C2–C4
- Inversion C0–C1 and/or C1–C2
- C4–C5, C5–C6, C6–C7

Extension Starting From a Flexed Position   Extension of the spine always begins in the caudal part of the cervical spine, in C6–C7 or C5–C6, but never in C4–C5. It proceeds from the caudal to the cranial end. The motion segments C2–C4 show little consistency in their behavior, but

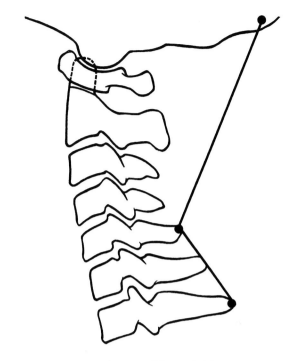

Figure 16–14   Funicular part of the nuchal ligament.

in general, movement in C2–C4 generally precedes the involvement of the C0–C2 block. As soon as the vector moves from the center of gravity of the head to a position parallel to the longitudinal axis of the C0–C2 block, the segment C1–C2 becomes involved in the movement and inversion occurs in segment C0–C1. When the extension in the segment C1–C2 is almost complete, the involvement of segment C0–C1 begins. This segment makes its greatest contribution at the moment when the center of gravity of the head reaches a position vertically above the instantaneous axis of movement of C0–C1 and the dorsal border of the body of C7. Extension ends in the caudal part of the cervical spine, of which segment C6–C7 is generally the last to be involved. The sequence of movements can be summarized as follows:

- C6–C7, C5–C6, C4–C5
- C2–C4
- C1–C2, inversion in C0–C1
- C0–C1
- C4–C5, C5–C6, C6–C7

Movement Sequence as an Assessment Parameter

Van Mameren's study (1988) shows that the range of segmental movement in the cervical spine in the sagittal plane, measured from static X-ray pictures, does not offer a reliable criterion for identifying pathology or for measuring the effects of therapy. The extent to which the sequence of movements he identified in healthy participants can be used as an objective parameter will depend on further studies of patients suffering from complaints arising from functional disturbances of the cervical spine. If these patients were to show a deviant movement sequence that was restored to normal following effective treatment, this would demonstrate that van Mameren had identified a reliable parameter that could be used for diagnostic and therapeutic purposes.

Cervical Segmental Instability

As described earlier, the cervical disks show small tears in childhood that progress to a total horizontal cleft in later life. Once this process is complete, the disks can make little contribution to cervical stability; more important factors at that stage are the concavity of the cranial endplates of vertebrae C3–C7, the uncovertebral joints, the ligaments that span the segment, and the extensive musculature. The stabilizing muscles are the intrinsic segmental musculature (innervated by the dorsal ramus of the cervical spinal nerve); the scalene muscles (ventral ramus, C1–C4); the longus colli muscle (ventral ramus, C2–C7); the sternocleidomastoid muscle (accessory nerve and spinal nerve), the trapezius muscle (accessory nerve and spinal nerve C3–C4); and the levator scapulae muscle (thoracodorsal nerve and ventral ramus C4).

From a biomechanical point of view, the cervical spine without the muscles would be an unstable system. The sternocleidomastoid muscle and the longus colli muscle work closely together to stabilize it (Lanser 1988). Both muscles are active during coughing and when carrying burdens on the head. Their activity also increases during movements such as spinal flexion against resistance and rising from a supine position. The stabilizing effect of these muscles is important primarily for segment C5–C6. Because of their position in the cervical curve, the joint surfaces of these segments are more or less horizontal. As a result, translation in the anterior-posterior plane encounters little resistance from the joint facets and depends heavily on the musculature. The longus colli muscle, as the only muscle that lies ventral to the vertebral column, exerts a compressive force on the cervical spine. This is especially important for segments C4–C6, the ligaments of which are the least strongly developed.

As already described in the context of lumbar segmental instability, instability leads to changes in arthrokinetic reflex activity. Under normal circumstances, the arthrokinetic reflexes bring about a subtle pattern of tension in the paravertebral musculature. Changes in the segmental pattern of movement cause changes in nonphysiologic stimulation of the mechanoreceptors in the intervertebral joints. This results in a changed nonphysiologic pattern of muscular tension.

Because of the increase in road traffic, the number of accidents has multiplied greatly. The cervical spine is one of the most vulnerable regions, so cases of cervical trauma form a relatively high proportion of the total. Injuries to the neck often cause segmental instability, which means that particular attention must be paid to this disorder. For details of history-taking and appropriate tests, please see the section titled "Instability Examination" later in this chapter.

Muscles That Influence the Cervical Spine

Muscle	Bilateral		Unilateral		
				Rotation	
	Flexion	Extension	Sidebending	Ipsilateral	Contralateral
Superior longus colli	X		X	X	
Inferior longus colli	X		X		X
Longus capitis	X			X	
Anterior scalene muscle	X		X		X
Middle scalene muscle			X		X
Posterior scalene muscle			X		X
Platysma muscle	X				
Sternocleidomastoid muscle	X	X	X		X
Splenius cervicis		X	X	X	
Splenius capitis		X	X	X	
Descending part of trapezius muscle		X	X		X
Levator scapulae		X	X	X	
Iliocostalis cervicis muscle		X	X		
Longissimus cervicis muscle		X	X		
Longissimus capitis muscle		X	X	X	
Spinalis cervicis		X			
Spinalis capitis		X			
Semispinalis cervicis		X			X
Semispinalis capitis		X			X
Multifidus muscles			X		X
Rotatores muscles		X			X
Interspinales muscle		X			
Intertransverse muscles			X		

Motor and Sensory Connections

Brachial Plexus

This consists of the following components, medial to lateral:

- Ventral rami (C5–C8)
- Superior trunk (C5–C6), middle trunk (C7), inferior trunk (C8–Th1) of the brachial plexus
- Ventral and dorsal parts
- Posterior, lateral, and medial fascicles

Peripheral Nerves of the Shoulder and Trunk

Segment	Nerve	Origin	Motor	Sensory
C5–C7	Long thoracic nerve	Ventral ramus	Serratus anterior	
C5	Dorsal scapular nerve	Ventral ramus	Levator scapulae Rhomboid minor Rhomboid major	
C5–C6	Subclavian nerve	Superior trunk	Subclavius	
C5–C6	Suprascapular nerve	Superior trunk	Supraspinatus Infraspinatus	
C5–T1	Pectoral nerve	Superior trunk Middle and inferior trunk	Pectoralis major Pectoralis minor	
C5–C6	Subscapular nerve	Posterior fascicle	Subscapularis Teres major	
C5–C6	Axillary nerve	Posterior fascicle	Deltoid Teres minor	*Superior lateral cutaneous brachial nerve:* caudal aspect skin deltoid
C6–C8	Thoracodorsal nerve	Posterior fascicle	Latissimus dorsi	
C8–T1	Medial cutaneous antebrachial nerve	Medial fascicle		*Anterior ramus:* 2/3 portion ventromedial aspect upper arm, ventro-ulnar aspect forearm, and hypothenar *Posterior ramus:* 1/3 portion dorsomedial upper arm, dorso-ulnar aspect forearm, upper dorsolateral aspect hand
C8–T1	Medial cutaneous brachial nerve	Medial fascicle		*Anterior ramus:* ventromedial aspect upper arm *Posterior ramus:* dorsomedial aspect upper arm

Peripheral nerves that supply the upper limbs

Segment	Nerve	Motor	Sensory
C5–C7	Musculocutaneous nerve	Coracobrachialis Brachialis Biceps brachii	*Lateral cutaneous brachial nerve:* ventroradial side of forearm and thenar
C5–T1	Radial nerve	triceps brachii brachioradialis muscle extensor carpi radialis longus extensor digitorum communis extensor carpi radialis brevis extensor carpi ulnaris supinator extensor digiti minimi extensor pollicis longus extensor pollicis brevis abductor pollicis longus extensor indicis	*Posterior cutaneous brachial nerve* *Inferior lateral cutaneous brachial nerve* *Posterior cutaneous antebrachial nerve:* dorsolateral aspect upper arm and dorsal aspect forearm *Superficial nerve:* dorsolateral aspect hand
C5–T1	Median nerve	Pronator teres Flexor carpi radialis Palmaris longus Flexor digitorum superficialis Pronator quadratus Flexor digitorum profundus Flexor pollicis brevis Abductor pollicis brevis Opponens pollicis Lumbricals	*Common palmar digital nerve:* palmar side thumb, radial side hand and 2nd, 3rd, and radial 4th finger; dorsal side distal 2/3 of 2nd, 3rd, and radial 4th finger
C8–T1	Ulnar nerve	Flexor digitorum profundus Flexor carpi ulnaris Flexor pollicis brevis Flexor pollicis Opponens digiti minimi Flexor digiti minimi brevis Abductor digiti minimi Palmaris brevis Interossei Lumbricals III, IV	*Palmar cutaneous branch* *Superficial branch proper palmar digital nerves:* ventro-ulnar side of wrist, hypothenar, 5th finger, and ulnar half 4th finger *Dorsal ramus of dorsal digital nerves:* dorso-ulnar aspect wrist, dorsum of the hand, 5th finger, proximal aspect 3rd and 4th finger, medial-distal portion 4th finger

REGIONAL EXAMINATION

Active-Assisted Regional Examination: Cervical

For more information, see the section titled "Active-Assisted Regional Examination: Cervicothoracic/cervical" in Chapter 15.

Regional Provocation Tests: Cervical

For more information, see the section titled "Regional Provocation Tests: Cervicothoracic/Cervical" in Chapter 15.

SEGMENTAL EXAMINATION

Segmental Tissue–Specific Examination: Cervical

For the assessment criteria, please see the section titled "Segmental Tissue–Specific Examination: Lumbar" in Chapter 14.

Pinwheel Sensory Examination

Examination position, patient: Prone, with forehead resting on the examination table.

Starting position, therapist: Standing beside the patient.

Procedure: The pinwheel is held between the thumb and the index finger. The skin segment of the level to be examined is tested directly adjacent to the spinous process for superficial sensitivity to pain. (See **Figure 16–15**.)

Remarks: This procedure tests the function of the medial branch of the dorsal ramus.

Kibler Test

Examination position, patient: Prone, with forehead resting on the examination bench.

Starting position, therapist: Standing beside the patient.

Procedure: The therapist takes the skin at the level to be examined, on one or both sides, between the thumb and index finger of both hands and produces a skin rolling movement. (See **Figure 16–16**.)

Palpation of Muscle Tone

Examination position, patient: Prone.

Starting position, therapist: Standing by the patient's head.

Procedure: The index fingers are placed one at either side of the spinous process on the muscles that span the segment to be examined. The muscle tone is palpated and compared with that in neighboring segments. (See **Figure 16–17**.)

Schöps et al. (2000) reported on the interrater agreement for palpation for muscle tone. The reported κ values for the left and right scalenes were 0.39 and 0.35; for the left and right sternocleidomastoid, 0.37 and 0.22; for the left and right trapezius, 0.30 and 0.20; for the left and right levator scapulae, 0.23 and 0.16; and for the left and right semispinalis capitis, 0.35 and 0.23, respectively.

Segmental Coordination Test

Examination position, patient: Supine

Starting position, therapist: Standing by the patient's head.

Procedure: The index fingers are placed on both sides on the lamina of the upper vertebra of the level to be examined. The patient is asked to resist light pressure exerted by the therapist on one or both sides. (See **Figure 16–18**.)

Remarks: The therapist should alternate pressure and release evenly, thereby producing a rhythmic stabilizing examination.

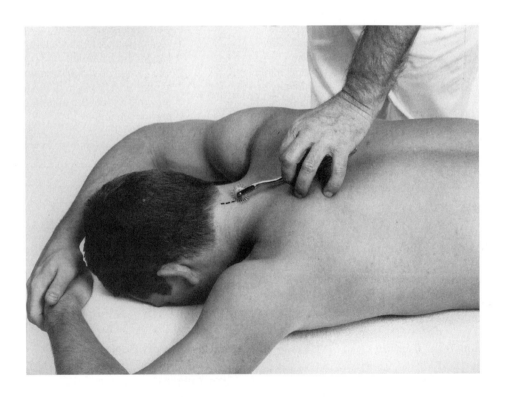

Figure 16–15

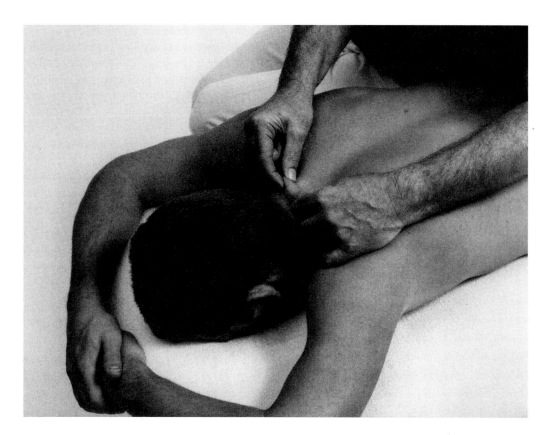

Figure 16–16

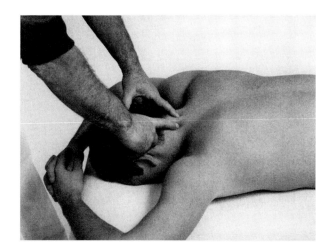

Figure 16–17

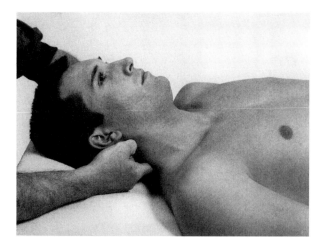

Figure 16–18 ⇅

Palpation of Specific Pain Points

Examination position, patient: Prone.

Starting position, therapist: Standing by the patient's head.

Procedure: The therapist places an index finger on the pain point associated with the level to be examined and exerts light pressure. (See **Figures 16–19, 16–20, 16–21**.)

Remarks: Depending on the type of pain point, the patient experiences local or radiating pain.

Bertilson et al. (2003) studied interrater reliability of palpation for tenderness at the C1–C3 and C4–C7 spinal processes and reported 80% ($\kappa = 0.6$) and 72% ($\kappa = 0.42$) agreement, respectively. Palpation for tenderness at the C1–C3 and C4–C7 joints yielded 66% ($\kappa = 0.32$) and 76% ($\kappa = 0.34$) agreement, respectively. Schöps et al. (2000) reported on the interrater agreement for palpation for tenderness at the C2–C7 facet joints: κ values left ranged from 0.32–0.61 and right from 0.30–0.66. Schöps et al. also reported on the interrater agreement for palpation for muscle tenderness. The reported κ values for the left and right scalenes were 0.37 and 0.23; for the left and right sternocleidomastoid, 0.63 and 0.46; for the left and right trapezius 0.37 and 0.31; for the left and right levator scapulae 0.45 and 0.26; and for the left and right semispinalis capitis, 0.69 and 0.52, respectively.

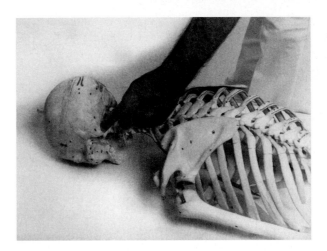

Figure 16–19

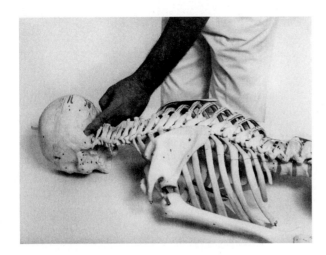

Figure 16–20

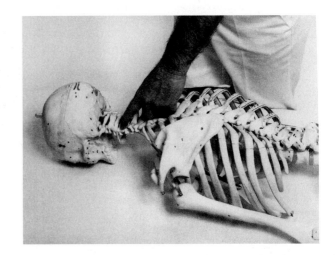

Figure 16–21

Segmental Provocation Tests: Cervical

For assessment criteria, see the section titled "Segmental Provocation Tests: Lumbar" in Chapter 14.

Segmental Springing Test

Examination position, patient: Prone, with forehead resting on the examination table.

Starting position, therapist: Standing by the patient's head.

Procedure: The therapist places his or her thumbs on the spinous process or on the lamina or lower facets of the upper vertebra. The therapist's fingers encircle the cervical spine from the ventral side, above the level to be examined, and produce a springing movement in a ventral direction. (See **Figure 16–22**.)

Remarks: Alternatively, the two thumbs can be used to support each other on one side on the lamina or lower facet of the upper vertebra (**Figure 16–23**).

Cleland et al. (2006) reported on interrater agreement for the prone C2–C7 springing test; these authors also provided interrater agreement data with regard to absence or presence of pain for this test. **Table 16–1** provides data on interrater percentage agreement (PA) and weighted κ values for the prone springing test.

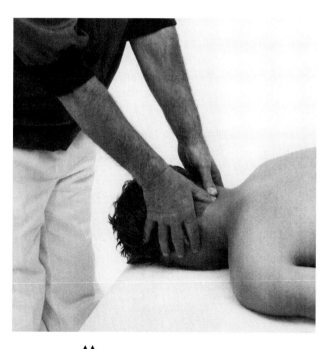

Figure 16–22 ⬆⬇

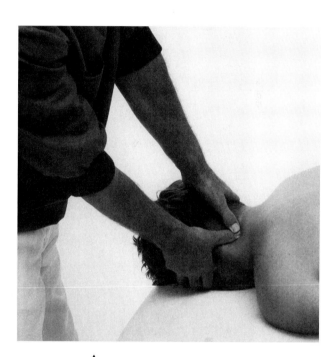

Figure 16–23 ⬆

Table 16–1 Data on Interrater Agreement Prone C2–C7 Springing Test

Level	K_w, 95% CI (mobility)	PA (mobility)	K_w, 95% CI (pain)	PA (pain)
C2	0.01 (−0.35–0.38)	67%	0.13 (−0.04–0.31)	50%
C3	0.10 (−0.25–0.44)	55%	0.13 (−0.21–0.47)	59%
C4	0.10 (−0.22–0.4)	55%	0.27 (−0.12–0.67)	64%
C5	0.10 (−0.15–0.35)	46%	0.12 (−0.09–0.42)	55%
C6	0.01 (−0.2–0.24)	41%	0.55 (0.22–0.88)	77%
C7	0.54 (0.2–0.88)	77%	0.90 (0.72–1.0)	95%

McGregor et al. (2001) questioned the validity of cervical springing tests as a method for segmental motion assessment: using MRI, they noted minimal if any intervertebral motion when a therapist applied a springing test motion to C2 or C6; rather, they reported soft tissue deformation.

Segmental Traction Test

Examination position, patient: Sitting on the long side of the examination table with the lower legs hanging down.

Starting position, therapist: Standing beside the patient.

Stabilization: The stabilizing hand maintains the position of the lower vertebra of the level to be examined; the thumb and index finger are placed on the lamina of the vertebra.

Procedure: The manipulating hand and arm surround the patient's head and cervical spine. The therapist places his or her little finger on the bow of the upper vertebra of the level to be examined and exerts traction. (See **Figure 16–24**.)

Remarks: Prior to the actual traction test, if the spine above the level to be examined is brought into the locked position, traction can be exerted at each level via the head.

Active-Assisted Segmental Examination: Cervical (C2–C7)

When the cervical spine is flexed, the action of the funicular part of the nuchal ligament causes upper cervical counterdirectional movement (van Mameren, 1988) (**Figure 16–25**). For this reason, when flexion in the middle and lower cervical spine is to be examined, extension is introduced in the upper cervical spine. This is consistent with Penning's theory (1978), according to which the alar ligaments and the apical ligament of the dens exert a flexion force on segment C2–C3 during extension of the upper cervical spine (**Figure 16–26**).

For practical reasons, the upper cervical spine is kept in the neutral position during examination of extension in the middle and lower cervical spine. This is possible because

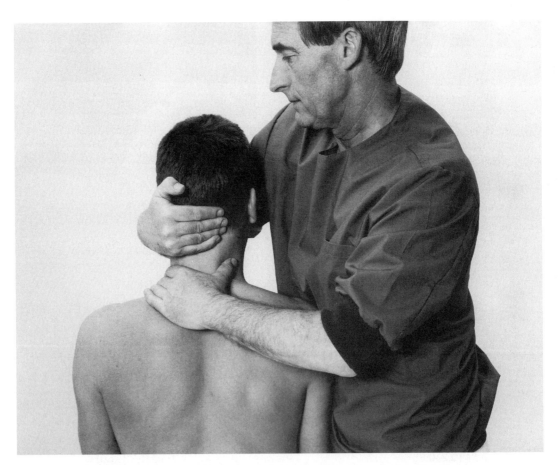

Figure 16–24

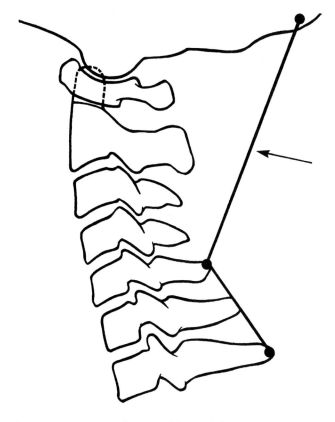

Figure 16–25 Funicular part of the nuchal ligament.

the neutral position of the upper cervical spine does not limit middle and lower cervical extension.

According to Penning (1978), upper cervical rotation causes contralateral sidebending because of the action of the contralateral alar ligament. It follows that during three-dimensional ipsilateral movements of the middle and lower cervical spine, a contralateral sidebending should be introduced in the upper cervical region.

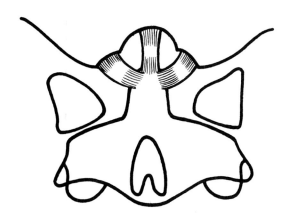

Figure 16–26 Upper cervical guiding ligaments.

Similarly, extension should be introduced in the upper cervical region during three-dimensional movements of the middle and lower cervical spine in which the sagittal component is flexion. If the sagittal component is extension, the upper cervical region is kept in the neutral position.

With the intent of localizing our examination techniques to the lower and mid-cervical spine, the table below provides the starting position of C0–C2 during middle and lower cervical examination:

Middle and Lower Cervical	Upper Cervical
Flexion	Extension
Flexion, sidebending, ipsilateral rotation	Extension, rotation, contralateral sidebending
Flexion, sidebending, contralateral rotation	Extension, sidebending, contralateral rotation
Extension	Neutral position
Extension, sidebending, ipsilateral rotation	Neutral position, rotation, contralateral sidebending
Extension, sidebending, contralateral rotation	Neutral position, sidebending, contralateral rotation

For assessment criteria, see the section titled "Active-Assisted Segmental Examination: Lumbar (L1 to L5)" in Chapter 14.

Flexion, Weight-Bearing

Examination position, patient: Sitting on the short side of the examination table with the lower legs hanging down. The upper cervical spine is brought into extension and the cervical spine into flexion as far as the level to be examined.

Starting position, therapist: Standing beside the patient.

Stabilization: The therapist stretches the thumb and finger of the stabilizing hand across the lamina of the lower vertebra at the level to be examined and holds the vertebra in position.

Procedure: The patient's head rests against the therapist's upper arm. The manipulating hand and arm surround the upper vertebra of the level to be examined and introduce flexion. (See **Figure 16–27**.)

Flexion, Sidebending, Ipsilateral Rotation, Weight-Bearing

Examination position, patient: Sitting on the short side of the examination table with the lower legs hanging down.

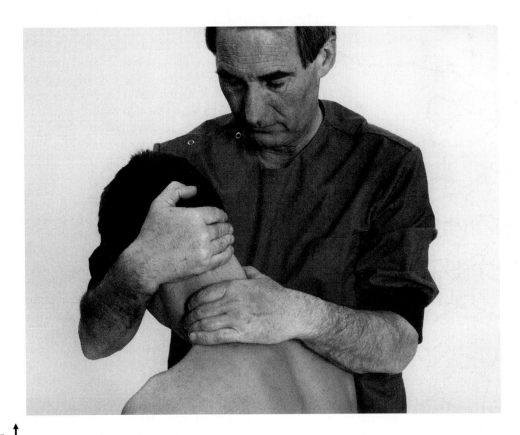

Figure 16–27 ↑

The upper cervical spine is brought into extension, rotation, and contralateral sidebending; the cervical spine is brought into flexion, sidebending, and ipsilateral rotation as far as the level to be examined.

Starting position, therapist: Standing beside the patient at the side to be examined.

Stabilization: The therapist spans the lamina of the lower vertebra of the level to be examined with the thumb and finger of the stabilizing hand and holds the vertebra in position.

Procedure: The patient's head rests against the therapist's upper arm. The manipulating hand and arm surround the contralateral lamina of the upper vertebra at the level to be examined and introduce flexion, sidebending, and ipsilateral rotation. (See **Figure 16–28**.)

Flexion, Sidebending, Contralateral Rotation, Weight-Bearing

Examination position, patient: Sitting on the short side of the examination table with the lower legs hanging down.

The upper cervical spine is brought into extension, sidebending, and contralateral rotation; the cervical spine is brought into flexion, sidebending, and contraexternal rotation as far as the level to be examined.

Starting position, therapist: Standing beside the patient at the side to be examined.

Stabilization: The therapist spans the lamina of the lower vertebra at the level to be examined with the thumb and index finger of the stabilizing hand and holds the vertebra in position.

Procedure: The patient's head rests against the therapist's upper arm. The manipulating hand and arm surround the contralateral lamina of the upper vertebra of the level to be examined and introduce flexion, sidebending, and contralateral rotation. (See **Figure 16–29**.)

Extension, Weight-Bearing

Examination position, patient: Sitting on the short side of the examination table with the lower legs hanging down. The upper cervical spine is brought into the neutral

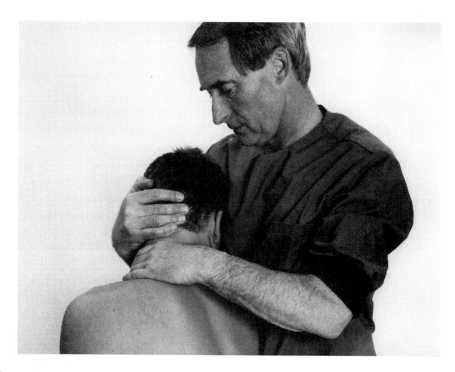

Figure 16–28

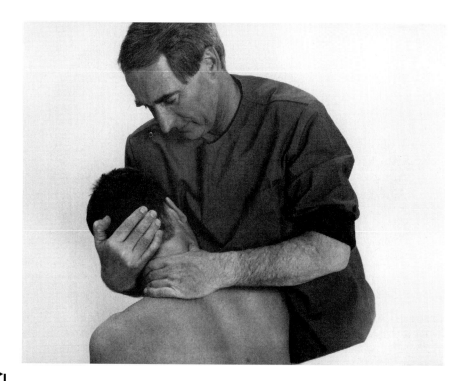

Figure 16–29

position; the cervical spine is brought into extension as far as the level to be examined.

Starting position, therapist: Standing beside the patient.

Stabilization: The therapist spans the lamina of the lower vertebra at the level to be examined with the thumb and index finger of the stabilizing hand and holds the vertebra in position.

Procedure: The patient's head rests against the therapist's upper arm. The manipulating hand and arm surround the upper vertebra of the level to be examined and introduce extension. The therapist uses his or her upper arm for support. (See **Figure 16–30**.)

Extension, Sidebending, Ipsilateral Rotation, Weight-Bearing

Examination position, patient: Sitting on the short side of the examination table with the lower legs hanging down. The upper cervical spine is brought into the neutral position, rotation, and contralateral sidebending; the cervi-

cal spine is brought into extension, sidebending, and ipsilateral rotation as far as the level to be examined.

Starting position, therapist: Standing beside the patient at the side to be examined.

Stabilization: The therapist spans the lamina of the lower vertebra at the level to be examined with the thumb and index finger of the stabilizing hand and holds the vertebra in position.

Procedure: The patient's head rests against the therapist's upper arm. The manipulating hand and arm surround the contralateral lamina of the upper vertebra of the level to be examined and introduce extension, sidebending, and ipsilateral rotation. The therapist uses his or her upper arm for support. (See **Figure 16–31**.)

Bronemo and Van Steveninck (1987) reported on the reliability of a seated C2–C7 segmental mobility test in an oblique posterior-lateral direction thereby similar to the test described here. They reported 88.2–94.7% average intrarater and 84.4% interrater agreement.

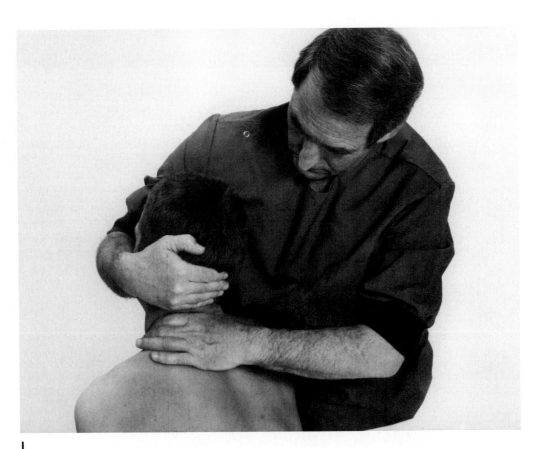

Figure 16–30

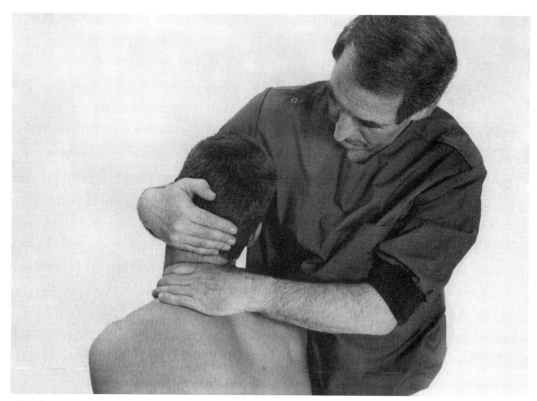

Figure 16–31

Extension, Sidebending, Contralateral Rotation, Weight-Bearing

Examination position, patient: Sitting on the short side of the examination table with the lower legs hanging down. The upper cervical spine is brought into the neutral position, sidebending, and contraexternal rotation; the cervical spine is brought into extension, sidebending, and contralateral rotation as far as the level to be examined.

Starting position, therapist: Standing beside the patient at the side to be examined.

Stabilization: The therapist spans the lamina of the lower vertebra at the level to be examined with the thumb and index finger of the stabilizing hand and holds the vertebra in position.

Procedure: The patient's head rests against the therapist's upper arm. The manipulating hand and arm surround the contralateral lamina of the upper vertebra of the level to be examined and introduce extension, sidebending, and contralateral rotation. The therapist uses his or her upper arm for support. (See **Figure 16–32**.)

Flexion, Non-Weight-Bearing

Examination position, patient: Lying on one side with the hips and knees flexed. The upper cervical spine is brought into extension; the cervical spine is brought into flexion as far as the level to be examined.

Starting position, therapist: Standing in front of the patient.

Stabilization: The therapist spans the lamina of the lower vertebra at the level to be examined with the thumb and index finger of the stabilizing hand and holds the vertebra in position.

Procedure: The manipulating hand and arm surround the upper vertebra of the level to be examined and introduce flexion. (See **Figure 16–33**.)

Remarks: **Figure 16–34** shows a patient being examined in the supine position.

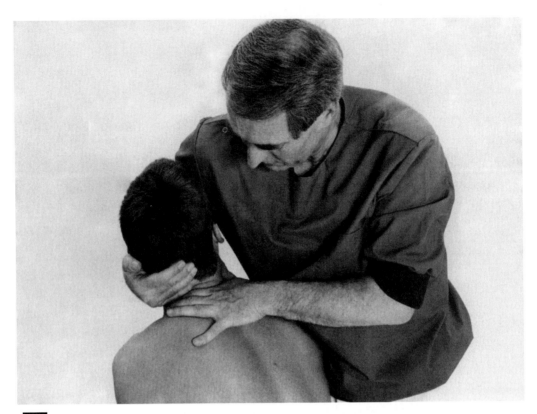

Figure 16–32

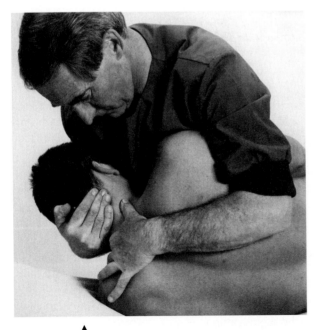

Figure 16–33

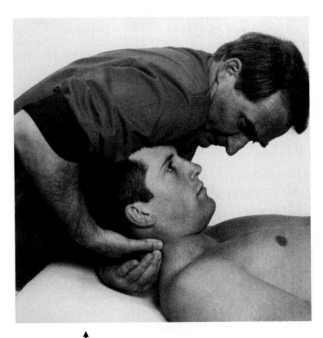

Figure 16–34

Flexion, Sidebending, Ipsilateral Rotation,
Non-Weight-Bearing

Examination position, patient: Lying on one side with the hips and knees flexed. The upper cervical spine is brought into extension, rotation, contralateral sidebending; the cervical spine is brought into flexion, sidebending, and ipsilateral rotation as far as the level to be examined.

Starting position, therapist: Standing in front of the patient.

Stabilization: The therapist spans the lamina of the lower vertebra at the level to be examined between the thumb and index finger of the stabilizing hand and holds the vertebra in position.

Procedure: The patient's head rests against the therapist's upper arm. The manipulating hand and arm surround the contralateral lamina of the upper vertebra of the level to be examined and introduce flexion, sidebending, and ipsilateral rotation. (See **Figure 16–35**.)

Remarks: **Figure 16–36** shows a patient being examined in the supine position.

Schöps et al. (2000) reported on interrater agreement for a C2–C3 flexion-sidebending-ipsilateral rotation test: interrater κ values were 0.04 and 0.34 for the right and left, respectively, when rated dichotomously for mobility. When rated for pain, these values were 0.43 and 0.52, respectively.

Flexion, Sidebending, Contralateral Rotation,
Non-Weight-Bearing

Examination position, patient: Lying on the side with the hips and knees flexed. The upper cervical spine is brought into extension, sidebending, and contraexternal rotation; the cervical spine is brought into flexion, sidebending, and contralateral rotation as far as the level to be examined.

Starting position, therapist: Standing in front of the patient.

Stabilization: The therapist spans the lamina of the lower vertebra at the level to be examined with the thumb and index finger of the stabilizing hand and holds the vertebra in position.

Procedure: The patient's head rests against the therapist's upper arm. The manipulating hand and arm surround the contralateral lamina of the upper vertebra of the level to be examined and introduce flexion, sidebending, and contralateral rotation. (See **Figure 16–37**.)

Remarks: **Figure 16–38** shows a patient being examined in the supine position.

Extension, Non-Weight-Bearing

Examination position, patient: Lying on the side with hips and knees flexed. The upper cervical spine is brought into

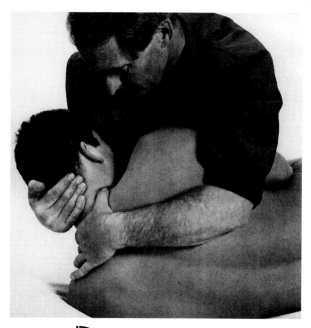

Figure 16–35

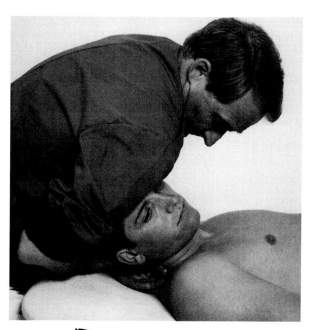

Figure 16–36

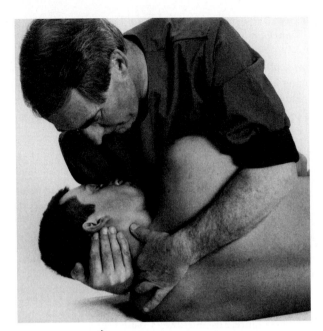

Figure 16–37

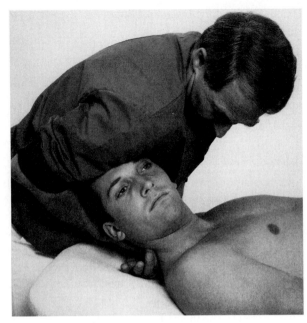

Figure 16–38

the neutral position; the cervical spine is brought into extension as far as the level to be examined.

Starting position, therapist: Standing in front of the patient.

Stabilization: The therapist spans the lamina of the lower vertebra at the level to be examined with the thumb and index finger of the stabilizing hand and holds the vertebra in position.

Procedure: The patient's head rests against the therapist's upper arm. The manipulating hand and arm surround the upper vertebra of the level to be examined and introduce extension. The therapist uses his or her upper arm for support. (See **Figure 16–39**.)

Remarks: **Figure 16–40** shows a patient being examined in the supine position.

Extension, Sidebending, Ipsilateral Rotation, Non-Weight-Bearing

Examination position, patient: Lying on the side with hips and knees flexed. The upper cervical spine is brought into the neutral position, rotation, and contralateral sidebending; the cervical spine is brought into extension, sidebending, and ipsilateral rotation as far as the level to be examined.

Starting position, therapist: Standing in front of the patient.

Stabilization: The therapist spans the lamina of the lower vertebra of the level to be examined with the thumb and index finger of the stabilizing hand and holds the vertebra in position.

Procedure: The patient's head rests against the therapist's upper arm. The manipulating hand and arm surround the contralateral lamina of the upper vertebra of the level to be examined and introduce extension, sidebending, and ipsilateral rotation. The therapist uses his or her upper arm for support. (See **Figure 16–41**.)

Remarks: **Figure 16–42** shows a patient being examined in the supine position.

Bronemo and Van Steveninck (1987) reported on the reliability of a supine C2–C7 segmental mobility test in an oblique posterior-lateral direction similar to the supine test variant described here. They reported 88.2–94.7% average intrarater and 84.8% interrater agreement.

Extension, Sidebending, Contralateral Rotation, Non-Weight-Bearing

Examination position, patient: Lying on the side with hips and knees flexed. The upper cervical spine is brought into the neutral position, sidebending, and contraexternal rotation; the cervical spine is brought into extension,

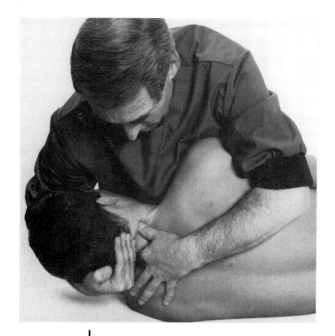

Figure 16–39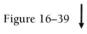

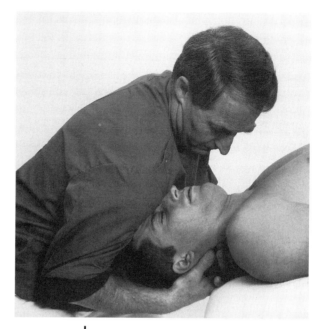

Figure 16–40 ↓

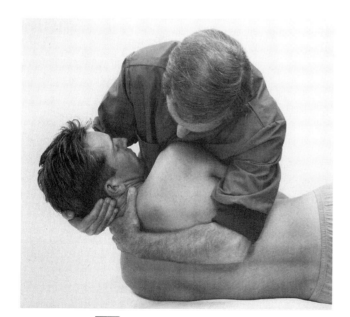

Figure 16–41

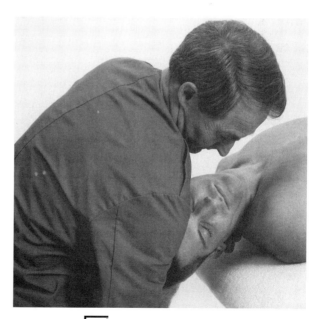

Figure 16–42

sidebending, and contralateral rotation as far as the level to be examined.

Starting position, therapist: Standing in front of the patient.

Stabilization: The therapist spans the lamina of the lower vertebra of the level to be examined with the thumb and index finger of the stabilizing hand and holds the vertebra in position.

Procedure: The patient's head rests against the therapist's upper arm. The manipulating hand and arm surround the contralateral lamina of the upper vertebra of the level to be examined and introduce extension, sidebending, and contralateral rotation. The therapist uses his or her upper arm for support. (See **Figure 16–43**.)

Remarks: **Figure 16–44** shows a patient being examined in the supine position.

INSTABILITY EXAMINATION: CERVICAL

As with the history and examination findings of patients with lumbar instability, the symptoms and signs proposed for the identification of patients with cervical instability lack specificity and are based on authority-based knowledge and anecdotal evidence.

Significant Features in the Patient's History

Symptoms proposed as indicative of cervical instability include:

- Pain during activities performed in endrange positions
- Pain on maintaining a particular position for a long period
- Pain after prolonged sleep
- Pain when writing or typing
- Pain when carrying heavy weights
- Pain when riding a bicycle with low handlebars

Clinical Signs

Signs proposed as indicative of cervical instability include:

- Disturbed course of active movements
- Disturbance of the rhythm of active movements
- Pain on palpation of the ligaments that span the segment
- Hyperesthesia of the dorsal ramus of the segment

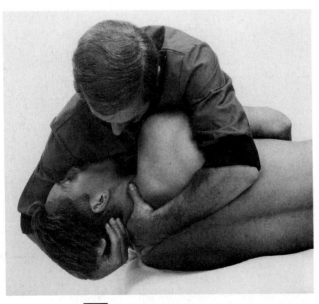

Figure 16–43

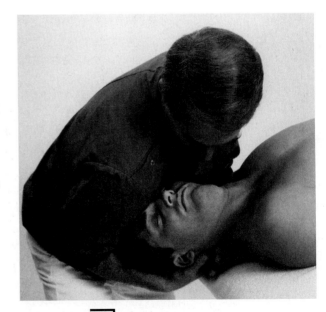

Figure 16–44

- Reduced reflex activity in the muscles innervated from the segment
- Reduced strength in the segmental muscles
- Reduced endurance in the segmental muscles
- Muscular guarding and pain during passive segmental movement

Instability Tests

- In cases of flexion instability, if the *lower* vertebra is stabilized during flexion in a ventrocaudal direction, and if pressure is applied in a dorsal direction during active movement—which accentuates the angular component—the pain occurs at a later stage or not at all (**Figure 16–45**).
- Where there is extension instability, if the *upper* vertebra is supported in a ventral direction during extension, and if pressure is applied in a ventral direction during active movement—which accentuates the angular component—the pain occurs at a later stage or not at all (**Figure 16–46**).

Coordination Test

With the patient in the supine position, resistance is applied with two fingers to the lamina of the upper vertebra of the unstable segment. If this provokes no response, and if the impulse is not detected, the test result is positive (Lanser, 1988) (**Figure 16–47**).

Additional Test Options

In the supine position, test options are as follows:

- Cervical flexion position
- Cervical ipsilateral three-dimensional flexion position

In the prone position, test options are as follows:

- Cervical extension position
- Cervical ipsilateral three-dimensional extension position

Lying on the side, the test options are as follows:

- Cervical sidebending position
- Cervical ipsilateral three-dimensional sidebending position

The preceding positions should be held for 10 seconds, separated by 10-second pauses. Each position should be repeated 10 times.

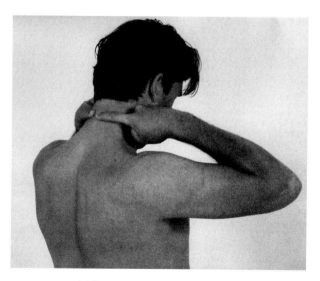

Figure 16–45

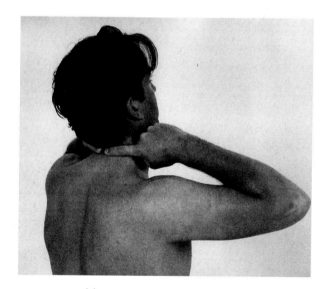

Figure 16–46

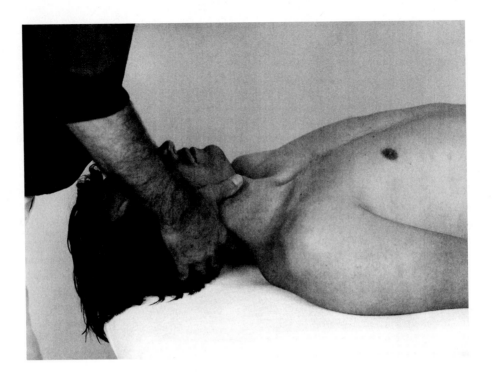

Figure 16–47 ⬆

Muscles That May Be Involved

The following muscles in the global muscle system may be involved:

- Sternocleidomastoid muscle
- Scalene muscle
- Suprahyoid muscle
- Infrahyoid muscle
- Splenius muscle
- Longissimus muscle
- Iliocostalis muscle
- Upper trapezius muscle
- Levator scapulae muscle

The following muscles in the local muscle system may be involved:

- Longus capitis muscle
- Longus colli muscle
- Rectus capitis anterior muscle

- Rectus capitis lateralis muscle
- Semispinalis muscle
- Spinalis muscle

The following muscles in the segmental muscle system may be involved:

- Multifidus muscle
- Interspinalis muscle
- Intertransverse muscle
- Rectus capitis posterior major muscle
- Rectus capitis posterior minor muscle
- Obliquus capitis superior muscle
- Obliquus capitis inferior muscle

Chronic neck pain leads to reduced sensorimotor function. The first four muscles in the local system are the first to lose strength in patients with chronic neck pain. Attention should also be paid to the mobility and stability of the cervicothoracic transitional area, the shoulder girdle, and the muscles that are important to these regions.

CHAPTER **17**

Examination of the Upper Cervical Spine

FUNCTIONAL ASPECTS OF THE UPPER CERVICAL SPINE C0–C2 (C3)

The upper cervical spine consists of the atlanto-occipital joint (a), the atlantoaxial joint (b), with additional articular surfaces between the anterior lamina of the atlas and the dens, and those between the transverse ligament and the dens (c) (see **Figure 17–1**).

The upper cervical spine differs from the lower part with regard to its structure, the absence of disks and uncovertebral joints, its specific ligamentous connections, and the presence of muscles that enable the segments to move independently (**Figure 17–2**). An example of this is rotation in C1–C2 produced by contraction of the obliquus capitis inferior muscle.

In addition to the nuchal ligament, the posterior longitudinal ligament, and the tectorial membrane, which connect the head and the cervical spine, extra ligaments in the up-

per cervical region stretch between the occiput and the axis. These are the apical ligament of the dens, the alar ligaments, and the vertical part of the cruciate ligament. The atlas is included in the upper cervical complex because it functions as a ball bearing between the head and the cervical spine (**Figure 17–3**).

Many researchers have done scientific studies of the upper cervical region because of the frequency with which it is damaged by trauma or infections. The research carried out by Penning (1968), Huguenin (1984), and Dvorak and Panjabi (1987) have led to a better understanding of function of the alar ligaments. The following are the findings of three specific studies of the alar ligaments.

Penning (1968) reports that the alar ligaments connect the upper back surface of the dens of the second cervical vertebra and the condyles of the occiput. The ligaments course in a lateroventrocranial direction between the back surface of the dens of the axis and the occipital condyles.

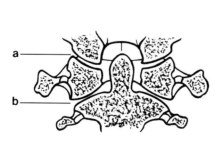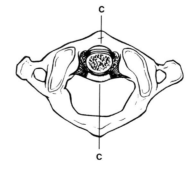

Figure 17–1   Upper cervical joints.

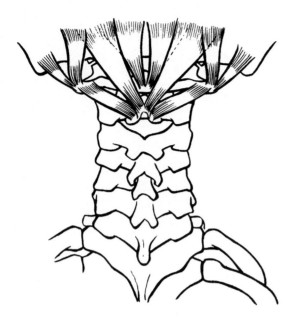

Figure 17–2   Upper cervical muscles that enable independent movement.

Penning (1968) also states that one of the most important functions of the alar ligaments is to maintain the position of the dens midway between the occipital condyles. The ways in which this influences physiologic movements are listed as follows:

- Extension of C0–C1 causes the dens of C2 to tilt forward because of the displacement of the C0 condyles in a ventral direction.
- Sidebending in C0–C1 causes ipsilateral rotation of C2 and relative contralateral rotation in C0–C1

because of the displacement of the contralateral condyle of C0 in a contralateral direction.
- Rotation of C0 and C1–C2 causes contralateral sidebending in C0–C1 because of the relative shortening of the contralateral alar ligament, which winds round the dens.

Huguenin (1984) agrees with Ludwig (1952) that the alar ligaments are attached to both the ventral and the dorsal aspects of the upper two-thirds of the dens of the axis. The posterior alar ligaments, with the upper horizontal fibers and the lower oblique fibers that run in a cranial direction, course between the dens and the condyles of the occiput (**Figure 17–4**). The anterior alar ligaments, together with horizontal fibers and the oblique fiber bundles that run cranially, also run from the dens to the lateral masses of the atlas, the joint capsule of C0–C1, and the occipital condyles (**Figure 17–5**).

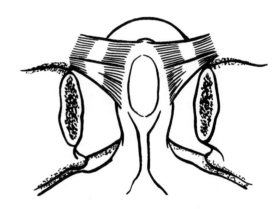

Figure 17–4   Dorsal aspect of the alar ligaments.

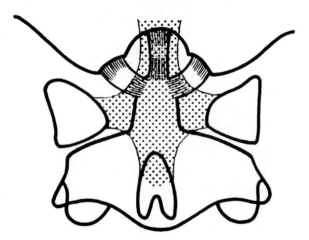

Figure 17–3   The ligamentous connections between C0–C2.

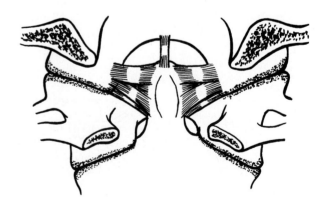

Figure 17–5   Ventral aspect of the alar ligaments.

Huguenin (1984) lists the following functions for the alar ligaments:

- Keeping the dens of the axis in its proper position relative to the atlas and the foramen magnum of the occiput.

- Guiding the rotation of C2 during sidebending of C0–C1. The alar ligament is supported in this by the Y-shaped ligament, which runs obliquely in a cranial direction and connects the base of the dens with the lateral mass of the atlas and the condyle of the occiput (**Figure 17–6**).

- Guiding and limiting the rotation of C0 and C1–C2 (**Figure 17–7**). The contralateral posterior alar ligament initiates and guides rotation of C2. The contralateral anterior alar ligament and the ipsilateral posterior alar ligament are the elements that limit the rotation of C2, whereas the ipsilateral anterior alar ligament relaxes.

- Setting the final limit on flexion and extension.

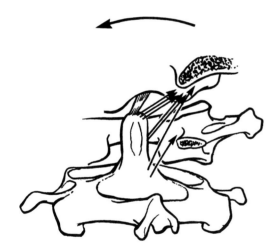

Figure 17–6 Sidebending right C0–C1, ipsilateral rotation C2.

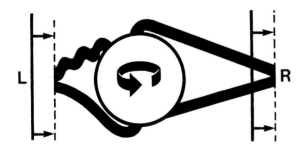

Figure 17–7 Function of alar ligaments during sidebending C0–C1 left.

Tearing of the transverse ligament can result in ventral displacement (5–8 mm) of the anterior arch of the atlas relative to the ventral aspect of the dens of the axis. If the alar ligaments are also torn, this displacement can increase by 2 to 3 mm (Huguenin, 1984).

Dvorak and Panjabi (1987) regard the alar ligament as consisting of two parts, an occipital part and an atlantal part. The occipital alar ligament courses between the dorsal and lateral aspects of the dens and the occipital condyle on the same side. Its average length is 11 mm. The atlantal alar ligament runs obliquely in a caudal direction from the ventral aspect of the dens to the lateral mass of the atlas. It has an average length of 3 mm.

The occipital alar ligaments are arranged parallel to each other. This ligament can withstand tensile stresses of about 200 N. For purposes of comparison, the transverse ligament, the fibers of which lie at an angle of 30°, the vertical part of the cruciate ligament, and the flaval ligament can withstand tensile stresses of 350 N, 436 N, and 113 N, respectively. The occipital alar ligaments, which course between the dens and the condyles of the occiput, lie in a straight line or form an obtuse angle of 150–170° opening toward the ventral side. In the frontal plane, they may run horizontally or in a cranial or caudal direction, depending on the position of C0 relative to the height of the dens. In the frontal plane, the atlantal alar ligaments run obliquely in the caudal direction from the ventral aspect of the dens to the lateral masses of the atlas.

Dvorak and Panjabi (1987) see the following as the primary functions of the alar ligaments:

- Guiding and limiting the rotation of C0 and C1–C2 (**Figure 17–8**). During rotation, the ipsilateral atlantal alar ligament and the contralateral occipital alar ligament are tensed, while the contralateral atlantal alar ligament and the ipsilateral occipital alar ligament relax. The lower fibers of the occipital alar ligament are tensed first, and the upper fibers at a later stage. If the occipital alar ligament is severed at one side, contralateral rotation of C0–C1 increases by 3.5° (9.4 to 5.9) and of C1–C2 by 5.8° (37.2 to 31.4) (Dvorak, Schneider, Saldinger, and Rahn, 1988). This indicates that lesions of the alar ligament will cause rotatory instability in the upper cervical region. The increase in rotation can have a significant effect on blood flow in the vertebral artery. The symptoms to which this can give rise are described in the section titled "Vertebrobasilar Insufficiency" in Chapter 7.

- Limiting sidebending and guiding the accompanying ipsiexternal rotation of the axis (**Figure 17–9**). During sidebending, the atlas moves ipsilaterally without the occurrence of rotation, and the occipital condyles

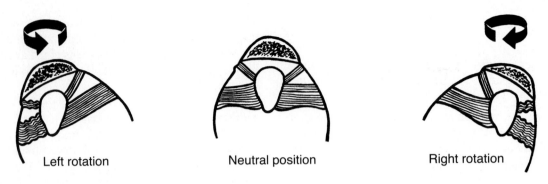

Figure 17–8   Left rotation; neutral position; right rotation.

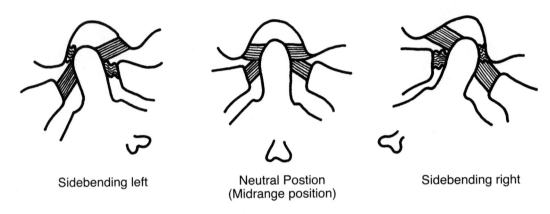

Figure 17–9   Left sidebending; neutral position; right sidebending

move in the contralateral direction. The result is that the ipsilateral atlantal alar ligament and the contralateral occipital alar ligament are tensed, while the contralateral atlantal alar ligament and the ipsilateral occipital alar ligament relax. The ligaments that are tensed limit sidebending and initiate ipsilateral rotation of the axis. The position of the joint facets in segment C2–C3 may also contribute to the rotation. The alar ligaments have a stabilizing function both in the transverse plane and in the frontal plane.

- Setting the final limit on flexion. Upper cervical flexion is limited by the nuchal ligament, the tectorial membrane, the posterior longitudinal ligament, the vertical part of the cruciate ligament, and the transverse ligament. The alar ligaments are only involved at the limit of movement.

- Limiting extension. Extension is limited in part by the ligaments that span the front of the upper cervical spine, but mainly by the alar ligaments.

According to Dvorak and Panjabi (1987), combined rotation and flexion exert the greatest tensile force on the alar ligaments. It is in this position, therefore, that they are most vulnerable.

In addition to the alar ligaments, Dvorak and Panjabi (1987) describe other ligaments that connect the atlas with the dens and the two condyles of the occiput with the dens. These ligaments were only present in a proportion of the persons examined. The anterior atlantodental ligament (**Figure 17–10**) forms a connection between the anterior arch of the atlas and the ventral aspect of the base of the dens. The function of this ligament is thought to be to support the transverse ligament. The transverse atlantal ligament (**Figure 17–11**) spans the two condyles of C0 and has a partial insertion on the dens.

The conclusions drawn from these studies indicate that there are differences of opinion with regard to the origin, the insertion, the course, and the components of the alar ligaments. However, there is a high level of consensus about their function.

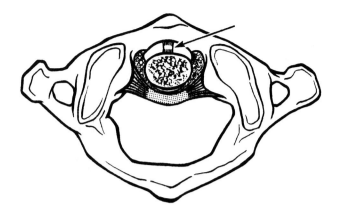

Figure 17–10   The anterior atlantodental ligament.

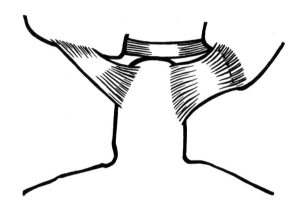

Figure 17–11   The transverse atlantal ligament.

Movement of C0 affects C2 directly and C1 and C3 indirectly via the ligamentous connections. The essential part of the movement occurs between C0 and C2 and is regulated by C1. Optimal efficiency of the upper cervical spine depends on the functioning of the individual segments C0–C1–C2–C3.

According to Putz (1981), the particular way in which the second cervical vertebra is attached to the third is an essential factor in the complex and differentiated mobility of the upper cervical spine. The structure of the third cervical vertebra is unusual compared with that of the cervical vertebrae below it. The angle of inclination of the upper intervertebral articular surfaces is greater and their opening angle is smaller. The distance between the vertebral body and the intervertebral articular surfaces is the same as that found in the seventh cervical vertebra. The distance between the intervertebral articular surfaces is relatively small. The load-bearing triangle is higher than in the other cervical vertebrae.

Because of this atypical structure, flexion–extension and rotation in C2–C3 are limited in comparison with the mobility of other vertebrae (Virchow, 1909; Markuske, 1971; Putz, 1981). Penning confirms this for ventral/extension (Penning 1964, 1968, 1978).

Penning (1978) also finds that the extent of rotation is greater than in all the lower segments of the cervical spine. With regard to the musculature, Penning (1978) points out the central position of the strongly developed spinous processes of C2, from which the small upper cervical muscles diverge cranially, and the semispinalis muscle and others diverge caudally (**Figure 17–12**).

The muscles that are attached caudal to C2 are interwoven to such an extent that independent segmental movement is impossible: every muscle activates several segments.

According to Minne et al. (1970), Mestdagh (1976), and Putz (1981), the structure of the third vertebra, combined with its muscular connections, makes it more or less a stable basis for the upper cervical joints. The upper cervical part (C0–C3) forms a functional unit, with C3 as its base, which enables the upper cervical joints to make finely coordinated movements (Putz, 1981).

Flexion C0–C2

The essential part of the movement takes place between C0 and C2 and is regulated by the atlas. Penning (1978)

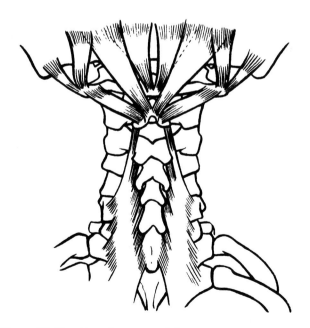

Figure 17–12   Central position of the spinous processes of C2 between cranially and caudally diverging muscles.

states that during flexion and extension, the position of the atlas is relatively independent of the relationship between the occiput and C2 at that moment.

Theoretically, C2 can move with C1 without changing the position of C0. C1 can also move with C0 while its position relative to C2 remains constant. In practice, in every position of the craniocervical joint, the posterior arch of the atlas can be located "somewhere" between the occiput and the spinous process of C2. It need not necessarily be exactly midway between the occiput and the spinous process of C2 (**Figure 7–13**). During flexion of the whole cervical spine,

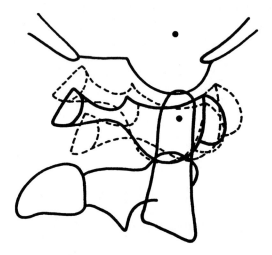

Figure 17–13   Relative independence of the position of the atlas during flexion–extension.

the posterior arch of the atlas sometimes seems to be closer to the occiput than during extension of the whole cervical spine (Penning, 1978).

During ventral nodding movements of the upper cervical spine (chin tuck), the distances between the posterior arch of the atlas and the occiput, and between the posterior arch of the atlas and the spinous process of C2, appear to be greater than in flexion of the whole cervical spine (**Figure 7–14**). These differences are a result of the fact that during flexion of the whole cervical spine, the funicular part of the nuchal ligament is tensed in a particular phase of the movement, which causes upper cervical inversion or counterdirectional movement (van Mameren, 1988). During specific upper cervical flexion (nodding), this limiting factor is not present, and the upper cervical spine can assume its optimal flexed position. During ventral nodding, C0 slides in a dorsocranial direction relative to C1. C1 rolls in the ventral direction relative to C2, and in the process it slips a little dorsally. The biconvexity of the joint cartilage in the lower articular surfaces of C1 and the upper ones of C2 causes the ventral low parts of the joint surfaces to approximate each other. As a result, the distance between C0 and C2 decreases ventrally, while the tension increases in the ligamentous structures behind the axis of movement. The axis of flexion in C0–C1 lies in the skull, in the center of the circles traced by the articular surfaces of C1 (**Figure 17–15**). The axis of flexion in C1–C2 lies in the top of the odontoid (**Figure 17–16**). It is determined not by the articular surfaces, but by the fibro-osseous ring of the anterior arch of the atlas and the transverse ligament (Penning, 1978). The apical lig-

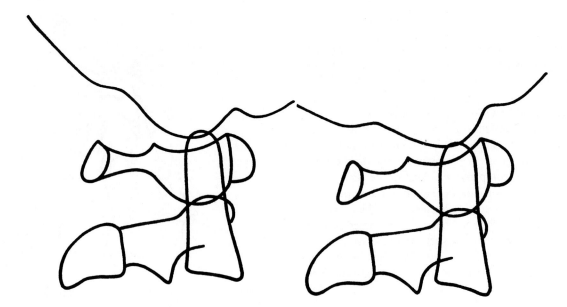

Figure 17–14   Ventral nodding, ventral flexion.

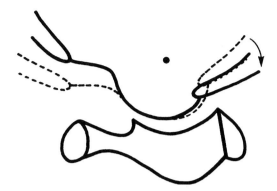

Figure 17–15   Axis C0–C1 during flexion–extension.

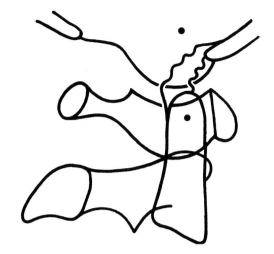

Figure 17–17   Relaxation of ligaments during ventral nodding.

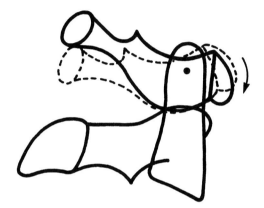

Figure 17–16   Axis C1–C2 during flexion–extension.

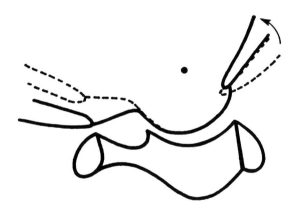

ament of the dens and the alar ligaments relax somewhat during flexion (nodding) (**Figure 17–17**). For C0–C1 and C1–C2, the average extent of movement during extension–flexion is 30° (Penning, 1978).

Figure 17–18   Dorsal nodding C0–C1.

Extension C0–C2

The positions of the axes of movement are the same as for flexion (**Figures 17–18** and **17–19**).

During extension, C0 glides in a ventrocranial direction relative to C1. The alar ligaments, which course in a ventro-laterocranial direction between C2 and C0, are tensed when the neck is bent backward; this is because of the cranioventral movement of C0, and it causes the odontoid to tilt in a ventral direction. Optimal upper cervical extension is, therefore, partly dependent on normal functioning in the segment C2–C3 (**Figure 17–20**).

During upper cervical extension, C1 rolls in a dorsal direction relative to C2 and slips somewhat ventrally. Because

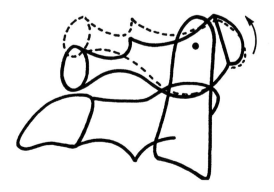

Figure 17–19   Dorsal nodding C1–C2.

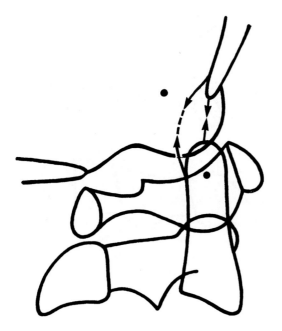

Figure 17–20   Influence of the ligaments on the movement of C2 during dorsal nodding.

of the biconvexity of the joint cartilage of the lower articular surfaces of C1 and the upper ones of C2, the posterior low parts of the articular surfaces approximate each other. As a result, the distance between C0 and C2 decreases dorsally, while tension increases in the ligamentous structures ventral to the axis of movement in C0–C1 and dorsal to that of C1–C2. The factors that limit extension are dorsal bony compression and the ligaments that lie both dorsal and ventral to the axes of movement.

Sidebending C0–C2

During upper cervical lateral bending, the movement of the atlas has a predetermined course influenced by the lateral mass, which broadens in a lateral direction. The attachment of the two alar ligaments to the condyles of C0 means that the odontoid process remains in the middle between the condyles. The odontoid process follows the movements of the occiput.

In upper cervical sidebending, the condyles of C0 slide toward the convex side, which causes the spaces between C0 and C2 to increase on the convex side and to decrease on the concave. This makes it possible, or even necessary, for the atlas to move in the concave direction because of the broad lateral mass. Sidebending of the atlanto-occipital segment is, therefore, always accompanied by ipsilateral sidebending of the atlantoaxial segment.

The lateral slide of the condyle on the convex side causes tension in the contralateral alar ligament, which runs from the posterior side of the odontoid in a cranioventrolateral direction toward the condyle of C0. The tensing of this ligament brings about ipsiexternal rotation of C2. We may, therefore, conclude that upper cervical sidebending is associated with ipsiexternal rotation of C2 and relative contraexternal rotation of C0 and C1 (**Figure 17–21**).

During sidebending of the whole cervical spine, with the head held in the anterior/ posterior position, C1–C2 makes a counter-rotation of about 35°. Because of the biconvexity of the joints in segment C1–C2, the distance between C0 and C2 decreases by 2 to 3 mm (see the section titled "Rotation C0–C2," which follows).

The axis of sidebending in C0–C1 runs through the skull (**Figure 17–22**). That of sidebending in C1–C2 lies in the middle cervical spine (**Figure 17–23**). During sidebending of C0–C2 with C2 fixated (Penning fixates C0), the C0–C2 axis of movement lies in the top of the odontoid, which is fixed against the occiput by the alar ligaments (Penning, 1978) (**Figure 17–24**). The factors that inhibit lateral bending are the impact on the concave side and the ligaments that lie on the convex side of the axis of movement. The average extent of sidebending of C0–C2 to one side is about 5°.

Rotation C0–C2

Rotation in C0–C1 is very limited according to some authors and completely absent according to others. Kapandji

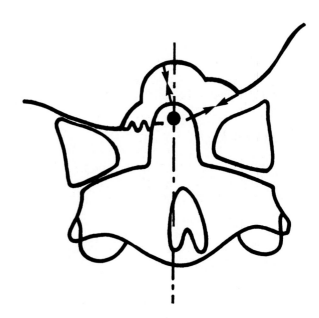

Figure 17–21   Sidebending left C0–C2 with synkinetic left rotation C2, that is, right rotation C0 and C1.

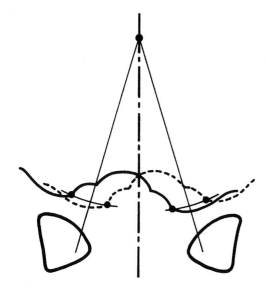

Figure 17–22   Axis of sidebending C0–C1.

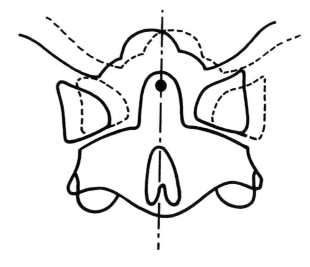

Figure 17–24   Axis of sidebending C0–C2.

(1974) is one who believes that limited rotation is possible. Rotation in the atlantoaxial segment accounts for about half of total cervical rotation, which is about 35°. The axis of rotation lies at the back of the odontoid in the transverse ligament (Penning, 1978) (**Figure 17–25**).

In a particular phase of the movement trajectory, rotation of C0–C2 is accompanied by ipsiexternal rotation of C2 and contralateral sidebending of C0–C1. This is the result of tension developing in the contralateral alar ligament.

During left rotation of C0–C2 (a in **Figure 17–26**), a small left rotation takes place in segment C0–C1. This causes the left condyle to move slightly in a dorsal direction relative to the upper left facet of C1 and the right condyle to move slightly in a ventral direction relative to the upper right facet of C1. The greatest coupled movement that occurs in segment C0–C1 is right, or contralateral, sidebending (b). Because of the tension in the contralateral alar ligament, both condyles move in an ipsilateral direction, that is, to the left, relative to the upper facets of C1.

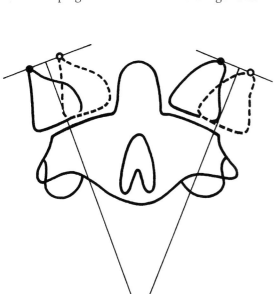

Figure 17–23   Axis of sidebending C1–C2.

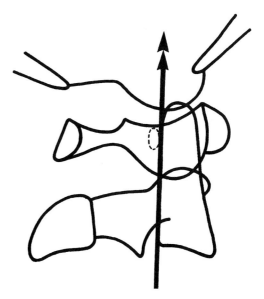

Figure 17–25   Axis of rotation C1–C2.

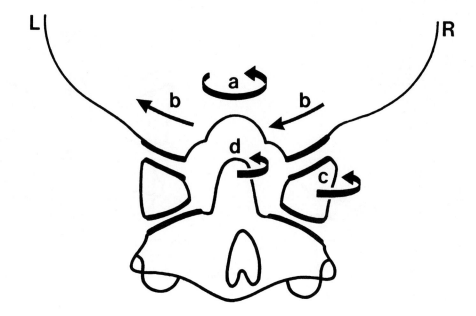

Figure 17–26   Movements during left rotation C0–C2.

In segment C1–C2, an ipsilateral or left rotation (c) takes place in which the ipsilateral or left lower facet of C1 moves in a dorsal direction relative to the left upper facet of C2. The contralateral or right lower facet of C1 moves in a ventral direction relative to the right upper facet of C2.

Rotation in C0–C2 also causes movement in segment C2–C3. Gutmann (1956) describes this as an ipsilateral, that is, left rotation of C2 (d), while Penning (1978) sees the movement as a contralateral displacement of the odontoid. The two authors agree, however, that tension in the contralateral alar ligament is responsible for the movement. When C0 and C1 rotate relative to C2, the contralateral alar ligament, which is attached dorsal to the odontoid, is twisted around the latter, thus becoming functionally shorter (**Figure 17–27**).

According to Henke (1863), Fick (1911), Strasser (1913) and others, the atlas sinks with a spiral-like movement relative to the axis. Putz and Pomaroli (1972) state that for the first 20°, the atlas remains in the same position in the transverse plane, but that it sinks 2 to 3 mm on further rotation. This phenomenon can be explained by the biconvexity of the joint surfaces in C1–C2. During left rotation, the anterior low part of the lower left articular surface of C1 approximates the posterior low part of the upper left articular surface of C2. The pattern in the right articular surfaces is the mirror image. This reduces the distance between

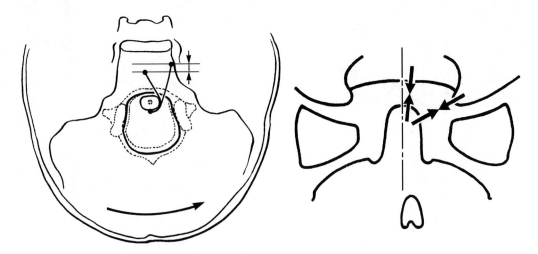

Figure 17–27   Increase in tension in contralateral alar ligament during C0–C2 rotation.

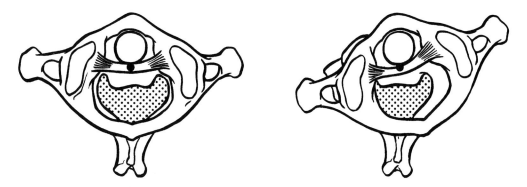

Figure 17–28   Relation axis of rotation C1–C2 and changes in diameter of the vertebral canal.

C0–C2, which decreases the tension in the ligaments. The structures that limit upper cervical rotation are the capsular ligaments and all the other ligaments involved. The average extent of movement to one side is 35°.

The position of the axis of rotation has the advantage that the vertebral canal is narrowed little or not at all during rotation: at the level of the atlas and axis, the vertebral canal is part of a cylinder having the axis of rotation at its center (**Figure 17–28**).

OCCIPITALIZATION OF THE ATLAS

Occipitalization of the atlas means that no movement is possible between the atlas and the occiput. The atlas loses its function as a ball bearing between C0 and C2 (**Figure 17–29**).

Extension and flexion remain possible between C1 and C2. Maximum flexion creates maximum tension in the ligaments that span the occiput and odontoid because this is the position in which they are stretched the most.

Sidebending between C1 and C2 is almost impossible because it requires sidebending of a few degrees between C0 and C1. The ipsilateral alar ligament is stretched during even the smallest sidebending in C1–C2.

Rotation is possible in C1–C2. However, it cannot reach its fullest extent because contralateral sidebending is not possible in C0–C1.

As with the other movements, abnormal stretching can occur in the ligaments that span the occiput and the odontoid. Overstretching may lead ultimately to atlantoaxial dislocation, which is often found in later life in people with this anomaly (Penning, 1978).

Muscular Influences on the Upper Cervical Spine

All the muscles that connect the ribs, the thoracic/lower/middle cervical spine, and the occiput affect upper cervical functioning. However, only those that are responsible for independent upper cervical movement are described here (**Figure 17–30**). The description assumes the axes of

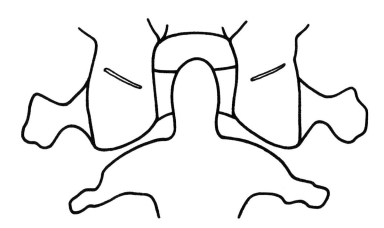

Figure 17–29   Occipitalization of C0–C1.

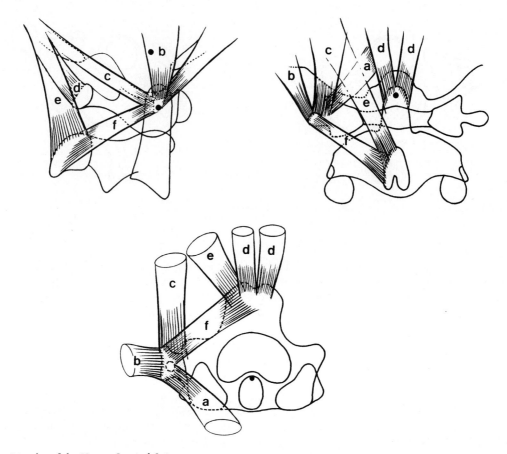

Figure 17–30   Muscles of the Upper Cervical Spine.

movement that are described by Penning (1964, 1968, and 1978), namely, the extension–flexion axis of C0–C1 and C1–C2, the sidebending axis of C0–C2, and the rotation axis of C1–C2 (see "Functional Aspects of the Upper Cervi-cal Spine C0–C2 (C3)"). Penning (1978) provides the infor-mation on functions provided in **Table 17–1** based on the direction in which the muscles run relative to the axes of movement.

Table 17–1   Functions

Figure	Muscle	Segment	Flexion	Extension	Sidebending		Rotation	
					Left	Right	Left	Right
a	Rectus capitis anterior	C0–C1	+	−	−	+	..	..
b	Rectus capitis lateralis	C0–C1	−	−	+	−	..	..
c	Obliquus capitis superior	C0–C1	−	+	−	−	..	..
d	Rectus capitis posterior minor	C0–C1	−	+	−	−	..	..
e	Rectus capitis posterior major	C0–C2	−	+	(+)	−	(−)	−
f	Obliquus capitis inferior	C1–C2	−	−	−	+	+	−

Motor-Sensory Relationships

Knowledge of the motor and sensory innervation of the upper cervical and head region is an important prerequisite for optimal clinical reasoning during evaluation and diagnosis.

Cervical Plexus

The cervical plexus (**Table 17–2**) consists of the ventral rami of the upper four cervical segments and contains both motor and sensory nerves.

Table 17–2

Segment	Nerve	Motor	Sensory
C0	Suboccipital nerve	Rectus capitis muscle Obliquus capitis muscle Semispinalis capitis muscle	
C1	Greater occipital nerve	Obliquus capitis inferior muscle Semispinalis muscle Longissimus capitis muscle Splenius capitis and cervicis muscles	Parts of occiput and neck
C2	Third occipital nerve	Longissimus capitis and cervicis muscles Semispinalis capitis and cervicis muscles Splenius capitis and cervicis muscles	Small portion of skull and neck
C2–C3	Lesser occipital nerve		Skin lateral occipital part of skull, mastoid and upper medial part of external ear
C2–C4	Transversus colli nerve		Ventrolateral part of neck, sternum to chin
C2–C3	Greater auricular nerve		Lower part of external ear, skin above parotid gland, and angle of the jaw
C3–C4	Medial, intermediate, and lateral supraclavicular nerve	Motor compartment consisting of lateral and medial branches supplies deep cervical musculature, diaphragm, and the infrahyoid muscle. The lateral branches, together with the accessory nerve, innervate the trapezius and the sternocleidomastoid muscles. Together with the thoracodorsal nerve, they innervate the levator scapulae muscle.	Skin above clavicle, lateral-most part of neck, upper part of deltoid muscle region, and thorax as far as third rib
C1–C2–C3	Ansa cervicalis Radix superior Radix inferior	Thyrohyoid muscle Geniohyoid muscle Sternohyoid muscle Sternothyroid muscle Omohyoid muscle	

(continued)

Table 17–2   *(Continued)*

Segment	Nerve	Motor	Sensory
C(3)–4(5)	Phrenic nerve		Small, sensitive branches, the accessory phrenic nerves accompany the motor nerve and run to the diaphragm, the pericardium, and parts of the pleura.
C1–C4	Small motor branches	Rectus capitis anterior muscle Longus colli muscle Longus capitis muscle Anterior scalene muscle Middle scalene muscle Rectus capitis lateralis muscle Sternocleidomastoid muscle Trapezius muscle Intertransversarii posterior cervicis muscle Levator scapulae muscle	
C1–C4	Dorsal rami	Intrinsic neck muscles	
C4–T1	Dorsal rami	Iliocostalis cervicis muscle Longissimus capitis and cervicis muscles Semispinalis capitis and cervicis muscles Multifidus muscles	Parts of neck and back

EXAMINATION SEQUENCE C0 TO C3

Because of the ligamentous attachments among the segments C0–C2, they form a functional unit of which C3 is the base. This unit should first be examined as a whole, both in the sagittal plane and in three-dimensional movements. Unlike the three-dimensional examinations of other spinal regions, that of the upper cervical spine is carried out mainly in contralateral movement combinations because of the ligamentous control mechanisms.

If there is an overall dysfunction in the upper cervical region, the therapist will try to identify the segment responsible. He or she will need to choose a sequence in which to perform the different parts of the examination. This is not a simple matter because segment C0–C1 cannot function at its best unless segments C1–C2–C3 are working normally, and C1–C2 cannot work properly if there is any dysfunction C0–C1 or C2–C3.

For C0–C1 to function well in the endrange position, there must be freedom of movement in C1–C2 and C2–C3

The odontoid process must be able to tilt in the sagittal and frontal planes. Freedom of movement in segments C0–C1 and C2–C3 is required for optimal functioning of segment C1–C2 in the end position. Movements in the sagittal plane depend on segment C0–C1 being able to slide in the dorsal and ventral directions and on extension–flexion in segment C2–C3. Movement in the transverse plane depends on segment C0–C1 being able to slide laterally or on rotation in C2–C3.

Segment C2–C3 is not attached to C0 or C1 by separate controlling ligaments, so full functioning is not biomechanically dependent on normal movement in segments C0–C1 and C1–C2. This also means that rotation in C1–C2 can also be examined over a reasonable trajectory without fear of overloading the ligaments. To reach the end phase of movement, there must be free contralateral sidebending in C0–C1. This movement must also be unobstructed during the rotational maneuver of C0–C1. If rotation in C1–C2 appears abnormal in the end phase, and if no contralateral sidebending occurs in segment C0–C1, then movement in segment C0–C1 must be examined, including sidebending.

In conclusion, it may be said that the most convenient segmental examination sequence is from caudal (C3) to cranial (C0). The examination should cover the following movements:

C2–C3: Flexion, extension, and the three-dimensional movements.

C1–C2: Rotation, with support by contralateral sidebending in segment C0–C1. It should be emphasized here that if rotation to both sides is normal, movements in the sagittal plane will also be normal.

C0–C1: Flexion (dorsal glide), extension (ventral glide), sidebending (contralateral glide), and the three-dimensional movements.

Segment C0–C1 can be examined with C3 stabilized, or with C1 to C7 in a three-dimensional locked position. In both cases, the lower segments must be non-impaired so that pain, ligamentous obstruction, and/or defensive muscle spasm do not hinder the examination of segment C0–C1.

When segment C0–C1 is being examined with the cervical spine locked, the locking position is important. When flexion in C0–C1 is being examined, the part of the cervical spine below that level should be brought into extension to ensure that the funicular part of the nucal ligament does not obstruct full movement in C0–C1. When extension is being examined in C0–C1, the cervical spine should be brought into flexion so that the dens of C2 can move in a ventral direction. When segment C0–C1 is being examined for optimal three-dimensional function with the cervical spine in a locked position, the locking must be arranged so that the coupled movement of C0–C2 is not impeded. This means that the movement component in the sagittal plane is in the direction opposite to that of physiologic examination in segment C0–C1, and the sidebending and rotation components are in the same direction as that of the examination.

REGIONAL EXAMINATION

The regional examination of the upper cervical region consists of the instability tests, the active-assisted regional examination, and the regional provocation tests.

Instability Examination: Upper Cervical

If instability is suspected at level C1–C2, the segment must be tested before the upper cervical region is examined further. Passive stability in the upper cervical region is largely dependent on the transverse and alar ligaments. Where a disorder of an inflammatory nature is present, such as rheumatoid arthritis or cervical trauma, in which case these ligaments could be damaged, the therapist should be especially alert to possible instability in segment C1–C2.

Lateral Translation Test, Non-Weight-Bearing

Examination position, patient: Supine.

Starting position, therapist: Standing by the patient's head.

Stabilization: The stabilizing hand maintains the position of the axis; the index finger is placed against the ipsilateral lamina of the axis.

Procedure: The index finger of the manipulating hand is placed against the contralateral lamina of the atlas, the thenar eminence against the lateral part of the back of the head, and the thumb on the maxilla. The hand introduces a contralateral gliding movement of C0 and C1 relative to C2. (See **Figure 17–31**.)

Assessment: Lateral translation between C1 and C2, which is not normally observed.

Remarks: The test is carried out first between C1–C2. To prevent the movement from being obstructed by the head if C0–C1 is blocked, C0 is included in the movement. The test should be carried out in both directions.

Cattrysse et al. (1997) reported 54.5–83.3% intrarater agreement ($\kappa = 0.09$–0.67) for this test. Pairwise interrater agreement ranged from 18.2–72.7 % ($\kappa = -0.64$–0.45).

Upper Cervical Flexion Test, Non-Weight-Bearing

Examination position, patient: Supine.

Starting position, therapist: Standing by the patient's head.

Stabilization: The stabilizing hand maintains the position of the axis; the thumb and index finger are placed around the arch of the axis.

Procedure: With the manipulating hand, the therapist holds the patient's head from behind, resting his or her shoulder against the patient's forehead, and gently introduces flexion (**Figure 17–32**).

Assessment: Laxity of the ligaments in the atlantoaxial joints and possible cord signs.

Cattrysse et al. (1997) reported 63.6–100.0% intrarater agreement ($\kappa = -0.27$–1.00) for this test. Pairwise interrater agreement ranged from 75–100% ($\kappa = 0.50$–1.00).

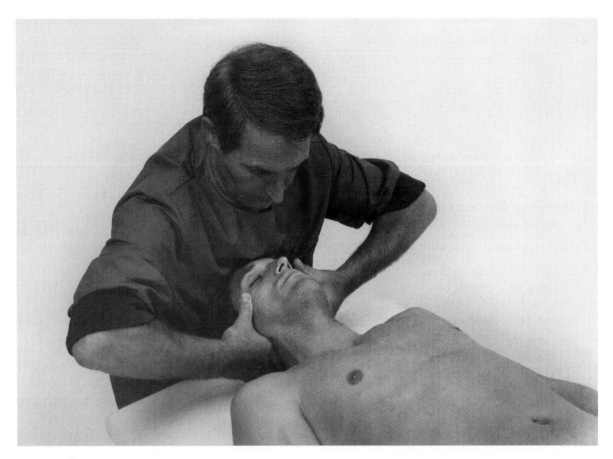

Figure 17–31

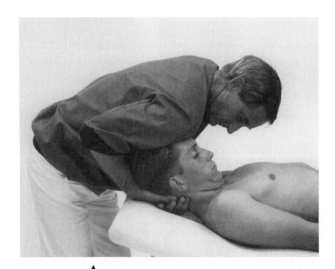

Figure 17–32

Sharp-Purser Test, Weight-Bearing

Examination position, patient: Sitting with the neck muscles relaxed and the head slightly bent.

Starting position, therapist: Standing beside the patient.

Stabilization: The stabilizing hand maintains the position of the axis, with the index finger on its spinous process.

Procedure: The palm of the manipulating hand is placed on the patient's forehead and light pressure is applied in a dorsal direction (**Figure 17–33**).

Assessment: Reduction or disappearance of the symptoms.

Cattrysse et al. (1997) reported 54.5–83.3% intrarater agreement (κ = 0.29–0.67) for this test. Pairwise interrater agreement ranged from 54.5–83.3% (κ = 0.09–0.67). Research by Uitvlugt and Indenbaum (1988) indicates that

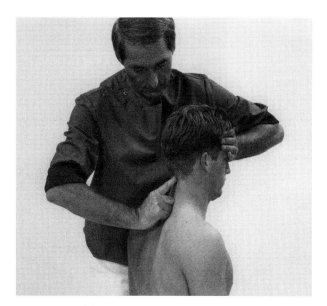

Figure 17–33 ⇧⇩

where in patients with rheumatoid arthritis there is ligamentary laxity of more than 4 mm, this test scores 88% for specificity and 96% for sensitivity.

Active-Assisted Regional Examination: Upper Cervical

For examination criteria, see the section titled "Active-Assisted Regional Examination: Lumbar" in Chapter 14.

Flexion, Weight-Bearing

Examination position, patient: Sitting on the short side of the examination table with the lower legs hanging down.

Starting position, therapist: Standing beside the patient.

Stabilization: The therapist spans the arch of C3 with the thumb and index finger of the stabilizing hand and holds the vertebra in position.

Procedure: The patient's head rests against the therapist's upper arm. The therapist places his or her manipulating hand and arm around the back of the patient's head, with the ulnar side against the inferior nuchal line, and introduces flexion, during which his or her upper arm supports the dorsocranial gliding movement of C0 (**Figure 17–34**).

Flexion, Sidebending, Contralateral Rotation, Weight-Bearing

Examination position, patient: Sitting on the short side of the examination table with the lower legs hanging down.

Starting position, therapist: Standing beside the patient at the side to be examined.

Stabilization: The therapist spans the arch of C3 with the thumb and index finger of the stabilizing hand and holds the vertebra in position.

Procedure: The patient's head rests against the therapist's upper arm. The therapist places his or her manipulating hand and arm around the back of the patient's head, with the ulnar side against the inferior nuchal line, and introduces flexion, sidebending, and contralateral rotation, during which his or her upper arm supports the dorsocranial gliding movement of C0 (**Figure 17–35**).

Extension, Weight-Bearing

Examination position, patient: Sitting on the short side of the examination table with the lower legs hanging down.

Starting position, therapist: Standing beside the patient.

Stabilization: The therapist spans the arch of C3 with the thumb and index finger of the stabilizing hand and holds the vertebra in position.

Procedure: The patient's head rests against the therapist's upper arm. The therapist places his or her manipulating hand and arm around the back of the patient's head, with the ulnar side against the inferior nuchal line, and introduces extension, during which the ulnar side of the hand supports the ventrocranial gliding movement of C0 (**Figure 17–36**).

Extension, Sidebending, Contralateral Rotation, Weight-Bearing

Examination position, patient: Sitting on the short side of the examination table with the lower legs hanging down.

Starting position, therapist: Standing beside the patient at the side to be examined.

Stabilization: The therapist spans the arch of C3 with the thumb and index finger of the stabilizing hand and holds the vertebra in position.

Procedure: The patient's head rests against the therapist's upper arm. The therapist places his or her manipulating hand and arm around the back of the patient's head, with the ulnar side against the inferior nuchal line, and introduces extension, sidebending, and contralateral

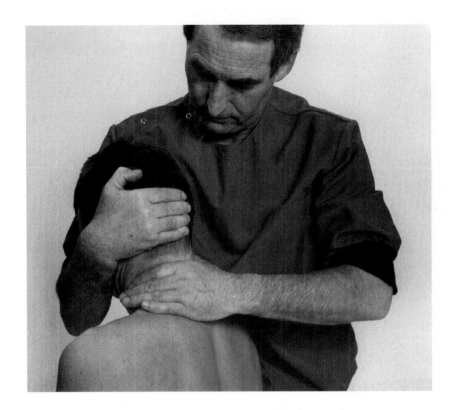

Figure 17–34

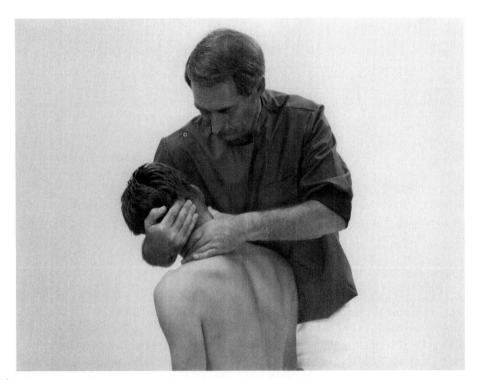

Figure 17–35

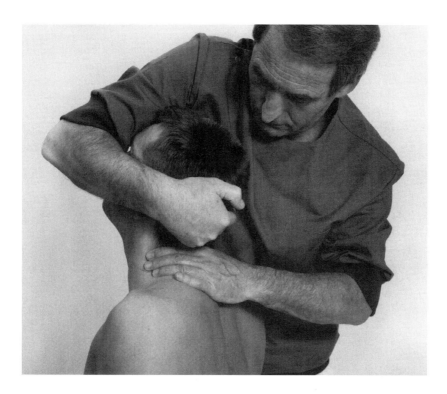

Figure 17–36

rotation, during which the ulnar side of the hand supports the ventrocranial gliding movement of C0 (**Figure 17–37**).

Examination Position for Non-Weight-Bearing Regional Examination

The non-weight-bearing active-assisted regional examination can be performed with the patient either lying on the side or supine. Because the non-weight-bearing regional examination of the cervical spine was described with the patient lying on his or her side, the non-weight-bearing regional examination of the upper cervical spine is described here with the patient in the supine position. With the patient supine, the examination can be done either with or without stabilization. Both situations are shown in the photographs, but only examination without stabilization is described.

Flexion, Non-Weight-Bearing

Examination position, patient: Supine, with the cervical spine in the extended position over the edge of the examination table, or in the neutral position on the table.

Starting position, therapist: Standing by the patient's head.

Procedure: The therapist places one hand on the patient's chin and the other on the back of his or her head and uses both hands to introduce flexion (**Figure 17–38**).

Remarks: **Figure 17–39** shows examination with stabilization of C3.

Flexion, Sidebending, Contralateral Rotation, Non-Weight-Bearing

Examination position, patient: Supine, with the cervical spine in extension, sidebending, and contraexternal rotation.

Starting position, therapist: Standing by the patient's head.

Procedure: The therapist places one hand on the patient's chin and the other on the back of his or her head and uses both hands to introduce flexion, sidebending and contralateral rotation (**Figure 17–40**).

Remarks: **Figure 17–41** shows examination with stabilization of C3.

Extension, Non-Weight-Bearing

Examination position, patient: Supine, with the cervical spine flexed.

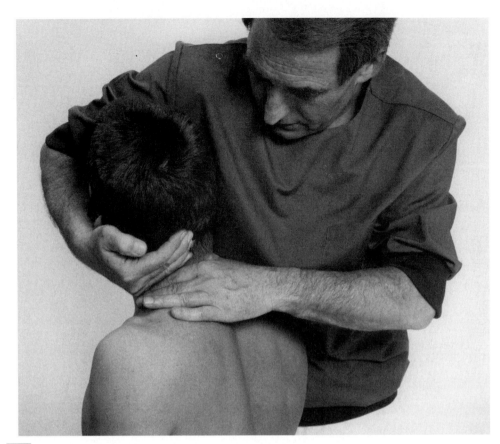

Figure 17–37

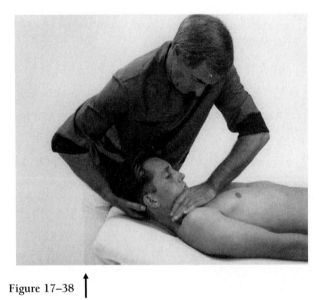

Figure 17–38

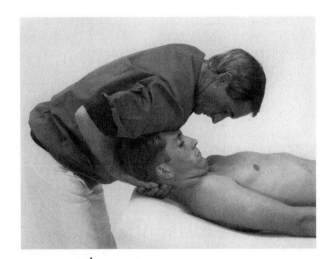

Figure 17–39

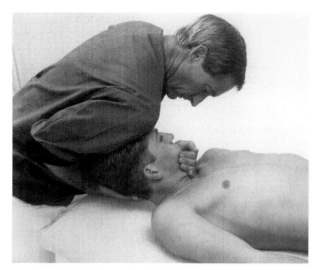

Figure 17–40

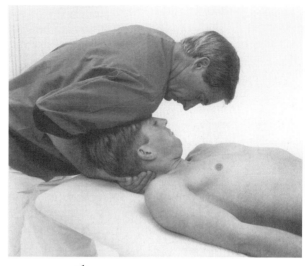

Figure 17–41

Starting position, therapist: Standing by the patient's head.

Procedure: The therapist places one hand on the patient's chin and the other on the back of his or her head and uses both hands to introduce extension (**Figure 17–42**).

Remarks: **Figure 17–43** shows examination with stabilization of C3.

Extension, Sidebending, Contralateral Rotation, Non-Weight-Bearing

Examination position, patient: Supine, with the cervical spine in flexion, sidebending, and contralateral rotation.

Starting position, therapist: Standing by the patient's head.

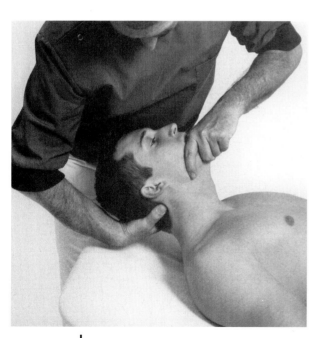

Figure 17–42

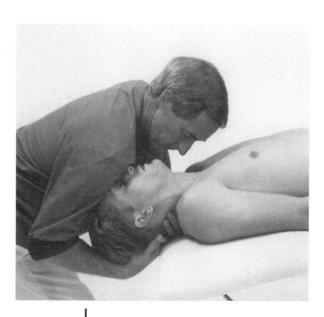

Figure 17–43

Procedure: The therapist places one hand on the patient's chin and the other on the back of his or her head and uses both hands to introduce extension, sidebending, and contralateral rotation (**Figure 17–44**).

Remarks: **Figure 17–45** shows examination with stabilization of C3.

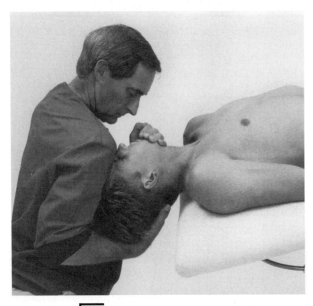

Figure 17–44

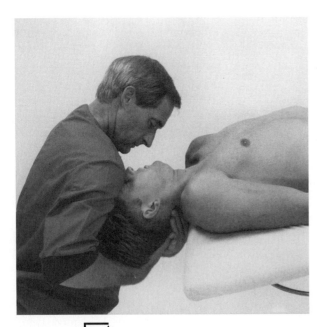

Figure 17–45

Regional Provocation Tests: Upper Cervical

For the upper cervical regional provocation tests the reader is referred to the section titled "Regional Provocation Tests: Cervicothoracic/Cervical" in Chapter 15.

SEGMENTAL EXAMINATION

As in other regions the segmental examination of the upper cervical spine entails a segmental tissue-specific examination, segmental provocation tests, and an active-assisted segmental examination.

Segmental Tissue-Specific Examination: Upper Cervical

For the upper cervical tissue-specific examination, please see the section titled "Segmental Tissue–Specific Examination: Cervical" in Chapter 16. When examining this region, the therapist should pay special attention to the upper cervical trigger points as described by Dvorak and Dvorak (1983) (**Figure 17–46**) and to the upper cervical segment points on the linea nuchae, as described by Sell (1969) (**Figure 17–47**).

Piva et al. (2006) reported 93% interrater agreement ($\kappa = 0.83$; 95% CI: 0.74–0.92) for tenderness to palpation over the transverse process of C1. Schöps et al. (2000) reported on the interrater agreement for palpation for tender-

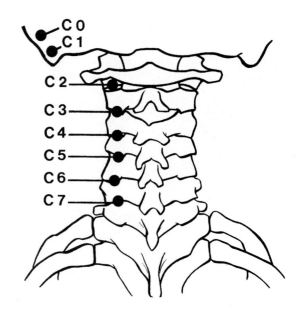

Figure 17–46

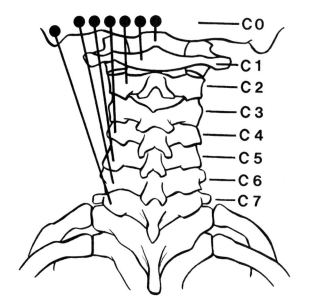

Figure 17–47

ness at the C1–C2 facet joints: $\kappa = 0.39$ for the right and $\kappa = 0.28$ for the left joint. Aprill et al. (2002) noted a 60% positive predictive value for occipital headaches originating in the C1–C2 joint with the combination of reported pain in the (sub) occipital region, tenderness to palpation over the C1–C2 joint, and restricted C1–C2 rotation.

Segmental Provocation Tests: Upper Cervical

See the section titled "Segmental Provocation Tests: Cervical" in Chapter 16. Although admittedly less relevant to the use of these tests as provocation tests, using a dichotomous rating scale for mobility of normal versus not normal, Hanten et al. (2002) reported on intra- and interrater agreement of upper cervical springing tests. Data are provided in **Table 17–3**.

Active-Assisted Segmental Examination: Upper Cervical

For assessment criteria, see the section titled "Active-Assisted Segmental Examination: Lumbar (L1 to L5)" in Chapter 14. The examination sequence for the upper cervical segments is as discussed in the section "Examination Sequence C0 to C3"C2–C3, C1–C2, and C0–C1.

Active-Assisted Segmental Examination: C2–C3

For a description and illustrations of active-assisted segmental examination of C2–C3, please see the section titled "Active-Assisted Segmental Examination: Cervical (C2–C7)" in Chapter 16.

Rotation C1–C2, Weight-Bearing

Examination position, patient: Sitting on the short side of the examination table with the lower legs hanging down.

Starting position, therapist: Standing beside the patient at the side to be examined.

Stabilization: The stabilizing hand holds C2 in position with the thumb against the contralateral spinous process or the ipsilateral lamina of the vertebra.

Procedure: The patient's head rests against the therapist's upper arm. The therapist uses the manipulating hand and arm to introduce rotation, with the little finger around the contralateral lamina of C1 (**Figure 17–48**).

Smedmark et al. (2000) reported 87% ($\kappa = 0.28$) interrater agreement for seated C1–C2 rotation using a

Table 17-3 Reliability Upper Cervical Springing Tests

Technique	Intrarater Reliability	Interrater Reliability
Central C1	85% ($\kappa = 0.50$)	90% ($\kappa = -0.053$)
Central C2	75% ($\kappa = 0.375$)	85% ($\kappa = 0.583$)
Unilateral C1 right	70% ($\kappa = 0.211$)	85% ($\kappa = 0.483$)
Unilateral C1 left	85% ($\kappa = 0.659$)	85% ($\kappa = -0.071$)
Unilateral C1 right via TP	90% ($\kappa = 0.0737$)	95% ($\kappa = 0.857$)
Unilateral C1 left via TP	85% ($\kappa = 0.687$)	85% ($\kappa = 0.318$)
Unilateral C2 right	75% ($\kappa = 0.432$)	70% ($\kappa = 0.400$)
Unilateral C2 left	60% ($\kappa = 0.208$)	85% ($\kappa = 0.706$)

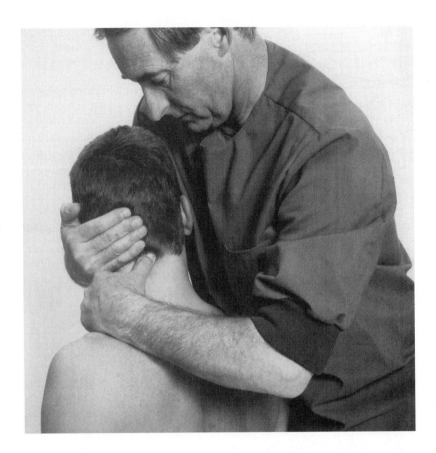

Figure 17–48 C

dichotomous rating scale of hypomobile versus normal or hypermobile.

Rotation, Non-Weight-Bearing and Variation

Examination position, patient: Supine.

Starting position, therapist: Standing by the patient's head.

Stabilization: The therapist spans the arch of C2 with the thumb and index finger of the stabilizing hand, or places the thumb on the contralateral side against the spinous process of C2, and holds the vertebra in position.

Procedure: The patient's head rests against the therapist's upper arm. The therapist encircles the patient's head, with the index finger on the ipsilateral lamina of C1, and introduces rotation (**Figure 17–49**).

Remarks: Contralateral sidebending in C0–C1 must not be impeded.

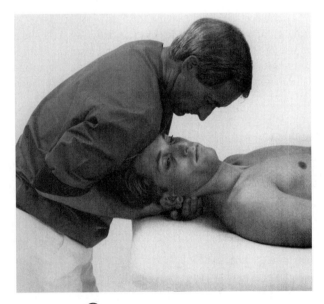

Figure 17–49 C

Variation

Examination position, patient: Supine, with the whole of the cervical spine from C0 in rotation, and contralateral sidebending.

Procedure: The therapist places one hand on the patient's chin and encircles the patient's head with the other, placing the index finger on the contralateral lamina of C1, and introduces rotation (**Figure 17–50**).

Flexion, C0–C1, Weight-Bearing

Examination position, patient: Sitting on the short side of the examination table with the lower legs hanging down.

Starting position, therapist: Standing beside the patient.

Stabilization: The therapist spans the arch of C1 with the thumb and index finger of the stabilizing hand and holds the vertebra in position.

Procedure: The therapist places the ulnar side of the manipulating hand against the inferior nuchal line, the upper part of the manipulating arm against the patient's forehead, and introduces flexion (**Figure 17–51**).

Remarks: The upper arm supports the dorsocranial gliding movement of C0.

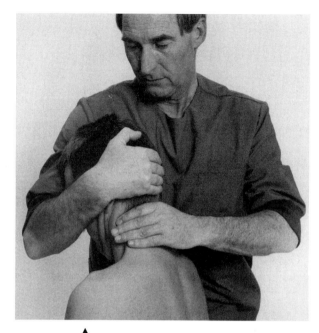

Figure 17–51 ↑

Flexion, Sidebending, Contralateral Rotation, Weight-Bearing

Examination position, patient: Sitting on the short side of the examination table with the lower legs hanging down.

Starting position, therapist: Standing beside the patient at the side to be examined.

Stabilization: The therapist spans the arch of C1 with the thumb and index finger of the stabilizing hand and holds the vertebra in position.

Procedure: The therapist places the ulnar side of the manipulating hand against the inferior nuchal line, the upper part of the manipulating arm against the patient's forehead, and introduces flexion, sidebending, and contralateral rotation (**Figure 17–52**).

Extension, Weight-Bearing

Examination position, patient: Sitting on the short side of the examination table with the lower legs hanging down.

Starting position, therapist: Standing beside the patient.

Stabilization: The therapist spans the arch of C1 with the thumb and index finger of the stabilizing hand and holds the vertebra in position.

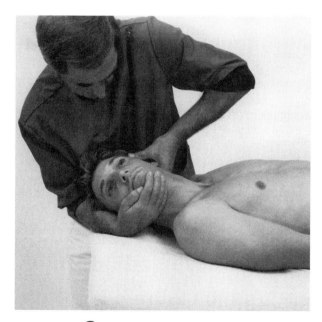

Figure 17–50 C

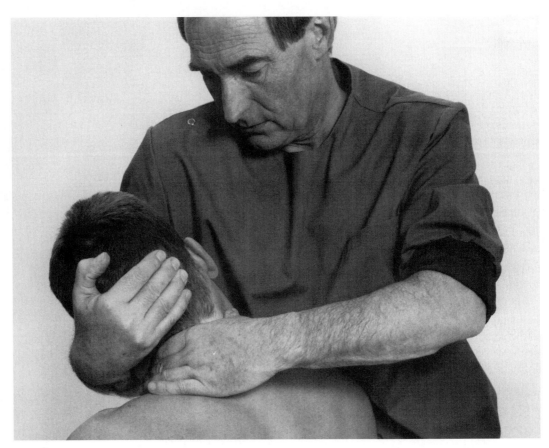

Figure 17–52

Procedure: The therapist places the ulnar side of the manipulating hand against the inferior nuchal line, the upper part of the manipulating arm against the patient's forehead, and introduces extension (**Figure 17–53**).

Remarks: The ulnar side of the hand supports the ventrocranial gliding movement of C0.

Extension, Sidebending, Contralateral Rotation, Weight-Bearing

Examination position, patient: Sitting on the short side of the examination table with the lower legs hanging down.

Starting position, therapist: Standing beside the patient at the side to be examined.

Stabilization: The therapist spans the arch of C1 with the thumb and index finger of the stabilizing hand and holds the vertebra in position.

Procedure: The therapist places the ulnar side of the manipulating hand against the inferior nuchal line, the upper

part of the manipulating arm against the patient's forehead, and introduces extension, sidebending, and contralateral rotation (**Figure 17–54**).

Examination Position and Procedure for Segmental Examination of C0–C1, Non-Weight-Bearing

The non-weight-bearing examination of segment C0–C1 can be performed with or without stabilization. It is described here with stabilization.

When the non-weight-bearing examination is carried out without stabilization, the therapist places his or her hands on each side of the patient's head and moves the cervical spine in the opposite direction in the sagittal plane.

Flexion, Non-Weight-Bearing

Examination position, patient: Supine, with the head over the edge of the examination table.

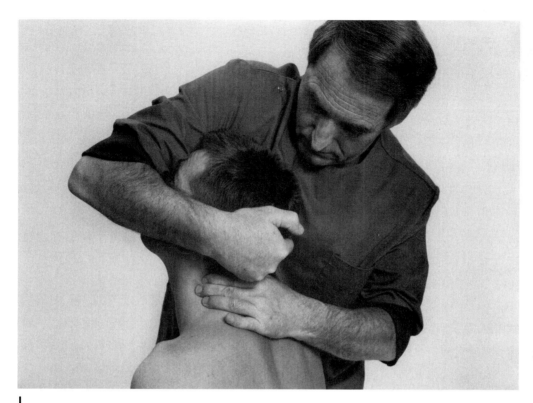

Figure 17–53

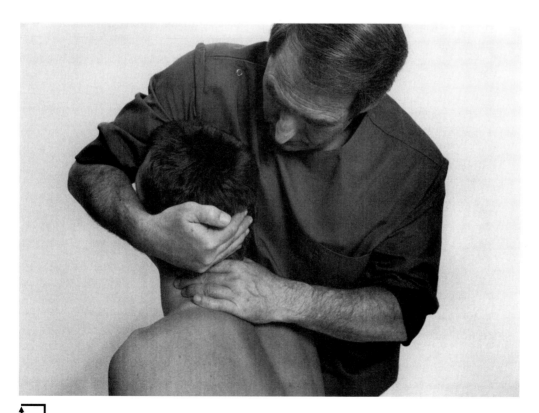

Figure 17–54

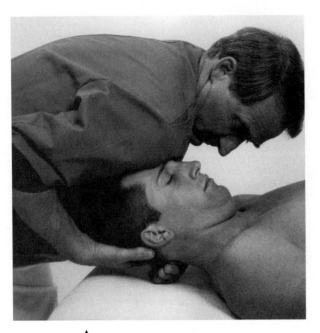

Figure 17–55

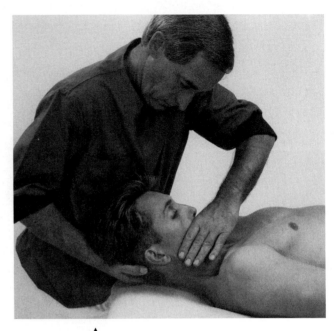

Figure 17–56

Starting position, therapist: Standing by the patient's head.

Stabilization: The therapist spans the lamina of C1 between the thumb and index finger of the stabilizing hand, or places the hand below C1, and holds the vertebra in position.

Procedure: The therapist places the ulnar side of the manipulating hand against the inferior nuchal line, the upper part of the manipulating arm against the patient's forehead, and introduces flexion (**Figure 17–55**).

Remarks: **Figure 17–56** shows the non-weight-bearing examination without stabilization.

Using a dichotomous rating scale of limited or not limited, Pool et al. (2004) reported 77% interrater agreement for the non-weight-bearing C0–C1 flexion test; the associated κ value was 0.29. Interrater agreement on pain provoked during this test using an 11-point pain rating scale yielded an ICC of 0.73.

Flexion, Lateral Flexion, Contralateral Rotation, Non-Weight-Bearing

Examination position, patient: Supine, with the head on the examination table or extending over the edge.

Starting position, therapist: Standing at the patient's head.

Stabilization: The thumb and index finger of the stabilizing hand span the lamina of C1 and hold the vertebra in position.

Procedure: The radial side of the manipulating hand is placed against the inferior nuchal line and the upper arm on the patient's forehead. The therapist introduces flexion, lateral flexion, and contralateral rotation (**Figure 17–57**).

Remarks: Non-weight-bearing, without stabilization, see **Figure 17–58**.

Extension, Non-Weight-Bearing

Examination position, patient: Supine, with the head extending over the edge of the examination table.

Starting position, therapist: Standing at the patient's head.

Stabilization: The thumb and index finger of the stabilizing hand span the lamina of C1 and maintain the vertebra in position.

Procedure: The radial side of the manipulating hand is placed against the inferior nuchal line and the upper arm on the patient's forehead. The therapist introduces extension (**Figure 17–59**).

Remarks: Non-weight-bearing, without stabilization, see **Figure 17–60**.

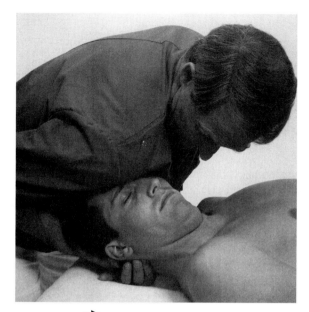

Figure 17–57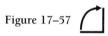

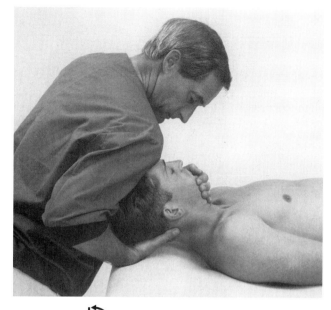

Figure 17–58

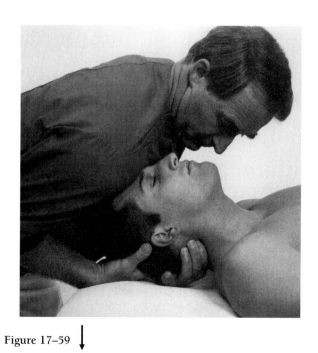

Figure 17–59

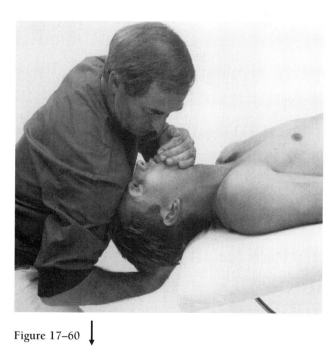

Figure 17–60

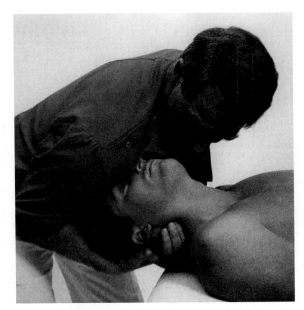

Figure 17–61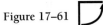

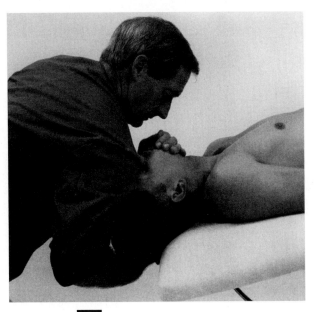

Figure 17–62

Extension, Lateral Flexion, Contralateral Rotation, Non-Weight-Bearing

Examination position, patient: Supine, with the head extending over the edge of the examination table.

Starting position, therapist: Standing at the patient's head.

Stabilization: The thumb and index finger of the stabilizing hand span the lamina of C1 and maintain the vertebra in position.

Procedure: The radial side of the manipulating hand is placed against the inferior nuchal line and the upper arm on the patient's forehead. The therapist introduces extension, lateral flexion, and contralateral rotation (**Figure 17–61**).

Remarks: Non-weight-bearing, without stabilization, see **Figure 17–62**.

CHAPTER 18

Examination of the Temporomandibular Joints

THE TEMPOROMANDIBULAR JOINT

If a patient presents with pain, dysfunction, and sensory disturbances in the craniocervical region, the function of the temporomandibular joint needs to be examined during the process of differential diagnosis and to plan appropriate manual therapy. The treatment should be aimed at dysfunctions that are reversible. Arthrogenic disturbances are of central interest to the manual diagnostician, though to obtain the full picture, neurogenic, viscerogenic, and psychogenic factors must be taken into account.

The various functions performed by the head and neck region are coordinated by a number of regulating mechanisms. Dysfunction in one element in the whole complex can affect the functioning of another element; the structure and functioning of the temporomandibular joint, and its relationships with the whole of the masticatory system are, therefore, described in this chapter.

Anatomic Features

The temporomandibular joint is part of the masticatory system, a functional unit consisting of the two temporomandibular joints, the tongue, and the cheeks, together with the associated musculature, innervation, vascularization, and dentition, and the larynx, pharynx, and the hyoid bone. From a functional point of view, one can include the cervicocephalic transitional area, the cervical spine, and the shoulder girdle (Rocabado, 1985).

The temporomandibular joints are a pair of joints that work as a unit. They form a mobile attachment between the mandibular bone and the skull. Each joint is divided into two chambers by a biconcave articular disk, the upper chamber formed by the disk and the temporal bone.

The disk consists of the following structures:

- Anterior band (A)
- Intermediate zone (i)
- Posterior band (P)
- Bilaminary zone: inferior and superior stratum (B_i and B_s) (Rees, 1954) (**Figure 18–1**)

Ventrally, the disk is connected directly to the capsule and indirectly to the superior part of the lateral pterygoid muscle (MPL). It is attached laterally to the mandibular head by a medial and a lateral collateral ligament. The more dorsal part is the bilaminary zone, which has a loose structure and a rich supply of nerves and blood vessels. The three-dimensional network of collagen fibers in the disk is a

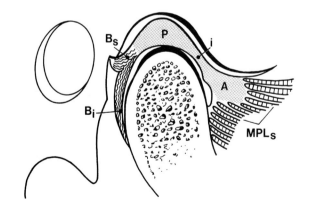

Figure 18–1 Disk temporomandibular joint.

solid construction capable of absorbing the shearing forces exerted on the disk.

The mandibular head is 15–20 mm long, ellipsoid in shape, and curved at the ventral side. The articulating component points toward the cranium (Kraus, 1988). The articular fossa of the temporal bone, which is covered with fibrous cartilage, joins the articular tubercle ventrally; it is biconcave and points in a dorsal and caudal direction. The roof of the fossa is one of the thinnest parts of the skull. The capsule is strengthened laterally by the temporomandibular ligament, while the fibers that run vertically prevent the articular surfaces from separating. Caudal to the temporomandibular joint lie the sphenomandibular and stylomandibular ligaments.

Musculature

The masticatory musculature (**Figure 18–2**) consists of the following structures:

- The masseter muscle (1)
- The temporal muscle (2)
- The medial pterygoid muscle (3)
- The lateral superior (4) and inferior (5) pterygoid muscles

The following are other groups of muscles that play a part in the masticatory system:

- Suprahyoid musculature:
  Anterior and posterior digastric muscles
  Mylohyoid muscle
  Geniohyoid muscle
  Stylohyoid muscle
- Infrahyoid musculature:
  Thyrohyoid muscle

Sternohyoid muscle
Superior and inferior omohyoid muscles

- Mimic musculature and the platysma (Honnée and Naeije, 1980; Kraus, 1988).

Innervation

Like the other synovial joints, the temporomandibular joint is doubly innervated. The primary innervation, responsible for articulation, is via the auriculotemporal nerve, which is a branch of the mandibular nerve. This contains both myelinated and unmyelinated fibers, varying in diameter between 1 and 12 Ìm. The secondary innervation is via accessory branches of the masticatory musculature (temporal, pterygoid, and masseter nerves).

An important function of the nerves that supply the masticatory system is to regulate the position of the lower jaw and control its movements. Four kinds of receptors are involved in these functions:

- Mechanoreceptors in the mucosa
- Mechanoreceptors in the paradontium
- Mechanoreceptors in and around the temporomandibular joint
- Muscle spindles and Golgi receptors in the masticatory muscles

The first two types have a low threshold and activate closing muscles when pressure is exerted on them (Honnée and Naeije, 1980).

Mechanoreceptors (Wyke's Classification as discussed in chapter 7 under "Sensory Examination")

Receptors of types I, II, III, and IV as described by Wyke (1976) are present in the capsule of the temporomandibular

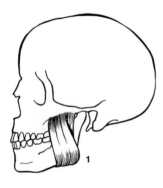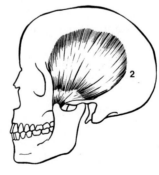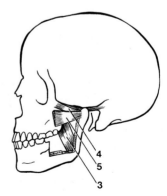

Figure 18–2   Masticatory musculature.

joint, type II receptors being present in an especially high density.

In the temporomandibular joint, these four types serve mechanosensory and nociceptive functions. The mechanoreceptors play a part in regulating the position and movement of the lower jaw; movement can occur both reflexively and under conscious control.

The type IV nociceptors only become active when there is tissue damage, mechanical overloading, or chemical irritation. With regard to nociception, there is a close association between the masticatory system and the upper cervical segments. Neuroanatomic connections exist between the afferent fibers of the trigeminal, glossopharyngeal, hypoglossal, and vagus nerves and the afferent fibers from the upper cervical segments (Bogduk, 1987). These afferent fibers are connected via the spinal tract of the trigeminal nerve with the spinal nucleus of the trigeminal nerve, the medullary end of which reaches as far down as the level of C3 (Duus, 1980) (**Figure 18–3**).

Muscle Spindles

Accessory branches from the muscles surrounding the temporomandibular joint provide its secondary innervation. The ratio of the muscle spindles in the opening muscles to those in the closure muscles is 1:10 (opening musculature 0–15, closure musculature 155–217) (Honnée and Naeije, 1980).

The sensory neurons of the muscle spindles are located in the mesencephalic nucleus of the trigeminal nerve, which is situated in the brain stem (Duus, 1980). The motor nucleus of the trigeminal nerve lies caudal to the mesencephalic tract nucleus of the same nerve and is directly connected with it by a lateral branch of the trigeminal nerve. The masseter reflex appears to function via this branch (Duus).

The axons that run from the motor nucleus of the trigeminal nerve via the mandibular nerve supply the masseter, temporalis, and medial and lateral pterygoid muscles. The mylohyoid muscles and the anterior part of the digastric muscle are also innervated from this motor ganglion (**Figure 18–4**).

Sympathetic Innervation

The tissue structures associated with the temporomandibular joint are richly innervated by the sympathetic system. The direct sympathetic innervation from the trigeminal ganglion proceeds via postganglionic fibers in the trigeminal nerve and reaches the effector organs via this route. The indirect sympathetic innervation of the tissues of the masticatory system proceeds via the external carotid artery from a perivasal plexus that surrounds the maxillary artery (Oostendorp, 1988). The preganglionic neurons of the head and the upper cervical area are located at levels C8–T3.

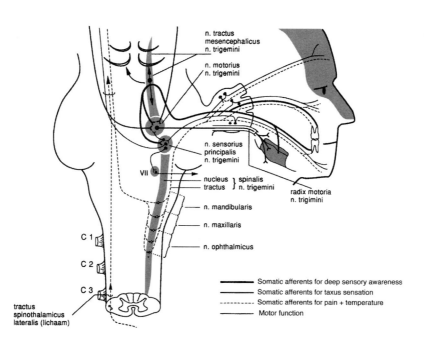

Figure 18–3 Trigeminal nuclei with afferent and efferent connections.

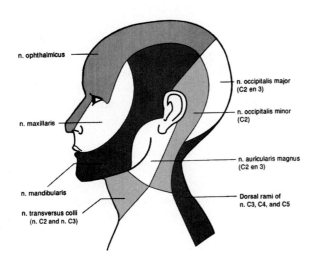

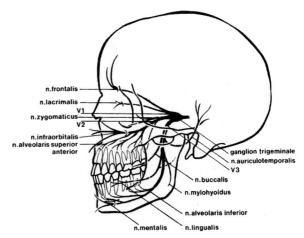

Figure 18–4   Innervation of head area.

Circulation

Circulation involves the following arteries (**Figure 18–5**):

External carotid artery (1)

Maxillary artery (2)

A. auricularis profunda (3)

A. meningea media (4)

A. alveolaris superior posterior (5)

A. temporalis profunda (6)

A. buccalis (7)

A. sphenopalatina (8)

A. palatina descendens (9)

A. alveolaris inferior (10)

A. infraorbitalis (11)

and the following veins (**Figure 18–6**):

V. temporalis superficialis (1)

V. auricularis posterior (2)

Maxillary vein (3)

V. retromandibularis (4)

V. facialis (5)

External jugular vein (6)

Internal jugular vein (7)

Anterior jugular vein (8)

Functional Aspects

In cases of temporomandibular joint dysfunction, a thorough and effective examination is often best made by a dentist and a manual therapist working closely together. To

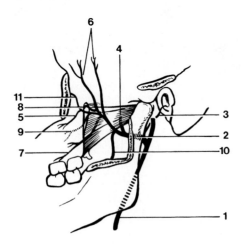

Figure 18–5   Arterial circulation.

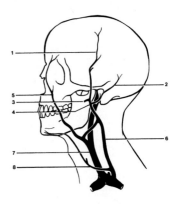

Figure 18–6   Venous circulation.

facilitate communication, a number of dentistry terms are defined in the following subsection.

Dental Terminology

Relation: The position of the mandible relative to the skull.

Rest position (RP): The most important of the relations. It is the position of the mandible in which the Frankfurt plane (the plane passing through the upper margin of the external auditory canal and the lower margin of the orbit) is horizontal and the oral muscle groups are in a state of minimal activity. This is known as the *loose-packed position.* In this position, there is *free way space* of 2 to 3 mm.

Central position: The relation between the mandible and the skull in which the Frankfurt plane is horizontal and the head of the mandible is in the unforced dorsal position.

Occlusion: Static contact between one or more teeth in the lower and upper jaws (Derksen, 1970). The number of contacts is greatest during maximal occlusion (MO).

Central maximal occlusion: The maximal occlusion in which the lower jaw is in a central relation.

Anterior close-packed position: The maximal end position with the mouth open. It is the most ventral position of the disk and head of the mandible on the articular eminences of the temporal bones. All structures are in a state of tension.

Intercuspidal contact position (ICP): The occlusion position in which the occlusal surfaces of the elements of the maxilla and the mandible are maximally congruent.

Maximum protruded contact position (PP): The most ventral position of the mandible with preservation of element contacts (**Figure 18–7**). The range of movement from ICP to PP = 7–10 mm (Posselt, 1958).

Maximal retruded contact position (RCP): The most dorsal position of the head of the mandible with preservation of element contact. In this position, which is the same as posterior *close-packed position,* the ligaments are in a state of maximal contraction. The range of movement from ICP to RCP = 0–22 mm (Posselt, 1958).

Loose-packed position: Every position between the anterior and posterior *close-packed positions* in which the soft structures are more or less relaxed.

Movements of the Joints

Depression–Elevation Movements that start from the rest position all begin with the capsular ligaments and the

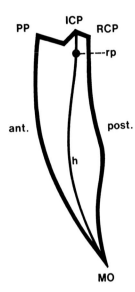

Figure 18–7 Sagittal view of the movements of the mandible.

superior and inferior pterygoid muscles in a relaxed state (Rocabado, 1985).

$$\text{Functional opening} = \text{Rotation} - \text{Translation}$$

See **Figure 18–8**.

The rotation component is responsible for about 50% of the depression of the mandible and takes place throughout the first half of the movement. The articular surface of the mandibular condyle rolls in an anterior direction in the lower joint compartment, while the disk slides in a posterior direction relative to the condyle. At the same time, the inferior lateral pterygoid muscle contracts, while the superior lateral pterygoid muscle and the dorsal capsule relax. Rotation ends when the lateral ligaments are tensed. Before opening, a small translation component is added to the rotation. During the translation, the mandibular condyle and the disk slide in the upper joint compartment in a ventral direction relative to the articular eminence until the dorsal capsule comes under tension. The superior and inferior lateral pterygoid muscles contract to guide the condyle and the disk.

Additional Translation The jaws are fully opened by an additional ventral and caudal translatory movement of the disk and mandibular condyle in the upper joint compartment. The articular surface of the maxillary articular eminence guides the movement. As the translatory movement continues, the lateral pterygoid muscle continues to contract, while tension increases in the capsule and ligaments.

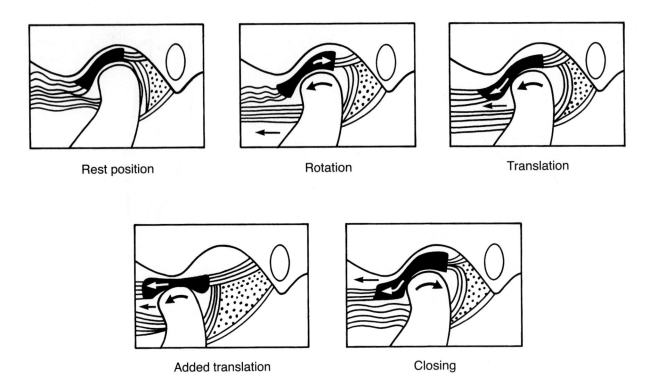

Rest position   Rotation   Translation

Added translation   Closing

Figure 18–8   Opening and closing the mouth.

Elevation   During this movement, the inferior lateral pterygoid muscle relaxes, the mandibular condyle rolls in a dorsal direction, and the disk slides in a ventral direction relative to it. As the movement continues toward the functional rest position, the disk is brought into its rest position as a result of the viscoelasticity of the capsule and ligaments.

Maximal Opening   The temporomandibular joint reaches its end position during maximal opening. In adults, the distance between the incisors is 53 to 59 mm. Maximal opening of the mouth is greater in men than in women (Rocabado, 1985).

Functional Opening   This is the extent of opening that is sufficient for all normal functions; it is 70% to 80% of maximal opening. If someone has a maximal mouth opening of 54 mm and a functional opening of 40.5 mm (75%), the rotation component will be responsible for 27 mm (50% of maximal mouth opening) and the translatory component for 13.5 mm (25% of maximal mouth opening).

Laterotrusion   Laterotrusion is a lateral movement of the mandibula relative to the skull, with or without maintenance of tooth contact. During laterotrusion to the right, the left articular condyle moves in a ventral-caudal-medial direction, and rotation occurs in the right articular condyle,

accompanied by a small movement in a lateral-ventral direction because its axis lies just posterior to the ipsilateral condyle (Hansson, Honnée, and Hesse, 1985). In laterotrusion where tooth contact is maintained, the range of movement is 10–15 mm (Agerberg, 1974).

Protrusion   Protrusion is a movement of the mandible in a ventral direction relative to the skull, with or without maintenance of tooth contact. Both mandibular heads make a translatory movement along the dorsal slope of the maxillary eminence in a ventral-caudal direction. When the end-to-end position is reached, the ligaments are under maximal tension and the anterior close-packed position results.

Retrusion   Retrusion is a displacement of the mandible in a dorsal direction relative to the skull, with or without maintenance of tooth contact. The two mandibular heads make a translatory movement in a dorsal direction and end in the dorsal contact position, or dorsal close-packed position.

Cranio-Cervical-Mandibular Functional Unit

The functions of the cranio-cervical-mandibular system are closely interrelated neurologically and biomechanically. They are also related viscerogenically because the abdominal organs have certain reflex influences on segments C2 to

C4 via the phrenic nerve (Hansen and Schliack, 1962). Stimuli from the thoracic and abdominal organs can also reach the brain stem via the vagus nerve. The fact that the nucleus of the vagus nerve reaches as far caudally as the C2 segment may explain the appearance of head and neck symptoms in patients with internal disorders.

The nociceptive relationship between the upper cervical region and the trigeminal area was described at an earlier point in this book. The relationship between the cervicothoracic transitional area and the head–neck region has also been discussed in the context of the origin of sympathetic innervation. A prolonged increase in tonic sympathetic activity at the cervicothoracic level can lead to specific changes in the tissues that receive their sympathetic innervation from this area. Disturbance in one element in the cranio-cervical-mandibular functional unit may upset the autonomic balance within the system.

The upper cervical spine, together with the eyes and the vestibular system, plays an important part in maintaining posture. The vestibular proprioceptors, the nuclei of the external eye muscles, and the mechanoreceptors of the upper cervical vertebral joints and muscles are connected via the vestibular nuclear complex. They interact allowing us to determine the position of the head in space (Duus, 1980; Kraus, 1988).

The position of the cervical spine, the head, the mandible, and the hyoid bone are important factors within the system of biomechanical relationships. They are discussed in greater detail because disturbance of the functional relationships among them can lead to craniomandibular dysfunction.

Rocabado (1985) points out that the positions of the cervical spine and the head in the sagittal plane affect the position of the mandibular joint. In the physiologically upright state, it seems that only a small contractile force is needed in the elevator muscles to keep the mandibular joint in the rest position (Rugh and Drago, 1981). Flexion of the head and the cervical spine leads to an increase in tone in the elevation–retrusion muscles because of the increase in tensile forces on the closing muscles (Kraus, 1988). Extension of the head and cervical spine exerts increased tensile force on the structures responsible for depression and retrusion. This leads to an increase in tone in the muscles responsible for elevation and retrusion (Kraus). When the head is in a forward head position as a result of increased thoracic kyphosis and cervical lordosis, there is tension in the ventral submandibular soft tissue structures. This leads to an increase in tone in the closing muscles, so the elevation-retrusion force on the mandible is increased (Rocabado, 1985).

The position of the hyoid bone is another important factor in the system of cranio-cervical-mandibular relationships (Rocabado, 1983). This bone has muscular, ligamen-

tous, and fascial connections with the pharynx, mandible, cranium, cervical spine, sternum, and scapula. The suprahyoid musculature, which stretches between the hyoid and the mandible, can exert a depressive force on the mandible if the hyoid bone is fixated. Given that occlusion and articulation are satisfactory, correct static relationships between the head, cervical spine, and hyoid are a necessary condition for optimal functioning of the temporomandibular joint (Rocabado, 1983) (**Figure 18–9**).

In adults, the base of the hyoid should be at the level of the lower anterior angle of C3, and its posterior horns at the level of disk C2–C3. The position of the hyoid depends on the tension in its muscular, ligamentous, and fascial connections with the styloid process, the mandibular symphysis, the sternum, the scapula, and C3.

Using a technique developed by Bibby (1981), Rocabado (1983) established some criteria for determining the proper positions for the cranium, cervical spine, hyoid bone, and mandible (**Figure 18–10**). The position of the cranium is determined by the angle between the line that joins the lower anterior corner of the odontoid and the apex of the odontoid, and that which joins the basi-occiput and the posterior nasal bone (McGregor's plane, MGP). This angle should be 100°, plus or minus 5°. The distance between the basi-occiput and the posterior arch of the atlas is also measured. It should be between 4 and 9 mm. The position of the cervical spine is determined by measuring the distance between the midcervical spine and the tangent to the apex of the thoracic curve. With the head in a normal position, this distance should be about 6 cm.

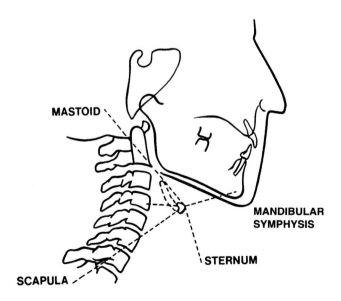

Figure 18–9 Forces in relation to head, cervical spine, mandible, and hyoid region.

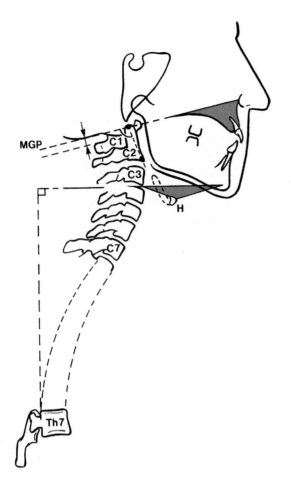

Figure 18–10 Spatial relationships with normal head and neck position.

The position of the hyoid bone is determined by the hyoid triangle. This is formed by joining the anterior lower edge of C3, the lowest dorsal point of the mandibular symphysis, and the highest and most ventral point on the hyoid bone. If cervicocephalic relations and cervical lordosis are normal, the triangle is said to be a positive one, that is, the hyoid bone lies below the line that joins C3 and the mandibular symphysis. If the cervicocephalic or cervical relationships are abnormal, the hyoid bone is displaced in a cranial direction. If it lies above the line joining C3 and the mandibular symphysis, the triangle is a negative one.

The following conclusions may be drawn from this summary of the functional relationships in the cranial-cervical-mandibular system:

- Dysfunction of the mandibular joint affects all the tissues that belong to the joint as part of a functional and trophic unit.
- Dysfunction of the upper cervical region can lead to dysfunction in the masticatory system.

- If the craniocervical region is in a position that deviates from the physiologic upright posture, the position of the mandible can be changed, leading to possible craniomandibular dysfunction.

Pathologies

Based on the segmental relationships of the mandibular joint as described, pathologic conditions may be assigned to one of two groups:

- Local dysfunctions
- Segmental dysfunctions

Local Dysfunctions

Local dysfunctions of the temporomandibular joint (Carlsson, 1980) are mandibular dysfunction, neuromuscular disturbance, osteoarthrosis, and the following degenerative conditions:

- Erosive arthritis
- Traumatic arthritis
- Immobilization-related arthritis
- Infections
- Rheumatoid arthritis
- Arthritis of unknown etiology

Dysfunctions internal to the joint are as follows:

- Luxation of the disk
- Perforation of the disk
- Disk deformities

Luxation of the disk can occur in any direction, that is, dorsally, ventrally, medially, or laterally. Sudden dorsal luxation is rare, as are medial and lateral displacement; if it does occur, however, it causes problems with the movements involved in closing the mouth. Ventral luxation of the disk is more frequent and may or may not be amenable to reduction. In cases where it can be reduced, the clicking phenomenon occurs both when the mouth is opened and when it is closed. The clicking noise during opening occurs when the condyle slides from its position under the posterior band of the disk into the concave part. The precise point when the opening click occurs appears to be related to the distance by which the disk is displaced ventrally. During the closing movement, the clicking noise occurs when the condyle slides from the concave part of the disk to the position below the posterior band (**Figure 18–11**).

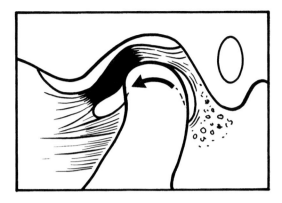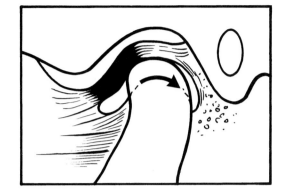

Figure 18–11 Opening/closing click.

When the disk lies permanently in front of the head of the mandible and the luxation cannot be reduced, this is described as a *closed lock* situation (**Figure 18–12**). The opening movement is limited and painful, and the mandible deviates toward the ipsilateral side. If the permanent luxation of the disk is chronic in nature, the disk may be deformed (Koole, 1989). The changed shape of the disk may slowly increase the mobility of the joint. The disk may also be perforated, permitting direct contact between the condyle and the tuberculum. In these cases, crepitation can be heard when the mouth opens and closes.

The usual causes of temporomandibular dysfunction are endogenous factors such as anomalies of the teeth and exogenous factors such as trauma and psychogenic influences.

Segmental Dysfunctions

The masticatory system has neural links with the upper cervical spine and autonomic links with segments C8 to T3 (see earlier). Dysfunctions of the temporomandibular joint can, therefore, spread to the upper cervical region and, under certain circumstances, to the tissues innervated from segments C8 to T3 (Oostendorp et al., 1986). Conversely, disorders of the upper cervical region can lead to dysfunction of the temporomandibular joint. An abnormal position of the cervical spine can also biomechanically lead to disturbances of the joint (Schmitt and Gerrits, 1989).

Manual diagnosis is based on a biopsychosocial model; familiarity with the relationships and the potential interactions just described is, therefore, essential to differential diagnosis. The therapist must be able to identify local dysfunctions and biomechanical and neural relationships to identify the primary cause of disorders.

Muscles That Control the Temporomandibular Joint

To allow for clinical reasoning during evaluation and diagnosis, it is important to be familiar with the functional roles of various muscles on temporomandibular joint movements (**Table 18–1** and **18–2**).

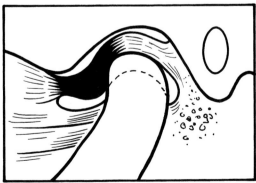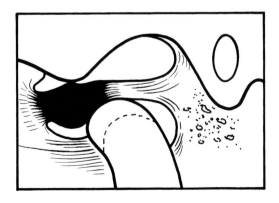

Figure 18–12 Closed lock.

Table 18–1   Muscles Acting on the Temporomandibular Joint

Muscle	Depression	Elevation	Protrusion	Retrusion	Laterotrusion
Masseter					
Pars superior		+++	+++		++
Pars profundus		+++		+++	
Medial pterygoid		+++	+++		
Lateral pterygoid					
Pars superior	+++		+++		+++
Pars inferior	+++		+++		+++
Temporalis					
Pars anterior		+++	+++		+
Pars medius		+++	+	+	+
Pars posterior		+++		+++	

Muscles That Control the Hyoid, Mandible, and Thyroid

Hyoid   *Mandible*   *Thyroid*

Table 18–2   Muscular Influence on Hyoid Bone, Mandible, and Thyroid Cartilage

Muscle	Hyoid depression	Hyoid elevation	Hyoid anterior	Hyoid posterior	Mandible depression	Thyroid elevation	Thyroid depression
Suprahyoidal muscles							
Digastic muscle							
Pars anterior		+	+		+		
Pars posterior		+		+			
Mylohyoid		+			+		
Geniohyoid		+			+		
Stylohyoid		+		+			
Infrahyoidal muscles							
Thyrohyoid	+					+	
Sternohyoid	+						
Sternothyroid							+
Omohyoid							
Pars superior	+						
Pars inferior	+						
Platysma					+		

Table 18-3

Nerve	Motor	Sensory
Trigeminal nerve (cranial nerve V)	Masseter	Face, mouth, eye Upper and lower jaws
Masticatory nerve	Medial pterygoid Lateral pterygoideus Pars inferior and superior Temporalis	
Inferior alveolar nerve	Anterior digastric Mylohyoid	
Facial nerve (cranial nerve VII)	Posterior digastric	
Digastric ramus	Stylohyoid	
Ansa cervicalis 1, 2	Geniohyoid Thyrohyoid	
Ansa cervicalis 1, 2, 3	Sternohyoid	
Facial nerve (cranial nerve VII)	Sternothyroid	
Ramus colli	Omohyoid	
Accessory nerve	Platysma	
Plexus cervicalis	Sternocleidomastoid	

Motor-Sensory Relationships

Knowledge of motor and sensory innervation of the temporomandibular region is a prerequisite for clinical reasoning in the evaluation and diagnosis of patients with complaints in this region (**Tables 18–2** and **18–3**).

Referred Pain Originating in the Temporomandibular Muscles

Within the context of clinical reasoning in the evaluation and diagnosis of patients with complaints in the temporomandibular region it is relevant to also be familiar with referral patterns originating in myofascial trigger points of the temporomandibular musculature. The reader is referred to Chapter 11. Palpatory Examination for illustrations of the following referral patterns (Travell, 1981).

Temporal muscle: Temporal bone, upper jaw

Masseter muscle: Lower jaw, cheek, ear, lateral part of occiput, and teeth

Pterygoid muscle: Ear and temporomandibular joint

Digastric muscle: Neck and throat

OBSERVATION

The cranio-cervical-mandibular functional unit is inspected dorsally, ventrally, and laterally (illustrations in Chapter 10 under the heading "Observation"). **Table 18–4** lists the points of observation.

Table 18–4   Observation of the Cranio-Cervical-Mandibular Region

Part	Assessment	Criteria
Dorsal		
Cervical spine	Position	Side bending, rotation, lateral shift
	Shape	Scoliosis
	Musculature	Atrophy, hypertrophy, swelling
Shoulder girdle	Position	Depression, elevation, unequal shoulder height
	Musculature	Atrophy, hypertrophy, swelling
Scapulae	Position	Alata, rotation, medial border position, neck-shoulder line–upper trapezius, asymmetry
Ventral		
Head	Shape of face	Symmetry, convergence of eye–mouth lines
	Masticatory muscles	Atrophy, hypertrophy, swelling
	Bite	Occlusion, contact between elements, symptoms of parafunctional activities
	Shape	Symmetry, deviation of mandible
Cervical spine	Position	Side bending, rotation, lateral shift
Lateral		
Head	Position	Anterior–posterior position, flexion–extension
Mandible	Position	Protrusion/retrusion
Cervical spine	Position	Flexion–extension, ventral and dorsal shift
Shoulder girdle	Position	Protraction–retraction
Scapulae	Position	Elevated

ACTIVE EXAMINATION

During active examination of the temporomandibular joint, three functional movements are inspected from the ventral and lateral viewpoints. To check whether any signs and symptoms are reproducible, the movements should be repeated several times. Protusion–retrusion and laterotrusion should be repeated with tooth contact, and the horizontal and vertical overbite measured.

Depression–Elevation 50%

See **Figures 18–13** and **18–14**.

- Start of the movement
- Course of the movement (rotation component)
- Deviation

Depression–Elevation 100%

See **Figures 18–15** and **18–16**.

- Course of the movement (sliding component)
- Deviation
- Measurement of interincisal mouth opening

Protrusion–Retrusion

See **Figures 18–17** and **18–18**.

- Course of the movement
- Deviation

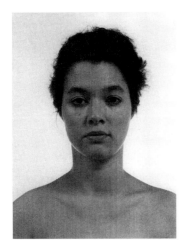

Figure 18–13 ↕

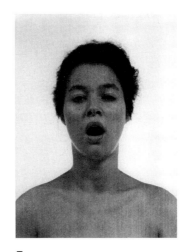

Figure 18–14 ↑↓

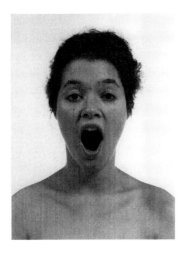

Figure 18–15 ↓

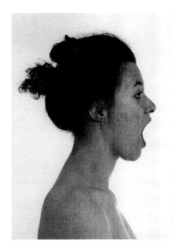

Figure 18–16 ↓

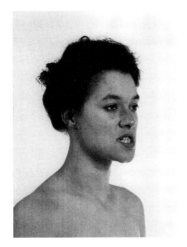

Figure 18–17 ↕↑

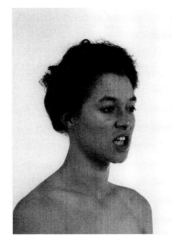

Figure 18–18 ↑↓

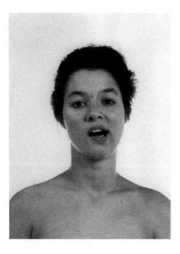

Figure 18–19   ⟵

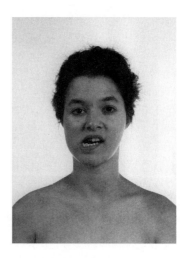

Figure 18–20   ⟶

Laterotrusion Left–Right

See **Figures 18–19** and **18–20**.

- Course of the movement
- Interincisal measurement

Additional Criteria for Active Examination

The following are additional criteria to use in the active exam:

- Stiffness
- Pain and the moment when it appears
- Crepitation (using a stethoscope)
- Click when the mouth opens or closes

If there is a click on opening, the point where it occurs should be noted because this helps with determining the location of the disk.

Using a ruler to establish range of motion during active movements of the temporomandibular joints in patients with temporomandibular joint dysfunction, Walker et al. (2000) reported an intrarater ICC = 0.94 and interrater ICC = 0.99 for full mouth opening. Laterotrusion right yielded ICC = 0.75–0.82 and ICC = 0.96 for intra- and interrater agreement, respectively; for laterotrusion left these values were 0.85–0.92 and 0.94, respectively. Intrarater agreement for protrusion yielded an ICC = 0.89–0.93, and interrater agreement yielded an ICC = 0.98.

de Wijer et al. (1995) reported interrater agreement for the presence of joint sounds during mouth opening (κ = 0.59); laterotrusion right (κ = 0.57); laterotrusion left (κ = 0.50), and protrusion (κ = 0.47). Interrater agreement for the presence of pain on opening, laterotrusion right and left, and protrusion yielded κ values of 0.28, 0.28, 0.28, and 0.36, respectively (de Wijer et al.).

Restriction of mouth opening by > 6 mm carried a sensitivity of 0.26, a specificity of 0.97, a positive likelihood ratio of 8.67, and a negative likelihood ratio of 0.76 in the identification of patients with temporomandibular disorders based on a gold standard of patient self-report of temporomandibular joint pain (Cacchiotti et al., 1991). The presence of crepitus during auscultation with joint motion had a sensitivity of 0.70, specificity of 0.43, positive likelihood ratio of 1.23, and a negative likelihood ratio of 0.70 for the diagnosis of temporomandibular dysfunction compared to a gold standard of arthroscopic visualization (Israel et al., 1998). Visscher et al. (2000) reported a sensitivity of 0.87, specificity of 0.67, positive likelihood ratio of 2.64, and a negative likelihood ratio of 0.19 for the presence of pain with maximal mouth opening, protrusion, and bilateral laterotrusion compared to a gold standard of patient-reported temporomandibular joint pain.

ACTIVE-ASSISTED BILATERAL EXAMINATION

Whereas the preceding active examination provides preliminary information with regard to movement pattern and reproduction of complaints, the active-assisted examination allows the clinician to assess endfeel and confirm deviations of mobility as well as symptom reproduction.

Depression–Elevation, Protrusion–Retrusion, Laterotrusion

Examination position, patient: Sitting on the short side of the examination table with the lower legs hanging down.

Starting position, therapist: Standing beside the patient.

Stabilization: The stabilizing hand and arm surround the patient's head and hold it in position; the palpating index finger is placed on the temporomandibular joint.

Hand positions:

Depression: The index finger is placed on the lower teeth and the thumb against the upper teeth (**Figures 18–21** and **18–22**).

Elevation: The patient's chin is held between the therapist's thumb and index finger (**Figures 18–23** and **18–24**).

Protrusion: The thumb is placed behind the lower teeth and the index finger under the lower jaw (**Figures 18–25** and **18–26**).

Retrusion: The patient's chin is held between the thumb and index finger (**Figures 18–27** and **18–28**).

Laterotrusion: The thumb is placed on the lower contralateral molars, the middle fingers surround the lower jaw, and the index finger is placed against the horizontal ramus of the mandible (**Figures 18–29** and **18–30**).

Procedure: The manipulating hand introduces depression–elevation, protrusion–retrusion, and laterotrusion to left and right.

Assessment: Endfeel and pain.

Remarks: The hand that makes oral contact is gloved.

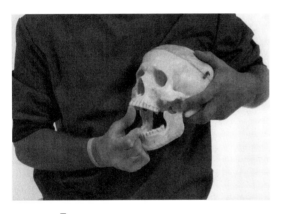

Figure 18–21 ⤓

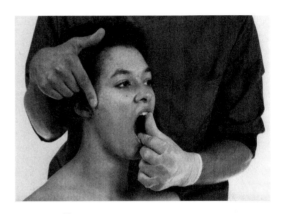

Figure 18–22 ⤓

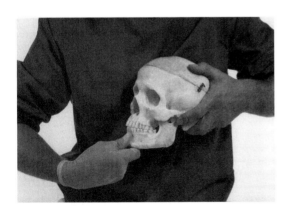

Figure 18–23 ⤒

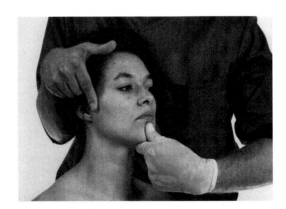

Figure 18–24 ⤒

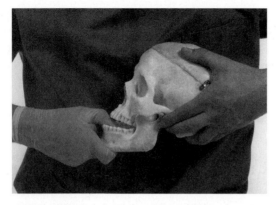

Figure 18–25 ⇕

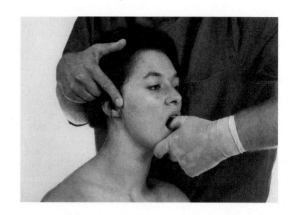

Figure 18–26 ⇕

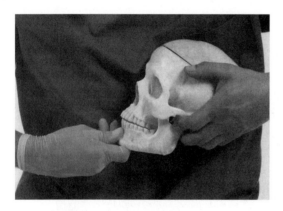

Figure 18–27 ⇓

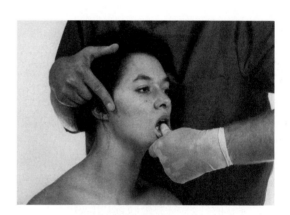

Figure 18–28 ⇓

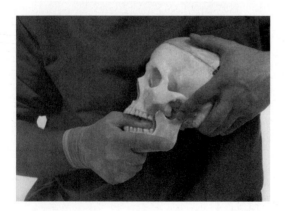

Figure 18–29 ⟵

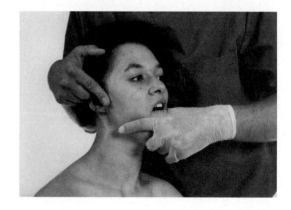

Figure 18–30 ⟶

Lobbezoo-Scholte et al. (1994) reported κ = 0.34 for agreement on the presence of pain on active-assisted mouth opening. Visscher et al. (2000) reported a sensitivity of 0.80, specificity of 0.64, positive likelihood ratio of 2.22, and a negative likelihood ratio of 0.31 for the presence of pain upon therapist-applied gentle overpressure during maximal mouth opening compared to a gold standard of patient-reported temporomandibular joint pain.

RESISTANCE TESTS

Examination position, patient: Sitting on the short side of the examination table with the lower legs hanging down.

Starting position, therapist: Standing beside or behind the patient.

Stabilization: When resistance is being tested at one side only, the stabilizing hand and arm surround the patient's head and hold it in position, while the palpating index finger is placed on the temporomandibular joint.

Hand positions:

Depression: The fingers of both hands are placed beneath the lower jaw (**Figure 18–31**).

Elevation: The fingers of both hands are placed on the lower jaw (**Figure 18–32**).

Protrusion: The second and third fingers of both hands are placed ventrally against the lower jaw (**Figure 18–33**).

Retrusion: The hypothenars of both hands are placed dorsally against the ascending branches of the lower jaw (**Figure 18–34**).

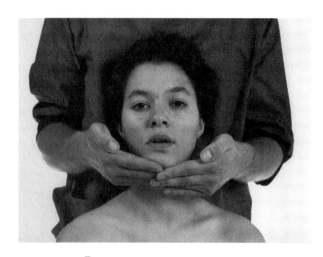

Figure 18–31 ↑

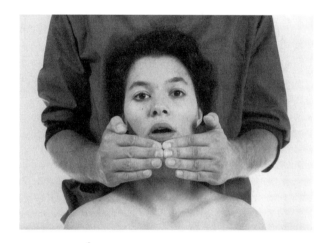

Figure 18–32 ↑

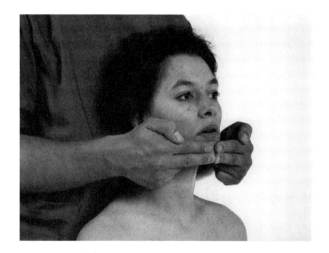

Figure 18–33 ↑↓

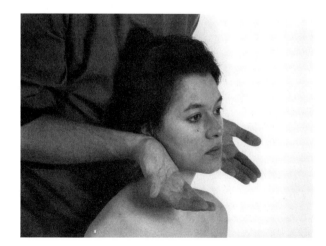

Figure 18–34 ↑↓

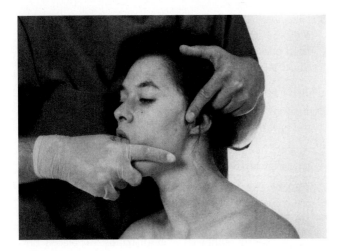

Figure 18–35 ⟵

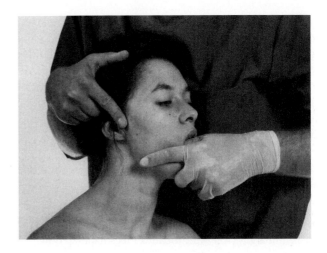

Figure 18–36 ⟶

Laterotrusion: The thumb is placed on the contralateral lower molars and the fingers surround the lower jaw. The index finger is placed against the horizontal ramus of the mandible (**Figures 18–35** and **18–36**).

Procedure: The therapist uses one or both hands to apply graded resistance to depression–elevation, protrusion–retrusion, and left and right laterotrusion.

Assessment: Strength, coordination, endurance, muscular stability, and pain.

de Wijer et al. (1995) reported interrater agreement for the presence of pain during isometric resistance tests for mouth opening ($\kappa = 0.24$), closing ($\kappa = 0.30$), laterotrusion right ($\kappa = 0.28$), laterotrusion left ($\kappa = 0.26$). Visscher et al. (2000) reported a sensitivity of 0.63, specificity of 0.93, positive likelihood ratio of 0.90, and a negative likeli-

hood ratio of 0.40 for the presence of pain during manually resisted mouth opening, closing, protrusion, and bilateral laterotrusion compared to a gold standard of patient-reported temporomandibular joint pain.

TISSUE-SPECIFIC EXAMINATION

This examination includes palpation of the temporomandibular joint and of the musculature. The head of the mandible is palpated via the external ear canal. During functional movements, it is palpated at the ventral side of the ear (**Figure 18–37**).

The most important masticatory muscles to be palpated are the masseter, temporalis, and lateral pterygoid muscles (**Figures 18–38, 18–39,** and **18–40**). They are palpated for

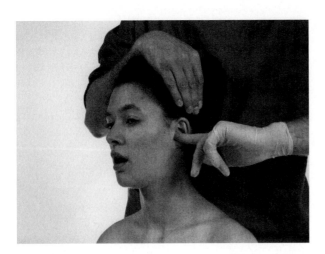

Figure 18–37

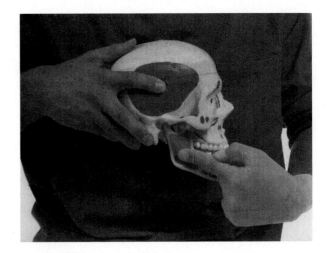

Figure 18–38

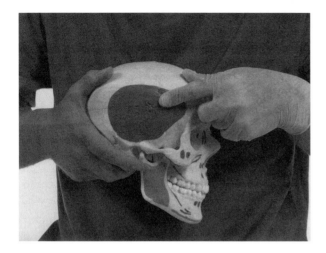

Figure 18–39

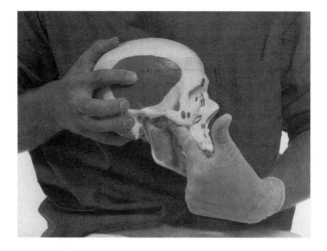

Figure 18–40

tone and for specific pain points; this may evoke local pain, with or without referral.

de Wijer et al. (1995) reported interrater agreement for the presence of pain during palpation of the masseter muscle ($\kappa = 0.33$), temporalis ($\kappa = 0.42$), and the medial pterygoid at its attachment ($\kappa = 0.23$). Lobbezoo-Scholte et al. (1994) reported identical κ values for pain on palpation of the same muscles. Palpation of the lateral aspect of the temporomandibular joint externally and the dorsal aspect via the external auditory meatus yielded an interrater κ value of 0.33 (Lobbezoo-Scholte et al.; de Wijer et al.). If the patient reports pain with this type of palpation or with active movement, this carries a sensitivity of 0.92, specificity of 0.21, positive likelihood ratio of 1.16, and a negative likelihood ratio of 0.38 in the diagnosis of temporomandibular joint synovitis when compared to a gold standard of arthroscopic findings (Israel et al., 1998). Visscher et al. (2000) reported a sensitivity of 0.75, specificity of 0.67, positive likelihood ratio of 2.27, and a negative likelihood ratio of 0.37 for the presence of pain upon palpation of the lateral and posterior joint, the masseter, and the temporalis muscle compared to a gold standard of patient-reported temporomandibular joint pain.

PROVOCATION TESTS

Distraction

Examination position, patient: Sitting on the short side of the examination table with the lower legs hanging down.

Starting position, therapist: Standing beside the patient at the side not being examined.

Stabilization: The stabilizing hand and arm surround the patient's head and hold it in position; the palpating index finger is placed on the temporomandibular joint.

Procedure: The thumb of the manipulating hand is placed on the back lower molars at the side to be examined, the index finger against the horizontal ramus of the mandible, and the other fingers surround the lower jaw. The therapist introduces distraction in a caudal direction, toward the mandibular ramus (**Figures 18–41** and **18–42**).

Assessment: Mobility, endfeel, pain.

de Wijer et al. (1995) reported κ values of -0.08 and 0.25 for the interrater agreement on the presence of pain during right and left traction, respectively. They also reported κ values of -0.03 and 0.08 for interrater agreement on restriction of motion during joint play and κ values of -0.05 and 0.20 for interrater agreement on endfeel for right and left traction, respectively.

Compression

Examination position, patient: Sitting on the short side of the examination table with the lower legs hanging down.

Starting position, therapist: Standing beside the patient at the side not being examined.

Stabilization: The stabilizing hand and arm surround the patient's head and hold it in position; the palpating index finger is placed on the temporomandibular joint.

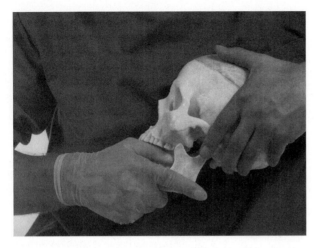

Figure 18–41 ↕

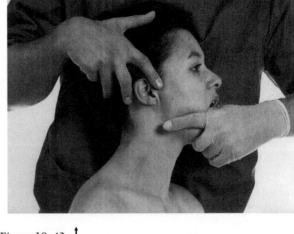

Figure 18–42 ↕

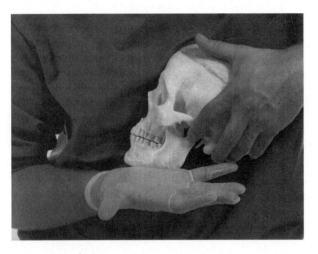

Figure 18–43 ↕

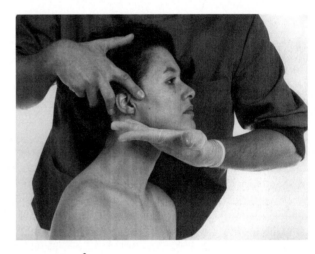

Figure 18–44 ↕

Procedure: The hypothenar of the manipulating hand is placed on the lower jaw at the level of the angle. Graded pressure is applied in a cranial direction (**Figures 18–43 and 18–44**).

Assessment: Pain.

Lobbezoo-Scholte et al. (1994) reported κ = 0.40 for interrater agreement on the presence of pain with compression and κ = 0.66 for the presence of crepitus or clicking with compression. de Wijer et al. (1995) reported κ values of 0.19 and 0.47 for interrater agreement on pain with joint compression right and left, respectively.

PASSIVE UNILATERAL TRANSLATORY EXAMINATION

Anterior Translation

Examination position, patient: Sitting on the short side of the examination table with the lower legs hanging down.

Starting position, therapist: Standing beside the patient at the side not being examined.

Stabilization: The stabilizing hand and arm surround the patient's head and hold it in position; the palpating index finger is placed on the temporomandibular joint.

Procedure: The thumb of the manipulating hand is placed on the lower back molars at the side to be examined, and the index finger at the back of the ascending ramus of the mandible. The remaining fingers surround the horizontal ramus of the mandible. Anterior translation is introduced (**Figure 18–45**).

Assessment: Mobility, endfeel, pain.

Posterior Translation

Examination position, patient: Sitting on the short side of the examination table with the lower legs hanging down.

Starting position, therapist: Standing beside the patient at the side not being examined.

Stabilization: The stabilizing hand and arm surround the patient's head and hold it in position; the palpating index finger is placed on the temporomandibular joint.

Procedure: The thumb of the manipulating hand is placed on the lower back molars at the side to be examined and the index finger on the ascending ramus of the mandibula. The remaining fingers surround the horizontal ramus of the mandibula. Posterior translation is introduced (**Figure 18–46**).

Assessment: Mobility, endfeel, pain.

Medial Translation

Examination position, patient: Sitting on the short side of the examination table with the lower legs hanging down.

Starting position, therapist: Standing beside the patient at the side not being examined.

Stabilization: The stabilizing hand and arm surround the patient's head and hold it in position; the palpating index finger is placed on the temporomandibular joint.

Procedure: The thumb of the manipulating hand is placed on the lower back molars at the side to be examined and the index finger on the ascending ramus of the mandible. The remaining fingers surround the horizontal ramus of the mandible. Medial translation is introduced (**Figure 18–47**).

Assessment: Mobility, endfeel, pain.

de Wijer et al. (1995) reported κ values of 0.50 and 0.28 for the interrater agreement on the presence of pain during right and left mediolateral translation, respectively. They also reported κ values of -0.05 and -0.1 for interrater agreement on restriction of motion during joint play and κ values of -0.05 and 0.13 for interrater agreement on endfeel for right and left translation, respectively.

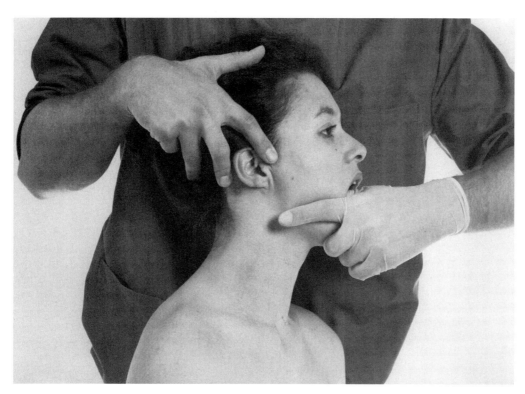

Figure 18–45

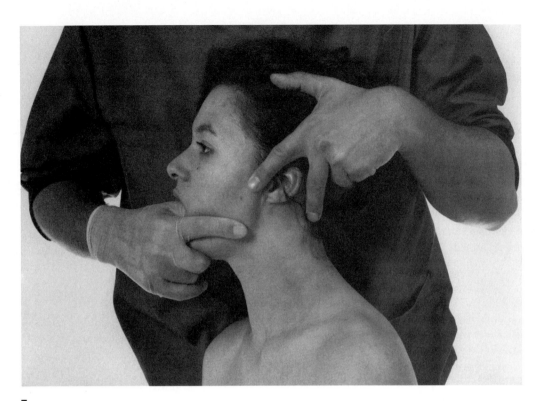

Figure 18–46

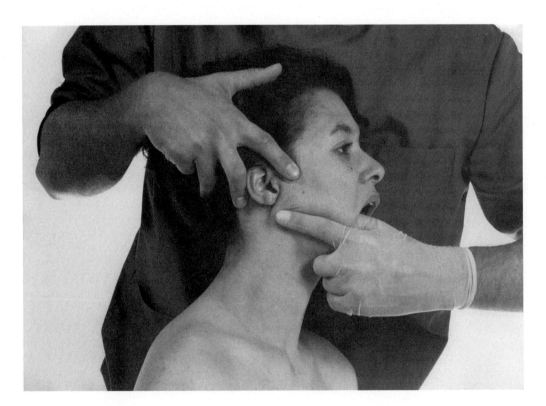

Figure 18–47

ADDITIONAL EXAMINATIONS OF THE UPPER CERVICAL, CERVICAL, AND UPPER THORACIC SPINE

The biomechanical and neurological relationships within the thoracic-cervical-cranio-mandibular functional unit have been described. It is clear from that description that where there is dysfunction of the temporomandibular joint, the upper cervical, cervical, and upper thoracic spine should also be examined. A correct diagnosis can be made only when all the data on signs and symptoms in the whole functional unit have been gathered. For details of examination of the cervical and upper thoracic spine, please see Chapters 15 through 17.

References

Abbott JH, McCane B, Herbison P, Moginie G, Chapple C, Hogarty T. Lumbar segmental instability: a criterion-related validity study of manual therapy assessment. *BMC Musculoskel Disord.* 2005;6:56.

Abbott JH, Mercer SR. Lumbar segmental hypomobility: criterion-related validity of clinical examination items. *New Zealand J Physiother.* 2003;31:3–9.

Adson AW. Cervical ribs; symptoms, differential diagnosis and indications for section of the insertion of the scalenus anticus muscle. *J Int Coll Surg.* 1951;16:546.

Agerberg G. On mandibular dysfunction and mobility. *Umea Univ Odontol Diss.* 1974;abstract 3.

Albert H, Godskesen M, Westergaard J. Evaluation of clinical tests used in classification procedures in pregnancy-related pelvic joint pain. *Eur Spine J.* 2000;9:161–166.

American Physical Therapy Association. *Guide to Physical Therapist Practice.* 2nd ed. Alexandria, Va: American Physical Therapy Association *Phys Ther;* 2001:9–744.

Aprill C, Axinn MJ, Bogduk N. Occipital headaches stemming from the lateral atlanto-axial (C1–C2) joint. *Cephalalgia.* 2002;22:15–22.

Arkin AM. The mechanism of rotation in combination with lateral deviation in the normal spine. *J Bone Joint Surg [Am]* 1950;32:180–188.

Arlen A. Die "paradoxale Kippbewegung des Atlas" in der Funktionsdiagnostik der Halswirbelsäule. *Man Med.* 1977; 15:16–22.

Arnold C, Bourassa R, Langer T, Stoneham G. Doppler studies evaluating the effect of a physical therapy screening protocol on vertebral artery blood flow. *Man Ther.* 2004;9:13–21.

Aufdemkampe G. Meetinstrumenten en manuele therapie I t/m IV. *T v Man Ther.* 1990;9(1):4.

August B, Miller FB. Clinical value of the palmomental reflex. *JAMA.* 1952;148:120–121.

Ausman JJ, Shrontz CE, Pearce JE, Diaz FG, Crecelius JL. Vertebrobasilar insufficiency: a review. *Arch Neurol.* 1985; 42:803–808.

Azevedo I, Soares da Silva P. Are fibroblasts adrenergically cells? *Bloodvessels.* 1981;18:330–332.

Barber R. Treatment for chronic low back pain. *Proc Fourth Int Congr Phys Med* (Paris). 1964.

Barker D, Saito M. Autonomic innervation of receptors and muscle fibers in cat skeletal muscle. *Proc R Soc Lond.* 1981; 212:317–322.

Barré J. Sur un syndrome sympathique cervical posterior et sa cause frequente: l'arthrite cervical. *Rev Neurol.* 1926;1:1246.

Basbaum AI, Fields HL. Endogenous pain control systems: brainstem spinal pathways and endorphin circuitry. *Ann Rev Neurosci.* 1984;7:309–338.

Basmajian JVMD. *Primary Anatomy.* 7th ed. Baltimore, Md: Williams & Wilkins; 1976.

Batson OV. The vertebral vein system. *Amer J Roentgenol.* 1957;78:195–212.

Batterham AM, George KP. Reliability in evidence-based clinical practice: a primer for allied health professionals. *Phys Ther Sport.* 2003;4:122–128.

Baur R. Zum Problem der Neugliederung der Wirbelsäule. *Acta Anat.* 1969;72:321–356.

Beaudry M, Spence JD. Motor vehicle accidents: the most common cause of traumatic vertebrobasilar ischaemia. *Can J Neurol Sci.* 2003;30:320–325.

Beighton P, Horan F. Orthopaedic aspects of Ehlers-Danlos syndrome. *J Bone Joint Surg [Am].* 1969;51:444–453.

Benini A. *Das kleine Gelenk der Lendenwirbelsäule.* Bern, Switzerland: Huber; 1978.

Benninghoff A, Goerttler K. *Lehrbuch der Anatomie des Menschen, 1e Band: Algemeine Anatomie und Bewegungsapparat.* 8th ed. München, Germany: Urban & Schwarzenberg, 1961.

Bergsmann OM, ed. *Thoracale Funktionsstörungen.* Heidelberg, Germany: Haug Verlag; 1977.

Bernards ATM. Fysiologie en pathofysiologie van nocisensoriek. In: van Zutphen HCF, van Sambeek HWR, eds. *Nederlands Leerboek der Fysische Therapie in Engere Zin, Deel 1.* Utrecht, The Netherlands: Wetenschappelijke uitgeverij Bunge; 1991: 34–100.

Bernards ATM. Trainbaarheid van een individuele sporter. *Geneeskunde en Sport.* 1997;30(1):5–9.

Bernards JA, Oostendorp RAB. De Fysiologie van de gewrichtsfunctie. *Tijdschrift Verz Gen.* 1988;25:17–20.

Bertilson BC, Bring J, Sjoblom A, Sundell K, Strender LE. Inter-examiner reliability in the assessment of low back pain (LBP) using the Kirkaldy-Willis Classification (KWC). *Eur Spine J.* 2006;15:1695–1703.

Bertilson BC, Grunnesjö M, Strender LE. Reliability of clinical tests in the assessment of patients with neck/shoulder problems: impact of history. *Spine.* 2003;28:2222–2231.

Beurskens AJHM, Vet HCW, Köke AJA. Responsivenes of functional status in low back pain. A comparison of different instruments. *Pain.* 1996:65:71–76.

Bibby RE. The hyoid triangle. *Am J Orthod.* July 1981;80(1).

Blumberg H, Jänig W. Changes of reflexes in vasoconstrictor neurons supplying the cat hindlimb following chronic nerve lesions: a model for studying mechanisms of reflex sympathetic dystrophy. *J Autonom Sys.* 1983;7:399–411.

Blunt SB, Galton C. Cervical carotid or vertebral artery dissection. *BMJ.* 1997;314:243.

Bogduk N. Cervical causes of headache and dizziness. In: Grieve GP, ed. *Modern Manual Therapy of the Vertebral Column.* Edinburgh, UK: Churchill Livingstone; 1987.

Bogduk N. *Biomechanics of the Cervical Spine.* Amsterdam, The Netherlands: Unpublished lecture NVMT Congress; 1990.

Bogduk N, Twomey LT. *Clinical Anatomy of the Lumbar Spine.* 2nd ed. Edinburgh, UK: Churchill Livingstone; 1991.

Boline PD, Keating JC, Brist J, Denver G. Interexaminer reliability of palpatory evaluations of the lumbar spine. *Am J Chiropr Med.* 1988;1:5–11.

Bolton JE. Never certain, only confident. *Clin Chiropr.* 2007; 10:50–52.

Bopp HH. *Orthop Praxis.* 1971;10:261.

Bos JW. *Functionele Aspecten van Steunweefsel.* Amersfoort, The Netherlands: SOMT, 1999.

Bourdiol RJ. *Pied et Statique.* Masson, France: Maissonneuve Editeur; 1980.

Bowman C, Gribble R. The value of the forward flexion tests and three tests of leg length changes in the clinical assessment of movement of the sacroiliac joint. *J Orthop Med.* 1995:17:66–67.

Braus H, Elze C. *Anatomie des Menschen.* Berlin, Germany: Springer Verlag; 1921.

Braus H, Elze C. *Anatomie des Menschen.* 3rd ed. Berlin, Germany: Springer Verlag; 1954.

Brismée JM, et al. Interrater reliability of palpation of 3-dimensional segmental motion of the lumbar spine. *J Man Manipulative Ther.* 2005;13:216–221.

Brismée JM, et al. Interrater reliability of a passive physiological intervertebral motion test in the mid-thoracic spine. *J Manipulative Physiol Ther.* 2006;29:368–373.

Broadhurst NA, Bond MJ. Pain provocation tests for the assessment of sacroiliac joint dysfunction. *J Spinal Disord.* 1998;11:341–345.

Bronemo L, van Stevenick J. *A comparison of the inter- and intra-examiner reliability of motion palpation of the lower cervical spine (C2–C7) in the oblique-posterior-lateral direction in sitting and supine positions.* Doctoral thesis; Anglo-European College of Chiropractic, Bournemouth, UK; 1987.

Bronisch FW. *Die Reflexe und ihre Untersuchung in Klinik und Praxis.* Stuttgart, Germany: Georg Thieme Verlag; 1973.

Brown MD. Degenerative spondylolisthesis. *AAOS Instr Course Lecture.* 1983;32:162.

Brüegger A. Vertebrale radikulaire und pseudoradikulaire Syndrome. *Acta Rheum.* 1969;18.

Brüegger A. *Die Erkrankungen des Bewegungsapparates und seines Nervensystems.* Stuttgart, Germany: Fischer; 1977.

Brüegger A, Rhonheimer CH. *Pseudoradikulaire Syndrome des Stammes.* Bern, Switzerland: Verlag Hans Huber; 1965.

Buckwalter JA. Articular cartilage: injuries and potential for healing. *J Orthop Sports Phys Ther.* 1998;28(4):192–202.

Bumke O, Foerster O. *Handbuch der Neurologie. Rückenmark, Hirnstamm Kleinhirn.* Vol. 5. Berlin, Germany: J. Springer Verlag; 1936.

Burgerhout WG, Mook CA, de Morree JJ, Zijlstra WG. *Fysiologie: Leerboek voor Paramedische Opleidingen.* Utrecht, The Netherlands: Wetenschappelijke uitgeverij Bunge; 1995.

Cacchiotti DA, Plesh O, Bianchi P, McNeill C. Signs and symptoms in samples with and without temporomandibular disorders. *J Craniomandib Disord.* 1991;5:167–172.

Cannon WB. Stresses and strains of homeostasis *Am J Med Sci.* 1935;189:1–14.

Carlsson GE. Mandibular dysfunction and temporomandibular joint pathosis. *J Prostet Dent.* 1980;43:658.

Cassidy JD, et al. Risk of vertebrobasilar stroke and chiropractic care. *Spine.* 2008;33:S176–S183.

Cattrysse EHM, Swinkels RAHM, Oostendorp RAB, Duquet W. Upper cervical stability: are clinical tests reliable. *Man Ther.* 1997:2:91–97.

Childs JD, Flynn TW. Spinal manipulation for low back pain. *Ann Intern Med.* 2004;140:665.

Childs JD, et al. A clinical prediction rule to identify patients with low back pain most likely to benefit from spinal manipulation: a validation study. *Ann Intern Med.* 2004a;141:920–928.

Childs JD, Fritz JM, Piva SR, Whitman JM. Proposal of a classification system for patients with neck pain. *J Orthop Sports Phys Ther.* 2004b;34:686–696.

Childs JD, Piva SR, Fritz JM. Responsiveness of the Numeric Pain Rating Scale in patients with low back pain. *Spine.* 2005;30:1331–1334.

Christensen HW, et al. Palpation of the upper thoracic spine: an observer reliability study. *J Manipulative Physiol Ther.* 2002;25:285–292.

Christensen HW, et al. Palpation for muscular tenderness in the anterior chest wall: an observer reliability study. *J Manipulative Physiol Ther.* 2003;26:469–475.

Chusid JG. *Correlative Neuroanatomy and Functional Neurology.* 18th ed. Los Altos, Calif: Lange Medical Publications; 1982.

Clara M. *Das Nervensystem des Menschen.* 3rd ed. Leipzig, Germany: JA Barth; 1959.

Cleland JC. *Orthopaedic Clinical Examination: An Evidence-Based Approach for Physical Therapists.* Carlstadt, NJ: Icon Learning Systems; 2005.

Cleland JC, Childs JD, Fritz JM, Whitman JM. Interrater reliability of the history and physical examination in patients with mechanical neck pain. *Arch Phys Med Rehabil.* 2006;87:1388–1395.

Cleland JC, Childs JD, Fritz JM, Whitman JM, Eberhart SL. Development of a clinical prediction rule for guiding treatment of a subgroup of patients with neck pain: use of thoracic spine manipulation, exercise, and patient education. *Phys Ther.* 2007;87:9–23.

Cleland JC, Fritz JM, Brennan GP. Predictive validity of initial fear avoidance beliefs in patients with low back pain receiving physical therapy: is the FABQ a useful screening tool for identifying patients at risk for a poor recovery. *Eur Spine J.* 2008:17:70–79.

Clemens HJ. *Die Venensysteme der menschlichen Wirbelsäule.* Berlin, Germany: De Gruyter; 1961.

Clemens HJ. Die Vaskularisation der Wirbelsäule und des Rückenmarks. In: Trostdorf E, St. Stender H, eds. *Wirbelsäule und Nervensystem.* Stuttgart, Germany: Thieme; 1970.

Clemens HJ. Die anatomischen Grundlagen der Schmerzempfindung an den einzelnen Wirbelsäulenstrukturen. *Die Wirbelsäule in Forschung und Praxis.* 1971;52:39–46.

Clemens HJ, Noeske K, Roll D. Die arterielle Versorgung der menschlichen Wirbelsäule und des Rückenmarkes. In: Heine KH, ed. *Zur funktionellen Pathologie und Therapie der Wirbelsäule.* Berlin, Germany: Verlag für Prakt. Medizin; 1957.

Clemente CD, ed. *Gray's Anatomy.* 30th American ed. Baltimore, Md: Williams & Wilkins; 1985.

Cohen PC, Foster RJ, Mow VC. Composition and dynamics of articular cartilage: structure, function, and maintaining healthy state. *J Orthop Sports Phys Ther.* 1998;28(4):203–215.

Cook CE, Hegedus EJ. *Orthopaedic Physical Examination Tests: An Evidence-Based Approach.* Upper Saddle River, NJ: Prentice Hall; 2008.

Côté P, et al. The validity of the extension-rotation test as a clinical screening procedure before neck manipulation: a secondary analysis. *J Manipulative Physiol Ther.* 1996;19:159–164.

Cramer A. Funktionelle Merkmale der Wirbelsäulestastik. In: *Wirbelsäule in Forsch. und Praxis.* Vol. 5. Stuttgart, Germany: Hippokrates; 1958.

Cramer K. Ueber Rückgratsverkrümmung bei lumbosacralen Assimilationsbecken. *Z Orthop Chir.* 1908;22.

Culav EM, Clark CH, Merrilees MJ. Connective tissues: matrix composition and its relevance to physical therapy. *Phys Ther.* 1999;79(3):308–319.

Currier DP, Nelson RM. *Dynamics of Human Biologic Tissues.* Philadelphia, Pa: FA Davis; 1992.

Cyriax J. *Textbook of Orthopaedic Medicine. Vol. 1: Diagnosis of Soft Tissue Lesions.* London, UK: Bailliere Tindall and Cassell; 1947.

Damen L, Buyruk HM, Gueler-Ysal F, Lotgering FK, Snijders CJ, Stam HJ. The prognostic value of asymmetric laxity of the sacroiliac joints in pregnancy-related pelvic pain. *Spine.* 2002;27:2820–2824.

Davidson JM. Wound repair. *J Hand Ther.* 1998;11(2):80–94.

Davidson M. The interpretation of diagnostic tests: a primer for physiotherapists. *Aust J Physiother.* 2002;48:227–233.

Davis RC. Response patterns. *Trans NY Acad Sci.* 1957;19:731–739.

de Kleyn A. Some remarks on vestibular nystagmus. *Confin Neurol.* 1938; 2:257.

de Kleyn A, Nieuwenhuyse P. Schwindelanfälle und Nystagmus bei einer bestimmten Stellung des Kopfes. *Acta Ato-Laryngol.* 1927;11:155.

de Kleyn A, Niuewenhuyse AC. Schwindelanfälle bei einer bestimmten Stellung des Kopfes. *Acta Otolaryngologica.* 1927;11:155–157.

de Morree JJ. *Dynamiek van het Menselijk Bindweefsel.* Utrecht, The Netherlands: Bohn, Scheltema, Holkema; 1989.

de Morree JJ. Heeft bindweefsel wel een reflextonus nodig? *Nederlands Tijdschrift voor Fysiotherapie.* 1991;101(6):127–131.

de Morree JJ. *Dynamiek van het Menselijk Bindweefsel*. 2nd revised edition: Houten/Zaventem, The Netherlands: Bohn Stafleu Van Loghum, 1993.

de Palma A, Rothman RH. *The Intervertebral Disc*. Philadelphia, Pa: Saunders; 1970.

de Sèze S, Levernieux J. Use of vertebral tractions. *Rev Rhum Mal Osteoartic* 1951;17:303–304.

de Sèze S. L'épaule douloureuse et l'épaule bloque—une étude anatomique et arthrografique. *Ann Med Can.* 1961.

de Wijer A, Lobbezoo-Scholte AM, Steenks MH, Bosman F. Reliability of clinical findings in temporomandibular disorders. *J Orofac Pain.* 1995;9:181–191.

Delitto A, Erhard RE, Bowling RW. A treatment-based classification approach to low back syndrome: identifying and staging patients for conservative treatment. *Phys Ther.* 1995;75:470–485.

Delmas A. Fonction sacro-iliaque et statique du corps. *Rev Rhum Mal Osteoartic* 1950:17:475–481.

Delmas A, Ndjaga-Mba M, Vannareth T. Le cartilage articulare de L4–L5 et L5–S1. *C. R. Ass. Anat. 55e Congr* 1970: 230–234.

Derksen AAD. *Inleiding tot de Bouw en Functie van het Kauwstelsel*. Utrecht, The Netherlands: Bohn, Scheltema & Holkema; 1970.

Detsky ME, McDonald DR, Baerlocher MO, et al. Does this patient with headache have a migraine or need neuroimaging? *JAMA.* 2006;296:1274–1283.

Deville W, van der Windt D, Dzaferagic A, Bezemer P, Bouter L. The test of Lasegue: systematic review of the accuracy in diagnosing herniated discs. *Spine.* 2000;25: 1140–1147.

Deyo RA, Rainville J, Kent DL. What can the history and physical examination tell us about low back pain? *JAMA.* 1992;268:760–765.

Di Fabio RP. Manipulation of the cervical spine: risks and benefits. *Phys Ther.* 1999;79:50–65.

Dimnet J et al. Radiographic studies of lateral flexion in the lumbar spine. *J Biomech.* 1978;11(3):143–150.

Doerr M, Thoden U. Zervikal ausgelöste Augenbewegungen. In: Wolf HD, ed. *Die Sonderstellung des Kopfgelenkbereichs hrsgb*. Berlin, Germany: Springer Verlag; 1988.

Donatelli R, Owens-Brukhart H. Gevolgen van immobilisering op de rekbaarheid van periarticulair bindweefsel. *Stimulus pag.* 1982:325–330. Trans in: *J Orthop Sports Phys Ther.* 1981;3(2):67–72.

Donelson R. *Rapidly Reversible Low Back Pain: An Evidence-Based Pathway to Widespread Recoveries and Savings*. Hanover, NH: Self Care First; 2007.

Dreyfuss P, Michaelsen M, Pauza K, McLarty J, Bogduk N. The value of medical history and physical examination in diagnosing sacroiliac joint pain. *Spine.* 1996;21: 2594–2602.

Drukker J, Jansen JC. *Compendium Anatomie*. Lochem, The Netherlands: De Tijdstroom; 1969.

Dunk NM, Sullivan Compton D, Callaghan JP. The reliability of quantifying upright standing postures as a baseline diagnostic clinical tool. *J Manipulative Physiol Ther.* 2004; 27:91–96.

Duus P. *Neurologisch-Topische Diagnostik*. Stuttgart, Germany: Georg Thieme Verlag; 1980.

Dvorak J, Dvorak V. *Manuelle Medizin Diagnostik*. Stuttgart, Germany: Georg Thieme Verlag; 1983.

Dvořák J, Grob D, Baumgartner H, Gschwend N, Grauer W, Larsson S. Functional evaluation of the spinal cord by magnetic resonance imaging in patients with rheumatoid arthritis and instability of upper cervical spine. *Spine.* 1989;14(10):1057–1064.

Dvořák J, Panjabi MM. Functional anatomy of the alar ligaments. *Spine.* 1987;12(2):183–189.

Dvořák J, Schneider E, Saldinger P, Rahn B. Biomechanics of the craniocervical region: the alar and transverse ligaments. *J Orthopaed Res.* 1988;6:452–461.

Dwyer A, Aprill C, Bogduk N. Cervical zygapophyseal joint pain patterns, I: a study in normal volunteers. *Spine.* 1990; 15:453–457.

Eigler J. Methodische Fehler bei Feststellung der Beinlänge und Beinlängen Differenzen. *Orthopäde.* 1972;1:14–20.

Eliasziw M, Young S, Woodbury M, Fryday-Field K. Statistical methodology for the concurrent assessment of interrater and intrarater reliability: using goniometric measurements as an example. *Phys Ther.* 1994;74:777–788.

Elvey RL. Brachial plexus tension test for the pathoanatomical origin of arm pain. In: Glasglow E, Twomey L, eds. *Aspects of Manipulative Therapy*. Melbourne, Australia: Lincoln Institute of Health Sciences; 1979:105–110.

Elvey RL. The need to test the brachial plexus in painful shoulder and upper quadrant conditions. *Proc Neck Shoulder Symp.* Manip Therapists Assoc.; Brisbane, Australia; October 8–9, 1983:39–52.

Elvey RL. Functional anatomy of the glenohumeral joint. *Proc Manip Ther Assoc.* Australian Fourth Biennial Conference, Brisbane, Australia; May 22–25, 1985: 234–243.

Elvey RL. Treatment of arm pain conditions when they are accompanied by signs of abnormal brachial plexus tension. *Aust J Physiother.* 1986;32(4):225–230.

Emminger E. Die Gelenkdisci an der Wirbelsäule (eine mögliche Erklarung Wirbelsäuleabhangiger Schmerzzustande). *Hefte Unfallheilk.* 1954;48:142–148.

Emminger E. *Die Anatomie und Pathologie des blockierten Wirbelgelenkes*. Stuttgart, Germany: Hippokrates; 1967.

Erdmann H. Die Verspannung des Wirbelsockels im Beckenring. In: *Wirbelsäule in Forsch. u. Praxis.* Vol. 1. Stuttgart, Germany: Hippokrates; 1956:51–62.

Erdmann H. Möglichkeiten und Grenzen in der Röntgen-Diagnostik der Wirbelsäule. *Die Wirbelsäule in Forschung und Praxis.* 1964;28:9–22.

Erdmann H. Vergleichend anatomische Untersuchungen zum Verständnis der Statik und Dynamik von Becken- und Lendenwirbelsäule bei verschiedenen Beckentypen. *Asklepios.* 1965;6:1–4.

Erdmann H. Grundzüge einer funktionellen Wirbelsäulen-betrachtung. 1. *Teil Man Med.* 1967;6:32–37.

Erdmann H. Grundzüge einer funktionellen Wirbelsäulen-betrachtung. 2. *Teil Man Med.* 1968a;5:55–63.

Erdmann H. Grundzüge einer funktionellen Wirbelsäulen-betrachtung. 3. *Teil Man Med.* 1968b;6:78–90.

Ernst E. Manipulation of the cervical spine: a systematic review of case reports of serious adverse events, 1995–2001. *Med J Aust.* 2002;176:376–380.

Evans P. The healing process at cellular level: a review. *Physiotherapy.* 1980;66(8):256–259.

Fedorak C, Ashworth N, Marshall J, Paull H. Reliability of the visual assessment of cervical and lumbar lordosis: how good are we? *Spine.* 2003;28:1857–1859.

Ferguson WR. Some observations on the circulation in foetal and infant spines. *J Bone Joint Surg.* 1950;32-A: 640–648.

Fernández-de-las-Peñas C, Cleland JA, Cuadrado ML, Pareja JA. Predictor vartiables for identifying patients with chronic tension type headache who are likely to achieve short-term success with muscle trigger point therapy. *Cephalalgia.* 2008;28:264–275.

Fick R. Ueber die Form der Gelenkflächen. *Arch Anat Physiol.* 1890;1:391–402.

Fick R. Spezielle Gelenk- und Muskelmechanik. In: *Handbuch der Anatomie und Mechanik der Gelenke.* III. Teil [Part 3]. Jena, Germany: Fischer; 1911.

Fischer LP, Garret JP, Gonon GP, Sayfi Y. La vascularisation de l'axis. *Médicine.* 1977:335–346.

Fleisch A. La régulation de la circulation periphérique. *Acta Neurovegetativa.* Vol. 14, Wien, Austria: Springer Verlag; 1956: 88–93.

Flynn T, et al. A clinical prediction rule for classifying patients with low back pain who demonstrate short-term improvement with spinal manipulation. *Spine.* 2002;27: 2835–2843.

Foerster O. Die *Leitungsbahnen des Schmerzgefühls und die chirurgische Behandlung der Schmerzzustände.* Berlin, Germany: Urban & Schwarzenberg; 1922.

Foerster O. *Handbuch der Neurologie, Ergänzungsband.* Part 2. Von Bumke OV, Foerster O, eds., Berlin, Germany: Springer Verlag; 1929:1256–1258.

Folkman S, Lazarus RS. An analysis of coping in a middle-aged community sample. *J Health Soc Behav.* 1980;21: 219–239.

Fortin JD, Dwyer AP, West S, Pier J. Sacroiliac joint: pain referral maps upon applying a new injection/arthrography technique, part I: asymptomatic volunteers. *Spine.* 1994a; 19:1475–1482.

Fortin JD, Aprill CN, Ponthieux B, Pier J. Sacroiliac joint: pain referral maps upon applying a new injection/arthrography technique, part II: clinical evaluation. *Spine.* 1994b;19:1483–1489.

Freeman ML, Raaphorst GP, Hopwood LE, Dewey WC. The effect of pH on cell lethality induced by hyperthermia treatment. *Cancer* (Philadelphia). 1980;45:2291.

Freyette H. A discussion of the physiological movements of the spine. In: *Principles of Osteopathic Technic.* Newark, OH: Academy of Applied Osteopathy, 1954.

Frick H, Leonhardt H, Starck D. *Allgemeine Anatomie, Spezielle Anatomie I.* Stuttgart, Germany: Thieme; 1977.

Frisch H. *Programmierte Untersuchung und Programmierte Therapie des Bewegungsapparats: Chirodiagnostik.* Berlin, Germany: Springer-Verlag; 1977.

Fritz JM. *A Research-Based Approach to Low Back Pain.* Presented at: Distinguished Lectures in Sports Medicine Series; October 12, 1999; Holland, Mich.

Fritz JM, Brennan GP, Clifford SN, Hunter SJ, Thackeray A. An examination of the reliability of a classification algorithm for subgrouping patients with low back pain. *Spine.* 2006;31:77–82.

Fritz JM, Childs JD, Flynn TW. Pragmatic application of a clinical prediction rule in primary care to identify patients with low back pain with a good prognosis following a brief spinal manipulation intervention. *BMC Family Prac.* 2005a;6:29.

Fritz JM, et al. Is there a subgroup of patients with low back pain likely to benefit from mechanical traction? *Spine.* 2007;32:E793–E800.

Fritz JM, Piva SR, Childs JD. Accurcacy of the clinical examination to predict radiographic instability of the lumbar spine. *Eur Spine J.* 2005b;14:743–750.

Fritz JM, Whitman JM, Childs JD. Lumbar segmental mobility assessment: an examination of validity for determining intervention strategies in patients with low back pain. *Arch Phys Med Rehabil.* 2005c;86:1745–1752.

Fritz JM, Whitman JM, Flynn TW. Factors related to the inability of individuals with low back pain to improve with a spinal manipulation. *Phys Ther.* 2004;84:173–190.

Frymoyer JW. *The Adult Spine: Principles and Practice.* Vol. II. New York, NY: Raven Press; 1996.

Fuiks DM, Crayson Ch E. Vacuum pneumarthography and the spontaneous occurence of gas in the joint spaces. *J Bone Joint Surg [Am].* 1963;45:873.

Fujita K, Nakagawa T, Hirabayashi K, Nagai Y. Neutral proteinases in human intervertebral disc. *Spine.* 1993; 18(13).

Garfin SR, Rydevik BL, Braun RA. Compressive neuropathy of spinal nerve roots: a mechanical or biological problem? *Spine.* 1991;2:162–167.

Gertzbein SD, et al. Determination of a locus of instantaneous centers of rotation of the lumbar disc by Moiré fringes: a new technic. *Spine.* 1984;9:409–413.

Gertzbein SD, et al. Centrode patterns and segmental instability in degenerative disc disease *Spine.* 1985;10:257–261.

Gerweck LE, Gillette EL, Dewey WC. Killing of Chinese hamster cells in vitro by heating under hypoxic or aerobic conditions. *Eur J Cancer.* 1974;10:691.

Ghazwinian R, Kramer J. Optimale Lagerung bei der Operation des Lumbalen Bandscheibenvorfalls. *Z Orthop.* 1974;112:815.

Gillard J, et al. Diagnosing thoracic outlet syndrome: contribution of provocative tests, ultrasonography, electrophysiology, and helical computed tomography in 48 patients. *Joint Bone Spine.* 2001;68:416–424.

Glaser J, Cure J, Bailey K, Morrow D. Cervical spinal cord compression and the Hoffman sign. *Iowa Orthop J.* 2001;21:49–52.

Gosh P. *The Biology of the Intervertebral Disc.* Boca Raton, Fla: CRC Press; 1988.

Gray H. *Gray's Anatomy.* 35th ed. Norwich, UK: Longmans Gr. Ltd, Jarrold and Sons Ltd; 1973.

Graziano DL, Nitsch W, Huijbregts PA. Positive cervical artery testing in a patient with chronic whiplash syndrome: clinical decision making in the presence of diagnostic uncertainty. *J Man Manipulative Ther.* 2007;15:E45–E63.

Gregerson G, Lucas DB. An in vivo study of the axial rotation of the human thoracolumbar spine. *J Bone Joint Surg.* 1967;49-A:247–262.

Grieve GP. Manipulation. *Physiotherapy.* 1975;6(1):11–18.

Grieve GP. *De Wervelkolom.* Lochem, The Netherlands: Uitgeverij De Tijdstroom; 1984.

Grieve GP, ed. *Common Vertebral Joint Problems.* Edinburgh, UK: Churchill Livingstone; 1981.

Grieve GP, ed. *Modern Manual Therapy of the Vertebral Column.* Edinburgh, UK: Churchill-Livingstone; 1986.

Grimm RJ. Inner ear injuries in whiplash. *J Whiplash Rel Disord.* 2002;1:65–75.

Guillon B, et al. Infection and the risk of spontaneous cervical artery dissection. *Stroke.* 2003;34:e79–e81.

Guntz E. Kritische Bemerkungen zum Problem der statischen und funktionellen Störungen der Wirbelsäule mit therapeutischen Rückschlüssen aus der Blickrichtung des Orthopäden sowie Demonstrationen zur Arthrosis deformans der kleine Wirbelgelenke. *Die Wirbelsäule in Forschung und Praxis* 1956;1:126–132.

Gutmann G. Einführung in die statischfunktionelle Röntgendiagnostik der Wirbelsäule unter besonderer Berücksichtigung der Kopfgelenke und Halswirbelsäule. *Die Wirbelsäule in Forschung und Praxis* 1956;1:70–72.

Gutmann G. Zur Frage der Konstruktionsgerechten Beanspruchung von Lendenwirbelsäule und Becken beim Menschen. *Asklepios.* 1965;6:263–269.

Gutmann G. Schulkopfschmerz und Kopfhaltung. Ein Beitrag der Pathogenese des Anteflexions-Kopfschmerzes und zur Mechanik der Kopfgelenke. *Z Orthop.* 1968;105:497–515.

Gutmann G. *Plaats en Doel van de Manuele Therapie in het Kader van de Hedendaagse Geneeskunde.* Lecture, 1970.

Gutmann G. Chirotherapie, Grundlagen, Indikationen, Gegenindikationen und Objektivierbarkeit. *Med Welt.* 1978;29:653.

Gutmann G. Zum Problem des Vasospasmus im A. Vertebralis Basilaris-Gefäsebereich. In: von Gutmann G, ed. *Arteria Vertebralis.* Berlin, Germany: Springer Verlag; 1985.

Gutmann G, Biedermann H. *Funktionelle Pathologie und Klinik der Wirbelsäule, Band 1: Die Halswirbelsäule (Teil 2).* Stuttgart, Germany: Gustav Fischer Verlag; 1984.

Gutmann G, Vélé F. Die Gelenke der oberen Halswirbelsäule und ihre Einwirkung auf motorische Stereotypen. In: Wolff HB, ed. *Manuelle Medizin und ihre wissenschaftliche Grundlagen.* Heidelberg, Germany: Physikalische Medizin, 1970:1–31.

Gutzeit K. Wirbelsäule als Krankheitsfactor. *Dtsch Med Wschr.* 1951;76.

Guyton AC. *Textbook of Medical Physiology.* New York, NY: Saunders; 1986.

Haas M. Statistical methodology for reliability studies. *J Manipulative Physiol Ther.* 1991;14:119–132.

Hagenaars LHA. Fysiotherapeutische benaderingswijzen bij spierfunctiestoornissen. *Geneeskunde en Sport.* 1987;20(2):78–86.

Hagenaars LHA. *Vertebrobasilaire Insufficiëntie.* Rotterdam, The Netherlands: Niet gepubliceerde lezing; 1989.

Hagenaars LHA, Bernards ATM, Bos JM, Oostendorp RAB. Heeft bindweefsel een reflextonus? De noodzaak van fundamenteel onderzoek voor de fysiotherapie. *Nederlands Tijdschrift voor Fysiotherapie.* 1991;101(1):11–14.

Hagenaars LHA, Bernards ATM, Oostendorp RAB. *Het Meerdimensioneel Belasting-belastbaarheidsmodel.* Amersfoort, The Netherlands: Nederlands Paramedisch Instituut; 1996.

Hagenaars LHA, Dekker LJ, van der Plaats J, Bernards ATM, Oostendorp RAB. Effecten van het orthosympatische zenuwstelsel op de dwarsgestreepte spier. *Ned. T. v. Fysiother.* 1985;95(4):77–88.

Haher Th, et al. Instataneous axis of rotation as a function of the three columns of the spine. *Spine.* 1992;17:s149–s154.

Haldeman S, et al. Unpredictability of cerebrovascular ischaemia with cervical spine manipulation therapy: a review of sixty-four cases after cervical spine manipulation. *Spine*. 2002;27:49–55.

Haneline MT, Cooperstein R, Young MD, Ross J. Determining spinal level using the inferior level of the scapula as a reference landmark: a retrospective analysis of 50 radiographs. *J Can Chiropr Assoc*. 2008;52:24–29.

Haneline MT, Lewkovich G. Identification of internal carotid artery dissection in chiropractic practice. *J Can Chiropr Assoc*. 2004:48:206–210.

Haneline M, Triano J. Cervical artery dissection: a comparison of highly dynamic mechanisms: manipulation versus motor vehicle collision. *J Manipulative Physiol Ther*. 2005; 28:57–63.

Hansen K, Schliack H. *Segmentale Innervation, ihre Bedeutung fur Klinik und Praxis*. Stuttgart, Germany: Georg Thieme Verlag; 1962.

Hansson T, Honnée W, Hesse J. *Craniomandibulaire Dysfunctie*. Alphen aan de Rijn/Brussel, The Netherlands/Belgium: Samsom Stafleu; 1985.

Hanten WP, Olsen SL, Ludwig GM. Reliability of manual mobility testing of the upper cervical spine in subjects with cervicogenic headache. *J Man Manipulative Ther*. 2002;10:76–82.

Hardy M, Woodall W. Therapeutic effects of heat, cold, and stretch on connective tissue. *J Hand Ther*. 1998;11(2): 148–156.

Harff EG. *Algemene en Speciële Pathologie*. Vierde, herziene druk. Lochem, The Netherlands: De Tijdstroom; 1998.

Haswell K, Williams M, Hing W. Interexaminer reliability of symptom-provoking active sidebend, rotation, and combined movement assessments of patients with low back pain. *J Man Manipulative Ther*. 2004;12:11–20.

Hautant A. Rapport sur l'étude clinique de l'examen functionel de l'appareil vestibulaire. *Rev Neurol*.1927;1: 909–976.

Haynes MJ. Vertebral arteries and cervical movement: Doppler ultrasound velocimetry for screening before manipulation. *J Manipulative Physiol Ther*. 2002;25: 556–567.

Haynes MJ, Cala LA, Melsom A, Mastaglia FL, Milne N, McGeachie JK. Vertebral arteries and cervical rotation: modeling and magnetic resonance angiography studies. *J Manipulative Physiol Ther*. 2002;25:370–383.

Heerkens YF. *Cursusdictaat Syndesmologie*. Eindhoven, The Netherlands: Stichting Opleiding Manuele Therapie; 1987.

Heerkens YF. Gewrichtskraakbeen. *Nederlands Tijdschrift voor Fysiotherapie*. 1989;97(10):224–230.

Heijmans WFGJ, Hendriks HJM, Van der Esch M, et al. *Guideline: Manual Therapy for Low Back Pain*. Amersfoort, The Netherlands: Koninklijk Nederlands Genootschap voor Fysiotherapie (KNGF), 2002.

Heine KH. Ueber Bewegungs- und Haltungseinstellungen der Wirbelsäule. In: Heine KH, ed. *Zur funktionelle Pathologie und Therapie der Wirbelsäule*. Berlin, Germany: Verlag für praktische Medizin; 1957.

Henke JW. *Handbuch der Anatomie und Mechanik der Gelenke*. Leipzig-Heidelberg, Germany: CF. Wintersche Verlagshandlung, 1863.

Henneman E. Organization of the motoneuron pool: the size principle. In: Mountcastle VB, ed. *Medical Physiology*. St. Louis, Mo: Mosby; 1980.

Hernandez Conesa MJ, Argote ML. *A Visual Aid to the Examination of Nerve Root*. London, UK: Bailliere Tindall; 1976.

Heylings DJA. Supraspinous and interspinous ligaments of the human lumbar spine. *J Anat* (London). 1978;125: 127–131.

Hicks GE, Fritz JM, Delitto A, Mishock J. Interrater reliability of clinical examination measures for identification of lumbar segmental instability. *Arch Phys Med Rehabil*. 2003; 84:1858–1864.

Hicks GE, et al. Preliminary development of a clinical prediction rule for determining which patients with low back pain will respond to a stabilization exercise program. *Arch Phys Med Rehabil*. 2005;86:1753–1762.

Hillen B, Fonville F. De invloed van bewegingen van het hoofd op de doorstroming van de A. vertebralis. *Nederlands Tijdschrift voor Geneeskunde*. 1980;124:172.

Hisaw FL. The influence of the ovary on the resorption of the pubic bones. *J Exper Zool*. 1925;23:661.

Holstege G. *Descending Motor Pathways and Spinal Motor System: Limbic and Non-limbic Components*. New York, NY: Elsevier; 1991.

Honnée W, Naeije M. *Inleiding tot de Functieleer van het Kauwstelsel*. Course material, Universiteit van Amsterdam; 1980.

Hoogland P. *Nieuwe inzichten in de Morphologie en Functie van de Cervicale Discus Intervertebralis*. Lecture Conference Dutch Manual Therapy Association. The Hague, The Netherlands: 1988.

Hoogland R. *Specifieke Pijnpunten*. Ede, The Netherlands: Niet gepubliceerde lazing; 1987.

Hoppenfeld S. *Physical Examination of the Spine and Extremities*. Norwalk, Conn: Appleton Century Crofts; 1976.

Huguenin F. Der intrakanalikuläre Bandapparat des zerviko-okzipitalen Ueberganges. Eine klinische und diagnostische Studie seiner Funktion und seiner Verletzungen. *Manuelle Medizin*. 1984;22:25–29.

Huijbregts PA. Spinal motion palpation: a review of reliability studies. *J Man Manipulative Ther*. 2002;10:24–39.

Huijbregts PA. Invited commentary: evidence-based diagnosis and treatment of the painful sacroiliac joint. *J Man Manipulative Ther*. 2008;16:153–154.

Huijbregts PA, Hobby M, Salmas P. Scaphoid fracture: a case report illustrating evidence-based diagnosis and discussing measures of reliability and concurrent criterion-related validity. *Interdivisional Rev.* January/February 2005;14:8.

Hülse M. *Die cervikalen Gleichgewichtsstörungen.* Berlin, Germany: Springer Verlag; 1983a.

Hülse M. Hör- und Gleichgewichtsstörungen im Rahmen der vertebrobasilären Insuffizienz und im Rahmen der funktionellen Kopfgelenksstörung. In: Hohmann D von, ed. *Neuro-orthopadie.* Vol. 1 Berlin, Germany: Springer Verlag; 1983b.

Huneke G. *Das Sekundenphenomen.* Stuttgart, Germany: Georg Fischer Verlag; 1954.

Hungerford BA, Gilleard W, Moran M, Emmerson C. Evaluation of the ability of physical therapists to palpate intrapelvic motion with the stork test on the support side. *Phys Ther.* 2007;87:879–887.

Hurwitz EL, et al. Manipulation and mobilization of the cervical spine: a systematic review of the literature. *Spine.* 1996;21:1746–1759.

Ingelmark BE, Lindström J. Asymmetries of the lower extremities and pelvis and their relations to lumbar scoliosis. *Acta Morph. Scand.* 1963;5:221–234.

Isakov E, Sazbon L, Costeff H, Luz Y, Najenson T. The diagnostic value of three common primitive reflexes. *Eur Neurol.* 1984;23:17–21.

Israel H, Diamond B, Saed-Nejad F, Ratcliffe A. Osteoarthritis and synovitis as major pathoses of the temporomandibular joint: comparison of clinical diagnosis with arthroscopic morphology. *J Oral Maxillofac Surg.* 1998;56:1023–1028.

Jaeschke R, Guyatt GH, Sackett DL. Users' guides to the medical literature. III. How to use an article about a diagnostic test. B. What are the results and will they help me in caring for my patients? The Evidence-Based Medicine Working Group. *JAMA.* 1994;271:703–707.

Janda V. *Muskelfunktionsdiagnostik, Muskeltest Untersuchung verkürzter Muskeln, Untersuchung der Hypermobilität.* Leuven, Belgium: Verlag Acco; 1979.

Jänig W. Systemic and specific autonomic reactions in pain: efferent, afferent and endocrine components. *Eur J Anaesth.* 1985;2:319–346.

Jellinger K. Zur *Orthologie und Pathologie der Rückenmarksdurchblutung.* Wien, Austria: Springer Verlag; 1966.

Jepsen JR, Laursen LH, Hagert CG, Kreiner S, Larsen AI. Diagnostic accuracy of the upper limb examination. Part I: inter-rater reproducibility of selected findings and patterns. *BMC Neurol.* 2006;6:8.

Josza L, Kannus P, Balint JB, Reffy A. Three-dimensional ultrastructure of human tendons. *Acta Anatomica* (Basel). 1991;142:306–312.

Jull GA, Stanton WR. Predictors of responsiveness to physiotherapy management of cervicogenic headache. *Cephalalgia.* 2005;25:101–108.

Junghanns H. Das Bewegungssegment der Wirbelsäule und seine praktische Bedeutung. *Arch. PUTTI chir. org.* 1954; 5:103–111.

Junqueira LC, Carneiro J, Kelley RO. *Basic Histology.* 8th ed. Norwalk, Conn: Appleton & Lange; 1995.

Kaltenborn FM. Manuelle Therapie der Extremitätengelenke. Technik spezieller Untersuchungsverfahren. *Mobilisationen und Manipulationen.* Course material, 1973.

Kapandji JA. *The Physiology of the Joints, Vol. 3. The Trunk and the Vertebral Column.* Edinburgh, UK: Churchill Livingstone; 1974.

Kawchuk GN, et al. The relationship between the spatial distribution of vertebral artery compromise and exposure to cervical manipulation. *J Neurol.* 2008;255:371–377.

Keating L, Lubke C, Powell V, Young T, Souvlis T, Jull G. Mid-thoracic tenderness: a comparison of pressure pain threshold between spinal regions in asymptomatic subjects. *Man Ther.* 2001;6:634–639.

Keessen W. Stiffness properties of the lumbosacral joint in the sagittal plane: a radiological in-vivo assessment. *Academic thesis Rijksuniversiteit Utrecht,* 1988.

Keijzer A. Het teken van Lhermitte. *Ned. Tijdschrift voor Manuele Therapie.* 1988;88(7(1)).

Kellgren A. *Technics of Ling's System of Manual Treatment.* Edinburgh, UK: Young J. Pentland; 1890.

Kelly AM. The minimal clinically significant difference in visual analog pain score does not differ with severity of pain. *Emerg Med J.* 2001;18:205–207.

Kendall HO, Kendall FC, Wadsworth GE. *Muscles: Testing and Function.* Baltimore, Md: Williams & Wilkins; 1971.

Kerr RSC, Cadoux-Hudson TA, Adams CBT. The value of accurate clinical assessment in the surgical management of the lumbar disc protrusion. *J Neurol Neurosurg Psychiat.* 1988;51:169–173.

Kerry R, Taylor AJ. Cervical arterial dysfunction assessment and manual therapy. *Man Ther.* 2006;11:243–253.

Kerry R, Taylor AJ, Mitchell J, McCarthy C, Brew J. Manual therapy and cervical arterial dysfunction, directions for the future: a clinical perspective. *J Man Manipulative Ther.* 2008;16:39–48.

Kirkaldy-Willis WH. Instability of the lumbar spine. *Clin Orthop.* 1982;165:110–123.

Kitano, et al. Biochemical changes associated with the symptomatic human intervertebral disc. *Clin Orthop.* 1993; 193:372–377.

Knuttson B. Comparative value of electromyographic, myelographic, and clinical-neurological examinations in diagnosis of lumbar root compression syndrome. *Acta Orthop Scand.* 1961;(suppl 49):19–49.

Knutsson F. The instability associated with disc degeneration in the lumbar spine. *Acta Radiol.* 1944;25:593–609.

Kobayashi S, Suzuki Y, Asai T, Yoshizawa H. Changes in nerve root motion and intraradicular blood flow during intraoperative femoral nerve stretch: Report of four cases. *J Neurosurg (Spine 3).* 2003;99:298–305.

Koch R, Gross D, Kaeser HE. *Sympathalgien des Nacken-Schulter -Arm -Bereiches, Nacken-Schulter- Armsyndrom, Schmerzstudien nr. 3.* Stuttgart, Germany: G. Fischer Verlag; 1980.

Köke AJA, Heuts PHTG, Vlaeyen JWS, Weber WEJ. *Meetinstrumenten Chronische Pijn. Deel 1 Functionele Status.* Maastricht, The Netherlands: Pijn Kennis Centrum; 1999.

Kokmeyer DJ, van der Wurff P, Aufdemkampe G, Fickenscher TCM. The reliability of multitest regimens with sacroiliac pain provocation tests. *J Manipulative Physiol Ther.* 2002;25:42–48.

Komandatow GL. Propriozeptieve Reflexe von Augen und Kopf bei Kaninchen. *Fiziol zurn.* 1945;31(2):62.

Koole R. In: Steenks MH, de Wijer A, eds. Diagnostiek bij pijn rond het kaakgewricht hfdst. *Cranio-mandibulaire Dysfunkties: vanuit Fysiotherapeutisch en Tandheelkundig Perspectief.* Lochem: De Tijdstroom, The Netherlands: 1989;8: 51–75.

Kopell HP, Thompson WAL. *Peripheral Entrapment Neuropathies.* Huntington, NY: Krieger; 1976.

Korr IM. Sustained sympaticotonia as a factor in disease. In: Korr IM, ed. *The Neurobiologic Mechanisms in Manipulative Therapy.* New York, NY: Plenum; 1978.

Kos J. Contribution à l'étude de l'anatomie et de la vascularisation des articulations intervertébrales. *Comptes rendus Ass. Anat. 5e Congr.* 1969:1088–1105.

Kos J, Wolf J. Die "Menisci" der Zwischenwirbelgelenke und ihre mögliche Rolle bei Wirbelblockierung. *Man Med.* 1972;10:105–114.

Krämer J. *Bandscheiben bedingte Erkrankungen, Ursachen, Diagnose Behandlung, Vorbeugung, Begutachtung.* Stuttgart, Germany: Georg Thieme Verlag; 1978.

Kraus SL, ed. *TMJ Disorders: Management of the Craniomandibular Complex.* New York, NY: Churchill Livingstone; 1988.

Kunert W. *Wirbelsäule, vegetatives Nervensystem und Innere Medizin.* 2nd ed. Stuttgart, Germany: Enke; 1975.

Landel R, Kulig K, Fredericson M, Li B, Powers C. Intertester reliability and validity of motion assessments during lumbar spine accessory motion testing. *Phys Ther.* 2008;88:43–49.

Langhout RFH, Wingbermühle RW. Discus intervertebralis. Interne publicatie SOMT; 1999.

Lanser K. Cervicale segmentale instabiliteit. *Nederlands Tijdschrift voor Manuele Therapie.* 1988;7(4).

Lantz CA. Application and evaluation of the kappa statistic in the design and interpretation of chiropractic clinical research. *J Manipulative Physiol Ther.* 1997;20: 521–528.

Laslett M. Evidence-based diagnosis and treatment of the painful sacroiliac joint. *J Manual Manipulative Ther.* 2008; 16:142–152.

Laslett M, Williams M. The reliability of selected pain provocation tests for sacroiliac joint pathology. *Spine.* 1994; 19:1243–1249.

Laslett M, Young SB, Aprill CN, McDonald B. Diagnosing painful sacroiliac joints: a validity study of a McKenzie evaluation and sacroiliac provocation tests. *Aust J Physiother.* 2003;49:89–97.

Laupacis A, Sekar N, Stiell I. Clinical prediction rules: a review and suggested modification of methodological standards. *JAMA.* 1997;277:488–494.

Lazorthes G. *Le système neurovasculaire.* Paris, France: Masson; 1949.

Lechtape-Grutter H, Zulch KJ. Gibt es einen Spasmus der Hirngefässe. *Radiologie.* 1971;11:429–435.

Lederman E. *Fundamentals of Manual Therapy.* New York, NY: Churchill Livingstone; 1997.

Lériche R. *Translation de la Chirurgie de la Douleur.* 3rd ed. Paris, France: Masson; 1949.

Lériche R. *Schmerzchirurgie.* Leipzig, Germany: Barth; 1958.

Levin U, Stenström CH. Force and time recording for validating the sacroiliac distraction test. *Clin Biomech.* 2003; 18:821–826.

Lewin T. Anatomical variations in lumbosacral synovial joints with particular reference to subluxation. *Acta Anat.* 1968a;71:229–248.

Lewin T. Foramen intervertebrale und Wirbelbogengelenke im Lendenabschnitt der Wirbelsäule. *Die Wirbelsäule in Forschung und Praxis.* 1968b;40:74–82.

Lewit K. *Manuelle Medizin im Rahmen der medizinischen Rehabilitation.* Munich, Germany: Urban & Schwarzenberg; 1977.

Lewit K. Bericht von der zwei gemeinsame Arbeitstagungen der Gesellschaft fur Physiotherapie der D.D.R., Sektion Manuelle Therapie und der Paedagogischen Hochschule "Karl Liebknecht" Potsdam, Wissenschaftsbereich Sportmedizin, von September 5–8, 1984, in Potsdam. *Manuelle Medizin.* 1984;24:135.

Lewit K. Kopfgelenke und Gleichgewichtsstörung. *Manuelle Medizin.* 1986;24:26–29.

Lewit K, Berger M. Zervikale Störungsmuster bei Schwindelpatienten. *Manuelle Medizin.* 1985;21:15–19.

Lewit K, Krausová L. Messungen von Vorund Rückbeuge in den Kopfgelenken. *Forsch. Röntg.* 1963;99:538–543.

Li G, Hahn G. A proposed operational model of thermotolerance based on effects of nutrients and the initial treatment temperature. *Cancer Research.* 1980;40: 4501–4508.

Licht PB, Christensen HW, Høilund-Carlsen PF. Vertebral artery volume flow in human beings. *J Manipulative Physiol Ther.* 1999;22:363–367.

Licht PB, Christensen HW, Høilund-Carlsen PF. Is there a role for premanipulative testing before cervical manipulation? *J Manipulative Physiol Ther.* 2000;23:175–179.

Licht PB, Christensen HW, Høilund-Carlsen PF. Carotid artery blood flow during premanipulative testing. *J Manipulative Physiol Ther.* 2002;25:568–572.

Linton SJ, Haldén BA. Can we screen for problematic backpain? A screening questionnaire for predicting outcome in acute and subacute back pain. *Clin J Pain.* 1998; 14:209–215.

Lysell E. Motion in the cervical spine: an experimental study on autopsy specimens. *Acta Orthop (Scandinavica).* 1969;suppl 123):1+.

Lobbezoo-Scholte AM, de Wijer A, Steenks MH, Bosman F. Interexaminer reliability of six orthopaedic tests in diagnostic subgroups of craniomandibular disorders. *J Oral Rehabil.* 1994;21:273–285.

Loesberg C, van Miltenburg JC, van Wijk R. Heat production of mammalian cells at different cell cycle phases. *J Thermal Biol.* 1982a;7:209–213.

Loesberg C, van Miltenburg JC, van Wijk R. Heat production of Reuber H35 rat hepatoma cells under normo- and hyperthermica conditions. *J Thermal Biol.* 1982b; 7:87–90.

Loeser JD. A definition of pain. *Medicine.* 1980;7:3.

Loeweneck H. *Ueber die sensible Innervation der Articulationes intervertebrales.* Dissertation. Munich, Germany; 1966.

Louis R. The anatomic basis of surgery on the thoracolumbar vertebral junction. *Anatomia Clinica.* 1978;1:73–80.

Lovett W. The mechanics of lateral curvature of the spine. *Boston Med Surg J.* 1900;142:622–627.

Lovett W. *Lateral Curvature of the Spine and Round Shoulders.* London, UK: Heinemann; 1916.

Ludwig KS. Über das Ligamentum alare dentis epistrophei des Menschen. *Anat. Entwicklungsgesch.* 1952;116:442–445.

Lumsden RM, Morris JM. An in vivo study of axial rotation and immobilization at the lumbosacral joint. *J Bone Joint Surg.* 1968;50:1591–1602.

Lundborg G. Structure and function of the intraneural microvessels as related to trauma, edema formation, and nerve function. *J Bone Joint Surg.* 1975;57:938–948.

Lurija AR. *Grondslagen van de Neuropsychologie.* Deventer, The Netherlands: Van Loghum Slaterus; 1982.

Luschka H. Die *Anatomie des Menschen.* Vol. I, Part 2. Tübingen, Germany: Laupp; 1862.

MacConnail MA, Basmajian JV. *Muscles and Movements: A Base for Human Kinesiology.* Baltimore, Md: Williams & Wilkins; 1969.

Magnus R. *Körperstellung.* Berlin, Germany: Springer Verlag; 1924.

Magnus R, de Kleyn A. Die Abhängigkeit des Tonus der Extremitätenmuskeln von der Kopfstellung. *Pflügers Arch. ges. Physiol.* 1912;145:455.

Magyar MT, Nam EM, Csiba L, Ritter MA, Ringelstein EB, Droste DW. Carotid artery auscultation: anachronism or useful screening procedure? *Neurol Res.* 2002;24:705–708.

Maher C, Adams R. Reliability of pain and stiffness assessments in clinical manual lumbar spine examination. *Phys Ther.* 1994;74:801–811.

Maigne JY, Aivaliklis A, Pfefer F. Results of sacroiliac joint double block and value of sacroiliac pain provocation tests in 54 patients with low back pain. *Spine.* 1996;21: 1889–1892.

Maigne R. *Douleurs d'Origine Vertébrale et Traitements par Manipulations.* Paris, France: Expansion Scientique; 1968.

Maigne R. Low back pain of thoracolumbar origin. *Arch Phys Med Rehabil.* 1980;61:389–395.

Manabu I, et al. A biomechanical definition of spinal segmental instability taking personal and disc level differences into account. *Spine.* 1993;18:2294–2304.

Marin R, Dillingham TR, Chang A, Belandres P. Extensor digitorum brevis reflex in normals and patients with radiculopathies. *Muscle Nerve.* 1995;18:52–59.

Markuske H. *Untersuchungen zur Statik und Dynamik der kindlichen Halswirbelsäule: Der Aussagewert seitlicher Röntgenaufnahmen. Die Wirbelsäule und Praxis.* Vol. 50. Stuttgart, Germany: Hippokrates; 1971.

Marsman J. *Unpublished Lecture.* Eindhoven, The Netherlands: 1981.

Mayer T, et al. *Functional Restoration for Spinal Disorders: The Sports Medicine Approach.* Philadelphia, Pa: Lea & Febinger; 1988.

McComas AJ. *Skeletal Muscle: Form and Function.* Champaign, Ill: Human Kinetics; 1996.

McCormick WE, Steinmetz MP, Benzel EC. Cervical spondylotic myelopathy: make the difficult diagnosis, then refer for surgery. *Cleveland Clin J Med.* 2003;70:899–904.

McCouch GP, Deering JD, Ling TH. Location of receptors for tonic neck reflexes. *J Neurophysiol.* 1951;14:191.

McEvoy J, Huijbregts PA. Reliability of myofascial trigger point palpation: a systematic review. In: Dommerholt J, Huijbregts PA, eds. *Myofascial Trigger Points: Pathophysiology and Evidence-Informed Diagnosis and Management.* Forest Grove, Ore: Otter Rock Press; 2008.

McGregor AH, Wragg P, Gedroyc WMW. Can interventional MRI provide an insight into the mechanics of a posterior-anterior mobilisation? *Clin Biomech.* 2001;16:926–929.

Melzack R. Myofascial trigger points: relation to acupuncture and mechanisms of pain. *Arch Phys Med.* 1981; 62:114.

Melzack R, Wall PD. Pain mechanisms: a new theory. *Science.* 1965;150:971–979.

Mens J. Bekken instabiliteit: oefentherapeutisch handelen. *Kwartaaluitgave NVOM* 1996;4.

Mens JMA, Stam HJ, Vleeming A, Snijders CJ. Active straight leg raising: a clinical approach to the load transfer functions of the pelvic girdle. In: Vleeming A, et al, eds. *Movement, Stability, and Low Back Pain.* New York, NY: Churchill Livingstone, 1997:425–432.

Mens JMA, Vleeming A, Snijders CJ, Stam HJ, Ginai AZ. The active straight leg raise test and mobility of the pelvic joints. *Eur Spine J.* 1999;8:468–473.

Mens JMA, Vleeming A, Snijders CJ, Ronchetti I, Stam HJ. Reliability and validity of hip adduction strength to measure disease severity in posterior pelvic pain since pregnancy. *Spine.* 2002;27:1674–1679.

Mens JMA, Vleeming A, Stoeckart R, Stam HJ, Snijders CJ. Understanding peripartum pelvic pain: implications of a patient survey. *Spine.* 1996;21:363–370.

Mestdagh H. Morphological aspects and biomechanical properties of the vertebroaxial joint (C2–C3). *Acta Morphol. Neerl. Scand.* 1976;14:19–30.

Miller TM, Johnston SC. Should the Babinski sign be part of the routine neurologic examination. *Neurology.* 2005;65:1165–1168.

Mink AJF, ter Veer HJ, Vorselaars JAC Th. *Extremiteiten. Functie-onderzoek en Manuele Therapie.* Eindhoven, The Netherlands: SOMT; 1978.

Minne J, Depreux R, Mestdagh H. Les mouvements de rotation du rachis cervical inférieur (de C3 à C7). *Bull. Ass. Anat. 55e Congr.* (Nancy). 1970:929–935.

Mitchell JA. Vertebral artery atherosclerosis: a risk factor in the use of manipulative therapy. *Physiother Res Int.* 2002;7:122–130.

Mitchell JA. Changes in vertebral artery blood flow following normal rotation of the cervical spine. *J Manipulative Physiol Ther.* 2003;26:347–351.

Mooney V, Snijders CJ, Dorman T, eds. Integrated function of the lumbar spine and sacroiliac joint. *Rotterdam European Conference Organizers* 1995;195:207–220.

Moore RJ, Vernon-Roberts B, Osti OL. Remodelling of vertebral bone after outer anular injury in sheep. *Spine.* 1996;21(8):936–940.

Morscher E. *Aetiologie und Klinik der Beinlängenunterschiede, Orthopäde 1.* Berlin, Germany: Springer Verlag; 1972:1–8.

Morscher E, Figner G. *Die Messung der Beinlängen, Orthopäde 1.* Berlin, Germany: Springer Verlag; 1972: 9–13.

Moser M. Zervikalnystagmus und seine diagnostische Bedeutung. *HNO.* 1974;22:350–355.

Müller W. Spaltbildungen an Gelenk- und Dornfortsätzen der Wirbelsäule auf der Basis von Umbauzonen. *Forschr. Röntgenstr.* 1931;44:644–648.

Mumenthaler M. *Neurologie.* Stuttgart, Germany: Georg Thieme Verlag; 1973.

Mumenthaler M, Schliack H. *Läsionen peripherer Nerven.* Stuttgart, Germany: Georg Thieme Verlag; 1973.

Mumenthaler M, Schliack H. *Läsionen periferer Nerven. Diagnostiek und Therapie.* 4th ed. Stuttgart, Germany: Georg Thieme Verlag; 1992.

Nachemson A. The load on lumbar discs in different positions of the body. *Clin Orthop.* 1966;45:107.

Nachemson AN, Jonsson E, eds. *Neck and Back Pain: The Scientific Evidence of Causes, Diagnosis and Treatment.* New York, NY: Lippincott Williams & Wilkins; 2000.

Naffziger HC, Grant T. Neuritis of the brachial plexus mechanical in origin. *Clin Orthop.* 1967;51:7.

Nakamura K, Saku Y, Torigoe R, Ibayashi S, Fujishima M. Sonographic detection of heamodynamic changes in a case of vertebrobasilar insufficiency. *Neuroradiology.* 1998;40:164–166.

Nathan PW. Pain and the sympathetic system. *J Auton Nerv Sys.* 1983;7:363–370.

Neuman HD. Scriptum zum Informationskurs der Deutschen Gesellschaft für Manuelle Medizin. Buhl, Germany: Deutschen Gesellschaft für Manuelle Medizin; 1978.

Newman AP. Articular cartilage repair. *Am J Sports Med.* 1998;26(2):309–324.

Oegema Th R. Biochemistry of the intervertebral disc. *Clin Sports Med.*1993;12:419–439.

Olesen J. The international classification of headache disorders. 2nd ed. *Cephalalgia.* 2004;24:1–150.

Olmarker K, Holm S, Rydevik B. Importance of compression onset rate for the degree of impairment of impulse propagation in experimental compression injury of the porcine cauda equina. *Spine.* 1990;15:416–419.

Olmarker K, Rydevik BL, Hansson T, Holm S. Compression-induced changes of the nutritional supply to the porcine cauda equina. *J Spinal Disord.* 1990;3:25–29.

Oostendorp RAB. Neurofysiologische aspecten van het bewegingsapparaat. In: Winkel D, ed. *Weke Aandoeningen van het Bewegingsapparaat, deel 2: Diagnostiek.* Utrecht-Antwerpen, The Netherlands/Belgium: Bohn, Scheltema en Holkema; 1984.

Oostendorp RAB. *Weefselspecifieke Reacties van het Houdings- en Bewegingsapparaat als Klinisch Teken van een Verhoogde Activiteit binnen het Orthosympatisch Zenuwstelsel.* Amersfoort, The Netherlands: Stichting Wetenschap en Scholing Fysiotherapie; 1985.

Oostendorp RAB. *Functionele Vertebrobasilaire Insufficiëntie: Onderzoek en Behandeling in de Fysiotherapie,* Nijmegen, The Netherlands: 1988.

Oostendorp RAB. Manual physical therapy in the Netherlands: reflecting on the past and planning for the future in an international perspective. *J Man Manipulative Ther.* 2007;15:133–141.

Oostendorp RAB, Bernards JA, Clarijs JP, Elvers JWH. Functional vertebrobasilar insufficiency: a physical effect research. *Ned. T. v. Fys.* 1990;90(6):181–186.

Oostendorp RAB, Bernards ATM, Querido C, Hagenaars LHA, Meldrum MA. Neurologie en manuele therapie, de vertebrale insufficiëntie, deel I, II, III en IV. *Ned. Tijdschrift voor Manuele Therapie.* 1984;84/3(3/4),1985; 85/4(2),1986;86/4(2/3).

Oostendorp RAB, Elvers JWH. Funktionele vertebrobasilaire insufficiëntie, een diagnostisch en therapeutisch concept. *Ned. T. v. Fys.* 1990;90(6):147–149.

Oostendorp RAB, et al. Dizziness following whiplash injury: a neuro-otological study in manual therapy practice and therapeutic implications. *J Man Manipulative Ther.* 1999; 7:123–130.

Oosterhuis HJG. *Klinische Neurologie.* 4th ed. Utrecht, The Netherlands: Bohn, Scheltema, Holkema; 1977.

Oosterveld WJ. *Diagnostiek van de Cervicale Duizeligheid.* Unpublished lecture, Zeist, The Netherlands, 1984.

Orvieto R, Achiron A, Ben-Rafael Z, Gelernter I, Achiron R. Low backpain of pregnancy. *Acta Obstet Gynecol Scan.* 1994;73:209–214.

Oshima H, Urban JPG. The effect of lactate and pH on proteoglycan and protein synthesis rates in intervertebral disc. *Spine.* 1992;17(9).

Osti OL, Vernon-Roberts B, Moore R, Fraser RD. Annular tears and disc degeneration in the lumbar spine. *J Bone Joint* Surg [Br]. 1992;74:678–682.

Ottoson A. *Sjukgymnasten-Vart Tog Han Vägen?* Doctoral dissertation; Historiska Institutionen, Göteborgs Universitet, Göteborg, Sweden; 2005.

Overbeek WJ, Stenvers JD. *5 Mobiliteitstesten van de Schouder.* Course material, Groningen, The Netherlands: 1977.

Paciaroni M, et al. Seasonal variability in spontaneous cervical artery dissection. *J Neurol Neurosurg Psychiatry.* 2006; 77:677–679.

Panjabi M, White A. A mathematical approach for three dimensional analysis of the mechanics of the spine. *J Biomech.* 1971;4:203–211.

Paris SV. Mobilization of the spine. *Phys Ther.* 1979;49: 988–995.

Paris S. *Onderzoekingen van de Lumbale Wervelkolom.* Course material, 1982.

Paris S. Physical signs of instability. *Spine.* 1985;10:277.

Passchier J, Trijsburg RW, de Wit R, Eerdmans-Dubbelt SLC. *Psychologie van Onbegrepen Chronische Pijn.* Assen, The Netherlands: Van Gorcum Comp. BV; 1998.

Patla C, Paris S. *The Endfeel.* Course material, 1982.

Pauwels F. *Biomechanics of the Normal and Diseased Hip.* New York, NY: Springer Verlag; 1976.

Pearcy MJ, et al. Instantaneous axis of rotation of lumbar intervertebral joints. *Spine.*1988;13:1033–1041.

Peeters GG, Aufdemkampe G, Oostendorp RA. Sensibility testing in patients with a lumbosacral radicular syndrome. *J Manipulative Physiol Ther.* 1998;21:81–88.

Penning L. *Funktioneel Röntgenonderzoek bij Degeneratieve en Traumatische Afwijkingen der Laag-cervicale Bewegingssegmenten.* Master's thesis; University van Groningen, Netherlands; 1960.

Penning L. Nonpathologic and pathologic relationships between the lower cervical vertebrae. *Am J Roentgenol.* 1964; 91:1036–1050.

Penning L. *Functional Pathology of the Cervical Spine.* Amsterdam, The Netherlands: Excerpta Medica Foundation; 1968.

Penning L. Normal movements of the cervical spine. *Am J Roentgenol.* 1978;130:317–326.

Penning L, Töndury G. Entstehung, Bau und Funktion der meniskoiden Strukturen in den Halswirbelgelenken. *Z. Orthop.* 1964;98:1–14.

Peret C, et al. Validity, reliability, and responsiveness of the fingertip-to-floor test. *Arch Phys Med Rehabil.* 2001;82: 1566–1570.

Phillips DR, Twomey LT. A comparison of manual diagnosis with a diagnosis established by a uni-level lumbar spinal block procedure. *Man Ther.* 1996;2:82–87.

Piva SR, Erhard RE, Childs JD, Browder DA. Inter-tester reliability of passive intervertebral and active movements of the cervical spine. *Man Ther.* 2006;11:321–330.

Plewa MC, Delinger M. The false-positive rate of thoracic outlet shoulder maneuvers in healthy patients. *Acad Emerg Med.* 1998;5:337–342.

Pool JJ, Hoving JL, de Vet HC, van Mameren H, Bouter LM. The interexaminer reproducibility of physical examination of the cervical spine. *J Manipulative Physiol Ther.* 2004;27:84–90.

Pope MH, Panjabi M. Biomechanical definitions of spinal instability. *Spine.* 1985;10:255–256.

Porchet F, Fankhauser H, de Tribolet N. Extreme lateral lumbar disc herniation: clinical presentation in 178 patients. *Acta Neurochir* (Wien). 1994;127(3–4):203–209.

Portney LG, Watkins MP. *Foundations of Clinical Research: Applications to Practice.* 3rd ed. Upper Saddle River, NJ: Prentice Hall; 2008.

Posselt U. Movement areas of the mandible. *J Prosthet Dent.* 1957;7:375–383.

Posselt U. Range of movement of the mandible. *J Am Dent Assoc.* 1958;56:10.

Potter NA, Rothstein JM. Intertester reliability for selected tests of the sacroiliac joint. *Phys Ther.* 1985;65:1671–1675.

Preece SJ, Willan P, Nester CJ, Graham-Smith P, Herrington L, Bowker P. Variation in pelvic morphology may prevent the identification of anterior pelvic tilt. *J Man Manipulative Ther.* 2008;16:113–117.

Putz R. Charakteristische Fortsätze - Processus uncinati - als besondere Merkmale des I. Brustwirbels. *Anat. Anz.* 1976; 139:442–454.

Putz R. Beitrag zur Morphologie und Funktion der kleinen Gelenke der Lendenwirbelsäule. *Verh. Anat. Ges.* 1977a; 71:1355–1359.

Putz R. Zur Morphologie und Rotationsmechanik der kleinen Gelenke der Lendenwirbel. *Z. Orthop.* 1977b; 114:902–912.

Putz R. *Funktionelle Anatomie der Wirbelgelenke.* Stuttgart, Germany: Georg Thieme Verlag; 1981.

Putz R, Pomaroli A. Form und Funktion der Articulatio Atlanto-axialis Lateralis. *Acta Anat.* 1972;83:333–345.

Qvistgaard E, Rasmussen J, Lætgaard J, Hecksher-Sørensen S, Bliddal H. Intra-observer and inter-observer agreement of the manual examination of the lumbar spine in chronic low back pain. *Eur Spine J.* 2007;16:272–282.

Ravelli A. Das Vakuum-Phänomen (R. FICK-sches Zeichnen). *Fortschr. Röntgenstr.* 1955;83:236–240.

Rees LA. The structure and function of the mandibular joint. *Br Dent J.* 1954;6:125–133.

Refshauge KM. Rotation: A valid premanipulative dizziness test? Does it predict safe manipulation? *J Manipulative Physiol Ther.* 1994;17:413–414.

Reichmann S. Motion of the lumbar articular processes in flexion-extension and lateral flexions of the spine. *Acta Morphol. Neerl* (Scandinavia). 1970–1971;8:261–272.

Reichmann S. The postnatal development of form and orientation of the lumbar intervertebral joint surfaces. *Z. Anat. Entw. Gesch.* 1971a;133:102–123.

Reichmann S. Longitudinal growth of the lumbar articular processes with reference to the development of clefts. *Z. Anat. Entw. Gesch.* 1971b;133:124–134.

Reichmann S. Tomography of the lumbar intervertebral joints. *Acta Radiol* (Stockholm). 1972;12:641–659.

Reichmann S, Berglund E, Lindgren K. Das Bewegungszentrum in der Lendenwirbelsäule bei Flexion und Extension. *Z. Anat. Entw. Gesch.* 1972;138:283–287.

Reinhardt K. Die Anatomie und Pathologie der kleine Wirbelgelenke im Röntgenbild. *Acta Radiol* (Stockholm). 1963;4:665–700.

Reishauer F. Wirbelsäule und Bandscheibenschäden. *Therapie-woche.* 1957;8:130.

Renner K. Statik und Anatomie an den kleinen Gelenken und der Kyphose der Brustwirbelsäule. Dissertation; Hamburg, Germany; 1956.

Reynolds DV. Surgery in the rat during electrical analgesia induced by focal brain stimulation. *Science.* 1969;164: 444–445.

Richter RR, Reinking MF. Evidence in practice. *Phys Ther.* 2005;85:589–599.

Richter T, Lawall J. Zur Zuverlässigkeit manualdiagnostischer Befunde. *Man Med.* 1993;31:1–11.

Riddle DL. Classification and low back pain: a review of the literature and critical analysis of selected systems. *Phys Ther.* 1998;78:708–737.

Riddle DL, Freburger JK, North American Orthopaedic Rehabilitation Research Network. Evaluation of the presence of sacroiliac region dysfunction using a combination of tests: a multicenter intertester reliability study. *Phys Ther.* 2002;82:772–781.

Ritossa F. A new puffing pattern induced by heat, shock and DNP in Drosophila. *Experientia.* 1962;18:571–573.

Rivett DA, Milburn PD, Chapple C. Negative premanipulative vertebral artery testing despite complete occlusion: a case of false negativity. *Man Ther.* 1998;3:102–107.

Rivett DA, Sharpless KJ, Milburn PD. Effect of premanipulative tests on vertebral artery and internal carotid artery blood flow: a pilot study. *J Manipulative Physiol Ther.* 1999; 22:368–375.

Roberts S, et al. Collagen types around cells of the intervertebral disc and cartilage endplate. *Spine.* 1991;16: 1030–1038.

Rocabado M. Biomechanical relationship of the cranial, cervical and hyoid regions. *J Craniomandib Prac.* June–August 1983;1(3).

Rocabado M. *Cursus Tandheelkunde en Fysiotherapie in een Multidiciplinaire Benadering van Dysfunctie van het Kauwstelsel.* Course notes; Amsterdam, The Netherlands; 1984.

Rocabado M. *Arthrokinematics of the Temporomandibular Joint: Clinical Management of Head, Neck and TMJ Pain and Dysfunction.* Philadephia, Pa: W B Saunders; 1985.

Rothwell DM, Bondy SJ, Williams JI. Chiropractic manipulation and stroke: a population-based case control study. *Stroke.* 2001;32:1054–1060.

Rubinstein SM, et al. A systematic review of the risk factors for cervical artery dissection. *Stroke.* 2005;36: 1575–1580.

Rugh JD, Drago CJ. Vertical dimension: a study of clinical rest position and jaw muscular activity. *J Prosthet Dent.* 1981;45:670.

Runge H, Zippel H. Untersuchungen zur Entwicklung des Wirbelbogens im Lumbosacralbereich. *Beitr. Orthop. Traum.* 1976;23:19–29.

Rydevik BL, Pedowitz RA, Hargens AR, Swenson MR, Meyers RR, Garfin SR. Effects of acute, graded compression on spinal nerve root function and structure: an experimental study of the pig cauda equina. *Spine.* 1991;2:487–494.

Sakaguchi M, et al. Mechanical compression of the extracranial vertebral artery during neck rotation. *Neurology.* 2003; 61:845–847.

Saxon-Bullock J. Postural alignment in standing: a repeatability study. *Aust J Physiother.* 1993;39:25–29.

Schadé JP. *The Peripheral Nervous System.* Amsterdam, The Netherlands: Elsevier; 1966.

Schiff DCM, Parke WW. The arterial supply of the odontoid process. *J Bone Joint Surg.* 1973;55-A:1450–1456.

Schlüter K. *Form und Struktur des normalen und des pathologisch veranderten Wirbels. Wirbelsäule in Forschung und Praxis.* Vol. 30. Stuttgart, Germany: Hippokrates; 1965.

Schmidt RF. *Fundamentals of Neurophysiology.* Berlin, Germany: Springer Verlag; 1978.

Schminke A, Santo E. Zur normalen und pathologischen Anatomie der Halswirbelsäule. *Zbl. Path.* 1932;55:369–372.

Schmitt MA, Gerrits M. Fysiotherapie bij patiënten met klachten in het kauwstelsel op grond van een arthrogene dysfunctie. Hfdst.8:134-148. In: Steenks MH, de Wijer A, eds. *Craniomandibulaire Dysfuncties vanuit Fysiotherapeutisch en Tandheelkundig Perspectief.* Lochem, The Netherlands: De Tijdstroom; 1989.

Schmorl G. Ueber Verlagerungen von Bandscheibengewebe und ihre Folgen. *Arch. Klin. Chir.* 1932;172:240.

Schmorl G, Junghanns H. *Die gesunde und kranke Wirbelsäule in Röntgenbild und Klinik.* 5th ed. Stuttgart, Germany: Thieme; 1968.

Schöps P, Pfingsten M, Siebert U. Reliabilität manualmedizinischer Untersuchungstechniken an der Halswirbelsäule. Studie zur Qualitätssicherung in der manuellen Diagnostik. *Z Orthop Ihre Grenzgeb.* 2000;138:2–7.

Schultz A, Galante J. A mathematical model for the study of the mechanics of the human vertebral column. *J Biomechanics.* 1970:13:405–416.

Schwarzer A, et al. Clinical features of patients with pain stemming from the lumbar zygapophyseal joint. *Spine.* 1994;19:1132–1137.

Schwarzer AC, Aprill CN, Bogduk N. The sacroiliac joint in chronic low back pain. *Spine.* 1995;20:31–37.

Scrimshaw SV, Maher C. Responsiveness of visual analogue and McGill pain scale measures. *J Manipulative Physiol Ther.* 2001;24:501–504.

Seidel A. Diagnostik der Wirbelschiefstand. *Man Med.* 1969; 7:1.

Sell K. Spezielle manuelle Segment-Technik als Mittel zur Abklärung spondylogener Zusammenhangsfragen. *Manuelle Med.* 1969;7:99.

Selye H. A syndrome produced by diverse nocuous agents. *Nature.* 1936:138:32.

Selye H. *Stress in Health and Disease.* Reading, Mass: Butterworths; 1976a.

Selye H. *The Stress of Life.* Rev. ed. New York, NY: McGraw-Hill; 1976b.

Selye H. *Stress.* Utrecht, The Netherlands: Het Spectrum; 1978.

Seroo JM, Hulsbosch A. *Literatuurstudie Driedimensionaal Bewegen van de Wervelkolom.* Eindhoven, The Netherlands: Internal report Stichting Manuele Geneeskunde; 1982.

Seroo JM, Penning L. Unpublished research into the location of the frontal plane axis of movement of the lumbar spine. TUE, RUG, SOMT (1981).

Seroo JM, Snijders CJ, Snijder JGN, Hahn HJ. Some results of the application of the stabilograph in the orthopaedic clinic: a preliminary report. *Agressologie.* 1976;17(D): 55–59.

Sesam Atlas van de anatomie dl. 1: Bewegingsapparaat 2nd ed. Georg Thieme Verlag, Nederl. Uitgave Bosch en Keuning n.v., Baarn, The Netherlands, 1982.

Sesam Atlas van de anatomie dl. 3: Zenuwstelsel en zintuigen. 2nd ed. Georg Thieme Verlag, Nederl. Uitgave Bosch en Keuning n.v., Baarn, The Netherlands, 1982.

Shahinfar S, Johnson LN, Madsen RW. Confrontation visual field loss as a function of decibel sensitivity loss on automated static perimetry: implications on the accuracy of confrontation visual field testing. *Ophthalmology.* 1995; 102:872–877.

Sicard A, Gerard Y. Les fractures isolées des apophyses articulaires lombaires. *J Chir* (Paris). 1955;71:469–491.

Sieglbauer F. *Normale Anatomie des Menschen.* 8th ed. Munich, Germany: Urban & Schwarzenberg; 1958.

Simons DG. Electrogenic nature of palpable bands and local twitch response associated with myofascial trigger points. In: Bonica JJ, Albe-Fessard D, eds. *Advances in Pain Research and Therapy.* Vol. I. New York, NY: Raven Press; 1976.

Simons DG, Travell JG, Simons LS. *Travell and Simons' Myofascial Pain and Dysfunction: The Trigger Point Manual.* 2nd ed. Vol. 1. Baltimore, Md: Williams & Wilkins; 1999.

Slipman CW, Jackson HB, Lipetz JS, Chan KT, Lenrow D, Vresilovic EJ. Sacroilac joint pain referral zones. *Arch Phys Med Rehabil.* 2000;81:334–338.

Smedmark V, Wallin M, Arvidsson I. Interexaminer reliability in assessing passive intervertebral motion of the cervical spine. *Man Ther.* 2000;5:97–101.

Smelik PG. De biologie van stress. *Hart Bulletin.* 1982.

Smith AR, Catlin PA, Nyberg RE. Intratester/intertester reliability of segmental motion testing of cervicothoracic forward bending in a symptomatic population. In: Paris SV, ed. *IFOMT Proceedings.* Vail, Colo: IFOMT; 1992:194.

Smith KF. The thoracic outlet syndrome. *Am J Orthoped Sports PhysTher.* 1979;1(2):89–99.

Snijders CJ, Snijder JGN, Schijvens AWN, Seroo JM. Die Anwendung des Stabilographen bei Schiefhaltung infolge Beinlängenunterschied. *Orthopadische Praxis Heft.* 1975;7(XI):493–500.

Snijder JGN, Snijders CJ, Seroo JM, Hahn HJ. Der Stabilograph als Hilfsmittel für die konservatieve Behandlung bei asymmetrischen Beckenstand. *Z. Orthop.* 1976;114: 444–447.

Spanner R. *Spalteholz-Spanner Handatlas der Anatomie des Menschen: Bewegungsapparat.* 16th ed. Amsterdam, The Netherlands: Scheltema & Holkema; 1960.

Spector WG. *An Introduction to General Pathology.* 2nd ed. Edinburgh, UK: Churchill Livingstone Medical Text; 1980.

Stahl C. *Experimentelle Untersuchungen zur Biomechanik der Hals-wirbelsäule.* Med. Dissertation; Dusseldorf, Germany; 1977.

Steenks MH, de Wijer A. *Craniomandibulaire Dysfuncties vanuit Fysiotherapeutisch en Tandheelkundig Perspectief.* Lochem, The Netherlands: De Tijdstroom; 1989.

Stenvers JD, Overbeek WJ. *Het Kissing Coracoid.* Lochem, The Netherlands: De Tijdstroom; 1981.

Stoddard A. *Manual and Osteopathic Technique.* London, UK: Hutchinson; 1961.

Stofft E. Beitrag zum Schmerzgeschehen im Halswirbelsäulebereich aus anatomisch physiologischer Sicht. *Phys. Med. Rehabil.* 1977;4:178–184.

Stofft E, Müller G. Eine vergleichende Analyse der Intervertebralgelenkflächen. *Anat. Anz.* 1971;66:355–363.

Stokes I, Frymoyer JW. Segmental motion and instability. *Spine.*1987;12:688–691.

Strasser H. *Lehrbuch der Muskel- und Gelenkmechanik.* Vol. II. Berlin, Germany: Springer Verlag; 1913.

Stratford P. Getting more from the literature: estimating the standard error of measurement from reliability studies. *Physiother Can.* 2004;56:27–30.

Stratford PW, Binkley JM, Riddle DL. Health status measures: strategies and analytic methods for assessing change scores. *Phys Ther.* 1996;76:1109–1123.

Strender LE, Sjoeblom A, Sundell K, Ludwig R, Taube A. Interexaminer reliability in physical examination of patients with low back pain. *Spine.* 1997;22:814–820.

Sunderland S. *Nerves and Nerve Injuries.* 2nd ed. Edinburgh, UK: Churchill Livingstone; 1978.

Sung RD, Wang JC. Correlation between a positive Hoffamn's reflex and cervical pathology in asymptomatic individuals. *Spine.* 2001;26:67–70.

Sutter M. Versuch einer Wesenbestimmung pseudoradikulärer Syndrome. *Schweizerische Rundschau Medizin* (Praxis). 1974;63:842–845.

Swaine BR, Desrosiers J, Bourbonnais D, Larochelle JL. Norms for 15- to 34-year-olds for different versions of the finger-to-nose tests. *Arch Phys Med Rehabil.* 2005a;86:1665–1669.

Swaine BR, Lortie E, Gravel D. The reliability of the time to execute various forms of the finger-to-nose test in healthy subjects. *Physiother Theory Pract.* 2005b;21:271–279.

Swinkels-Meewisse EJCM, Swinkels RAHM, Verbeek ALM, Vlaeyen JWS, Oostendorp RAB. Psychometric properties of Tampa Scale for kinesiophobia and the fear-avoidance beliefs questionnaire in acute low back pain. *Man Ther.* 2003;8:29–36.

Taillard W, Morscher E. *Beinlängenunterschiede.* Basel, Switzerland: Karger; 1965.

Terlouw TJA. Roots of physical medicine, physical therapy, and mechanotherapy in the Netherlands in the 19th century: a disputed area within the health care domain. *J Man Manipulative Ther.* 2007;15:E23–E41.

Terrett AGJ. Vertebrobasilar stroke following spinal manipulation therapy. In: Murphy DR, ed. *Conservative Management of Cervical Spine Syndromes.* New York, NY: McGraw-Hill; 2000:553–578.

Thiel HW. Gross morphology and pathoanatomy of the vertebral arteries. *J Manipulative Physiol Ther.* 1991;14:133–141.

Thiel H, Rix G. Is it time to stop functional pre-manipulation testing of the cervical spine? *Man Ther.* 2005;10:154–158.

Tilscher H. Die topischen Zusammenhänge zwischen Gesichtsschmertz und subokzipital Maximalpunkte. *Manuelle Medizin.* 1982;20:127–130.

Tissières A, Mitchell HK, Tracy UM. Protein synthesis in salivary glands of *D. melanogaster*: relation to chromosome puffs. *J Mol Biol.* 1974;84:389–398.

Töndury G. Beitrag zur Kenntnis der kleinen Wirbelgelenke. *Z. Anat. Entw. Gesch.* 1940;110:568–575.

Töndury G. *Entwicklungsgeschichte und Fehlbildungen der Wirbelsäule. Die Wirbelsäule in Forschung und Praxis.* Vol. 7. Stuttgart, Germany: Hippokrates; 1958.

Töndury G. *The Cervical Spine.* Bern, Switzerland: Huber; 1974.

Töndury R. (1958). Referenced in: Lang J. *Neuroorthopaedie 1.: Funktionelle Anatomie der Halswirbelsäule und des benachbarsten Nervensystems.* Berlin, Germany, 1983.

Travell J. Myofascial trigger points: clinical view. In: Bonica JJ, Albe-Fessard DG, eds. *Advances in Pain Research and Therapy.* Vol. I. New York, NY: Raven Press; 1976:199.

Travell J. Identification of myofascial trigger point syndromes: a case of atypical fascial neuralgia. *Arch Phys Med.* 1981;62:100.

Travell J, Rinzler SH. The myofascial genesis of pain. *Postgrad Med.* 1952;2:425.

Travell JG, Simons DG. *Myofascial Pain and Dysfunction: The Triggerpoint Manual.* Baltimore, Md: Williams & Wilkins; 1984.

Triano JJ, Kawchuk G. *Current Concepts: Spinal Manipulation and Cervical Arterial Incidents.* Clive, Iowa: NCMIC; 2006.

Tseng YL, Wang WTJ, Chen WY, Hou TJ, Chen TC, Lieu FK. Predictors for the immediate responders to cervical manipulation in patients with neck pain. *Man Ther.* 2006;11:306–315.

Tullberg T, Blomberg S, Branth B, Johnsson R. Manipulation does not alter the position of the sacroiliac joint: a Roentgen stereophotogrammetric analysis. *Spine.* 1998; 23:1124–1128.

Uchihara T, Furukawa T, Tsukagoshi H. Compression of the brachial plexus as a diagnostic test of cervical cord lesion. *Spine.* 1994;19:2170–2173.

Uitvlugt G, Indenbaum S. Clinical assessment of atlantoaxial instability using the Sharp-Purser test. *Arthritis Rheum.* July 1988;31(7).

Urban JP. De chemie van de tussenwervelschijf in verband met haar functie. In: Grieve GP, ed. *Grieve's. Moderne Manuele Therapie van de Wervelkolom, Deel 2.* Lochem, The Netherlands: De Tijdstroon, 1988.

Urban L. The straight-leg raising test, a review. *J Orthop Sports Phys Ther.* 1981;2:117–133.

Urban J, Hohn S, Maroudas A, Nachemson A. Diffusion of sulfate and proteoglycan turnover in discs of the dog. Referenced by Nachemson, 1976 (see above).

Urban J, Maroudas A. The chemistry of the intervertebral disc in relation to its physiological function and requirements. *Clin Rheum Dis.* 1980;6(1).

van Mameren H. *Motion Patterns in the Cervical Spine.* Doctoral Dissertation. Rijksuniversiteit Limburg; 1988.

van Meerwijk GM. Het Thoracic Outlet Compressie Syndroom. *Ned. T.v.Fysiotherapie.* 1986;96(6):122–127.

van Meerwijk GM. *Syllabus Onderzoeken en Behandelen, Orthopaedisch onderzoek.* Amsterdam, The Netherlands: Stichting Akademie voor Fysiother; 1979.

van Meerwijk GM. T.O.S. In: Winkel D, Fischer S, Vroege C, eds. *Weke-delen Aandoeningen van het Bewegingsapparaat, Deel 2: Diagnostiek.* Utrecht, The Netherlands: Bohn, Scheltema en Holkema; 1984.

van Stralen CJC. *Myofasciale Triggerpoints.* Amersfoort, The Netherlands: Unpublished lecture, Stichting Wetenschap en Scholing Fysiotherapie; 1985.

van Wijk R. Stress en ordening, een fundamenteel bioregulatie principe. *Integraal.* 1988.

van Zoest G. *Unpublished Research with regard to 3-Diemnsional Function of the Spine.* Amsterdam, The Netherlands: Vrije Universiteit Amsterdam; 1985.

van den Berg F. *Angewandte Physiologie: Das Bindegewebe des bewegungsapparates verstehen und beeinflussen.* Stuttgart, Germany: Georg Thieme Verlag; 1999.

van den Burgt M, Verhulst F. *Doen en Blijven Doen. Patiëntenvoorlichting in de Paramedische Praktijk.* Houten/Diegem, The Netherlands: Bohn Stafleu Van Loghum; 2003.

van den Hoogen HMM, Koes BW, Van Eijk JTM, Bouter LM. On the accuracy of history, physical examination, and erythrocyte sedimentation rate in diagnosing low back pain in general practice. *Spine.* 1995;20:318–327.

van der Bijl G Sr. Publicaties. *Tijdschrift voor Fysiotherapie.* 1969; July/August.

van der El A. *Mobilisatie, Stabilisatie en Coördinatie bij Rug- en Nekklachten (Mobilization, Stabilisation and Co-ordination in Complaints of Low Back and Cervical Spine).* Rotterdam, The Netherlands: Manthel; 2002:2.

van Dillen LR, et al. Reliability of physical examination items used for classification of patients with low back pain. *Phys Ther.* 1998;78:979–988.

van Faassen F. *Functioneel Anatomische Aspecten van de Wervelkolom.* Amsterdam, The Netherlands: Unpublished lecture, 1981.

van Kessel-Cobelens AM, Verhagen AP, Mens JM, Snijders CJ, Koes BW. Pregnancy-related pelvic girdle pain: intertester reliability of 3 tests to determine asymmetric mobility of the scaroiliac joints. *J Manipulative Physiol Ther.* 2008;31:130–136.

Vélè F. Wirbelgelenk und Bewegungssegment innerhalb des Steuerungssystems der Haltemuskulatur. *Man. Med.* 1968; 6:94–96.

Vidal P, Huijbregts P. Dizziness in orthopaedic physical therapy practice: history and physical examination. *J Man Manipulative Ther.* 2005;13:222–251.

Viidik A. Structure and function of normal and healing tendons and ligaments. In: Mow VC, Ratcliff A, Woo SLY, eds. *Biomechanics of Diarthrodial Joints.* Vol. I. New York, NY: Springer-Verlag; 1990:3–38.

Vincent-Smith B, Gibbons P. Inter-examiner and intra-examiner reliability of the standing flexion test. *Man Ther.* 1999;4:87–93.

Virchow H. *Sitzungsber. d. Ges. d. Naturf. Freunde,* Berlin, Germany: 1909:265–290.

Visscher CM, et al. Clinical tests in distinguishing between persons with or without craniomandibular or cervical spinal pain complaints. *Eur J Oral Sci.*2000;108: 475–483.

Vlaeyen JWS, Heuts PHTG. *Gedragsgeoriënteerde Behandeling bij lage Rugpijn.* Houten/Diegum, The Netherlands/Belgium: Bohn Stafleu Van Loghum; 2000.

Vlaeyen JWS, Kole-Snijders AMJ, van Eek H. *Cronische Pijn en Revalidatie. Praktijkreeks Gedragstherapie.* Houten, The Netherlands: Bohn Stafleu Van Loghum; 1996.

Vleeming A, Stoeckart R, Volkers ACW, Snijders CJ. Relation between form and function in the sacroiliac joint. Part II: biomechanical aspects. *Spine.* 1990;15:133–136.

Vogel G. *Experimentelle Untersuchungen zur Mobilität des Nucleus pulposus in lumbalen Bandscheiben.* Medical Dissertation; Dusseldorf, Germany; 1977.

Voorhoeve PE. *Leerboek der Neurofysiologie.* Amsterdam, The Netherlands: Elsevier; 1978.

Waddell G. Biopsychosocial analysis of low back pain. *Baillieres Clin Rheum.* 1992;6:523–557.

Waddell G, Waddell H. Social influences on neck and low back pain. In: Nachemson AN, Jonsson E, eds. *Neck and*

Back Pain: The Scientific Evidence of Causes, Diagnosis and Treatment. New York, NY: Lippincott Williams & Wilkins; 2000.

Wainner RS, Fritz JM, Irrgang JJ, Boninger ML, Delitto A, Allison S. Reliability and diagnostic accuracy of the clinical examination and patient self-report measures for cervical radiculopathy. *Spine*. 2003;28:52–62.

Walker JM. Pathomechanics and classification of cartilage lesions, facilitation of repair. *J Orthop Sports Phys Ther*. 1998;28(4):216–231.

Walker JM, Helewa A. *Physical Therapy in Arthritis*. Philadelphia, Pa: WB Saunders; 1996.

Walker N, Bohannon RW, Cameron D. Discriminant validity of temporomandibular joint range of motion measurements obtained with a ruler. *J Orthop Sports Phys Ther*. 2000;30:484–492.

Weiler PJ, et al. Analyses of sagittal plane instability of the lumbar spine in vivo. *Spine*. 1990;15:1300–1306.

Weir JP. Quantifying test-retest reliability using the Intraclass Correlation Coefficient and the SEM. *J Strength Cond Res*. 2005;19:231–240.

Weisl H. The movements of the sacroiliac joint. *Acta Anat*. 1955;23:80–91.

Wells P, Luttgens A. *Kinesiology: Scientific Basis of Human Motion*. Philadelphia, Pa: WB Saunders; 1976.

Werne S. Studies in spontaneous atlas dislocation. *Acta Orthop Scand*. 1957;23(suppl):1–150.

Westaway MD, Stratford P, Symons B. False negative extension/rotation pre-manipulative screening test on a patient with an atretic and hypoplastic vertebral artery. *Man Ther*. 2003;8:120–127.

White A. Analysis of the mechanics of the thoracic spine in man [Thesis]. *Acta Orthop Scand*. 1969;127(suppl).

White A. Kinematics of the normal spine as related to scoliosis. *J Biomech*. 1971;4:405–411.

White AA, Panjabi MM. *Clinical Biomechanics of the Spine*. 2nd ed. Philadelphia, Pa: JB Lippincott Company, 1990.

Wiesenfeld-Hallin Z, Hallin RG. Possible role of the sympathetic activity in abnormal behaviour of rats induced by lesion of the sciatic nerve. *J Auton Nerv Syst*. 1983;7:385–390.

Wingerden BAM van. *Bindweefsel in de revalidatie. Herziene uitgave*. Liechtenstein, Germany: Scipro Verlag Schaan; 1997.

Wlitse LL, Rothmann SLG. Spondylolisthesis: classification, diagnosis and natural history. *Semin Spine Surg*. 1989; 1:78.

Wolf J. *Die Chondrosynovialmembran und ihre Bedeutung fur die Herabsetzung der Reibung und Schutz der Gelenkflächer*. Stornik lek; 1946.

Wolf J. *Die Chondrosynovialmembran als einheitliche Auskleidungshaut der Gelenkhöhle mit Gleit und Barrierefunktion*. Heidelberg, Germany: 1970.

Wolff HD. Studien an der mittleren Halswirbelsäule. *Die Wirbelsäule in Forschung und Praxis*. 1963;26:78–84.

Wong TM, Leung HB, Wong WC. Correlation between magnetic resonance imaging and radiographic measurements of the cervical spine in cervical myelopathic patients. *J Orthop Surg*. 2004;12:239–242.

Woo SLY, Buckwalter JA, eds. *Injury and Repair of the Musculoskeletal Soft Tissue*. Park Ridge, Ill: American Academy of Orthopaedic Surgeons; 1991.

World Health Organization (WHO). *International Classification of Functioning, Disability and Health*. Geneva, Switzerland: WHO; 2001.

Wrisley DM, et al. Cervicogenic dizziness: a review of diagnosis and treatment. *J Orthop Sports Phys Ther*. 2000;30: 755–766.

Wyke BD. The neurology of joints. Presented at: Arris and Gale Lecture; February 17, 1966; Royal College of Surgeons of England, Neurological Laboratory, Department of Applied Physiology, Royal College of Surgeons of England.

Wyke BD. *The Neurology of Joints*. Ann R Coll Surg Engl. 1976;41:25–50.

Wyke BD. Neurology of the cervical spinal joints. *Physiotherapy* 1979;65(3):72–76.

Yi-Kai L, Yun-Kun Z, Cai-Mo L, Shi-Zhen Z. Changes and implications of blood flow velocity of the vertebral artery during rotation and extension of the head. *J Manipulative Physiol Ther*. 1999;22:91–95.

Youdas JW, Cary JR, Garrett TR. Reliability of measurements of cervical spine range of motion: comparison of three methods. *Phys Ther*. 1991;71:98–106.

Yu Che. The arteries of the human thoracic vertebrae. *Acta anat. sin*. 1966;9:301–308.

Zizina M. *La Douleur Contralateral dans la Sciatique*. Montpellier, France: These de Montpellier. 1910.

Zutphen NCF, van Sambeek HWR, Oostendorp RAB, van Rens PPThG, Bernards ATM. *Nederlands Leerboek der Fysische Therapie in Engere Zin*. Part 1, 4th ed. Utrecht, The Netherlands: Wetenschappelijke uitgeverij Bunge; 1991.

Index

Italicized page locators indicate a photo/figure; tables are noted with a *t*.